SURGICAL AND MEDICAL TREATMENT OF OSTEOPOROSIS

SURGICAL AND MEDICAL TREATMENT OF OSTEOPOROSIS

PRINCIPLES AND PRACTICE

Edited by

Peter V. Giannoudis

Professor and Chairman
Academic Department of Orthopaedic and Trauma Surgery
School of Medicine
University of Leeds
Leeds, United Kingdom

Thomas A. Einhorn

Professor of Orthopedic Surgery
New York University
Director of Clinical and Translational Research Development
NYU Hospital for Joint Disease
New York, New York, USA

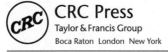

CRC Press
Taylor & Francis Group
Boca Raton London New York

CRC Press is an imprint of the
Taylor & Francis Group, an **informa** business

CRC Press
Taylor & Francis Group
6000 Broken Sound Parkway NW, Suite 300
Boca Raton, FL 33487-2742

First issued in paperback 2023

© 2020 by Taylor & Francis Group, LLC
CRC Press is an imprint of Taylor & Francis Group, an Informa business

No claim to original U.S. Government works

ISBN: 978-1-03-256976-5 (pbk)
ISBN: 978-1-4987-3224-6 (hbk)

DOI: 10.1201/9780429161087

Library of Congress Cataloging-in-Publication Data

Names: Giannoudis, Peter V., editor. | Einhorn, Thomas A., editor.
Title: Surgical and medical treatment of osteoporosis : principles and practice / [edited by] Peter V. Giannoudis, Thomas A. Einhorn.
Description: Boca Raton : CRC Press, [2020] | Includes bibliographical references and index. | Summary: "Osteoporosis is the most common bone disease and is associated with pathological fractures that can lead to significant morbidity. It represents an economic burden to the health care system, directly linked to an ageing population. Guidelines on osteoporosis prevention have been published but these do not provide the required specialised knowledge for the treating physician. This book 'fills the gap' and focuses on the principles of surgical and medical treatment of osteoporosis. It aims to improve education and provide answers based on current evidence, helping doctors follow best practice, improve patient care and outcomes, and minimise the complications of medical and surgical management"-- Provided by publisher.
Identifiers: LCCN 2019049209 (print) | LCCN 2019049210 (ebook) | ISBN 9781498732246 (hardback ; alk. paper) | ISBN 9780429161087 (ebook)
Subjects: MESH: Osteoporosis--surgery | Osteoporotic Fractures--surgery
Classification: LCC RC931.O73 (print) | LCC RC931.O73 (ebook) | NLM WE 250 | DDC 616.7/16--dc23
LC record available at https://lccn.loc.gov/2019049209
LC ebook record available at https://lccn.loc.gov/2019049210

**Visit the Taylor & Francis Web site at
http://www.taylorandfrancis.com**

**and the CRC Press Web site at
http://www.crcpress.com**

Contents

Preface   vii

Contributors   ix

1   Definition, risk factors, and epidemiology of osteoporosis   1
Enrique Guerado and Enrique Caso

2   Pathogenesis: Molecular mechanisms of osteoporosis   13
Anastasia E. Markatseli, Theodora E. Markatseli, and Alexandros A. Drosos

3   Osteoporosis: Biochemical investigations   35
Ippokratis Pountos and Peter V. Giannoudis

4   Diagnosis: Radiological investigations   43
David J. Hak and Rodrigo Banegas

5   Development of a fragility liaison service   49
Paul Andrzejowski and Peter V. Giannoudis

6   NICE guidelines for medical treatment of osteoporosis: An update   55
Katherine Lowery and Nikolaos K. Kanakaris

7   Role of bisphosphonates and denosumab   59
Blossom Samuels, Yi Liu, and Joseph Lane

8   The role of anabolic agents   69
Nifon K. Gkekas, Eustathios Kenanidis, Panagiotis Anagnostis, Michael Potoupnis,
Dimitrios G. Goulis, and Eleftherios Tsiridis

9   Current and emerging pharmacological agents in the treatment of osteoporosis   73
James X. Liu and Thomas A. Einhorn

10   Monitoring/surveillance of medical treatment   81
Konstantinos D. Stathopoulos and Andreas F. Mavrogenis

11   Systemic complications of osteoporosis medical treatment   91
Konstantinos G. Makridis and Stamatina-Emmanouela Zourntou

12   Complications of medical treatment: Atypical fractures   97
Owen Diamond, Natalie C. Rollick, and David L. Helfet

13   Biomechanical considerations for fixation of osteoporotic bone   107
Peter Augat and Christian von Rüden

14   The fix and treat principle: An update   117
Vasileios P. Giannoudis and Peter V. Giannoudis

15   Principles of management of osteoporotic fractures   121
Seth M. Tarrant and Zsolt J. Balogh

16   Can we accelerate the osteoporotic bone fracture healing response?   141
Martijn van Griensven and Elizabeth Rosado Balmayor

17   Management of osteoporotic proximal humeral fractures: An overview   149
J.P.A.M. Verbruggen

18 Distal humerus fractures in the elderly: To fix or to replace?   163
Jon B. Carlson, Craig S. Roberts, and David Seligson

19 Distal radius osteoporotic features: My preferred method of treatment   171
Donato Perretta and Jesse B. Jupiter

20 Management of osteoporotic pelvic fractures   177
Pol M. Rommens, Daniel Wagner, and Alexander Hofmann

21 Management of osteoporotic acetabular fractures: Fix or replace?   195
Peter V. Giannoudis and Panagiotis Douras

22 Management of osteoporotic proximal intertrochanteric/subtrochanteric femoral fractures   203
Avadhoot Kantak and George Tselentakis

23 Osteoporotic distal femoral fractures: When to fix and how   221
Cyril Mauffrey and Nicholas A. Alfonso

24 Osteoporotic distal femoral fractures: When to replace and how   235
Richard Stange and Michael J. Raschke

25 Osteoporotic long bone fractures: My preferred method of treatment   245
Sascha Halvachizadeh and Hans-Christoph Pape

26 Management of osteoporotic extra-articular proximal tibial fractures   251
Daniela Sanchez, Amrut Borade, and Daniel S. Horwitz

27 Osteoporotic ankle fractures: Principles of treatment   261
Theodoros H. Tosounidis and Michael G. Kontakis

28 Treatment of distal intra-articular/extra-articular tibial fractures   267
Vasileios P. Giannoudis and Peter V. Giannoudis

29 Osteoporotic os calcis fractures: How I manage them   275
Angus Jennings and Richard Buckley

30 Current trend in kyphoplasty for osteoporotic vertebral fractures   281
Kalliopi Alpantaki, Georgios Vastardis, and Alexander G. Hadjipavlou

31 Osteoporotic thoracolumbar fractures: My preferred method of nonoperative treatment   305
Terence Ong and Opinder Sahota

32 Augmentation of fracture fixation: An update   315
Peter V. Giannoudis and Panagiotis Douras

33 Complications of surgical treatment for osteoporotic fractures   327
Paul C. Baldwin III and Christian Krettek

34 Total shoulder replacement and osteoporosis: An Update   343
David Limb

35 Total hip replacement and osteoporosis: Current trends   349
Antonios Koutalos, Georgios Komnos, and Theofilos Karachalios

36 Total knee replacement and osteoporosis: An overview   357
Edward S. Holloway and Veysi T. Veysi

37 Rehabilitation of the osteoporotic patient: Is it different?   363
Theodoros H. Tosounidis and Amy Margot Lindh

Index   369

Preface

Osteoporosis, a common bone disorder characterized by disruption of bone microarchitecture and an increased risk of fracture, is on the rise in the elderly population. The World Health Organization (WHO) predicts that the number of people over the age of 65 years will increase by 88% over the next 25 years, and not surprisingly, therefore, osteoporosis has been labeled as a "new epidemic." Its medical and surgical treatment remains a challenge as a plethora of adverse sequelae can occur, including fragility fractures and their potentially fatal outcomes.

For optimum treatment, coordinated medical and surgical input is essential. Fixation of fragility fractures requires specific implants and reconstruction techniques to minimize the risk of failure and to support early patient mobilization. Similarly, prompt initiation of appropriate medical treatment can reduce future fracture risk, and as such, the "fix and treat principle" can produce substantial cost savings among other initiatives when it is applied successfully.

This book covers important aspects of both medical and surgical treatment of osteoporosis. It is hoped that every chapter is helpful to both physicians and surgeons, will improve their understanding of the disease process, and will provide a platform for a common language of communication for the issues to be addressed in managing this difficult cohort of patients.

Contributors

Nicholas A. Alfonso
Department of Orthopaedic Surgery
UCHealth University of Colorado Hospital
Aurora, Colorado
and
Department of Orthopaedics
University of Colorado
Denver, Colorado

Kalliopi Alpantaki
Department of Materials Science and Technology
University of Crete
Heraklion, Greece

Panagiotis Anagnostis
Center of Orthopaedic and Regenerative Medicine (C.O.RE.)
Center for Interdisciplinary Research and Innovation
Aristotle University of Thessaloniki (C.I.R.I.-AU.Th)
and
Unit of Reproductive Endocrinology
Department of Obstetrics and Gynecology
Medical School, Aristotle University of Thessaloniki
Thessaloniki, Greece

Paul Andrzejowski
Academic Department of Orthopaedic and Trauma Surgery
School of Medicine
University of Leeds
Leeds, United Kingdom

Peter Augat
Institute of Biomechanics
Berufsgenossenschaftliche Unfallklinik
Murnau, Germany

and

Institute of Biomechanics
Paracelsus Medical University
Salzburg, Austria

Paul C. Baldwin III
Department of Orthopaedics
Saint Francis Hospital and Medical Center
Hartford, Connecticut
and
Fleming Island, Florida

Elizabeth Rosado Balmayor
Department of Instructive Biomaterial Engineering (IBE)
MERLN Institute for Technology-Inspired Regenerative
  Medicine
Maastricht University
Maastricht, The Netherlands

Zsolt J. Balogh
Department of Orthopaedic Trauma Surgery
John Hunter Hospital
and
University of Newcastle
Newcastle, Australia

Rodrigo Banegas
Denver Health Medical Center
and
Department of Orthopaedic Surgery
University of Colorado
Denver, Colorado

Amrut Borade
Musculoskeletal Institute and Department of
  Orthopaedic Surgery
Geisinger Medical Center
Danville, Pennsylvania

Richard Buckley
Department of Orthopaedics
University of Calgary
Calgary, Canada

Jon B. Carlson
Department of Orthopaedic Surgery
University of Louisville School of Medicine
Louisville, Kentucky

Enrique Caso
Department of Orthopaedics
Hospital Universitario Costa del Sol
University of Malaga
Malaga, Spain

Owen Diamond
Department of Orthopaedics
Royal Victoria Hospital
Belfast, Northern Ireland

Panagiotis Douras
Academic Department of Orthopaedic and Trauma Surgery
School of Medicine
University of Leeds
Leeds, United Kingdom

Alexandros A. Drosos
Rheumatology Clinic
Department of Internal Medicine
Medical School, University of Ioannina
Ioannina, Greece

Thomas A. Einhorn
Professor of Orthopedic Surgery
New York University
Director of Clinical and Translational Research Development
NYU Hospital for Joint Disease
New York, New York

Peter V. Giannoudis
Academic Department of Orthopaedic and Trauma Surgery
School of Medicine
University of Leeds
Leeds, United Kingdom

Vasileios P. Giannoudis
Academic Department of Orthopaedic and Trauma Surgery
School of Medicine
University of Leeds
Leeds, United Kingdom

Nifon K. Gkekas
Academic Orthopaedic Department
Papageorgiou General Hospital
Aristotle University Medical School
and
Center of Orthopaedic and Regenerative Medicine (C.O.RE.)
Center for Interdisciplinary Research and Innovation
Aristotle University of Thessaloniki (C.I.R.I.-AU.Th)
Thessaloniki, Greece

Dimitrios G. Goulis
Center of Orthopaedic and Regenerative Medicine (C.O.RE.)
Center for Interdisciplinary Research and Innovation
Aristotle University of Thessaloniki (C.I.R.I.-AU.Th)
and
Unit of Reproductive Endocrinology
Department of Obstetrics and Gynecology
Medical School, Aristotle University of Thessaloniki
Thessaloniki, Greece

Enrique Guerado
Department of Orthopaedic Surgery and Traumatology
Hospital Universitario Costa del Sol
University of Malaga
Malaga, Spain

Alexander G. Hadjipavlou
Department of Orthopaedic Surgery and
 Rehabilitation
University of Texas Medical Branch
Galveston, Texas

David J. Hak
Denver Health Medical Center
and
Department of Orthopaedic Surgery
University of Colorado
Denver, Colorado

Sascha Halvachizadeh
Department of Orthopaedics Trauma
University of Hospital Zurich
University of Zurich
Zurich, Switzerland

David L. Helfet
Orthopaedic Trauma Service
Hospital for Special Surgery
and
New York Presbyterian Hospital
and
Weill Medical College
Cornell University
New York City, New York

Alexander Hofmann
Department of Orthopaedics and Traumatology
University Medical Centre
Johannes Gutenberg University
Mainz, Germany

Edward S. Holloway
Department of Orthopaedics
Leeds Teaching Hospitals NHS Trust
Leeds, United Kingdom

Daniel S. Horwitz
Musculoskeletal Institute and Department of Orthopaedic
 Surgery
Geisinger Medical Center
Danville, Pennsylvania

Angus Jennings
Department of Orthopaedics
University of Calgary
Calgary, Alberta, Canada

Jesse B. Jupiter
Orthopaedic Surgery
Harvard Medical School
and
Department of Orthopaedic Surgery
Division of Hand Surgery
Massachusetts General Hospital
Boston, Massachusetts

Nikolaos K. Kanakaris
Department of Orthopaedics and Trauma
Leeds Teaching Hospitals NHS Trust
Leeds, United Kingdom

Avadhoot Kantak
Department of Orthopaedics
East Surrey Hospital
Surrey, United Kingdom

Theofilos Karachalios
Orthopaedic Department
School of Health Sciences, Faculty of Medicine
General University Hospital of Larissa
Larissa, Greece

Eustathios Kenanidis
Academic Orthopaedic Department
Papageorgiou General Hospital
Aristotle University Medical School
and
Center of Orthopaedic and Regenerative
  Medicine (C.O.RE.)
Center for Interdisciplinary Research and Innovation
Aristotle University of Thessaloniki (C.I.R.I.-AU.Th)
Thessaloniki, Greece

Georgios Komnos
Orthopaedic Department
School of Health Sciences, Faculty of Medicine
General University Hospital of Larissa
Larissa, Greece

Michael G. Kontakis
Department of Orthopaedic Surgery
University Hospital of Heraklion
Crete, Greece

Antonios Koutalos
Orthopaedic Department
School of Health Sciences, Faculty of Medicine
General University Hospital of Larissa
Larissa, Greece

Christian Krettek
Department of Traumatology
Medizinische Hochschule Hannover (MHH)
Hannover, Germany

Joseph Lane
Metabolic Bone Disease Service
Hospital for Special Surgery
New York City, New York

David Limb
Department of Orthopaedics
Leeds Teaching Hospitals NHS Trust
Leeds, United Kingdom

Amy Margot Lindh
Department of Trauma and Orthopaedics
Leeds General Infirmary
Leeds, United Kingdom

James X. Liu
NYU Hospital for Joint Diseases
New York University Langone Medical Center
New York University School of Medicine
New York City, New York

Yi Liu
Metabolic Bone Disease Service
Hospital for Special Surgery
New York City, New York

Katherine Lowery
Leeds Teaching Hospitals
NHS Trust
Leeds, United Kingdom

Konstantinos G. Makridis
Iaso Thessaly, Private Hospital
and
Department of Orthopaedics
Medical School
University of Thessaly
Larissa, Greece

Anastasia E. Markatseli
Endocrinology Clinic
Department of Internal Medicine
Medical School, University of Ioannina
Ioannina, Greece

Theodora E. Markatseli
Rheumatology Clinic
Department of Internal Medicine
Medical School, University of Ioannina
Ioannina, Greece

Cyril Mauffrey
Department of Orthopaedics
Denver Health Medical Center
Denver, Colorado

Andreas F. Mavrogenis
First Department of Orthopaedics
School of Medicine
National and Kapodistrian University of Athens
Athens, Greece

Terence Ong
Department of General Medicine
Nottingham City Hospital
Nottingham, United Kingdom

Hans-Christoph Pape
Department of Trauma
University Hospital of Zurich
and
Department of Traumatology
University of Zurich
Zurich, Switzerland

Donato Perretta
Department of Orthopaedic Surgery
Division of Hand Surgery
Massachusetts General Hospital
Boston, Massachusetts

Michael Potoupnis
Academic Orthopaedic Department
Papageorgiou General Hospital
Aristotle University Medical School
and
Center of Orthopaedic and Regenerative Medicine (C.O.RE.)
Center for Interdisciplinary Research and Innovation
Aristotle University of Thessaloniki (C.I.R.I.-AU.Th)
Thessaloniki, Greece

Ippokratis Pountos
Academic Department of Orthopaedic and Trauma Surgery
School of Medicine
University of Leeds
Leeds, United Kingdom

Michael J. Raschke
Department of Trauma
Hand and Reconstructive Surgery
University Hospital Münster
Münster, Germany

Craig S. Roberts
Department of Orthopaedic Surgery
University of Louisville School of Medicine
Louisville, Kentucky

Natalie C. Rollick
Section of Orthopaedic Surgery
Department of Surgery
University of Calgary
Calgary, Alberta, Canada

Pol M. Rommens
Department of Orthopaedics and Traumatology
University Medical Centre
Johannes Gutenberg University
Mainz, Germany

Opinder Sahota
Department of Care of the Elderly
Nottingham University Hospital, NHS Trust
Nottingham, United Kingdom

Blossom Samuels
Metabolic Bone Disease Service
Hospital for Special Surgery
New York City, New York

Daniela Sanchez
Musculoskeletal Institute and Department of
 Orthopaedic Surgery
Geisinger Medical Center
Danville, Pennsylvania

David Seligson
Department of Orthopaedic Surgery
University of Louisville School of Medicine
Louisville, Kentucky

Richard Stange
Department of Regenerative Musculoskeletal Medicine
Institute of Musculoskeletal Medicine (IMM)
and
Department of Trauma
University Hospital Münster
Münster, Germany

Konstantinos D. Stathopoulos
First Department of Orthopaedics
School of Medicine
National and Kapodistrian University of Athens
Athens, Greece

Seth M. Tarrant
Department of Traumatology
John Hunter Hospital and University of Newcastle
Newcastle, Australia

Theodoros H. Tosounidis
Department of Orthopaedic Surgery
University Hospital of Heraklion
Crete, Greece

George Tselentakis
Department of Orthopaedics
East Surrey Hospital
Redhill, Surrey, United Kingdom

Eleftherios Tsiridis
Academic Orthopaedic Department
Papageorgiou General Hospital
Aristotle University Medical School
and
Center of Orthopaedic and Regenerative Medicine (C.O.RE.)
Center for Interdisciplinary Research and Innovation
Aristotle University of Thessaloniki (C.I.R.I.-AU.Th)
Thessaloniki, Greece

Martijn van Griensven
Department of Cell Biology-Inspired Tissue Engineering
 (cBITE)
MERLN Institute for Technology-Inspired Regenerative
 Medicine
Maastricht University
Maastricht, The Netherlands

Georgios Vastardis
Endoscopic and Minimally Invasive Spine Surgery Clinic
Iaso General Hospital
Athens, Greece

J.P.A.M. Verbruggen
Department of Trauma Surgery
Maastrict University
Maastricht, Holland

Veysi T. Veysi
Department of Orthopaedics
Leeds Teaching Hospitals NHS Trust
Leeds, United Kingdom

Christian Von Rüden
Department of Trauma Surgery
Berufsgenossenschaftliche Unfallklinik
Murnau, Germany

Daniel Wagner
Department of Orthopaedics and Traumatology
University Medical Centre
Johannes Gutenberg University
Mainz, Germany

Stamatina-Emmanouela Zourntou
Department of General Medicine
Iaso Thessaly, Private Hospital
Larisa, Greece

Definition, risk factors, and epidemiology of osteoporosis

ENRIQUE GUERADO and ENRIQUE CASO

DEFINITION

Osteoporosis is the x-ray image of osteopenia—a diminution of the bone mass volume. Although pathologic in younger people, osteoporosis is a normal physiologic situation in elderly persons, particularly women. Yet osteoporosis has always been considered to be pathologic, and the word *osteoporosis* is used every day in orthopedic clinics. A homogeneous diminution of bone density under x-ray can also be the product of a reduction of bone tissue calcification, a disease called *osteomalacia*, which is always a pathologic situation.

When we say that a patient has osteoporosis, we actually mean that she or he has osteopenia. In clinical practice, osteoporosis is retrospectively recognized when a patient experiences a low-energy trauma, provoking what is termed a "fragility fracture" (1). Therefore, the definition of osteoporosis is very much related to the reduction of bone strength (2), secondary to an abnormal bone architecture (3,4); in consequence, osteoporosis and fractures are commonly, but wrongly, studied as the same disease. However, since the sensitivity of the clinical presentation of osteoporosis or its visibility in a simple x-ray projection—requiring a diminution of up to 20% of the mineralized bone matrix for bone mass loss to be detectable—is very low, a more accurate definition is needed.

The World Health Organization's (WHO) definition of osteoporosis is based on densitometry findings. An individual with a bone mass index 2.5 standard deviations (SDs) or more below the average value for young healthy women would be considered to be osteoporotic (5). Although no alternative objective standard has been proposed, this definition is unrelated to the normal situation of elderly persons, for whom, in general, bone deterioration is just a part of overall body decline.

On the basis of the WHO definition, densitometry is considered by patients' associations to be the gold standard for the diagnosis of osteoporosis, even for older persons,

an attitude that has led some authors to criticize this definition, accusing pharmaceutical companies of sponsoring the characterization of diseases (6–8) and of systematically distorting both the evidence and evidence-based medicine and guidelines (9,10).

According to the industry, all persons presenting osteoporosis, under the WHO densitometry definition, should receive pharmaceutical treatment, and this recommendation is often at odds with the actual clinical situation (5). On the one hand, although all postmenopausal women will present osteoporosis, pharmaceutical companies assert that from a given age, the entire population should be pharmacologically treated for this disease. In consequence, for the majority of physicians and orthopedic surgeons, the elderly nontreated population are in fact undertreated patients. However, this outlook is not corroborated in clinical practice; as far as complications of osteoporosis are concerned, only a minority of elderly persons present "fragility fractures," according to technological evaluation agencies (11). In this respect, health technology agencies have published data obtained from five independent evaluations of the predictive performance of bone density measurements. Depending on the threshold values used and the assumed lifetime incidence of hip fracture, these studies have reported predictive values for positive results in bone mass index tests ranging from 8% to 36% (12). Similarly, recent systematic reviews have concluded that there is insufficient evidence to inform the choice of which bone turnover marker should be used in routine clinical practice to monitor the response to osteoporosis treatment (13).

In view of these considerations, the overriding research priority should be to identify promising treatment-test combinations for evaluation in methodologically rigorous randomized controlled trials (RCTs). In order to determine whether or not bone turnover marker monitoring actually improves treatment decisions, and ultimately impacts on patient outcomes in terms of reduced incidence of fracture, well-designed RCTs are needed (13). Such projects should also focus on the multifactor etiology (comorbidity, type and circumstances of trauma, polypharmacy, previous fractures, hereditary, menopause, etc.) of broken bones. International registries represent a major step toward achieving this approach and contribute to obtaining a more accurate definition of the disease.

There is often much confusion between the concept of a fracture patient with osteoporosis versus one with an "osteoporotic fracture." The definition of "osteoporotic fracture" arouses controversy, as osteoporosis is merely one of many independent variables—and in many instances not necessarily the most important one—also including age, dementia, and/or cataracts, in the clinical background of the disease. Obviously, when an elderly person is admitted to hospital with a hip fracture, and with concurrent cataracts that may provoke falls, this patient is not said to have suffered an "ophthalmic fracture," even though the origin of the fracture could be a fall caused by defective vision (14). Furthermore, although all elderly persons are osteopenic, only a small percentage of them will suffer a fall, and less than half of those who do will develop an injury as a result (15). Moreover, persons aged 65 years or older who have a fall are likely to suffer another one within a year but will not necessarily experience a fracture (16).

Today, it is fairly well established that falls are the main cause of hip fractures, and also that although osteoporosis provokes more severe fracture patterns than those found in nonosteoporotic bones, this disease is not the origin of hip or wrist fractures. Only with respect to the treatment provided, and not as regards the physiopathology, could the expression "osteoporotic fracture" be properly used. However, even in well-reputed standard textbooks, the terms *osteoporosis* and *fracture* in elderly patients are commonly confused (17).

EPIDEMIOLOGY

The epidemiology of osteoporosis is very difficult to determine, as osteopenia is always considered a disease. Therefore, such epidemiology must rely on its own definition. On the one hand, since osteopenia is the normal outcome of bone metabolism in aging people, particularly women after the onset of menopause, osteoporosis can be viewed as the "physiologic" situation reached by everyone, especially women aged 50 years or more. On the other hand, after the WHO (5) established a bone mineral density (BMD) cutoff point of 2.5 standard deviations below the average value for a young healthy person, measured in the spine or hip, among the elderly (and the not so elderly), osteoporosis has come to be categorized, rather than a physiologic situation, as a pathologic one.

Another problem hampering determination of the epidemiology of osteoporosis is that of a confusion between osteoporosis and fractures occurring in osteoporotic patients, generally attributed to this disease. It has been estimated that some 300,000 hip fractures occur each year in the United States, and 1.7 million in Europe (18,19),

while wrist fractures in the United States affect about 800 per 100,000 women (20), and almost one million women suffer postmenopausal vertebral fractures every year. All of these fractures are attributed to osteoporosis, although all elderly people present osteopenia, and only a small minority of the nearly 25 million U.S. citizens with BMD <2.5 SD will suffer an "osteoporotic fracture."

It is no coincidence that elderly people have more disabilities than younger ones and suffer more fractures (21). Studies of the treatment of disabilities, such as cataract surgery, have demonstrated that improvements in fall prevention diminish the incidence of these fractures (15), much more than any pharmacologic treatment for osteoporosis. Consequently, the use of fracture prevalence or incidence is a poor means of predicting/establishing the epidemiology of osteoporosis. Nevertheless, in many epidemiological studies, these two factors are often associated.

The expression "pathologic osteoporotic fractures," secondary to a primary disease or a surgical intervention, would be a closer approximation to the reality of a disease. Pathologic estrogen deficit—before the menopause—due to disease or medical intervention is the predominant pathophysiologic disorder of primary osteoporosis, together with the use of glucocorticoids.

Accordingly, it is essential to distinguish carefully between physiologic and pathologic osteoporosis, and also between their prevalence among women and men. In consequence, it is important to note that in addressing osteoporosis, age is a crucial variable; although osteoporosis secondary to disease or medical intervention exists throughout the population, it is encountered more frequently among the elderly. Male osteoporosis has received little research attention, although the Osteoporotic Fractures in Men (MrOS) study is expected to shed some light on this question (22).

The problems arising from an aging population are global and even affect emerging countries. In Brazil, it is estimated that by 2050, 23% of the population will be elderly and that children younger than 14 years will only account for 13% of the population. Accordingly, chronic diseases, including osteoporosis, will be of growing importance (23). Moreover, problems may arise in determining its prevalence, due to differences in study methods, the selection of the sample population, and the definition of diseases (23–25). Thus, while some studies have reported a prevalence ranging from 22.2% to 33.2%, depending on the bone evaluated (26), a telephone survey obtained a prevalence of 8% among persons aged 45–54 years, 19% among those aged 55–64 years, and 32.7% among women over 65 years (27). In 2010, the Brazilian Osteoporosis Study (BRAZOS) conducted a survey of nearly 1700 women and reported that among persons older than 40 years, 35% were premenopausal, and that the subjects' average age at the last menstrual period was 47 ± 5.1 years (28). The overall prevalence of osteoporosis was 15.1%, but among women older than 40 years, a dual-energy x-ray absorptiometry (DEXA) scan revealed a prevalence of up to 33% (29). Epidemiological problems in Brazil are very much related to social and race situations. Among the better-educated population, nonsmokers, those with a higher bone mass index, and those who are very active, the prevalence of osteoporosis is lower (27); in addition, non-Caucasian women appear to be less severely affected. Similar findings have been reported for other developing countries such as India and China (30,31).

In developed countries such as Germany, few cost studies have been undertaken in this field, but foreseeable demographic changes (32) lead us to believe that the costs arising from osteoporotic fractures will probably rise sharply in the relatively near future (33). In this context, four studies based on prevalence have been conducted, as well as one based on incidence, seeking to obtain an approximation of the lifetime costs provoked by hip fractures (34). In addition, a Markov-cohort model has been used to estimate the cumulative and annual osteoporosis-attributable costs of diverse fracture patterns (33). However, none of these investigations projected total numbers and costs for the major fractures that could occur during the patient's remaining lifetime. Moreover, the expected costs of specific subcategories, e.g., persons already suffering from osteoporosis, with a prevalent fracture, or living in a nursing home, were not analyzed (35). We emphasize that all of these studies address the relation between osteoporosis and fractures but not that between fractures and falls, or whether or not osteoporosis played a role in producing the fracture.

Northern European countries present higher rates of hip fractures than southern ones. In Spain, studies have demonstrated an incidence of 301–897/100,000 hip fractures among persons older than 65 years, a rate that is lower than elsewhere (36). With respect to people aged older than 50 years, the incidence is only 195 for women and 73 for men (37), one of the lowest in Europe. Nevertheless, this incidence varies over the years (38–41). What does seem clear is that the more southerly the country, the lower the incidence (38,41,42). This observation is corroborated by studies carried out in Greece, where the incidence is similar to that found in Spain (36,38,43) and in Finland, where it is higher (44).

In any case, studies in various developed countries, including Belgium and Italy, and in the European Union as a whole, have been undertaken considering that osteoporosis can easily provoke a fracture (45–47), a view that tends to underestimate the real value of epidemiology and to overestimate the need to treat osteoporosis in relation to senile fractures.

In this respect, studies have been conducted in the European Union and in the United States. In the European Union, a 2010 report predicted that 22 million women and 5.5 million men would have osteoporosis, according to the WHO diagnostic criteria. Incidence rates of hip fractures are readily accessible in most EU countries, but information on the incidence of forearm, vertebral, and other fractures is less commonly available. The latter study estimated that about 3.5 million fractures occurred each year in the European Union, including 620,000 of the hip; 520,000

affecting the spine; 560,000 the forearm; and 1,800,000 affecting other locations. Over 30% of all incident fractures were seen in women. Of those who sustained a hip fracture, over three million persons were aged 50 years or older, while an estimated 3.5 million men and women had prior spinal fractures with clinical symptoms. An estimated 43,000 deaths were apparently related to fractures. Among women, 50% of these deaths were provoked by hip fractures, 28% by clinical vertebral fractures, and 22% by other fractures. The corresponding figures for male deaths were 47%, 39%, and 14%, respectively (47). Despite the evident gravity of this situation, in the latter study, not only was nothing said about cognitive situations, patients' proclivity to fall, or the role played by the social situation (a factor shown to be essential in studies conducted in Brazil) (23,27–29), but the attribution of deaths to these fractures totally ignored the influence of concurrent diseases.

RISK OF OSTEOPOROSIS

Epidemiological risk

In clinical epidemiology, when we conclude that a disease or condition A has caused disease B, it is usually because we have reason to believe that the patient was previously at risk of developing disease B, because he or she already had disease/condition A. For example, when we see an elderly person (condition A), we suspect that he or she has osteoporosis (disease B) (Figure 1.1).

Moreover, once a patient has developed disease B, even if there is no evidence of disease/condition A, we will study him or her seeking indications of A, in the view that a subclinical situation A already exists or, if it is still undeveloped, could theoretically be prevented (Figure 1.2). Under the concept of a "causal loop," one situation sequentially provokes another. Thus, when a young patient suffers a complex fracture after a mild trauma, the presence of osteoporosis may be considered. But, as osteoporosis does not commonly occur in young patients, a more detailed study of the clinical circumstances should also be performed, seeking a lifestyle condition, or an endocrine or gastrointestinal disorder, or other likely explanation for the osteoporosis. However, such an investigation would probably never be conducted in the case of an elderly patient. Sometimes, a simple, easy consideration of the patient's clinical history may provide the solution to the problem.

Therefore, the epidemiological risk is the probability of a patient having disease B because disease/condition A is already present. Hence, conceptually it is very difficult to distinguish between secondary osteoporosis—when osteoporosis is the consequence B of exposure to disease/condition A—and the risk of having osteoporosis once disease A has developed. In the first case, osteoporosis is present, whereas in the second, it may appear in the future.

This reasoning corresponds to clinical epidemiology, which is based on statistics: the accumulation of many observations allows us to calculate a probability and

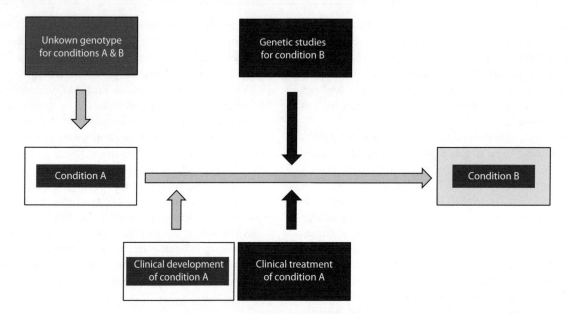

Figure 1.1 A condition A can cause a disease B (condition B): We believe that the patient was previously at risk of developing the disease (condition B), just because he or she already has the condition A. For example, when we see an elderly person (condition A), we suspect that he or she has osteoporosis (disease B) just because he or she is an elderly person.

therefore the strength of an expectation. Under this reasoning, osteoporosis would always be a secondary disease (Tables 1.1 through 1.3), and cases of primary osteoporosis, such as juvenile idiopathic osteoporosis, are classified as such merely because we do not know the first steps of the causal loop.

In clinical epidemiology, not only the fact of exposure but also its duration become a major issue. Since women now live for longer than before, their lifetime risk of having osteoporosis is greater than it used to be (48).

Genetic risk

The search for the origin of a lifestyle or a disease, in order to determine the beginning or end of a given causal loop, may be such a long process that it will ultimately lead nowhere (49). Nevertheless, this "nowhere" is what genetics studies are exploring today, seeking to understand an individual's backstory before a disease/condition occurs.

In this context, risk has basically been defined as the probability of disease/condition A provoking disease B

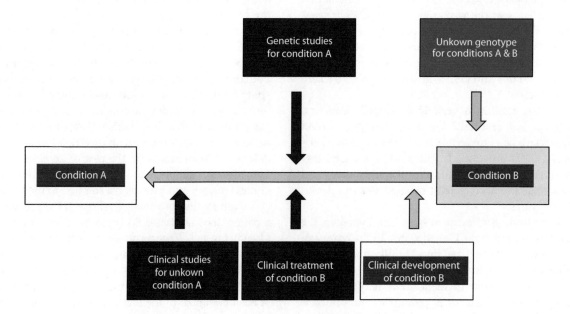

Figure 1.2 When a patient has developed a disease (condition B), even if there is no evidence of previously having the disease or condition A, we study him or her seeking hints of A. We assume that just because the patient has the condition B, a subclinical situation A already exists. Under the concept of a "causal loop," one situation sequentially provokes another.

Table 1.1 Risk diseases for osteoporosis

Risk factor	Condition or disease
Diseases of genetic origin	Cystic fibrosis
	Ehlers–Danlos syndrome
	Gaucher disease
	Glycogen storage disease
	Hemochromatosis
	Homocystinuria
	Hypophosphatasia
	Idiopathic hypercalciuria
	Marfan syndrome
	Menkes disease
	Osteogenesis imperfecta
	Porphyria
	Riley-Day syndrome
Endocrine and reproductive diseases	Androgen insensitivity and hypogonadism
	Athletic amenorrhea
	Hyperprolactinemia
	Panhypopituitarism
	Premature ovarian failure
	Turner syndrome
	Klinefelter syndrome
	Adrenal insufficiency
	Cushing syndrome
	Diabetes mellitus
	Primary hyperparathyroidism
	Thyrotoxicosis
	Metabolic bone disease
	Acromegaly
	Growth hormone deficiency
	Cushing syndrome (ACTH-dependent and independent)
	Mucopolysaccharidoses
	Galactosemia
Gastrointestinal diseases	Celiac disease
	Gastric bypass
	Inflammatory bowel disease
	Malabsorption
	Pancreatic disease
	Gastrointestinal surgery
	Biliary cirrhosis
Hematologic diseases	Hemophilia
	Leukemia and lymphomas
	Multiple myeloma
	Sickle cell disease
	Systemic mastocytosis
	Thalassemia major
Rheumatic and autoimmune disease	Ankylosing spondylitis
	Rheumatoid arthritis
	Systemic lupus erythematosus

(Continued)

Table 1.1 (Continued) Risk diseases for osteoporosis

Risk factor	Condition or disease
Neuromuscular disorders	Duchenne muscular dystrophy
	Rett syndrome
	Systemic sclerosis
Other diseases	Chronic metabolic acidosis
	Congestive heart failure
	Depression
	Anorexia nervosa and bulimia
	Emphysema
	End-stage renal disease
	Epilepsy
	Parenteral nutrition and malnutrition
	Sarcoidosis

Table 1.2 Lifestyle and conditions for osteoporosis

Lifestyle	Condition
Lifestyle	Alcohol
	Pregnancy and lactation-associated osteoporosis
	Aluminium (antacids intake excess)
	Excess of vitamin A intake
	Caffeine intake excess
	Salt intake excess
	Little physical activity
	Low body mass index
	Low calcium intake
	Smoking
	Low vitamin D intake and blood levels

Table 1.3 Medicaments risks for osteoporosis

Medicament	
Medicament	Heparin and anticoagulants
	Anticonvulsants
	Aromatase inhibitors
	Barbiturates
	Chemotherapeutic agents
	Cyclosporine A
	Depo-Provera (medroxyprogesterone)
	Glucocorticoids
	Gonadotropin-releasing hormone agonists
	Lithium
	Oral hypoglycemics
	Proton pump inhibitors
	Tacrolimus
	Selective serotonin reuptake inhibitors

(in the case in question, osteoporosis). However, in the future, genetics may anticipate a diagnosis of B even if A has not yet been diagnosed or observed. This potential is especially useful with respect to disease C, for example, which is less likely to provoke the development of B (in

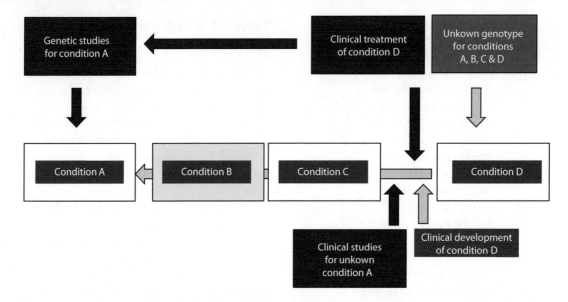

Figure 1.3 Risk has basically been defined as the probability of disease/condition A provoking disease B (in this example, osteoporosis). However, in the future, genetics may anticipate a diagnosis of disease/condition B even if disease/condition A has not yet been diagnosed or observed. This potential is especially useful with respect to disease C, for example, which is less likely to provoke the development of B (in contrast to A, which is an almost infallible forerunner of osteoporosis). Moreover, in subclinical condition D, which is also a risk factor for B, genetics is especially important since (as yet) there is no indication of B. Strangely enough, in these cases, genetic studies can enable us to detect the risk (genotype) before the disease (phenotype).

contrast to A, which is an almost infallible forerunner of osteoporosis). Moreover, in subclinical condition D, which is also a risk factor for B, genetics is especially important since (as yet) there is no indication of B. Strangely enough, in these cases, genetic studies can enable us to detect the risk (genotype) before the disease (phenotype) (Figure 1.3).

Consequently, the term *primary osteoporosis* includes those forms of osteopenia of unknown origin, while secondary osteoporosis is part of a specific disease. Since definitions are just a convention of terminology, as we obtain a better understanding of the causes of osteoporosis, many cases of primary osteoporosis will become, in fact, secondary. That is, they will be secondary to a genetic disorder, even if no clinical abnormality is yet apparent.

MOLECULAR AND GENETIC RISK FACTOR PREDICTORS

Epidemiological studies have sought to identify osteoporosis at an early stage, in order to prevent severe fracture patterns. Therefore, a better understanding of molecular pathways, gene expression regulators, and gene expression profiles related to osteoporosis would enable us to foster and implement novel therapeutic approaches under the concept of "personalized medicine" (50–52).

Genome-wide association studies (GWAS) and whole-exome sequencing in osteoporosis and bone mass disorders (50) have highlighted the importance of screening for nonsyndromic gene mutations (51), low-frequency noncoding variants (EN1, WNT16) with clinical impact on BMD and fracture (52), as has been shown in primary hypertrophic osteoarthropathy (53), inclusion-body myopathy (IBM) with Paget disease of bone (PDB) (54), Hajdu-Cheney syndrome (55), osteogenesis imperfecta

(56), vertebral compression fractures (57), and also osteoporosis (58). New-generation sequencing (NGS) analysis, therefore, constitutes a tool that adds value and speed and enables us to evaluate the process of osteoporosis, to identify biomarkers and targets for drugs, and to develop new therapies based on tissue engineering and personalized medicine. Faster and more cost-effective testing to acquire a better understanding of how the genotype regulation of molecular pathways modulates the coupling of bone-forming and bone-destroying cells will enable us to apply these studies to larger groups of people and thus raise the epidemiology and the risk calculation of osteoporosis to a new dimension and a more precise scientific level.

MOLECULAR PATHWAYS

Cell interactions for bone remodeling are mediated by molecular factors clustered mainly in three key molecular pathways; the receptor activator of nuclear factor-κB–osteoprotegerin(RANK-OPG), Wnt proteins, and bone morphogenetic proteins (BMPs). The RANKL-OPG (receptor activator of nuclear factor–κB ligand–osteoprotegerin) pathway modulates the balance of bone formation and bone resorption by regulating progenitor osteoclasts through RANK, CD4, CD11b, and cFms factors (Figure 1.4). Receptor activator RANKL binds to RANK, inducing osteoclast differentiation into mature cells, expressing specific osteoclast activity factors such as tartrate-resistant acid phosphatase (TRAP), calcitonin receptors, cathepsin K, matrix metalloproteinase 9 (MMP9) and α, and β3-integrin chains. RANKL, when competitively bound to OPG secreted by osteoblasts, induces the inhibition of osteoclastogenesis (59).

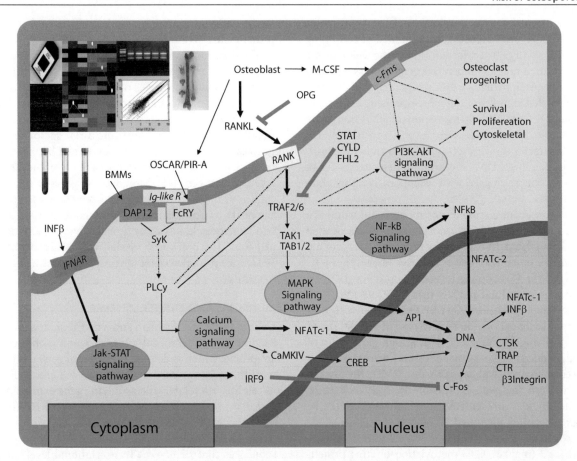

Figure 1.4 Osteoclast differentiation signaling pathways. In osteoclast progenitor, the activation and inhibiting signals (M-CSF, OPG, RANKL, BMMs, OSCAR/PIR-A, INFβ) are driven from cell membrane to nuclear DNA to modulate the transcription and expression of specific genes (NFTAc-1, INFb CTSK, TRAP, CTR, β3-integrin) expressed by mature osteoclast. Interconnected intracellular signaling pathways involved in the osteoclast differentiation process mainly include MAPK, NF-κB, PI3-AkT, calcium, and Jak-STAT cytoplasmic signaling pathways. RANKL-RANK interaction, at cell membrane, activates TNF receptor associated factors 6 and 2 (TRAF6/2), which function as signal transducers in MAPK, NF-κB, and PI3k-AkT signaling pathways. It also interferes with the calcium signaling pathway. TRAF is inhibited by STAT, CYLD, and FHL and also by osteoprotegerin (OPG) throughout inhibition of the RANL-RANK interaction.

The Wnt pathways enhance the osteoblast differentiation of bone marrow mesenchymal stem cells (MSCs) and the proliferation and differentiation of osteoblast progenitors by binding the Wnt ligand to its membrane receptor complex. The receptor is a complex of specific Frizzled (FZD) proteins and the low-density lipoprotein receptor-related protein 5/6 (LRP-5/6). Activated membrane ligand-receptor complexes release and stabilize β-catenin (OPG inhibitor) as intracellular signaling to regulate the Runx2 and Osterix gene coding proteins at the nuclei level, together with transcription factor 4 (TCF-4) or lymphoid enhancer binding factor 1 (LEF-1). Wnt signaling also reduces bone resorption by the competitive binding of secreted Frizzled-related protein 1 (Sfrp1) to RANKL expressed in osteoclast activity. Other regulators of this pathway include insulin-like growth factor 1 (IGF-1), Notch, and Sclerostin. BMPs are cytokines belonging to the transforming growth factor-beta (TGF-β) superfamily, which stimulates the phosphorylation of R-Smads (Samd1, Smad5, and Smad8), which, in turn, form complexes with Co-Smad (Smad4) modulating gene expression at the nuclei level, and thus increase osteogenesis. In this pathway, Runx2 regulates the gene expression of osteopontin (OPN), bone sialoprotein (BSP), osteocalcin (OCN), and PI3K/Akt and the activation of Smads.

Other abundant factors in bone tissue include members of the histone deacetylase (HDAC) family (HDAC1, HDAC3, HDAC5, and HDAC9), whereas HDAC5 inhibits Runx2 activity and HDAC9 inhibits peroxisome proliferator-activated receptor gamma (PPAR-γ) and RANKL-reducing osteoclastogenesis. Other factors modulating Runx2 expression are fibroblast growth factors (FGFR2s) and HOXA10 (59).

DIFFERENTIAL GENE EXPRESSION

The development of "-omics" technologies, enabling the large-scale, rapid study of genomes, exomes, proteomes, and differential gene expression, has expanded our understanding of the molecular processes involved in multifactorial diseases. New areas of research such as the genome, transcriptome, metabolome, and interactome constitute a challenge for translational research and an area of immense promise for the development of systems medicine. In this respect, studies have obtained encouraging results, improving our understanding of the osteoporotic process. Thus, a major comparative gene expression study of 13,463 genes in patients with osteoporosis and osteoarthritis revealed significant differences in gene expression profiles in 241 CpG methylation regions of DNA from bone (60). The affected 228 genes were associated with cell differentiation factors and bone transcription embryogenesis. Moreover, the lower DNA methylation detected in 217 of these genes was associated with osteoporosis rather than osteoarthritis.

In a Japanese population of postmenopausal women, a study of single nucleotide polymorphism (SNP) associated with BMD reported the existence of an increased risk of hip fractures in women with one or two risk phenotypes (GG and AG) of the 98 coupling receptor G protein (GPR98) (61). Studies in animal models using GPR98 knockout mice have explained these data by reference to a significant impairment of bone characteristics such as BMD and mechanical fragility, together with a high expression of RANKL-induced osteoclastogenesis and osteoclasts (61). In postmenopausal women with low BMD, the results obtained from the gene expression analysis of B cells, confirmed by real-time polymerase chain reaction (PCR) gene amplification, identified 29 repressed genes, including estrogen receptor 1 (ESR1), mitogen-activating protein kinase 3 (mapk3), CpG methylation-binding protein 2 (MECP2), phosphatase-interacting protein 1 (PSTPIP1), Scr-like-adapter (SLA), serine/threonine kinase 11 (STK11), WNK lysine-deficient protein kinase 1 (WNK1), and zinc finger protein 446 (ZNF446) (62).

These findings support the idea that new mechanisms for the pathogenesis of osteoporosis should be considered; by determining these molecular pathways, the risk of the disease developing can be more easily detected. A subsequent differential gene expression analysis of the same population of postmenopausal women identified 3 out of 70 differentially expressed genes (signal transducer and activator of transcription 1 [STAT1]; guanylate binding protein 1 [GBP1]; and chemokine [C-X-C motif] ligand 10 CXCL10) as playing a significant role in osteoclastogenesis (63). Other less well-known mechanisms of osteoblast differentiation may also be involved in osteoporosis as a polymorphic variant of the sulfide quinone reductase-like (SQRDL) gene coding for a mitochondria protein, which catalyzes the conversion of sulfide to persulfides and has been associated with the susceptibility factor for osteoporosis in postmenopausal women (64).

As a result of differential gene expression microarray analysis of B cells in postmenopausal women, new mechanisms have been suggested for osteoporosis, with the participation of several genes controlling the balance between osteoclastogenesis and osteoblastogenesis (62). Among these identified genes are ESR1, MAPK3, methyl CpG binding protein 2 (MECP2), proline-serine-threonine phosphatase interacting protein 1 (PSTPIP1), Scr-like-adaptor (SLA), serine/threonine kinase 11 (STK11), WNK

lysine-deficient protein kinase 1 (WNK1), and zinc finger protein 446 (ZNF446).

The determination of gene expression levels is of major importance for the early detection of disease risk in clinical practice. In fact, low levels of circulating mRNA of estrogen receptor alpha (ERα) gene, detected by quantitative real-time reverse-transcription polymerase chain reaction (QRT-PCR), appear to constitute a risk factor for osteoporosis in menopausal women and are a better indicator of clinical outcome than the patient's age and/or serum levels of estrogens (65). Moreover, no gene-by-sex interaction or sex-specific effects have been shown to influence the BMD, as demonstrated by genome-wide meta-analysis in a large population study (greater than 50,000 individuals) (66). The bone area needed with which to measure BMD for optimal skeletal phenotype studies has yet to be determined.

microRNAs AND TRANSCRIPTOME

Cells of the same organism and with the same genome can become very different cell types depending on their transcriptome, which is defined as the set of gene coding proteins that are expressed in a given cell at a precise moment of cell life. Therefore, when studying gene expression profiles, it is important to analyze at messenger RNA (mRNA) level the expression of its regulator molecules, called microRNAs (miRNAs). These are small noncoding RNA sequences that silence the transcriptional levels of genes coding for proteins involved in general biological processes and cell functions, from organogenesis to tissue differentiation and, therefore, the differentiation and functions of osteoblasts and osteoclasts. Up to 30% of human mRNAs are regulated by over 400 identified miRNAs, covering the expression of up to 4% of human genes; it has been suggested that the total number of miRNAs may exceed 800. The organ specificity, stability, and efficiency of the miRNAs in controlling mRNA transcription are aspects that help identify tissue-specific expression profiles and may lead to these molecules being considered as potential therapeutic targets.

These single-stranded RNA sequences of 20–22 nucleotides induce mRNA degradation in the cytoplasm or prevent protein translation by induction of the silencing complex activity, which is mediated by the RNA-RISC protein complex (import DICER and Argonaute proteins). The functionality of miRNAs arises from their interaction with the mRNA, forming mRNA-miRNA (MRM) modules with alternative regulatory mechanisms (*cis* and *trans*) involved in transcription factor (TF) mRNA interactions/TF gene (5'-3') targets for TF. While mRNA expression profiles are inversely related to the miRNA controlling their degradation, this simple relationship is not held by the miRNAs that mediate transcriptional inhibition. In this case, both the overexpression and the repression of miRNAs can induce the direct inhibition of multiple mRNA target transcription. This gives rise to significant differences between the expression levels of mRNAs depending on whether or not they are subjected to transcriptional control by multiple miRNAs, inducing a further degradation of mRNAs with multiple binding sites for miRNAs.

The role played by miRNAs in the genesis of osteoblasts and osteoclasts has been studied by Sun et al. (59). Several specific miRNAs (miR-20a, miR-29a, miR-15b, miR-210, miR-216a, miR-2861, miR-3960, and miR-2861) exert a regulatory effect in enhancing osteogenesis. Other miRNAs have inhibitory effects on osteoblasts (miR-204, miR-705, miR-3077-5p, miR-338-3P, miR-125b, miR-637, miR-188, miR-141-3p, miR-138, miR-138-5p, miR-675-5p, and miR-675-5p) or on osteoclastogenesis (miR-503, miR-148a, miR-9, and miR-181a). A dual effect is also produced by some miRNAs, enhancing osteoblast differentiation and inhibiting osteoclastogenesis (miR-34a, miR-26a) or inhibiting osteoblast differentiation and enhancing osteoclastogenesis (miR-214). Therefore, the determination of miRNA expression is a question of great interest, as molecular markers for risk and subclinical determination and for assessing clinical outcomes. High circulating levels of one miRNA (miR-194-5p) (79) determined by microarray analysis and QRT-PCR are associated with osteoporosis (64,67). Differences in expression levels of miRNAs have been observed in postmenopausal women with low BMD (miR-422a and miR-133a) (68), patients with osteoporosis and hip fractures (miR-122-5p, miR-125b-5p, miR-21-5p, miR-21, miR-23a, miR-24, miR-25, miR-100, and miR-125b) (69,70), and patients with osteoporosis and vertebral fractures (miR-106b and miR-19b) (59).

GENOTYPE

The analysis of SNPs in specific mRNA regions (3′UTRs), which are targets for miRNAs, in patients with osteoporosis, has identified three polymorphisms for fibroblast growth factor-2 (FGF2), which are regulated by nine miRNAs and significantly associated with bone density. These findings suggest that this mechanism may be a cause of increased susceptibility to osteoporosis (71). Therefore, analysis of the miRNAs involved in the regulation of the most important pathologic processes, driving the progression of osteoporosis, would be a key step in designing targeted and customized therapies for osteoporosis.

The integration of SNPs, transcription arrays, expression profiles, and GWASs has confirmed previously reported associations of gene variants and osteoporosis.

Association studies between BMD variation and fracture susceptibility, carried out by a meta-analysis of GWAS genotyping studies (72), have revealed a set of 32 new loci associated with BMD, some of which are clustered within specific signaling pathways, including the Wnt, endochondral ossification mesenchymal stem cell differentiation, and RANK-RANKL-OPG.

The TNFRSF11B/OPG gene encoding a member of the TNF-receptor superfamily is an osteoblast-secreted decoy receptor that functions as a negative regulator of bone resorption and has been associated with osteoporosis (73). This protein specifically binds to its ligand, osteoprotegerin ligand, and both of these are key extracellular regulators of osteoclast development.

The integration of these technologies has also enabled the identification of new chromosomal (Chr) locations associated with osteoporosis such as previously unknown bone-related loci, for instance (72), 18p11.21 (C18orf19), 7q21.3 (SLC25A13), 11q13.2 (LRP5), 4q22.1 (MEPE), 2p16.2 (SPTBN1), 10q21.1 (DKK1), Chr.1p13.2 for RAP1A, a member of the RAS oncogene family, Chr.2q11.2 for TBC1 domain family member 8 (TBC1D8), and Chr.18q11.2 for OSBPL1A, an oxysterol binding protein like 1A.

New candidates associated with BMD have also been suggested, including wntless Wnt ligand secretion mediator (GPR177) genes, and SRY-box 6 (SOX6), a transcriptional activator that is required for normal development of chondrogenesis and maintenance of skeletal muscle cells (73). A panel of more than 25 genes has been associated with BMD by GWAS analysis in postmenopausal women, including ARHGAP1, CLCN7, CTNNB1, ESR1, FAM3C, FLJ42280, FOXL1, GALNT3, GPR177, HDAC5, IBSP, JAG1, LRP5, LTBP3, MARK3, MEF2C, MEPE, OPG, RANK, RANKL, RSPO3, SOST, SOX4, SOX6, SP7 (Osterix), TARD3NL, and ZBTB40 (74).

The recent development and use of NGS technologies open up the possibility of determining the genotype response to drugs, through mass sequencing processes that provide great versatility for genotyping (GWAS, WES, RNA-seq, niRNA-seq, methyl-seq). This, in the short/medium term, will enable the implementation in clinical practice of routine screening and treatment response studies. By means of these technologies, a better epidemiological map of disease distribution and genomic risk, both potential and diagnosed, of the osteoporotic patient will be achievable.

IMPORTANCE OF DETERMINING EPIDEMIOLOGICAL AND GENETIC RISKS

Since the significance of osteoporosis is not so much the condition but the associated risk of severe events occurring, such as wrist or hip fractures, there is a danger of erroneous reasoning being made regarding its causal loop (14). As observed previously, the most common error in this regard is to assume that hip or wrist fractures in the elderly are caused by osteoporosis. Whether or not the term *osteoporotic fracture* was in fact coined by the pharmaceutical industry (14), the fact is that most physicians and orthopedic surgeons believe that a hip or wrist fracture is indeed an osteoporotic fracture, even though osteoporosis is simply one of many variables; although it can make the fracture pattern more severe, it is not the cause of the fracture (14).

Therefore, in our quest to prevent the occurrence of hip fractures, the causal loop must be redefined. Hip fractures are provoked by falls, which in turn are caused by cognitive defects. The latter can take various forms, the risk of which may be gauged by genetic studies. Nevertheless, although the main cause of hip fracture is not osteoporosis, this disease does contribute to fracture pattern complexity, and more detailed knowledge of the risk of its occurrence would also be very useful.

As hip fractures are usually caused by falls, by identifying the population with a genetic propensity to suffer a fall, i.e., persons with a sensory or cognitive problem aggravating the risk of a fall, and then providing proper treatment for such problems, both falls and hip fractures could be prevented. However, to date, genetic studies aimed at preventing fractures have focused exclusively on osteoporosis (14).

It has been reported that two specific gene variants of basic biological proteins can heighten the risk of osteoporosis and, consequently, of osteoporotic fracture. The joint consequence of these risk alleles on fractures is analogous to that of most well-replicated environmental risk factors. They exist in over 20% of Caucasian individuals, and therefore, screening might be useful (75). The latter authors studied the risk of osteoporosis but did not contemplate the risk of bone fracture or of falls.

Finally, great care should be taken to differentiate osteoporosis epidemiology and risk, on the one hand, from the incidence of hip, spine, or wrist fracture, on the other. Research should be focused on osteoporosis and on fall prevention as separate questions, so that new findings regarding the human genome, transcriptome, and metabolomics, if correctly addressed, would remove issues such as epidemiology, the risk of elderly people suffering falls, and the incidence of osteoporosis from the sphere of market interest (14,76–78).

REFERENCES

1. Pietschmann P, Rauner M, Sipos W, Kerschan-Schindl K. Osteoporosis: An age-related and gender-specific disease—A minireview. *Gerontology.* 2009;55:3–12.
2. Rachner TD, Khosla S, Hofbauer LC. New horizons in osteoporosis. *Lancet.* 2011;377:1276–87.
3. Guerado E, Cruz E, Cano JR et al. Mineralization: Effects on hip fractures. *Injury.* 2015;47(Suppl 1):S21–24.
4. The National Institutes of Health (NIH) Consensus Development Panel on Osteoporosis Prevention Diagnosis, and Therapy. Osteoporosis prevention, diagnosis, and therapy. *JAMA.* 2001;285:785–95.
5. The World Health Organization (WHO). Assessment of fracture risk and its application to screening for postmenopausal osteoporosis. Report of a WHO study group. *World Health Organ Tech Rep Ser.* 1994;843:1–129.
6. Morgan DJ, Wright SM, Dhruva S. Update on medical overuse. *JAMA.* 2015;175:120–4.
7. Moynihan R, Cassels A. *Selling sickness: How the World's Biggest Pharmaceutical Companies Are Turning Us All into Patients.* New York, NY: Nation Books, 2005.
8. Tiner R. The pharmaceutical industry and disease mongering. The industry works to develop drugs, not diseases. *BMJ.* 2002;325:216.
9. Spencer D. Evidence based medicine is broken. *BMJ.* 2014;348:g22.
10. Upshur RE, Tracy CS. Is evidence-based medicine overrated in family medicine? Yes. *Can Fam Physician.* 2013;59:1160–1.
11. Gotzsche PC. *Deadly Medicines and Organised Crime. How Big Pharma Has Corrupted Healthcare.* London, UK: Radcliffe Publishing, 2013.
12. Moynihan R, Heath I, Henry D. Authors' reply. *BMJ.* 2002;325:216.
13. Burch J, Rice S, Yang H et al. Systematic review of the use of bone turnover markers for monitoring the response to osteoporosis treatment: The secondary prevention of fractures, and primary prevention of fractures in high-risk groups. *Health Technol Assess.* 2014;18:1–180.
14. Guerado E, Sandalio RM, Caracuel Z, Caso E. Understanding the pathogenesis of hip fracture in the elderly, osteoporotic theory is not reflected in the outcome of prevention programs. *World J Orthop.* 2016;7:218–28.
15. To KG, Meuleners L, Bulsara M et al. A longitudinal cohort study of the impact of first- and both-eye cataract surgery on falls and other injuries in Vietnam. *Clin Interv Aging.* 2014;9:743–51.
16. To KG, Meuleners LB, Fraser ML et al. Prevalence and visual risk factors for falls in bilateral cataract patients in Ho Chi Minh City, Vietnam. *Ophthalmic Epidemiol.* 2014;21:79–85.
17. Lindsay R, Cosman F. Osteoporosis. In Kasper DL, Fauci AS, Hauser S, Longo D, Jameson JL, Loscalzo J, eds. *Harrison's Principles of Internal Medicine.* New York, NY: McGraw-Hill, 2015, pp. 2488–504. Vol 2. Section 4, Chapter 425.
18. Cooper C, Campion G, Melton LJ. Hip fractures in the elderly: A worldwide projection. *Osteoporosis Int.* 1992;2:285–9.
19. The European Commission. *Report on Osteoporosis in the European Community—Action for Prevention.* Brussels, 1998. Available from: http://ec.europa.eu/health/state/docs/eu-report-1998.pdf
20. DeLaet CEDH, Pols HAP. Fractures in the elderly: Epidemiology and demography. *Bailliere Best Pract Res Clin Endocrinol Metab.* 2000;14:171–9.
21. Ross PD. Clinical consequences of vertebral fractures. *Am J Med.* 1997;103:42S–35.
22. Genetic Factors for Osteoporosis Consortium (GEFOS). The Osteoporotic Fractures in Men (MrOS) Study—USA. http://www.gefos.org/?q=content/osteoporotic-fractures-men-mros-study-usa-0 (date last accessed January 2016)
23. Baccaro LF, Conde DM, Costa-Paiva L, Mendes Pinto-Nieto A. The epidemiology and management of postmenopausal osteoporosis: A viewpoint from Brazil. *Clin Interv Aging.* 2015;10:583–91.
24. Baccaro LF, de Souza Santos Machado V, Costa-Paiva L, Sousa MH, Osis MJ, Pinto-Neto AM. Factors associated with osteoporosis in Brazilian women: A population-based household survey. *Arch Osteoporos.* 2013;8:138.

25. Wright NC, Looker AC, Saag KG et al. The recent prevalence of osteoporosis and low bone mass in the United States based on bone mineral density at the femoral neck or lumbar spine. *J Bone Miner Res.* 2014;29:2520–6.

26. Camargo MB, Cendoroglo MS, Ramos LR et al. Bone mineral density and osteoporosis among a predominantly Caucasian elderly population in the city of São Paulo, Brazil. *Osteoporos Int.* 2005;16:1451–60.

27. Martini LA, Moura EC, Santos LC, Malta DC, Pinheiro Mde M. Prevalence of self-reported diagnosis of osteoporosis in Brazil, 2006. *Rev Saúde Pública.* 2009;43:107–16.

28. Pinheiro MM, Ciconelli RM, Jacques Nde O, Genaro PS, Martini LA, Ferraz MB. The burden of osteoporosis in Brazil: Regional data from fractures in adult men and women—The Brazilian Osteoporosis Study (BRAZOS). *Rev Bras Reumatol.* 2010;50:113–27.

29. Pinheiro MM, Reis Neto ET, Machado FS, Omura F, Yang JH. Risk factors for osteoporotic fractures and low bone density in pre- and postmenopausal women. *Rev Saúde Pública.* 2010;44:479–85.

30. Khadilkar AV, Mandlik RM. Epidemiology and treatment of osteoporosis in women: An Indian perspective. *Int J Womens Health.* 2015;7:841–50.

31. Lin X, Xiong D, Peng YQ et al. Epidemiology and management of osteoporosis in the People's Republic of China: Current perspectives. *Clin Interv Aging.* 2015;10:1017–33.

32. Statistisches Bundesamt [The Federal Statistical Office]. *Bevölkerung Deutschland bis 2060: Ergebnisse der 12. Koordinierten Bevölkerungsvorausbrechnung [Population in Germany up to the Year 2060: Results of the 12th Coordinated Projection of Population].* Wiesbaden, Germany: Federal Statistical Office, 2009.

33. Bleibler F, Konnopka A, Benzinger P, Rapp K, König HH. The health burden and costs of incident fractures attributable to osteoporosis from 2010 to 2050 in Germany—A demographic simulation model. *Osteoporos Int.* 2013;24:835–47.

34. Weyler EJ, Gandjour A. Sozioökonomische bedeutung von hüftfrakturen in Deutschland [Socioeconomic burden of hip fractures in Germany]. *Gesundheitswesen.* 2007;69:601–6.

35. Bleibler F, Rapp K, Jaensch A, Becker C, König HH. Expected lifetime numbers and costs of fractures in postmenopausal women with and without osteoporosis in Germany: A discrete event simulation model. *BMC Health Serv Res.* 2014;14:284.

36. Blanco JF, Díaz-Alvarez A, De Pedro JA, Borrego D, del Pino J, Cortés J. Incidence of hip fractures in Salamanca, Spain. Period: 1994–2002. *Arch Osteoporos.* 2006;1:7–12.

37. Ferrandez L, Hernandez J, Gonzalez-Orus A, Devesa F, Ceinos M. Hip fracture in the elderly in Spain. *Acta Orthop Scand.* 1992;63:386–8.

38. Serra JA, Garrido G, Vidán M, Marañon E, Brañas E, Ortiz J. Epidemiología de la fractura de cadera en ancianos en España. *An Med Interna.* 2002;19:389–95.

39. Sosa M, Segarra MC, Hernández D, Gonzalez A, Liminana JM, Betancor P. Epidemiology of proximal femoral fractures in Gran Canaria (Canary Islands). *Age Ageing.* 1993;22:285–8.

40. Díez A, Puig J, Martinez MT, Díez JL, Aubia J, Vivancos J. Epidemiology of fractures of the proximal femur associated with osteoporosis in Barcelona, Spain. *Calcif Tissue Int.* 1993;44:382–6.

41. Sanchez MI, Sangrador CO, Blanco IS, Prieto M, Lozano del Valle F, González TM. Epidemiología de la fractura osteoporótica de cadera en la provincia de Zamora. *Rev Esp Salud Pública.* 1997;71:357–67.

42. Herrera A, Martínez AA, Ferrandez L, Gil E, Moreno A. Epidemiology of osteoporotic hip fractures in Spain. *Int Orthop.* 2005;18:1–4.

43. Paspati I, Galanos A, Lyritis GP. Hip fracture epidemiology in Greece during 1977–1992. *Calcif Tissue Int.* 1998;62:542–7.

44. Kannus P, Niemi S, Parkkari J, Palvanen M, Vuori I, Jarvinen M. Hip fractures in Finland between 1970–1997 and predictions for the future. *Lancet.* 1999;353:802–5.

45. Body JJ, Bergmann P, Boonen S et al. Evidence-based guidelines for the pharmacological treatment of postmenopausal osteoporosis: A consensus document by the Belgian Bone Club. *Osteoporos Int.* 2010;21:1657–80.

46. Cianferotti L, Brandi ML. Guidance for the diagnosis, prevention and therapy of osteoporosis in Italy. *Clin Cases Miner Bone Metab.* 2012;9:170–8

47. Hernlund E, Svedbom A, Ivergård M et al. Osteoporosis in the European Union: Medical management, epidemiology and economic burden. A report prepared in collaboration with the International Osteoporosis Foundation (IOF) and the European Federation of Pharmaceutical Industry Associations (EFPIA). *Arch Osteoporos.* 2013;8:136.

48. Compston JL. Osteoporosis: Social and economic impact. *Radiol Clin N Am.* 2010;48:477–82.

49. Smith NJJ. "Time Travel." *Stanford Encyclopedia of Philosophy.* Available from https://plato.stanford.edu/entries/time-travel/ (30 January 2020).

50. Rivadeneira F, Mäkitie O. Osteoporosis and bone mass disorders: From gene pathways to treatments. *Trends Endocrinol Metab.* 2016;27:262–81.

51. Nishi E, Masuda K, Arakawa M et al. Exome sequencing-based identification of mutations in non-syndromic genes among individuals with apparently syndromic features. *Am J Med Genet A.* 2016;170:2889–94.

52. Zheng HF, Forgetta V, Hsu YH et al. Whole-genome sequencing identifies EN1 as a determinant of bone density and fracture. *Nature.* 2015;526:112–7.

53. Zhang Z, Xia W, He J et al. Exome sequencing identifies SLCO2A1 mutations as a cause of primary hypertrophic osteoarthropathy. *Am J Hum Genet.* 2012;90:125–32.

54. Gu JM, Ke YH, Yue H et al. A novel VCP mutation as the cause of atypical IBMPFD in a Chinese family. *Bone.* 2013;52:9–16.

55. Zhao W, Petit E, Gafni RI et al. Mutations in NOTCH2 in patients with Hajdu-Cheney syndrome. *Osteoporos Int.* 2013;24:2275–81.

56. Pyott SM, Tran TT, Leistritz DF et al. WNT1 mutations in families affected by moderately severe and progressive recessive osteogenesis imperfecta. *Am J Hum Genet.* 2013;92:590–7.

57. Fahiminiya S, Majewski J, Roughley P, Roschger P, Klaushofer K, Rauch F. Whole-exome sequencing reveals a heterozygous LRP5 mutation in a 6-year-old boy with vertebral compression fractures and low trabecular bone density. *Bone.* 2013;57:41–6.

58. Laine CM, Wessman M, Toiviainen-Salo S et al. A novel splice mutation in PLS3 causes X-linked early onset low-turnover osteoporosis. *J Bone Miner Res.* 2015;30:510–8.

59. Sun M, Zhou X, Chen L et al. The regulatory roles of MicroRNAs in bone remodeling and perspectives as biomarkers in osteoporosis. *Biomed Res Int.* 2016, Article ID 1652417, 11 pages. doi: 10.1155/2016/1652417.

60. Delgado-Calle J, Fernández AF, Sainz J et al. Genome-wide profiling of bone reveals differentially methylated regions in osteoporosis and osteoarthritis. *Arthritis Rheum.* 2013;65:197–205.

61. Urano T, Shiraki M, Yagi H et al. GPR98/Gpr98 gene is involved in the regulation of human and mouse bone mineral density. *J Clin Endocrinol Metab.* 2012;97:E565–574.

62. Xiao P, Chen Y, Jiang H et al. *In vivo* genome-wide expression study on human circulating B cells suggests a novel ESR1 and MAPK3 network for postmenopausal osteoporosis. *J Bone Miner Res.* 2008;23:644–54.

63. Lei SF, Wu S, Li LM et al. An *in vivo* genome wide gene expression study of circulating monocytes suggested GBP1, STAT1 and CXCL10 as novel risk genes for the differentiation of peak bone mass. *Bone.* 2009;44:1010–4.

64. Jin HS, Kim J, Park S et al. Association of the I264 T variant in the sulfide quinone reductase-like (SQRDL) gene with osteoporosis in Korean postmenopausal women. *PLOS ONE.* 2015;10(8):e0135285.

65. Chou CW, Chiang TI, Chang IC, Huang CH, Cheng YW. Expression levels of estrogen receptor α mRNA in peripheral blood cells are an independent biomarker for postmenopausal osteoporosis. *BBA Clin.* 2016;5:124–9.

66. Liu CT, Estrada K, Yerges-Armstrong LM et al. Assessment of gene-by-sex interaction effect on bone mineral density. *J Bone Miner Res.* 2012;27:2051–64.

67. Wang Y, Li L, Moore BT et al. MiR-133a in human circulating monocytes: A potential biomarker associated with postmenopausal osteoporosis. *PLOS ONE.* 2012;7(4):e34641.

68. Yang N, Wang G, Hu C et al. Tumor necrosis factor α suppresses the mesenchymal stem cell osteogenesis promoter miR-21 in estrogen deficiency-induced osteoporosis. *J Bone Miner Res.* 2013;28:559–73.

69. Panach L, Mifsut D, Tarín JJ, Cano A, García-Pérez MÁ. Serum circulating microRNAs as biomarkers of osteoporotic fracture. *Calcif Tissue Int.* 2015;97:495–505.

70. Seeliger C, Karpinski K, Haug AT et al. Five freely circulating miRNAs and bone tissue miRNAs are associated with osteoporotic fractures. *J Bone Miner Res.* 2014;29:1718–28.

71. Lei SF, Papasian CJ, Deng HW. Polymorphisms in predicted miRNA binding sites and osteoporosis. *J Bone Miner Res.* 2011;26:72–8.

72. Estrada K, Styrkarsdottir U, Evangelou E et al. Genome-wide meta-analysis identifies 56 bone mineral density loci and reveals 14 loci associated with risk of fracture. *Nat Genet.* 2012;44:491–501.

73. Hsu YH, Zillikens MC, Wilson SG et al. An integration of genome-wide association study and gene expression profiling to prioritize the discovery of novel susceptibility loci for osteoporosis-related traits. *PLOS Genet.* 2010;6(6):e1000977.

74. Duncan EL, Danoy P, Kemp JP et al. Genome-wide association study using extreme truncate selection identifies novel genes affecting bone mineral density and fracture risk. *PLOS Genet.* 2011;7:e1001372.

75. Richards JB, Rivadeneira F, Inouye M et al. Bone mineral density, osteoporosis, and osteoporotic fractures: A genome-wide association study. *Lancet.* 2008;371:1505–12.

76. Van Dijk FS, Zillikens MC, Micha D et al. PLS3 mutations in X-linked osteoporosis with fractures. *N Engl J Med.* 2013;369:1529–36.

77. Angell M. *The Truth about the Drug Companies.* New York, NY: Random House, 2004.

78. Dickinson JA. We cannot market the unsaleable. *Can Fam Physician.* 2007;53:1149–50.

79. Meng J, Zhang D, Pan N et al. Identification of miR-194-5p as a potential biomarker for postmenopausal osteoporosis. *PeerJ.* 2015;3: e971.

2

Pathogenesis: Molecular mechanisms of osteoporosis

ANASTASIA E. MARKATSELI, THEODORA E. MARKATSELI, and ALEXANDROS A. DROSOS

INTRODUCTION

Osteoporosis is a metabolic disease characterized by a disturbance in the quantity of bone tissue. In osteoporosis, in contrast with other metabolic disorders such as rickets and osteomalacia, the ratio of inorganic (hydroxyapatite crystals) to organic substance (matrix and collagen) is kept constant. Cancellous bone is affected to a greater extent compared to cortical bone, and this is due to the fact that 80% of the bone metabolism occurs in the cancellous bone, while the remaining 20% occurs in the cortical bone. In young adults and in premenopausal women, the formation and absorption of bone occur at the same rate, resulting in the maintenance of bone mass over time. Bone loss is a chronic process that starts after the fourth decade of life (1). The deficiency of estrogen and progesterone observed in menopause causes an increased rate of bone remodeling in which bone resorption predominates formation. Therefore, this negative balance results in bone mass loss and leads to postmenopausal osteoporosis (2,3). Particularly, an intensification in the loss of bone mass is observed the first 5–10 years after menopause (3–5).

Multiple genetic and environmental factors play a significant role in the determination of bone mass (6). Linkage analysis in families and candidate gene association analysis in the general population show that genetic factors account for up to 80% of the variance in bone mineral density (BMD) (7–11). Despite the fact that many studies have been conducted on the genetic background of osteoporosis, only a few genes have been identified (12–15).

The canonical Wnt signaling pathway is the major signaling pathway in osteoblasts, which plays an important role in the regulation of bone growth, in bone remodeling, and in fracture repair (16–18). Additionally, it may intervene in the regulation of osteoclastogenesis by altering the expression and secretion of osteoprotegerin (OPG) and receptor activator of nuclear factor–κB ligand (RANKL) from osteoblasts.

PHYSIOLOGY OF BONE TISSUE

Bone tissue

The bone tissue displays important functions in vertebrates that include the protection of vital organs and hematopoietic marrow, the support of muscles, and the storage and release of vital ions such as calcium. The bone tissue is a type of mesenchymal tissue. In the human body, there are two types of bone tissue: cortical and trabecular. The cortical bone represents 80% of the skeleton, while the trabecular bone the remaining 20%. The cortical tissue is found predominantly in the long bones. However, trabecular tissue is found in the central part of the epiphysis of long bones. Trabecular tissue outweighs the flat bones of the pelvis and the vertebrae and is coated in its surface of a cortical tissue layer. The major types of bone tissue cells are osteoblasts, osteoclasts, and osteocytes. We also distinguish organic and inorganic phases in bones. The organic phase includes type I collagen (90%), proteoglycans, and non-collagenous proteins. The organic phase constitutes one-third of bone mass. The inorganic phase comprises calcium salts in the form of hydroxyapatite crystals and constitutes two-thirds of bone mass (19).

Bone strength

Bones play a key role in skeletal support and movement. Osteocytes perceive mechanical forces applied on bones either through the piezoelectric effect or through the application of electrical charges (20,21). This initial process ensures that the adjustment of the mechanical strength of bones and the prevention of fractures will be achieved (22). The construction of bones (bone modeling) and bone remodeling are two functions that are inextricably linked and contribute to the adjustment of mechanical bone strength. The phenomenon of harmonious cooperation between osteoblasts and osteoclasts is called *conjugation* and leads to the maintenance, increase, or reduction of mechanical bone strength depending on the existing conditions (23,24). The factors that determine the mechanical strength of bones are divided into quantitative and qualitative. Bone density, size, and mass are considered quantitative factors (19,25,26). The micro- and macro-architecture of bones, microcracks, cell apoptosis, the rate of bone remodeling, and the properties of mineralized organic matrix are among the qualitative factors (20,27). In the term properties of mineralized organic matrix, the extent of mineralization, the size of hydroxyapatite crystals, and the proportion of collagen cross-links are included (21). Notably, cytokines and hormones also influence significantly the mechanical strength of bones (28).

Peak bone mass

The maximum bone mass that is acquired during life is called *peak bone mass*. The increase in bone mass during the period from birth till the onset of puberty shows no differences between the two sexes. The growth is faster during puberty, and then bone mass in the spine is doubled. The process of the increase in bone mass occurs 2 years earlier in girls than in boys. However, boys eventually achieve greater peak bone mass in the spine and hip (29,30). Bone mass acquires its maximum value during the third decade of life (30). Several factors contribute to the achievement and maintenance of peak bone mass. Among them are genetic, hormonal (levels of estrogens and androgens), nutritional (calcium intake from food), and mechanical factors (exercise) as well as exposure to various risk factors (31–37).

Bone remodeling

Unlike other resilient structures such as tendons, cartilage, and teeth, bone tissue, while it appears to be a "silent organ" that once ceases to grow, is actually a dynamic tissue that undergoes continuous remodeling in response to hormonal changes and mechanical stress. Bone remodeling occurs along with the development of the skeleton and is the main activity of bone tissue in adult life. Bone remodeling both plays a key role in the maintenance of the structure and the integrity of the skeleton and ensures maximum possible mechanical strength (23,24,38). It also regulates the levels of calcium concentration in serum (38).

Many researchers have made efforts to clarify the mechanisms involved in the homeostasis of bone tissue. Bone formation is mainly regulated by osteoblasts, which are derived from mesenchymal stem cells (39). Osteoblasts are small, cuboid, mononuclear cells. The mesenchymal stem cells first proliferate and then differentiate to osteoblast precursors (or preosteoblasts). Subsequently, preosteoblasts become mature osteoblasts that produce the organic substance of bone (proteins of the extracellular matrix). Thereafter, the genes, which are necessary for the

mineralization of the extracellular matrix, are expressed in osteoblasts. As a result, the crystals of hydroxyapatite are incorporated in the organic substance and mineralize it. Osteoblasts produce osteoid with which a bone cavity created by the action of osteoclasts will be filled (39).

Osteoclasts are primarily responsible for bone resorption. Osteoclasts are multinucleated giant cells derived from precursor cells of the monocyte-macrophage lineage (39,40). Mononuclear cells are attracted to the point of the bone surface that will be absorbed and proliferate and differentiate into preosteoclasts. The fusion of mononuclear preosteoclasts follows, which results in the creation of the multinucleated osteoclast. First, the mature osteoclast is firmly adhered to the bone with the help of specialized podosomes, which are rich in actin. Among the highly corrugated surface of the osteoclast and the bone surface, a closed cavity is formed. The osteoclast secretes proteolytic enzymes (cathepsin K) and hydrochloric acid (hydrogen ions) into the cavity (41). Proteolytic enzymes contribute to the fragmentation of the organic phase, while the hydrogen ions dissolve the inorganic phase. It should be noted that the carbonic anhydrase II is an enzyme found in the cytoplasm of the osteoclast and contributes to the production of hydrogen ions. Therefore, the main function of osteoclasts is the absorption of the matrix, which is achieved through the creation of absorption cavities (Howship lacunae) (40). The process of bone resorption is completed with the apoptosis of osteoclast. Throughout the absorption, osteoclasts release substances, and bone tissue also releases local factors that ultimately inhibit the action of osteoclasts and induce osteoblast activity (signals are transmitted to osteoblasts in order to present in the absorption cavities) (42).

At any given time, about 20% of the cortical bone and 80% of the cancellous bone undergo bone remodeling. Bone remodeling occurs in discrete units in the skeleton. These are called bone remodeling units (BRUs) (23,24). There are at least one million such tiny remodeling units at any given time in the adult skeleton (43). The transformation of an inactive bone surface to a surface capable of absorbing bone marks the onset of the bone remodeling cycle (23,24). It is believed that osteocytes communicate with osteoblasts and osteoclasts located on the bone surface by transferring to them local signals through a tubular system. Therefore, osteocytes mediate the onset of bone remodeling (44–47).

Each bone remodeling cycle substantially consists of six phases:

1. Activation phase of osteoclasts
2. Bone resorption phase
3. Reversal phase—activation of osteoblasts
4. Bone formation phase
5. Phase of osteoid mineralization
6. Quiescence phase

The phase of the activation of osteoclast precursors marks the onset of the bone remodeling cycle. In the bone resorption phase, osteoclast precursors differentiate into mature osteoclasts (39), while at the reversal phase, osteoclasts complete the process of resorption and produce signals that cause the onset of bone formation. In the bone formation phase, the mesenchymal cells differentiate into osteoblasts capable of synthesizing matrix (39). In the phase of osteoid mineralization, osteoblasts continue to produce and calcify the osteoid. Finally, in the quiescence phase, osteoblasts are either converted in resting bone lining cells or differentiate into osteocytes. It should be noted that the phase of bone resorption lasts about 2–4 weeks, while the bone formation phase lasts about 4–6 months. Therefore, the cycle of bone remodeling consists of an accelerated bone resorption phase that is followed by a slow bone formation phase (39).

The bone turnover rate is determined by the number of BRUs and the speed with which the functions of bone resorption by osteoclasts and bone formation by osteoblasts are performed.

Regulatory mechanisms of bone remodeling

The complex process of bone remodeling is regulated by heredity, age, as well as the combined effect of local and systemic agents.

With regard to local factors, studies have shown that OPG, RANKL, and receptor activator of nuclear factor-κB (RANK), which are members of the superfamily of ligands and receptors of tumor necrosis factor (TNF), play an essential role in the regulation of bone remodeling (48–50). It is noteworthy that both OPG and RANKL are produced by osteoblasts. In particular, RANKL affects the fusion of osteoclast precursors in order to create a multinuclear mature osteoclast. The mechanism by which this differentiation of osteoclasts is achieved is the activation of the expression of c-Fos by RANKL (51). In contrast, OPG inhibits osteoclast differentiation (52). Moreover, macrophage colony-stimulating factor (M-CSF) modulates the proliferation of osteoclast progenitors and their differentiation into mature osteoclasts (53). M-CSF is expressed by osteoblasts and contributes to the maintenance of the survival of osteoclast precursors as well as to the suppression of apoptosis of mature osteoclasts (54,55). Therefore, osteoblasts produce activators (RANKL, M-CSF) and inhibitors (OPG) of osteoclast differentiation.

Systemic factors regulating bone remodeling include cytokines, hormones, and growth and mechanical factors (56). Cytokines that play an important role in the increase of bone resorption are interleukins (IL) IL-1, IL-3, IL-6, IL-10, IL-11, IL-13, TNF-α, TNF-β, M-CSF, and granulocyte-macrophage colony-stimulating factor (GM-CSF). Hormones include estrogens, androgens, insulin, thyroxine, growth hormone, and glucocorticoids. Thyroxine and glucocorticoids increase bone resorption, while sex hormones reduce it. In regard to the calciotropic hormones (hormones that regulate calcium), 1,25-dihydroxycholecalciferol (1,25[OH]$_2$D$_3$) and parathyroid hormone (PTH) cause an increase in bone resorption, whereas calcitonin decreases it. Bone remodeling is also regulated by growth factors, such as transforming growth factor β (TGF-β), fibroblast growth factor (FGF), insulin-like growth factor

I and II (IGF-I, IGF-II), platelet growth factor (PGF), epidermal growth factor, and others. Notably, the family of bone morphogenetic protein (BMP), which belongs to the superfamily of TGF-β, prospers ectopic bone production *in vitro* and exerts a crucial role in the regulation of bone mass *in vivo* (57–59). Additionally, it has been reported that the family of IGF promotes the proliferation of osteoblasts *in vitro* (60) and increases the expression of the gene encoding the type I collagen (61). Mechanical factors influencing bone remodeling include mechanical stimuli and microfractures.

The fact that the canonical Wnt signaling pathway contributes to the regulation of osteoblast formation and function determines that this pathway is a regulator of bone remodeling (16,17,62–64).

CALCIUM, VITAMIN D, PARATHYROID HORMONE

Constant concentrations of calcium ions in the cytoplasm of the cell and into the extracellular space as well as the adequacy of vitamin D are essential prerequisites for ensuring skeletal health. This becomes readily apparent by the fact that both calcium deficiency (due to low calcium intake, due to impaired intestinal calcium absorption, or due to kidney loss) and vitamin D deficiency (65) may result in secondary hyperparathyroidism and thus in an accelerated bone mass loss. Vitamin D deficiency can also consecutively lead to neuromuscular impairment, bone instability, falls, and an increased risk of fractures (66–68).

Individuals take calcium from food. Calcium is absorbed from the intestine, and the amount of calcium that is not used to rebalance its concentration in the blood moves to the bone. There, together with phosphorus, it is converted to either amorphous calcium phosphate available for every need or the crystalline form of hydroxyapatite. Calcium that is not absorbed from the intestine will be expelled from the feces. Furthermore, a percentage of calcium that will be filtered in the renal tubules will be reabsorbed. This process is primarily regulated by the concentration of plasma calcium. Since the skeleton retains approximately 99% of the total calcium in the body, the processes of bone formation and resorption are reflected in the variations seen in plasma calcium concentrations and in urine-excreted calcium levels (69–71). Calcium not retained in the skeleton (1% of the total body calcium) remains mainly in the extracellular fluid. It is found in active ionized form by approximately 45% when the concentration of plasma proteins is normal.

PTH, vitamin D, and calcitonin are essential calciotropic hormones that regulate calcium homeostasis (72). PTH acts directly on bone and the kidneys and indirectly (through vitamin D) on the intestine. In bone tissue, PTH increases bone resorption and leads to the release of calcium and phosphate in the extracellular fluid (73–75). PTH acts on the kidneys in three ways: (a) increases calcium tubular reabsorption, (b) diminishes phosphate tubular reabsorption, and (c) increases the activity of the enzyme 1-hydroxylase and therefore stimulates the conversion of 25-hydroxycholecalciferol (25[OH]D$_3$) in the active form of vitamin D (1,25[OH]$_2$D$_3$) (74–77). In the intestine, PTH promotes the absorption of calcium obtained from food through vitamin D.

PTH acts specifically to target cells of the bone and the kidney. It binds to specific receptors of the cell membrane, through enzymes adenylcyclase and phospholipase C, with the aid of G proteins (78).

Vitamin D in the circulation is bound to the vitamin D binding protein. The inactive form 25(OH)D$_3$ is the circulating form of vitamin D whose levels are used to determine vitamin D status. Although the lower normal limit of 25(OH)D$_3$ is 20 ng/mL according to most laboratories, this limit is preferred to be set at 30 ng/mL, since it has been shown that levels of inactive vitamin D less than 30 ng/mL induce secondary hyperparathyroidism (79–81).

Active vitamin D acts in the following three ways: (a) it increases calcium absorption in the small intestine from 10%–15% to 30%–40%, and, in parallel, it augments phosphorus absorption from 60% to 80% (74–76). Calcium absorption is accomplished through the interaction of vitamin D with the vitamin D receptor-retinoic acid x-receptor complex (VDR-RXR), which in turn enhances the expression of the epithelial calcium channel TRPV6 and the calcium-binding protein calbindin 9K (82). (b) It increases the expression of RANKL in osteoblasts, and, consequently, it induces the maturation of osteoclast precursors to osteoclasts. This process of osteoclastogenesis mobilizes calcium stores from the skeleton to maintain calcium homeostasis. (c) It decreases the synthesis and secretion of PTH from the parathyroid glands (82).

Various studies have shown that the administration of vitamin D offers fracture protection when given at doses of about 800 IU/day and in combination with calcium supplements (83–87). This combination corrects secondary hyperparathyroidism, increases bone density and muscle strength, and reduces the risk of falls in elderly and institutionalized patients (83,88–90).

With regard to the genetic background, the gene encoding vitamin D receptor (VDR) was the first gene that was studied for its relationship with BMD. The association of *VDR* gene with BMD is highly controversial, since there are several studies that suggest a positive association of certain polymorphisms of *VDR* gene with BMD (91,92), while other studies detect a negative association (93). With regard to the gene encoding vitamin D binding protein (DBP), several researchers have shown that certain polymorphisms are correlated with either BMD or fractures (94–97). Polymorphisms in the gene encoding PTH have also been examined in terms of their relationship with BMD with conflicting results (98–100). A genome-wide association study that was recently conducted showed a clear association of the examined polymorphisms with BMD at the femoral neck (101). Another study suggested an association of polymorphisms with the risk of fracture (102). The gene encoding the type I receptor of PTH has also been implicated in osteoporosis (103).

ESTROGEN AND FOLLICLE-STIMULATING HORMONE

The normal function of the ovaries ceases after menopause, leading to an acute drop in circulating estrogen levels. Estrogen deficiency can lead to postmenopausal osteoporosis (104). In postmenopausal women, both the risk of developing osteoporosis and the fracture risk are inversely correlated with postmenopausal estrogen levels. Estrogen deficiency increases bone remodeling, but it is the osteoclastic rather than the osteoblastic side of the remodeling process that is more affected (105,106). However, the fact that estrogen deficiency-associated bone loss is not accompanied by an adequate increase in bone formation, as it ought to happen as a physiological reaction to mechanical load, indicates that bone formation is also decreased in menopause (107).

The exact mechanism at the cellular level responsible for the mediation of the skeletal estrogen effects has not yet been unequivocally clarified. Estrogen prevents bone marrow precursors to differentiate into osteoclasts (108,109). Notably, 17β-estradiol increases the expression of *TNFRSF11B* gene encoding OPG. This is supported by experiments performed in human osteoblastic cells (110). Moreover, there is strong evidence derived from *in vitro* studies that estrogen diminishes the release of pro-inflammatory cytokines with known osteoclastogenic action such as TNF-α, IL-1, and IL-6 from osteoblasts. This is also true for TNF-α production from T cells (111,112). Consequently, estrogen deficiency in menopause enhances TNF-α production. TNF-α modulates the actions of osteoclasts via the signaling pathway of the nuclear factor NF-κB. This pathway is considered to play a crucial role in the development of osteoporosis (113). There is no doubt that TNF-α is involved in postmenopausal osteoporosis (114). Interestingly, previous studies conducted *in vitro* and in cultures of bone marrow in humans and mice indicate that TNF-α induces bone resorption (115,116).

However, the bone loss observed after menopause cannot be attributed to estrogen deficiency alone. Otherwise, mice knockout for both estrogen receptors would be osteoporotic, which is not true according to the results of several experiments on mice models (117–119). It is also difficult for one to explain the observation that the bone loss following ovariectomy is attenuated in hypophysectomized rats (120,121). The follicle-stimulating hormone (FSH), which belongs to the glycoprotein hormone family and is synthesized in the anterior pituitary, seems to be the answer in this puzzle. In an eugonadal metabolism situation, the principle function of the gonadotropin FSH is the stimulation of the estrogen production from the ovaries (122). In postmenopausal women, an increase of FSH in serum is observed due to the abrupt decline of estrogen production. A remarkable stimulatory effect of these increased FSH levels on bone tissue has been described (123). Notably, FSH exerts a stimulatory action on osteoclast formation and thus on bone resorption (124). FSH's impact on osteoclastogenesis is mediated through the kinases Akt, Ik-Ba, and Erk (124). These kinases, which are found in osteoclasts and whose phosphorylation is enhanced by FSH, are also essential for the effects of RANKL on osteoclast formation (124). In other words, FSH and RANKL share common pathways in osteoclasts that lead to bone resorption. Furthermore, it was previously demonstrated that TNF-α production by the macrophage precursors in bone marrow is promoted by FSH (125). Thus, the feedback mechanism of the increase of FSH secretion from an intact pituitary gland after menopause constitutes an essential prerequisite for postmenopausal osteoporosis. FSH correlates better than estrogen with bone turnover markers in postmenopausal women (126).

FSH's biological effects are exerted through its binding to the FSH receptor (FSHR) (127). FSHR has been identified in the granulosa cells of the ovary, osteoclasts, osteoclast precursors, and mesenchymal stem cells (128). In addition, low FSHR levels are expressed by the endothelial cells of the ovaries. FSHR belongs to the subfamily of Gs protein–coupled receptors having seven transmembrane segments. FSHR comprises three domains: a large extracellular N-terminal domain (or ligand-binding domain), a transmembrane domain with seven transmembrane segments, and an intracellular C-terminal domain (128). The interaction between FSH and FSHR is due to the N-terminal domain of the receptor. The phosphorylation of cAMP response element-binding (CREB) and protein kinase A (PKA) is the signaling pathway that is mainly induced by FSH. However, the mitogen-activated protein kinase pathway has also been considered to be activated by FSH (129).

Since estradiol production from the ovaries suddenly stops after menopause, very low estradiol levels are detected in serum, which are mostly produced by the peripheral aromatization of androgenic precursors in non-endocrine tissues. Aromatization is carried out by aromatase, which belongs to the cytochrome P450 enzyme family. This enzyme catalyzes the conversion of androstenedione to estrone as well as the conversion of testosterone to estradiol. Of note, apart from the ovarian granulosa cells, other tissues such as adipose tissue and bone tissue express aromatase (130). The role of the adipose tissue in the estrogen biosynthesis after menopause has been documented. A number of investigators have previously detected an association between fat mass and estradiol levels in serum in postmenopausal women. An inverse relationship between osteoporosis and body weight has also been reported (131,132). Estradiol production in the adipose tissue may contribute to the regulation of bone loss after menopause. Additionally, there is substantial evidence that aromatase and other enzymes participating in steroid metabolism are expressed by the bone cells (130). Thus, estradiol may act locally on bone cells, with a paracrine or even an autocrine manner, as observed in other tissues (133). Estrogen acts through binding at two different estrogen receptors, ERα and ERβ. Unfortunately, the levels of estrogen derived from peripheral aromatization are remarkably lower than those that are necessary for the preservation of a physiological remodeling process.

With regard to the gene encoding ERα, several polymorphisms have been examined in terms of their relationship with BMD. The two most important polymorphisms are those that are recognized by the restriction enzymes XbaI and PvuII. These polymorphisms are located within intron 1 and regulate the transcription of the *ERa* gene (134). A meta-analysis that included more than 5000 women from 22 published studies (11 in Caucasians and 11 in Asians) revealed an association between polymorphism XbaI (rs9340799), BMD, and fractures (135). Another meta-analysis of data from 18,917 people at eight European centers confirmed the presence of a correlation of this polymorphism with an increased risk of fracture, but not with BMD (136). Regarding polymorphism PvuII (rs2234693), a meta-analysis recorded a weak association with BMD at the femoral neck (137). Other *ERa* gene polymorphisms have also been associated with either hip fractures (138) or with BMD (139,140). Polymorphisms of the gene encoding estrogen receptor ERb have been studied to a lesser extent compared to those of the *ERa* gene for their relation with BMD and fracture risk. Loss of function mutations of the *CYP19A1* gene, which encodes aromatase, have been identified in patients with osteoporosis (141,142). A recent study conducted in postmenopausal women recorded a significant correlation between polymorphisms of the *CYP19A1* gene and BMD. However, it is worth highlighting the important role of age in this study, because statistical significance was noted only in a subset of individuals at or above 67 years of age and not in younger individuals (143). In addition, two previous studies have documented an association between polymorphisms of the *CYP19A1* gene and BMD in early postmenopausal women (144,145). The *CYP17A1* gene plays an important role in the synthesis of estrogen and androgen. Loss of function mutations of the *CYP17A1* gene lead to osteoporosis and reduce skeleton growth (146).

RECEPTOR ACTIVATOR OF NUCLEAR FACTOR–κB LIGAND/RECEPTOR ACTIVATOR OF NUCLEAR FACTOR-κB/OSTEOPROTEGERIN SIGNALING AXIS

In 1981, Rodan and Martin proposed that the osteoblasts express factors capable of modulating bone resorption. These factors belong to the superfamily of ligands and receptors of TNF (43). An exciting advance in the understanding of the mechanisms involved in osteoclastogenesis and activation of osteoclasts was the discovery of OPG, RANKL, and RANK in the mid- to late 1990s. One of the key factors is the RANKL, which binds to the RANK receptor on the osteoclast surface. Subsequently, this binding stimulates the recruitment and differentiation as well as the activation of osteoclasts (147–150). OPG acts as a natural decoy receptor and binds to RANKL, disrupting the interaction of RANKL with RANK (52,151). Consequently, OPG inhibits bone resorption. Thus, bone tissue homeostasis is maintained because of the OPG/RANKL/RANK signaling axis. Interestingly, osteoblasts express OPG and RANKL, and preosteoclasts and other cells of this line

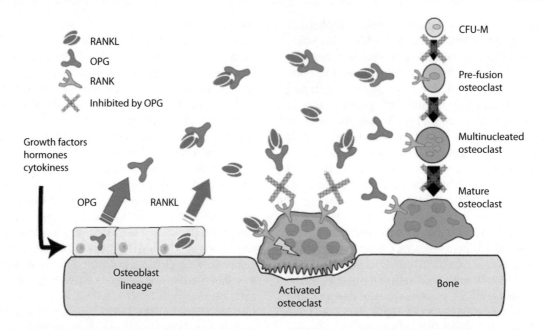

Figure 2.1   Receptor activator of nuclear factor–κB ligand (RANKL)/receptor activator of nuclear factor–κB (RANK)/osteoprotegerin (OPG) mechanism of action. Cells of the osteoblast lineage secrete RANKL, which binds to the RANK receptor on the osteoclast surface, stimulating the recruitment and differentiation as well as the activation of osteoclasts. OPG, which is also secreted by cells of the osteoblast lineage, acts as a natural decoy receptor that binds to RANKL, disrupting the interaction of RANKL with RANK (153). Colony-forming unit, megakaryote (CFU-M).

express RANK (152). The OPG/RANKL/RANK activation is shown in Figure 2.1.

Receptor activator of nuclear factor–κB ligand

RANKL belongs to the superfamily of the TNF receptor. Osteoblasts and activated T cells not only express but also secrete RANKL (153–155). RANKL is produced from the mammary gland, lungs, lymph nodes, and thymus at a high rate. The bone marrow and spleen express RANKL in a small percentage (154). It has been shown that RANKL plays a pivotal role in the activation of osteoclasts and function of dendritic cells (156). RANKL production from the synovial cells has been detected in inflammatory arthritis. RANKL acts simultaneously on bone resorption and hematopoiesis by inducing osteoclastogenesis and the release of hematopoietic stem cells in the bloodstream, respectively (157). It has also been reported that RANKL regulates bone metastases (158). The factors that regulate the expression of RANKL, RANK, and OPG are shown in Table 2.1. PTH, prostaglandin E2, and 1,25(OH)$_2$D$_3$ increase the expression of RANKL from osteoblasts and bone stromal cells. Interferon-γ (INF-γ) has also been shown to increase the expression of RANKL (153).

Receptor activator of nuclear factor-κB

RANK is a member of the superfamily of TNF receptors and a type I homotrimer transmembrane protein. RANK

Table 2.1   Regulators of osteoprotegerin, receptor activator of nuclear factor–κB ligand, and receptor activator of nuclear factor-κB expression (153)

	OPG	RANKL	RANK
1,25(OH)$_2$D$_3$	↑↓	↑	↑
Hormones			
Estrogen	↑	↓/—	
Testosterone	↑↓	—	
Glucocorticoid	↓	↑	
PTH	↓	↑	
PTHrP	↓	↑	
Cytokines			
IL-1	↑↓	↑	↑
IL-4			↓/—
IL-7		↑	
IL-13	↑	↓	—
IL-17	↓	↑	—
TNF-α		↑	
Interferon-γ	↑	↑	↑
Prostaglandin E2	↓	↑	
Growth factors			
TGF-β	↑	↑↓	—
Bone morphogenetic protein 2	↑		—

Abbreviations: ↑, increased expression; ↓, decreased expression; —, no change observed; IL, interleukin; OPG, osteoprotegerin; PTH, parathyroid hormone; RANK, receptor activator of nuclear factor–κB; RANKL, receptor activator of nuclear factor-κB ligand; TGF, transforming growth factor; TNF, tumor necrosis factor.

is expressed in osteoclasts (mature and precursors), dendritic cells, mature T cells, cells of the mammary gland, as well as hematopoietic progenitor cells (157,159). RANK's expression has been reported in breast cancer and primary and metastatic prostate cancer (160,161). RANK has been implicated to mediate the activation of T cells in the immune system (156). Notably, mutations in the gene encoding RANK affect the signal peptide of RANK causing familial expansile osteolysis (162).

Osteoprotegerin

OPG is also a member of the superfamily of TNF receptors and is a secretory glycoprotein (163). OPG production has been detected in bone, bone marrow, heart, liver, spleen, kidney, lungs, stomach, intestine, skin, and placenta (52,154). OPG binds either soluble RANKL (sRANKL) or RANKL, which is bound to the cell membrane, and by this way OPG inhibits osteoclastogenesis (52,164).

It has already been demonstrated that the Wnt/β-catenin signaling pathway, hormones, growth factors, and cytokines are the most important modulators of OPG expression (155,165). The role of the Wnt/β-catenin pathway in the formation of osteoblasts has been established (166). Additionally, the Wnt/β-catenin pathway prevents the differentiation of osteoblasts into chondrocytes (63). Table 2.1 summarizes the factors regulating the production of OPG. Interestingly, the increase in RANKL expression is associated with decreased expression of OPG (153,165).

RANKL/RANK/OPG signaling pathway

RANKL binds to the osteoclast cell-surface receptor RANK. Subsequently, RANK is trimerized and recruits a member of the TNF receptor-associated factors (TRAFs) at specific sites within its cytoplasmic domain (167). These factors are TRAF 2, 5, and 6. The most basic factor for osteoclasts (precursors and mature) seems to be TRAF 6 (56,168). The signaling pathways that are activated after the binding of RANK with TRAF are as follows:

- Four pathways that induce the formation of osteoclasts: (a) inhibitor of NF-κB kinase (IKK)/NF-κB), (b) nuclear factor of activated T cells (NFATc1), (c) c-Jun N-terminal kinase (JNK)/activator protein-1 (AP-1), and (d) c-myc.
- Three pathways that mediate activation ([a] MKK6/p38/MITF and [b] Src) and survival of osteoclasts ([a] kinase pathway regulated by extracellular signal and [b] Src pathway) (169). Figure 2.2a summarizes the signal transduction pathways after RANK.

The most important pathways in osteoclastogenesis are (a) IKK/NF-κB and (b) calcineurin/NFATc1. RANK's binding to TRAF 6 results in the activation of NF-κB and its transition to the nucleus. NF-κB induces the expression of the transcription factor c-Fos. NF-κB and c-Fos interact

with NFATc1 and thus promote the transcription of genes implicated in osteoclastogenesis. NFATc1 plays a significant role in the modulation of osteoclastogenesis (170). The bisphosphorylation of calcineurin is calcium dependent and also leads to the activation of NFATc1. C-Fos and RNA polymerase II contribute to the increase of the NFATc1 activation (171) (Figure 2.2b).

The Fc receptor common γ subunit (FcRγ) and DNAX-activating protein 12 (DAP12) constitute a signaling system that participates in the differentiation of osteoclasts. This system alone is not capable of increasing the transcription of NFATc1 and inducing the formation of osteoclasts. Therefore, it cooperates with the pathway induced by the binding of RANK to TRAF 6 (172). OPG binds to RANKL and inhibits its activity, blocking the interaction of RANKL with RANK and therefore osteoclastogenesis.

Association of OPG and RANKL with bone mineral density and bone metabolic markers

Various studies focused on the relationship between OPG and BMD, and inconsistency between the findings was found. Two reports in the literature showed that OPG was positively associated with BMD (173,174). In addition, some studies revealed a negative association (175–180), and in other studies no association was observed (181–183). Detailed analysis of a number of studies in which OPG was negatively correlated with BMD in osteoporotic postmenopausal women (175,177,178,180) suggests a beneficial effect of OPG on the prevention of accelerated bone loss observed after menopause (175). On the contrary, other investigators reported that the expression of OPG and RANKL was not associated with menopausal status (184). Moreover, another study showed that the concentration of RANKL in serum did not differ between the two sexes and did not depend on menopause (185).

The association of OPG with the markers of bone metabolism is surrounded by controversy. There are reports in the literature in which the concentration of OPG in serum was associated weakly with the markers of bone metabolism (173,174). However, other studies showed a positive association of OPG with these markers (175), while in other studies no correlation was detected (183). In another study, serum OPG levels were associated negatively with serum osteocalcin in elderly women (182). A study performed in women immediately after menopause showed a negative correlation between RANKL and 17β-estradiol in serum. RANKL levels were positively correlated with type I collagen N-terminal telopeptide (NTX-I) in urine and type I collagen C-terminal telopeptide (CTX-I) in serum in that study (186).

The controversy has arisen because OPG and RANKL are markers of bone metabolism but not specific ones. As already stated, OPG and RANKL are expressed in many tissues (52,154). Thus, it is possible that serum levels of OPG and RANKL are not representative of their activity in bone tissue. The conflicting results of the studies may

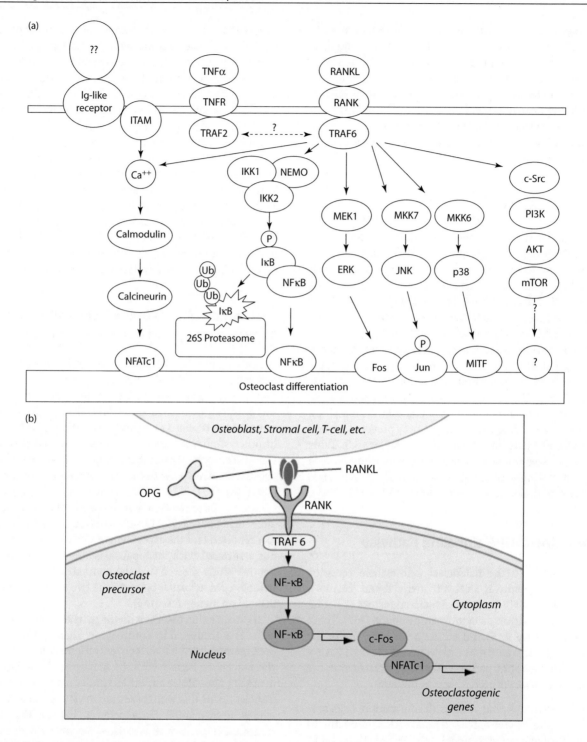

Figure 2.2 (a) Activation of multiple intracellular molecular pathways following the binding of RANKL to RANK (39). (b) The main RANKL/RANK-mediated intracellular pathway of osteoclast differentiation. RANKL's binding to RANK results in the activation of NF-κB through TRAF 6. NF-κB moves to the nucleus where it induces the expression of other transcription factors (c-Fos, NFATc1). Together, they promote the transcription of genes implicated in osteoclastogenesis (153).

also be due to differences in the measured fraction of OPG. Of note, there is an enzyme-linked immunosorbent assay (ELISA) method that detects all fractions of OPG (monomer OPG, homodimer OPG, and OPG bound to RANKL) (187). However, a polymerase chain reaction (PCR) technique detects only the homodimer OPG (188). Additionally, ELISA has a small capacity to detect sRANKL because of the relative instability of sRANKL in serum (189,190). The genetic and ethnic background, age, menopausal status, and renal function have a significant impact on OPG and RANKL measurements. Based on these data, there is a compelling need for further studies to establish the reliability of the measurement of OPG and RANKL in clinical practice.

Genetic variation in the RANKL/RANK/OPG signaling pathway: Association with bone mineral density and fractures

The *TNFRSF11B* gene encoding OPG has been mapped to chromosome 8q24.2 (191). Many researchers have examined the relationship of various polymorphisms of the *TNFRSF11B* gene with BMD particularly in postmenopausal women (192–207). The most frequently studied polymorphism of the *TNFRSF11B* gene is *G1181C*, which has been associated with an increase in BMD of the lumbar spine in postmenopausal women (192,194,196–199). However, there is disagreement with the results of other studies where *G1181C* polymorphism was not associated with BMD in postmenopausal women (200–202). In a recent meta-analysis, *G1181C* polymorphism was associated in Europeans with BMD at the lumbar spine, total hip, and femoral neck, and in Asians only with spinal BMD (208). The results of different studies are controversial because of the existence of national differences.

Several polymorphisms have also been identified in the promoter region of the *TNFRSF11B* gene. Due to their location in the promoter region, these polymorphisms may alter the binding of various transcription factors, thus affecting the transcription and the expression of the *TNFRSF11B* gene (209,210). However, the results of the studies that investigate the association of these polymorphisms with either BMD or fractures show a significant variation (192–196,198,203–205,211,212).

Polymorphisms of the *TNFRSF11* gene encoding RANKL have been studied for their relationship with BMD. Based on the studies' results, an association was recorded between the examined polymorphisms and BMD at the hip (213,214), the total body BMD (214), and the lumbar spine BMD (207,215,216).

With regard to the *TNFRSF11A* gene, which is located on chromosome 18q21–22 and encodes RANK, activating mutations have been associated with the following genetic disorders: early onset Paget's bone disease, familial extensive osteolysis, and extensive skeletal hyperphosphatasia (162). Additionally, several studies have examined the relationship between other polymorphisms of this gene with BMD. In the majority of these studies, the examined polymorphisms were associated with BMD at various skeletal sites (207,213,214,217,218).

CANONICAL Wnt SIGNALING PATHWAY

The large family of extracellular Wnt glycoproteins plays a cardinal role in the growth and differentiation of cells and tissues including bone tissue (16,219–222). Wnt proteins are also involved in embryogenesis (220,223,224), chondrogenesis (225), bone formation, function of osteoblasts and osteoclasts, bone remodeling, fracture repair (17,18,62–64,226–228), and tumor genesis (229,230).

Wnt proteins can activate three intracellular signaling pathways: (a) the planar cell polarity pathway, which plays a dominant role in embryogenesis; (b) the Wnt/Cα^{2+} pathway, which regulates cell migration; and (c) the canonical Wnt signaling pathway, which is involved in the bone remodeling as well as in the development and differentiation of organs in mammals (223,231–233). The canonical Wnt signaling pathway seems to play a crucial role in both osteoblast precursors and differentiated osteoblasts (227,234–238).

Steps of canonical Wnt signaling pathway

At the first step in the canonical Wnt signaling pathway, Wnt proteins bind to Frizzled receptors (Fzd) and to co-receptor LDL receptor-related protein 5 or 6 (LRP5 or LRP6) at the cell surface (Figure 2.3) (239). LRP5 is a transmembrane protein whose intracellular portion undergoes phosphorylation by an unknown kinase. Axin protein, which is a component of the protein complex β-catenin, Dishevelled (Dsh), and APC (Adenomatous polyposis coli), interacts with the phosphorylated site of the LRP5 protein (240,241). Therefore, glycogen synthase kinase 3β (GSK3β) is not connected to the cluster. Thus, β-catenin is not phosphorylated by GSK3β kinase and cannot undergo ubiquitination and proteasome degradation (242,243). Subsequently, the accumulation of β-catenin in the cytoplasm is followed by its translocation to the cell nucleus. There, it associates with transcription factors and specifically to lymphoid enhancer-binding factor/T-cell factor (Lef/Tcf) (220,226,244,245). This connection requires the creation of heterodimers between β-catenin and Lef/Tcf factors, and consequently, it leads to the activation of transcription and therefore to the expression of target genes that are necessary for bone formation, including the *Runx2* gene (220,226,234,244,246–249). Other target genes are repressed by the complex of Lef/Tcf-β-catenin.

When the signal in the Wnt pathway is absent, β-catenin binds to the complex consisting of the proteins axin, APC, Dsh, and GSK3β, and subsequently, β-catenin is phosphorylated by GSK3β kinase, resulting in reduced levels of free β-catenin in the cytoplasm. Phosphorylated β-catenin is degraded through the ubiquitin/proteasome pathway from the F-box protein and ligases E2 (250–252).

The antagonists of the canonical Wnt signaling are divided into intracellular and extracellular. The intracellular antagonists include APC3 protein and GSK3β kinase, whereas the extracellular antagonists include Dickkopfs (Dkks) and soluble Frizzled-related proteins (Sfrps). The Dkks antagonists are secretory proteins that bind to the LRP5 and LRP6 receptors on the cell membrane and bring them in contact with the Kremen proteins. Therefore, Dkks antagonists prevent the canonical Wnt signaling by decreasing the number of LRP5/6 receptors involved. Then, the cluster LRP5/6-Dkk-Kremen undergoes endocytosis and is transported to lysosomes for protein degradation or recycling (253,254). In regard to Sfrps, they are linked to free Wnt proteins in order to prevent their connection with Fzd receptors and co-receptors LRP5/6 (254,255).

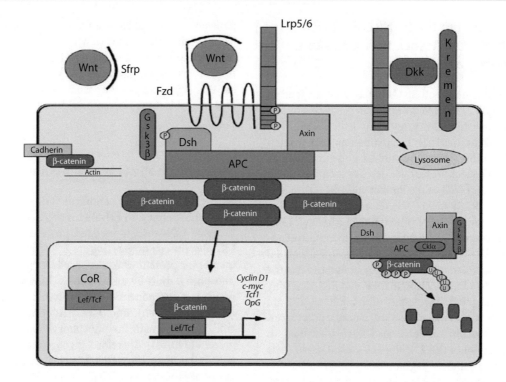

Figure 2.3 Canonical Wnt signaling pathway. Wnt proteins bind to Fzd and LRP5/6 proteins at the cell surface. The intracellular portion of LRP5 undergoes phosphorylation, and afterwards it interacts with axin protein, which is a component of the protein complex β-catenin, Dsh, and APC. Thus, β-catenin is not phosphorylated by GSK3β kinase and cannot undergo ubiquitination and proteasome degradation. Its accumulation in the cytoplasm is followed by its translocation to the cell nucleus, where it associates with transcription factors and leads to the expression of target genes that are necessary for bone formation (239).

Key players in the canonical Wnt signaling pathway

LRP5 and LRP6 proteins: Both LRP5 and LRP6 proteins belong to the LDLR receptor family. They both constitute transmembrane co-receptors for Wnt proteins and contribute to the activation of the canonical Wnt signaling pathway (240,256–258). They are composed of a large extracellular domain, a transmembrane domain, and an intracellular tail (257). LRP5 protein is detected in osteoblasts and plays an essential role in growth, differentiation, and proliferation of osteoblasts through interaction with Wnt proteins and subsequent activation of the canonical Wnt signaling pathway (64,223,234,240,248,259). It has been found that the *LRP5* gene includes a region of specific quantitative characteristics (quantitative trait locus) related to BMD and height in Caucasians (260,261). Experiments on mice have confirmed the role of LRP6 protein in the skeletal system (262).

β-catenin protein: It is known that β-catenin protein is expressed in osteoblasts. Using immunohistochemistry methods, β-catenin may be detected in the nucleus and in the cytoplasm of these cells (263). In experiments performed in mice, it was shown that in mature, fully differentiated osteoblasts, the activation of β-catenin results in a direct augmentation of the expression of OPG, which in turn inhibits the differentiation of osteoclasts, prevents bone resorption, and leads to increased bone mass (17,52).

The selective inhibition of the expression of β-catenin by osteoblasts contributes to a reduction in OPG expression and as a direct consequence in an increase of bone resorption and a decrease in bone mass. RANKL levels are not affected by the loss of β-catenin (17). In conclusion, the Wnt/β-catenin signaling in mature osteoblasts regulates the function and differentiation of osteoclasts through the OPG/RANKL signaling pathway (17,264,265).

Lef/Tcf transcription factors: Various isoforms of Lef/Tcf transcription factors have been described in the literature. The main isoforms expressed in osteoblasts are Tcf1 and Tcf4 (17,23). In the absence of Wnt signaling, Lef/Tcf factors are bound to transcriptional co-repressors (266–268). The activation of the canonical Wnt signaling pathway leads to the replacement of co-repressors by β-catenin and its binding to Lef/Tcf factors. Of note, several studies indicate that the activity of Lef/Tcf transcription factors is increased in areas of the skeleton that undergo bone remodeling (248,269–272).

Wnt proteins: Experiments conducted on mice have highlighted the role performed by Wnt proteins in osteoblastogenesis (273). Wnt are secretory glycoproteins that contain a high proportion of the amino acid cysteine. These amino acids of cysteine are linked to each other with disulfide bonds (219). The structure of Wnt proteins is insoluble (274). Since Wnt glycoproteins are secretory and are found in the extracellular matrix, their production site remains unknown.

Fzd proteins: The family of Fzd proteins is composed of various members. At least 10 Fzd proteins have been detected in humans (275). Fzd proteins are receptors for Wnt proteins. They are located on the cell surface (276). The interaction between Wnt and Fzd is ensured thanks to a domain that is located in the extracellular part of Fzd proteins and is rich in amino acid cysteine (cysteine-rich domain) (275). The Fzd receptors contain a KTxxxW motif that induces the canonical Wnt signaling (277). Conversely, Fzd1 and Fzd5 proteins lack the KTxxxW motif that explains the inhibition of the canonical Wnt signaling in mesenchymal cells by the Fzd1 protein (278). Fzd proteins regulate Wnt signaling in osteoblasts through a feedback mechanism. Several investigators suggested that the final differentiation of osteoblasts is achieved by the decrease in the expression of Fzd1 and Fzd8 (235), which regulate negatively the canonical Wnt signaling (278,279). The expression of Fzd proteins by osteoblasts is influenced by $1,25(OH)_2D_3$, epithelial growth factor (EGF), BMP-2 protein, and PTH (278,280). It is worth emphasizing that a small number of Fzd proteins do not take part in the canonical Wnt signaling pathway but contribute to the increase of the intracellular calcium through heterotrimeric G proteins (275).

Regulation of canonical Wnt signaling pathway

The canonical Wnt signaling pathway may be blocked at its initial steps. Sfrps and Wnt inhibitory factor 1 (Wif-1) block the interaction between Wnt proteins and Fzd proteins, while Dkks proteins and Sclerostin obstruct the binding of LRP5/6 with Wnt and Fzd, by binding to LRP5/6 receptors.

Sfrps bind to free Wnt proteins and prevent the formation of Wnt-Fzd-LRP5/6 complex (254). Of note, they contain a cysteine-rich domain, the sequence of which shows homology (approximately 50%) to the cysteine-rich domain of Fzd proteins. There are several known Sfrps such Sfrp1, Sfrp2, Sfrp3, and Sfrp4. Not all Sfrps negatively regulate bone formation by inhibiting the canonical Wnt signaling pathway. Sfrp1 is upregulated during the differentiation of preosteoblasts into preosteocytes (281). Sfrp1 not only inhibits the canonical Wnt signaling pathway, but it also increases the apoptosis rate of osteoblasts and osteocytes (281). Sfrp2 and Sfrp4 also block the canonical Wnt signaling pathway (281), while Sfrp3 inhibits the non-canonical Wnt5a-mediated signaling. Of note, it is likely that the secretion of Sfrp2 from the multiple myeloma cells may be the cause of osteoporosis observed in these patients (282). Furthermore, one could easily hypothesize a role of Sfrps in bone mineralization, since a high expression of Sfrp4 is detected in tumors associated with hypophosphatemia or osteomalacia, but also due to the increased excretion of phosphorus in urine through reduction of its reabsorption from the renal tubules by Sfrp4 (283).

With regard to Wif-1 factor, it is a secretory protein that binds to Wnt proteins and inhibits their activity (284). It is also believed that Wif-1 is involved in the differentiation of osteoblasts (285).

Dkks proteins are members of a family of secretory proteins (253) comprising Dkk1, Dkk2, Dkk3, and Dkk4 factors. A common feature of these factors is that they comprise a signal peptide as well as two domains that have a high content of the amino acid cysteine (286). Dkks factors are involved in high bone mass syndrome and multiple myeloma (287–289). Dkks play an important role in the canonical Wnt signaling pathway (290,291). All Dkks proteins apart from Dkk3 protein mediate the inhibition of Wnt signaling by binding to LRP5/6 and bring them into close proximity with Kremen 1 and Kremen 2 proteins (286,292). Then, the cluster LRP5/6-Dkk-Kremen undergoes endocytosis and transports to lysosomes for degradation or recycling (292). It has been shown that the Dkk3 protein does not affect the canonical Wnt signaling pathway (293). The expression of Dkk1 protein is increased by the administration of glucocorticoids and leads to the suppression of the canonical Wnt signaling pathway resulting in osteoporosis (294). Experiments conducted on mice led to the conclusion that the Dkk2 protein regulates the final differentiation of osteoblasts and helps the mineralization of the matrix (295).

Sclerostin is a secretory protein that is an antagonist of the canonical Wnt signaling pathway by binding to LRP5/6 and subsequently by inhibiting the interaction between LRP5/6 and Fzd (239,296). It is likely that sclerostin does not directly inhibit the canonical Wnt signaling pathway but prevents the subsequent signaling mediated by BMPs (297).

Apart from the inhibitors described previously, other intracellular or transmembrane molecules may also regulate the canonical Wnt signaling pathway. This category of regulators includes Kremen proteins, axin 2 protein, and receptor Ror 2.

Genetic variation in canonical Wnt signaling pathway: Association with bone mineral density and fractures

The *LRP5* gene plays an essential role in the regulation of bone mass. The pathogenetic mutations in the *LRP5* gene have been associated with a broad range of skeletal disorders, since their effect on osteoblasts results in an increase or a decrease in bone mass, while the activity of osteoclasts remains unchanged (234,248,298,299). Point mutations in the *LRP5* gene have been observed in patients with sclerosing bone dysplasias, such as autosomal dominant osteosclerosis, intraosseous hyperostosis, van Buchem disease, and osteopetrosis type I (300,301). Activating mutations of the *LRP5* gene cause the high bone mass syndrome (259,288), whereas inactivating mutations in the same gene lead to the appearance of the rare osteoporosis-pseudoglioma syndrome, which is characterized by skeletal deformities and osteoporotic fractures in childhood as well as by blindness (234). Similarly, transgenic mice expressing a mutated *LRP5* gene had an increased BMD (302), while mice with inactivating mutations of the *LRP5* gene or lack of LRP5 protein developed a low bone mass phenotype (248,303,304). These data show that the canonical Wnt signaling pathway through LRP5 protein plays an important role in the achievement of peak bone mass.

In addition to the aforementioned mutations, several polymorphisms of *LRP5* gene are also related to BMD (298,305–309). The most studied single-nucleotide polymorphisms are *V667M* and *A1330V*. The *V667M* polymorphism probably increases the binding affinity of LRP5 protein to Dkk1 (310), while *A1330V* seems to affect the interaction of LRP5 protein with its ligands (311,312). Both polymorphisms have been associated with an increased risk of low bone mass and fractures, but age, sex, and race seem to alter this risk (305–307,310,311,313).

The *Ile1062Val* polymorphism of the *LRP6* gene, which is the most frequently studied, has been associated with an increased risk of fractures (307). However, a recent meta-analysis did not detect a clear association of this polymorphism with either BMD or the risk of fracture (310).

The genes that encode the Wnt-16 protein (314), Fzd1 receptor (315), APC protein (316), Sfrp1 (317), Dkk2 protein (317), and the main transcription factor involved in the differentiation of osteoblasts RUNX2 (318–322) have also been associated with BMD. Of note, experiments on mice showed that the absence of RUNX2 transcription factor is associated with skeletal aplasia (323). Furthermore, mutations in the *SOST* gene encoding sclerostin are responsible for sclerosteosis. Of note, sclerosteosis is an autosomal disease characterized by an increase in BMD, which is due to the deficiency of the sclerostin protein (324).

REFERENCES

1. Kanis JA, Melton LJ 3rd, Christiansen C, Johnston CC, Khaltaev N. The diagnosis of osteoporosis. *J Bone Miner Res.* 1994;9(8):1137–41.
2. Kanis JA, Burlet N, Cooper C et al. European guidance for the diagnosis and management of osteoporosis in postmenopausal women. *Osteoporos Int.* 2008;19(4):399–428.
3. Kalu DN, Liu CC, Hardin RR. The aged rat model of ovarian hormone deficiency bone loss. *Endocrinology.* 1989;124(1):7–16.
4. Riggs BL, Khosla S, Melton LJ III. A unitary model for involutional osteoporosis: Estrogen deficiency causes both type I and type II osteoporosis in postmenopausal women and contributes to bone loss in aging men. *J Bone Miner Res.* 1998;13(5):763–73.
5. Recker R, Lappe J, Davies KM, Heaney R. Bone remodeling increases substantially in the years after menopause and remains increased in older osteoporosis patients. *J Bone Miner Res.* 2004;19(10):1628–33.
6. Ferrari S. Osteoporosis: A complex disorder of aging with multiple genetic and environmental determinants. In Simopoulos A, ed. *Nutrition and Fitness:* *Mental Health, Aging, and the Implementation of a Healthy Diet and Physical Activity Lifestyle.* Basel: Karger; 2005, pp. 35–51.
7. Deng HW, Livshits G, Yakovenko K et al. Evidence for a major gene for bone mineral density/content in human pedigrees identified via probands with extreme bone mineral density. *Ann Hum Genetics.* 2002;66(Pt 1):61–74.
8. Pocock NA, Eisman JA, Hopper JL, Yeates MG, Sambrook PN, Eberl S. Genetic determinants of bone mass in adults: A twin study. *J Clin Invest.* 1987;80(3):706–10.
9. Peacock M, Turner CH, Econs MJ, Foroud T. Genetics of osteoporosis. *Endocr Rev.* 2002;23(3):303–26.
10. Guéguen R, Jouanny P, Guillemin F, Kuntz C, Pourel J, Siest G. Segregation analysis and variance components analysis of bone mineral density in healthy families. *J Bone Miner Res.* 1995;10(12):2017–22.
11. Krall EA, Dawson-Hughes B. Heritable and life-style determinants of bone mineral density. *J Bone Miner Res.* 1993;8(1):1–9.
12. Efstathiadou Z, Tsatsoulis A, Ioannidis JP. Association of collagen I alpha 1 Sp1 polymorphism with the risk of prevalent fractures: A meta-analysis. *J Bone Miner Res.* 2001;16(9):1586–92.
13. Thakkinstian A, D'Este C, Eisman J, Nguyen T, Attia J. Meta-analysis of molecular association studies: Vitamin D receptor gene polymorphisms and BMD as a case study. *J Bone Miner Res.* 2004;19(3):419–28.
14. Ioannidis JP, Stavrou I, Trikalinos TA et al. Association of polymorphisms of the estrogen receptor alpha gene with bone mineral density and fracture risk in women: A meta-analysis. *J Bone Miner Res.* 2002;17(11):2048–60.
15. Liu YJ, Shen H, Xiao P et al. Molecular genetic studies of gene identification for osteoporosis: A 2004 update. *J Bone Miner Res.* 2006;21(10):1511–35.
16. Krishnan V, Bryant HU, Macdougald OA. Regulation of bone mass by Wnt signaling. *J Clin Invest.* 2006;116(5):1202–9.
17. Glass DA 2nd, Bialek P, Ahn JD et al. Canonical Wnt signaling in differentiated osteoblasts controls osteoclast differentiation. *Dev Cell.* 2005;8(5):751–64.
18. Gregory CA, Gunn WG, Reyes E et al. How Wnt signaling affects bone repair by mesenchymal stem cells from the bone marrow. *Ann N Y Acad Sci.* 2005;1049:97–106.
19. Compston J. Connectivity of cancellous bone. *Bone.* 1994;15(5):463–6.
20. Norman T, Wang Z. Microdamage of human cortical bone. *Bone.* 1997;20(4):375–9.
21. Myers E, Wilson S. Biomechanics of osteoporosis and vertebral fractures. *Spine.* 1997;22(Suppl 24):25S–31S.
22. Burr DB, Forwood MR, Fyhrie DP, Martin RB, Schaffler MB, Turner CH. Bone microdamage and skeletal fragility in osteoporotic and stress fractures. *J Bone Miner Res.* 1997;12(1):6–15.

23. Manolagas SC. Birth and death of bone cells: Basic regulatory mechanisms and implications for the pathogenesis and treatment of osteoporosis. *Endocr Rev.* 2000;21:115–37.

24. Manolagas SC. Cell number versus cell vigor: What really matters to a regenerating skeleton? *Endocrinology.* 1999;140(10):4377–81.

25. Rice JC, Cowi SC, Bowman JA. On the dependence of the elasticity and strength of cancellous bone on apparent density. *J Biomech.* 1988;21(2):155–68.

26. Seeman E. From density to structure: Growing up and growing old on the surfaces of bone. *J Bone Miner Res.* 1997;12(4):509–21.

27. Goldstein S, Goulet R, McCubbrey D. Measurement and significance of three-dimensional architecture to the mechanical integrity of trabecular bone. *Calcif Tissue Int.* 1993;53(Suppl 1):S127–33.

28. Manolagas SC, Kousteni S, Jilka RL. Sex steroids and bone. *Recent Prog Horm Res.* 2002;57:385–409.

29. Ruff CB, Hayes WC. Sex differences in age-related remodeling of the femur and tibia. *J Orthop Res.* 1988;6(6):886–96.

30. Lu PW, Cowell CT, LLoyd-Jones SA, Briody JN, Howman-Giles R. Volumetric bone mineral density in normal subjects, aged 5–27 years. *J Clin Endocrinol Metab.* 1996;81(4):1586–90.

31. Orwoll ES, Belknap JK, Klein RF. Gender specificity in the genetic determinants of peak bone mass. *J Bone Miner Res.* 2001;16(11):1962–71.

32. Belknap JJ, Dubay C, Crabbe JC et al. Mapping quantitative trait loci for behavioral traits in the mouse. In Blum K, Noble EP, eds. *Handbook of Psychiatric Genetics.* New York, NY: CRC Press; 1997, pp. 435–53.

33. Gunness M, Orwoll ES. Early induction of alterations in cancellous and cortical bone histology after orchiectomy in mature rats. *J Bone Miner Res.* 1995;10(11):1735–44.

34. Zhang XZ, Kalu DN, Erbas B, Hopper JL, Seeman E. The effect of gonadectomy on bone size, mass and volumetric density in growing rats may be gender-, site-, and growth hormone-dependent. *J Bone Miner Res.* 1999;14(5):802–9.

35. Aloia JF, Vaswani A, Yeh JK, Ross PL, Flaster E, Dilmanian FA. Calcium supplementation with and without hormone replacement therapy to prevent postmenopausal bone loss. *Ann Intern Med.* 1994;120(2):97–103.

36. Bassey EJ, Rothwell MC, Littlewood JJ, Pye DW. Pre- and post-menopausal women have different bone mineral density responses to the same high impact exercise. *J Bone Miner Res.* 1998;13(12):1805–13.

37. Welten DC, Kemper HC, Post GB et al. Weight-bearing activity during youth is a more important factor for peak bone mass than calcium intake. *J Bone Miner Res.* 1994;9(7):1089–96.

38. Riggs BL, Parfitt AM. Drugs used to treat osteoporosis: The critical need for a uniform nomenclature based on their action on bone remodeling. *J Bone Miner Res.* 2005;20(2):177–84.

39. Tanaka S. Signaling axis in osteoclast biology and therapeutic targeting in the RANKL/RANK/OPG system. *Am J Nephrol.* 2007;27(5):466–78.

40. Suda T, Takahashi N, Martin TJ. Modulation of osteoclast differentiation. *Endocr Rev.* 1992;13(1):66–80.

41. Teitelbaum SL, Ross FP. Genetic regulation of osteoclast development and function. *Nat Rev Genet.* 2003;4(8):638–49.

42. Vega D, Maalouf NM, Sakhaee K. The role of receptor activator of nuclear factor-κB (RANK)/RANK ligand/osteoprotegerin: Clinical implications. *J Clin Endocrinol Metab.* 2007;92(12):4514–21.

43. Boyce BF, Xing L. Biology of RANK, RANKL, and osteoprotegerin. *Arthritis Res Ther.* 2007;9(Suppl 1):S1.

44. Qiu S, Rao DS, Palnitkar S, Parfitt AM. Differences in osteocyte and lacunar density between Black and White American women. *Bone.* 2006;38(1):130–5.

45. Turner CH, Robling AG, Duncan RL, Burr DB. Do bone cells behave like a neuronal network? *Calcif Tissue Int.* 2002;70(6):435–42.

46. Burger EH, Klein-Nulend J, Smit TH. Strain-derived canalicular fluid flow regulates osteoclast activity in a remodelling osteon: A proposal. *J Biomech.* 2003;36(10):1453–9.

47. Huiskes R, Ruimerman R, van Lenthe GH, Janssen JD. Effects of mechanical forces on maintenance and adaptation of form in trabecular bone. *Nature.* 2000;405(6787):704–6.

48. Lacey DL, Timms E, Tan HL et al. Osteoprotegerin ligand is a cytokine that regulates osteoclast differentiation and activation. *Cell.* 1998;93(2):165–76.

49. Wong BR, Josien R, Choi Y. TRANCE is a TNF family member that regulates dendritic cell and osteoclast function. *J Leukoc Biol.* 1999;65(6):715–24.

50. Yasuda H, Shima N, Nakagawa N et al. Osteoclast differentiation factor is a ligand for osteoprotegerin/ osteoclastogenesis-inhibitory factor and is identical to TRANCE/RANKL. *Proc Natl Acad Sci USA.* 1998;95(7):3597–602.

51. Karsenty G, Wagner EF. Reaching a genetic and molecular understanding of skeletal development. *Dev Cell.* 2002;2(4):389–406.

52. Simonet WS, Lacey DL, Dunstan CR et al. Osteoprotegerin: A novel secreted protein involved in the regulation of bone density. *Cell.* 1997;89(2):309–19.

53. Tanaka S, Takahashi N, Udagawa N et al. Macrophage colony-stimulating factor is indispensable for both proliferation and differentiation of osteoclast progenitors. *J Clin Invest.* 1993;91(1):257–63.

54. Lagasse E, Weissman IL. Enforced expression of bcl-2 in monocytes rescues macrophages and partially reverses osteopetrosis in op/op mice. *Cell.* 1997;89(7):1021–31.

55. Yoshida H, Hayashi S, Kunisada T et al. The murine mutation osteopetrosis is in the coding region of the macrophage colony stimulating factor gene. *Nature.* 1990;345(6274):442–4.

56. Tanaka S, Nakamura I, Inoue J, Oda H, Nakamura K. Signal transduction pathways regulating osteoclast differentiation and function. *J Bone Miner Metab.* 2003;21(3):123–33.

57. Reddi AH. Bone morphogenetic proteins: An unconventional approach to isolation of first mammalian morphogens. *Cytokines Growth Factor Rev.* 1997;8(1):11–20.

58. Yoshida Y, Tanaka S, Umemori H et al. Negative regulation of BMP/Smad signaling by Tob in osteoblasts. *Cell.* 2000;103(7):1085–97.

59. Mundy G, Garrett R, Harris S et al. Stimulation of bones formation *in vitro* and in rodents by statins. *Science.* 1999;286(5446):1946–9.

60. Canalis E. Insulin like growth factors and the local regulation of bone formation. *Bone.* 1993;14(3):273–6.

61. Schmid C, Guler HP, Rowe D, Froesch ER. Insulin-like growth factor I regulates type I procollagen messenger ribonucleic acid steady state levels in bone of rats. *Endocrinology.* 1989;125(3):1575–80.

62. Day TF, Guo X, Garrett-Beal L, Yang Y. Wnt/beta-catenin signaling in mesenchymal progenitors controls osteoblast and chondrocyte differentiation during vertebrate skeletogenesis. *Dev Cell.* 2005;8(5):739–50.

63. Hill TP, Später D, Taketo MM, Birchmeier W, Hartmann C. Canonical Wnt/beta catenin signaling prevents osteoblasts from differentiating into chondrocytes. *Dev Cell.* 2005;8(5):727–38.

64. Westendorf JJ, Kahler RA, Schroeder TM. Wnt signaling in osteoblasts and bone diseases. *Gene.* 2004;341:19–39.

65. Prior JC. Perimenopause: The complex endocrinology of the menopausal transition. *Endocr Rev.* 1998;19(4):397–428.

66. Amling M, Grote HJ, Vogel M, Hahn M, Delling G. Three-dimensional analysis of the spine in autopsy cases with renal osteodystrophy. *Kidney Int.* 1994;46(3):733–43.

67. Lips P. Vitamin D deficiency and secondary hyperparathyroidism in the elderly: Consequences for bone loss and fractures and therapeutic implications. *Endocr Rev.* 2001;22(4):477–501.

68. Bischoff-Ferrari HA, Dawson-Hughes B, Willett WC et al. Effect of vitamin D on falls: A meta-analysis. *JAMA.* 2004;291(16):1999–2006.

69. Blaine J, Chonchol M, Levi M. Renal control of calcium, phosphate, and magnesium homeostasis. *Clin J Am Soc Nephrol.* 2015;10(7):1257–72.

70. Johnson JA, Kumar R. Renal and intestinal calcium transport: Roles of vitamin D and vitamin D-dependent calcium binding proteins. *Semin Nephrol.* 1994;14(2):119–28.

71. Felsenfeld A, Rodriguez M, Levine B. New insights in regulation of calcium homeostasis. *Curr Opin Nephrol Hypertens.* 2013;22(4):371–6.

72. Goodman WG, Quarles LD. Development and progression of secondary hyperparathyroidism in chronic kidney disease: Lessons from molecular genetics. *Kidney Int.* 2008;74(3):276–88.

73. Holick MF. Resurrection of vitamin D deficiency and rickets. *J Clin Invest.* 2006;116(8):2062–72.

74. Holick MF, Garabedian M. Vitamin D: Photobiology, metabolism, mechanism of action, and clinical applications. In Favus MJ, ed. *Primer on the Metabolic Bone Diseases and Disorders of Mineral Metabolism.* 6th ed. Washington, DC: American Society for Bone and Mineral Research; 2006, pp. 129–37.

75. Bouillon R. Vitamin D: From photosynthesis, metabolism, and action to clinical applications. In DeGroot LJ, Jameson JL, eds. *Endocrinology.* Philadelphia, PA: W.B. Saunders; 2001, pp. 1009–28.

76. DeLuca HF. Overview of general physiologic features and functions of vitamin D. *Am J Clin Nutr.* 2004;80(Suppl 6):1689S–96S.

77. Dusso AS, Brown AJ, Slatopolsky E. Vitamin D. *Am J Physiol Renal Physiol.* 2005;289(1):F8–F28.

78. Mannstadt M, Jüppner H, Gardella TJ. Receptors for PTH and PTHrP: Their biological importance and functional properties. *Am J Physiol.* 1999;277(5 Pt 2):F665–75.

79. Thomas MK, Lloyd-Jones DM, Thadhani RI et al. Hypovitaminosis D in medical inpatients. *N Engl J Med.* 1998;338(12):777–83.

80. Chapuy MC, Preziosi P, Maamer M et al. Prevalence of vitamin D insufficiency in an adult normal population. *Osteoporos Int.* 1997;7(5):439–43.

81. Holick MF, Siris ES, Binkley N et al. Prevalence of vitamin D inadequacy among postmenopausal North American women receiving osteoporosis therapy. *J Clin Endocrinol Metab.* 2005;90(6):3215–24.

82. Holick MF. Vitamin D deficiency. *N Engl J Med.* 2007;357(3):266–81.

83. Bischoff-Ferrari HA, Giovannucci E, Willett WC, Dietrich T, Dawson-Hughes B. Estimation of optimal serum concentrations of 25-hydroxyvitamin D for multiple health outcomes. *Am J Clin Nutr.* 2006;84(1):18–28.

84. Chapuy MC, Arlot ME, Duboeuf F et al. Vitamin D3 and calcium to prevent hip fractures in the elderly women. *N Engl J Med.* 1992;327(23):1637–42.

85. Dawson-Hughes B, Harris SS, Krall EA, Dallal GE. Effect of calcium and vitamin D supplementation on bone density in men and women 65 years of age or older. *N Engl J Med.* 1997;337(10):670–6.

86. Jackson RD, LaCroix AZ, Gass M et al. Calcium plus vitamin D supplementation and the risk of fractures. *N Engl J Med.* 2006;354(7):669–83.

87. Grant AM, Avenell A, Campbell MK et al. Oral vitamin D3 and calcium for secondary prevention of low-trauma fractures in elderly people (Randomised Evaluation of Calcium Or vitamin D, RECORD): A randomised placebo-controlled trial. *Lancet.* 2005;365(9471):1621–8.

88. Broe KE, Chen TC, Weinberg J, Bischoff-Ferrari HA, Holick MF, Kiel DP. A higher dose of vitamin D reduces the risk of falls in nursing home residents: A randomized, multiple-dose study. *J Am Geriatr Soc.* 2007;55(2):234–9.

89. Amling M, Grote HJ, Vogel M, Hahn M, Delling G. Three-dimensional analysis of the spine in autopsy cases with renal osteodystrophy. *Kidney Int.* 1994;46(3):733–43.

90. Lips P. Which circulating level of 25-hydroxyvitamin D is appropriate? *J Steroid Biochem Mol Biol.* 2004;89–90(1–5):611–4.

91. Thakkinstian A, D'Este C, Eisman J, Nguyen T, Attia J. Meta-analysis of molecular association studies: Vitamin D receptor gene polymorphisms and BMD as a case study. *J Bone Miner Res.* 2004;19(3):419–28.

92. Fang Y, van Meurs JB, d'Alesio A et al. Promoter and 3′-untranslated-region haplotypes in the vitamin D receptor gene predispose to osteoporotic fracture: The Rotterdam study. *Am J Hum Genet.* 2005;77(5):807–23.

93. Uitterlinden AG, Ralston SH, Brandi ML et al. The association between common vitamin D receptor gene variations and osteoporosis: A participant-level meta-analysis. *Ann Intern Med.* 2006;145(4):255–64.

94. Xiong DH, Shen H, Zhao LJ et al. Robust and comprehensive analysis of 20 osteoporosis candidate genes by very high-density single-nucleotide polymorphism screen among 405 white nuclear families identified significant association and gene-gene interaction. *J Bone Miner Res.* 2006;21(11):1678–95.

95. Al-oanzi ZH, Tuck SP, Mastana SS et al. Vitamin D–binding protein gene microsatellite polymorphism influences BMD and risk of fractures in men. *Osteoporos Int.* 2008;19(7):951–60.

96. Taes YE, Goemaere S, Huang G et al. Vitamin D binding protein, bone status and body composition in community-dwelling elderly men. *Bone.* 2006;38(5):701–7.

97. Lauridsen AL, Vestergaard P, Hermann AP, Moller HJ, Mosekilde L, Nexo E. Female premenopausal fracture risk is associated with GC phenotype. *J Bone Miner Res.* 2004;19(6):875–81.

98. Katsumata K, Nishizawa K, Unno A, Fujita Y, Tokita A. Association of gene polymorphisms and bone density in Japanese girls. *Bone Miner Metab.* 2002;20(3):164–9.

99. Deng HW, Shen H, Xu FH et al. Tests of linkage and/or association of genes for vitamin D receptor, osteocalcin, and parathyroid hormone with bone mineral density. *J Bone Miner Res.* 2002;17(4):678–86.

100. Gong G, Johnson ML, Barger-Lux MJ, Heaney RP. Association of bone dimensions with a parathyroid hormone gene polymorphism in women. *Osteoporos Int.* 1999;9(4):307–11.

101. Guo Y, Zhang LS, Yang TL et al. PTH and IL21R may underlie variation of femoral neck bone mineral density as revealed by a genome-wide association study. *J Bone Miner Res.* 2010;25(5):1042–8.

102. Tenne M, McGuigan F, Jansson L et al. Genetic variation in the PTH pathway and bone phenotypes in elderly women: Evaluation of PTH, PTHLH, PTHR1 and PTHR2 genes. *Bone.* 2008;42(4):719–27.

103. Duncan EL, Brown MA, Sinsheimer J et al. Suggestive linkage of the parathyroid receptor type 1 to osteoporosis. *J Bone Miner Res.* 1999;14(12):1993–9.

104. Kalu DN, Liu CC, Hardin RR, Hollis BW. The aged rat model of ovarian hormone deficiency bone loss. *Endocrinology.* 1989;124(1):7–16.

105. Ebeling PR, Atley LM, Guthrie JR et al. Bone turnover markers and bone density across the menopausal transition. *J Clin Endocrinol Metab.* 1996;81(9):3366–71.

106. Parfitt AM, Villanueva AR, Foldes J, Rao DS. Relations between histologic indices of bone formation: Implications for the pathogenesis of spinal osteoporosis. *J Bone Miner Res.* 1995;10(3):466–73.

107. Lee K, Jessop H, Suswillo R, Zaman G, Lanyon L. Endocrinology: Bone adaptation requires oestrogen receptor-alpha. *Nature.* 2003;424(6947):389.

108. Shevde NK, Bendixen AC, Dienger KM, Pike JW. Estrogens suppress RANK ligand-induced osteoclast differentiation via a stromal cell independent mechanism involving c-Jun repression. *Proc Natl Acad Sci USA.* 2000;97(14):7829–34.

109. Srivastava S, Toraldo G, Weitzmann MN, Cenci S, Ross FP, Pacifici R. Estrogen decreases osteoclast formation by down-regulating receptor activator of NF-kappa B ligand (RANKL)-induced JNK activation. *J Biol Chem.* 2001;276(12):8836–40.

110. Hofbauer LC, Khosla S, Dunstan CR, Lacey DL, Spelsberg TC, Riggs BL. Estrogen stimulates gene expression and protein production of osteoprotegerin in human osteoblastic cells. *Endocrinology.* 1999;140:4367–70.

111. Cenci S, Toraldo G, Weitzmann MN et al. Estrogen deficiency induces bone loss by increasing T cell proliferation and lifespan through IFN-gamma-induced class II transactivator. *Proc Natl Acad Sci USA.* 2003;100(18):10405–10.

112. Roggia C, Gao Y, Cenci S et al. Up-regulation of TNF-producing T cells in the bone marrow: A key mechanism by which estrogen deficiency induces bone loss *in vivo. Proc Natl Acad Sci USA.* 2001;98(24):13960–5.

113. Lorenzo J, Horowitz M, Choi Y. Osteoimmunology: Interactions of the bone and immune system. *Endocr Rev.* 2008;29(4):403–40.

114. Nanes MS. Tumor necrosis factor-α: Molecular and cellular mechanisms in skeletal pathology. *Gene.* 2003;321:1–15.

115. Cohen-Solal ME, Graulet AM, Denne MA, Gueris J, Baylink D, de Vernejoul MC. Peripheral monocyte culture supernatants of menopausal women can induce bone resorption: Involvement of cytokines. *J Clin Endocrinol Metab.* 1993;77(6):1648–53.

116. Li P, Schwarz EM, O'Keefe RJ et al. Systemic tumor necrosis factor mediates an increase in peripheral CD11bhigh osteoclast precursors in tumor necrosis factor α-transgenic mice. *Arthritis Rheum.* 2004;50(1):265–76.

117. McCauley LK, Tozum TF, Rosol TJ. Estrogen receptors in skeletal metabolism: Lessons from genetically modified models of receptor function. *Crit Rev Eukaryot Gene Expr.* 2002;12(2):89–100.

118. Lindberg MK, Alatalo SL, Halleen JM, Mohan S, Gustafsson JA, Ohlsson C. Estrogen receptor specificity in the regulation of the skeleton in female mice. *J Endocrinol.* 2001;171(2):229–36.

119. Windahl SH, Andersson G, Gustafsson JA. Elucidation of estrogen receptor function in bone with the use of mouse models. *Trends Endocrinol Metab.* 2002;13(5):195–200.

120. Yeh JK, Chen MM, Aloia JF. Ovariectomy-induced high turnover in cortical bone is dependent on pituitary hormone in rats. *Bone.* 1996;18(5):443–50.

121. Yeh JK, Chen MM, Aloia JF. Effects of 17 beta-estradiol administration on cortical and cancellous bone of ovariectomized rats with and without hypophysectomy. *Bone.* 1997;20(5):413–20.

122. Macklon NS, Fauser BC. Follicle development during the normal menstrual cycle. *Maturitas.* 1998;30(2):181–8.

123. Devleta B, Adem B, Senada S. Hypergonadotropic amenorrhea and bone density: New approach to an old problem. *J Bone Miner Metab.* 2004;22(4):360–4.

124. Sun L, Peng Y, Sharrow AC et al. FSH directly regulates bone mass. *Cell.* 2006;125(2):247–60.

125. Iqbal J, Sun L, Kumar TR, Blair HC, Zaidi M. Follicle-stimulating hormone stimulates TNF production from immune cells to enhance osteoblast and osteoclast formation. *Proc Natl Acad Sci USA.* 2006;103(40):14925–30.

126. Sowers MR, Greendale GA, Bondarenko I et al. Endogenous hormones and bone turnover markers in pre- and perimenopausal women: SWAN. *Osteoporos Int.* 2003;14(3):191–7.

127. Jiang X, Dias JA, He X. Structural biology of glycoprotein hormones and their receptors: Insights to signaling. *Mol Cell Endocrinol.* 2014;382(1):424–51.

128. Meduri G, Bachelot A, Cocca MP et al. Molecular pathology of the FSH receptor: New insights into FSH physiology. *Mol Cell Endocrinol.* 2008;282(1–2):130–42.

129. Hunziker-Dunn M, Maizels ET. FSH signaling pathways in immature granulosa cells that regulate target gene expression: Branching out from protein kinase A. *Cell Signal.* 2006;18(9):1351–9.

130. Enjuanes A, Garcia-Giralt N, Supervia A et al. Regulation of CYP19 gene expression in primary human osteoblasts: Effects of vitamin D and other treatments. *Eur J Endocrinol.* 2003;148(5):519–26.

131. Reid IR. Relationships among body mass, its components, and bone. *Bone.* 2002;31(5):547–55.

132. Simpson ER, Davis SR. Aromatase and the regulation of estrogen biosynthesis-some new perspectives. *Endocrinology.* 2001;142(11):4589–94.

133. Means GD, Mahendroo MS, Corbin CJ et al. Structural analysis of the gene encoding human aromatase cytochrome P-450, the enzyme responsible for estrogen biosynthesis. *J Biol Chem.* 1989;264(32):19385–91.

134. Herrington DM, Howard TD, Brosnihan KB et al. Common estrogen receptor polymorphism augments effects of hormone replacement therapy on E-selectin but not C-reactive protein. *Circulation.* 2002;105(16):1879–82.

135. Ioannidis JP, Stavrou I, Trikalinos TA et al. Association of polymorphisms of the estrogen receptor alpha gene with bone mineral density and fracture risk in women: A meta-analysis. *J Bone Miner Res.* 2002;17(11):2048–60.

136. Ioannidis JP, Ralston SH, Bennett ST et al. Differential genetic effects of ES1 gene polymorphisms on osteoporosis outcomes. *JAMA.* 2004;292(17):2105–14.

137. Wang CL, Tang XY, Chen WQ, Su YX, Zhang CX, Chen YM. Association of estrogen receptor alpha gene polymorphisms with bone mineral density in Chinese women: A meta-analysis. *Osteoporos Int.* 2007;18(3):295–305.

138. Wang JT, Guo Y, Yang TL et al. Polymorphisms in the estrogen receptor genes are associated with hip fractures in Chinese. *Bone.* 2008;43(5):910–4.

139. Styrkarsdottir U, Halldorsson BV, Gretarsdottir S et al. Multiple genetic loci for bone mineral density and fractures. *N Engl J Med.* 2008;358(22):2355–65.

140. Rivadeneira F, Styrkársdottir U, Estrada K et al. Twenty bone-mineral-density loci identified by large-scale meta-analysis of genome-wide association studies. *Nat Genet.* 2009;41(11):1199–206.

141. Morishima A, Grumbach MM, Simpson ER, Fisher C, Qin K. Aromatase deficiency in male and female siblings caused by a novel mutation and the physiological role of estrogens. *J Clin Endocrinol Metab.* 1995;80(12):3689–98.

142. Carani C, Qin K, Simoni M et al. Effect of testosterone and estradiol in a man with aromatase deficiency. *N Engl J Med.* 1997;337(2):91–5.

143. Riancho JA, Sañudo C, Valero C et al. Association of the aromatase gene alleles with BMD: Epidemiological and functional evidence. *J Bone Miner Res.* 2009;24(10):1709–18.

144. Salmen T, Heikkinen AM, Mahonen A et al. Relation of aromatase gene polymorphism and hormone replacement therapy to serum estradiol levels, bone mineral density, and fracture risk in early postmenopausal women. *Ann Med.* 2003;35(4):282–8.

145. Morón FJ, Mendoza N, Vázquez F et al. Multilocus analysis of estrogen-related genes in Spanish postmenopausal women suggests an interactive role of ESR1, ESR2 and NRIP1 genes in the pathogenesis of osteoporosis. *Bone.* 2006;39(1):213–21.

146. Yanase T, Simpson ER, Waterman MR. 17 alpha-hydroxylase/17, 20-lyase deficiency: From clinical investigation to molecular definition. *Endocr Rev.* 1991;12(1):91–108.

147. Matsuzaki K, Udagawa N, Takahashi N et al. Osteoclast differentiation factor (ODF) induces osteoclast-like cell formation in human peripheral blood mononuclear cell cultures. *Biochem Biophys Res Commun.* 1998;246(1):199–204.

148. Burgess TL, Qian Y, Kaufman S et al. The ligand for osteoprotegerin (OPGL) directly activates mature osteoclasts. *J Cell Biol.* 1999;145(3):527–38.

149. Blair JM, Zheng Y, Dunstan CR. RANK ligand. *Int J Biochem Cell Biol.* 2007;39(6):1077–81.

150. Hsu H, Lacey DL, Dunstan CR et al. Tumor necrosis factor receptor family member RANK mediates osteoclast differentiation and activation induced by osteoprotegerin ligand. *Proc Natl Acad Sci USA.* 1999;96(7):3540–5.

151. Bolon B, Carter C, Daris M et al. Adenoviral delivery of osteoprotegerin ameliorates bone resorption in a mouse ovariectomy model of osteoporosis. *Mol Ther.* 2001;3(2):197–205.

152. Fuller K, Wong B, Fox S, Choi Y, Chambers TJ. TRANCE is necessary and sufficient for osteoblast-mediated activation of bone resorption in osteoclasts. *J Exp Med.* 1998;188(5):997–1001.

153. Kearns AE, Khosla S, Kostenuik PJ. Receptor activator of nuclear factor κB ligand and osteoprotegerin regulation of bone remodeling in health and disease. *Endocr Rev.* 2008;29(2):155–92.

154. Wada T, Nakashima T, Hiroshi N, Penninger JM. RANKL-RANK signaling in osteoclastogenesis and bone disease. *Trends Mol Med.* 2006;12(1):17–25.

155. Takayanagi H. Osteoimmunology: Shared mechanisms and cross-talk between the immune and bone systems. *Nat Rev Immunol.* 2007;7(4):292–304.

156. Anderson DM, Maraskovsky E, Billingsley WL et al. A homologue of the TNF receptor and its ligand enhance T-cell growth and dendritic-cell function. *Nature.* 1997;390(6656):175–9.

157. Kollet O, Dar A, Shivtiel S et al. Osteoclasts degrade endosteal components and promote mobilization of hematopoietic progenitor cells. *Nat Med.* 2006;12(6):657–64.

158. Jones DH, Nakashima T, Sanchez OH et al. Regulation of cancer cell migration and bone metastasis by RANKL. *Nature.* 2006;440(7084):692–6.

159. Fata JE, Kong YY, Li J et al. The osteoclast differentiation factor osteoprotegerin-ligand is essential for mammary gland development. *Cell.* 2000;103(1):41–50.

160. Chen G, Sircar K, Aprikian A, Potti A, Goltzman D, Rabbani SA. Expression of RANKL/RANK/OPG in primary and metastatic human prostate cancer as markers of disease stage and functional regulation. *Cancer.* 2006;107(2):289–98.

161. Kim NS, Kim HJ, Koo BK et al. Receptor activator of NF-kappaB ligand regulates the proliferation of mammary epithelial cells via Id2. *Mol Cell Biol.* 2006;26(3):1002–13.

162. Hughes AE, Ralston SH, Marken J et al. Mutations in TNFRSF11A, affecting the signal peptide of RANK, cause familial expansile osteolysis. *Nat Genet.* 2000;24(1):45–8.

163. Yamaguchi K, Kinosaki M, Goto M et al. Characterization of structural domains of human osteoclastogenesis inhibitory factor. *J Biol Chem.* 1998;273(9):5117–23.

164. Yasuda H, Shima N, Nakagawa N et al. Identity of osteoclastogenesis inhibitory factor (OCIF) and osteoprotegerin (OPG): A mechanism by which OPG/OCIF inhibits osteoclastogenesis *in vitro. Endocrinology.* 1998;139(3):1329–37.

165. Theoleyre S, Wittrant Y, Tat SK, Fortun Y, Redini F, Heymann D. The molecular triad OPG/RANK/RANKL: Involvement in the orchestration of pathophysiological bone remodeling. *Cytokine Growth Factor Rev.* 2004;15(6):457–75.

166. Boyce BF, Xing L, Chen D. Osteoprotegerin, the bone protector, is a surprising target for beta-catenin signaling. *Cell Metab.* 2005;2(6):344–5.

167. Wong BR, Rho J, Arron J et al. TRANCE is a novel ligand of the tumor necrosis factor receptor family that activates c-Jun N-terminal kinase in T cells. *J Biol Chem.* 1997;272(40):25190–4.

168. Lomaga MA, Yeh WC, Sarosi I et al. TRAF6 deficiency results in osteopetrosis and defective interleukin-1, CD40, and LPS signaling. *Genes Dev.* 1999;13(8):1015–24.

169. Boyle WJ, Simonet WS, Lacey DL. Osteoclast differentiation and activation. *Nature.* 2003;423(6937):337–42.

170. Takayanagi H, Kim S, Koga T et al. Induction and activation of the transcription factor NFATc1 (NFAT2) integrate RANKL signaling in terminal differentiation of osteoclasts. *Dev Cell.* 2002;3(6):889–901.

171. Fretz JA, Shevde NK, Singh S, Darnay BG, Pike JW. Receptor activator of nuclear factor-kappaB ligand-induced nuclear factor of activated T cells (C1) autoregulates its own expression in osteoclasts and mediates the up-regulation of tartrate-resistant acid phosphatase. *Mol Endocrinol.* 2008;22(3):737–50.

172. Asagiri M, Takayanagi H. The molecular understanding of osteoclast differentiation. *Bone.* 2007;40(2):251–64.

173. Rogers A, Saleh G, Hannon RA, Greenfield D, Eastell R. Circulating estradiol and osteoprotegerin as determinants of bone turnover and bone density in postmenopausal women. *J Clin Endocrinol Metab.* 2002;87(10):4470–5.

174. Mezquita-Raya P, de la Higuera M, García DF et al. The contribution of serum osteoprotegerin to bone mass and vertebral fractures in postmenopausal women. *Osteoporos Int.* 2005;16(11):1368–74.

175. Yano K, Tsuda E, Washida N et al. Immunological characterization of circulating osteoprotegerin/osteoclastogenesis inhibitory factor: Increased serum concentrations in postmenopausal women with osteoporosis. *J Bone Miner Res.* 1999;14(4):518–27.

176. Kudlacek S, Schneider B, Woloszczuk W, Pietschmann P, Willvonseder R. Serum levels of osteoprotegerin increase with age in a healthy adult population. *Bone*. 2003;32(6):681–6.

177. Dai Y, Shen L. Relationships between serum osteoprotegerin, matrix metalloproteinase-2 levels and bone metabolism in postmenopausal women. *Chin Med J*. 2007;120(22):2017–21.

178. Grigorie D, Neacşu E, Marinescu M, Popa O. Circulating osteoprotegerin and leptin levels in postmenopausal women with and without osteoporosis. *Rom J Intern Med*. 2003;41(4):409–15.

179. Riggs BL, Khosla S, Atkinson EJ, Dunstan CR, Melton LJ 3rd. Evidence that type I osteoporosis results from enhanced responsiveness of bone to estrogen deficiency. *Osteoporos Int*. 2003;14(9):728–33.

180. Yano K, Shibata O, Mizuno A et al. Immunological study on circulating murine osteoprotegerin/osteoclastogenesis inhibitory factor (OPG/OCIF): Possible role of OPG/OCIF in the prevention of osteoporosis in pregnancy. *Biochem Biophys Res Commun*. 2001;288(1):217–24.

181. Liu JM, Zhao HY, Ning G et al. Relationships between the changes of serum levels of OPG and RANKL with age, menopause, bone biochemical markers and bone mineral density in Chinese women aged 20–75. *Calcif Tissue Int*. 2005;76(1):1–6.

182. Browner WS, Lui LY, Cummings SR. Associations of serum osteoprotegerin levels with diabetes, stroke, bone density, fractures, and mortality in elderly women. *J Clin Endocrinol Metab*. 2001;86(2):631–7.

183. Khosla S, Arrighi HM, Melton LJ 3rd et al. Correlates of osteoprotegerin levels in women and men. *Osteoporos Int*. 2002;13(5):394–9.

184. Seck T, Diel I, Bismar H, Ziegler R, Pfeilschifter J. Serum parathyroid hormone, but not menopausal status, is associated with the expression of osteoprotegerin and RANKL MRNA in human bone samples. *Eur J Endocrinol*. 2001;145(2):199–205.

185. Schett G, Kiechl S, Redlich K et al. Soluble RANKL and risk of nontraumatic fracture. *JAMA*. 2004;291(9):1108–13.

186. Eghbali-Fatourechi G, Khosla S, Sanyal A, Boyle WJ, Lacey DL, Riggs BL. Role of RANK ligand in mediating increased bone resorption in early postmenopausal women. *J Clin Invest*. 2003;111(8):1221–30.

187. Rogers A, Eastell R. Circulating osteoprotegerin and receptor activator for nuclear factor kappaB ligand: Clinical utility in metabolic bone disease assessment. *J Clin Endocrinol Metab*. 2005;90(11):6323–31.

188. Furuya D, Kaneko R, Yagihashi A et al. Immuno-PCR assay for homodimeric osteoprotegerin. *Clin Chem*. 2001;47(8):1475–7.

189. Hannon R, Eastell R. Preanalytical variability of biochemical markers of bone turnover. *Osteoporos Int*. 2000;11(Suppl 6):S30–44.

190. Hawa G, Brinskelle-Schmal N, Glatz K, Maitzen S, Woloszczuk W. Immunoassay for soluble RANKL (receptor activator of NF-κB ligand) in serum. *Clin Lab*. 2003;49(9–10):461–3.

191. Online Mendelian Inheritance in Man. Tumor necrosis factor receptor superfamily, member 11B; TNFRSF11B. Available from: http://omim.org/entry/602643.

192. Arko B, Prezelj J, Kocijancic A, Komel R, Marc J. Association of the osteoprotegerin gene polymorphisms with bone mineral density in postmenopausal women. *Maturitas*. 2005;51(3):270–9.

193. Arko B, Prezelj J, Komel R, Kocijancic A, Hudler P, Marc J. Sequence variations in the osteoprotegerin gene promoter in patients with postmenopausal osteoporosis. *J Clin Endocrinol Metab*. 2002;87(9):4080–4.

194. Langdahl BL, Carstens M, Stenkjaer L, Eriksen EF. Polymorphisms in the osteoprotegerin gene are associated with osteoporotic fractures. *J Bone Miner Res*. 2002;17(7):1245–55.

195. Yamada Y, Ando F, Niino N, Shimokata H. Association of polymorphisms of the osteoprotegerin gene with bone mineral density in Japanese women but not men. *Mol Genet Metab*. 2003;80(3):344–9.

196. García-Unzueta MT, Riancho JA, Zarrabeitia MT et al. Association of the 163A/G and 1181G/C osteoprotegerin polymorphism with bone mineral density. *Horm Metab Res*. 2008;40(3):219–24.

197. Choi JY, Shin A, Park SK et al. Genetic polymorphisms of OPG, RANK, and ESR1 and bone mineral density in Korean postmenopausal women. *Calcif Tissue Int*. 2005;77(3):152–9.

198. Kim JG, Kim JH, Kim JY et al. Association between osteoprotegerin (OPG), receptor activator of nuclear factor-kappaB (RANK), and RANK ligand (RANKL) gene polymorphisms and circulating OPG, soluble RANKL levels, and bone mineral density in Korean postmenopausal women. *Menopause*. 2007;14(5):913–8.

199. Zhao HY, Liu JM, Ning G et al. The influence of Lys3Asn polymorphism in the osteoprotegerin gene on bone mineral density in Chinese postmenopausal women. *Osteoporos Int*. 2005;16(12):1519–24.

200. Vidal C, Brincat M, Xuereb Anastasi A. TNFRSF11B gene variants and bone mineral density in postmenopausal women in Malta. *Maturitas*. 2006;53(4):386–95.

201. Wynne F, Drummond F, O'Sullivan K et al. Investigation of the genetic influence of the OPG, VDR (Fok1), and COLIA1 Sp1 polymorphisms on BMD in the Irish population. *Calcif Tissue Int*. 2002;71(1):26–35.

202. Ohmori H, Makita Y, Funamizu M et al. Linkage and association analyses of the osteoprotegerin gene locus with human osteoporosis. *J Hum Genet*. 2002;47(8):400–6.

203. Brändström H, Gerdhem P, Stiger F et al. Single nucleotide polymorphisms in the human gene for osteoprotegerin are not related to bone mineral density or fracture in elderly women. *Calcif Tissue Int*. 2003;74(1):18–24.

204. Chung H, Hwang C, Kang Y. Osteoprotegerin polymorphism contributes to urine calcium excretion in Korean postmenopausal women. *J Bone Miner Res*. 2000;15(Suppl 1):SU130.

205. Brändström H, Gerdhem P, Stiger F. Polymorphisms in the genes for vitamin D receptor and osteoprotegerin, relation to bone mineral density in Swedish women aged 75. *J Bone Miner Res*. 2000;15(Suppl 1):SA160.

206. Richards JB, Rivadeneira F, Inouye M et al. Bone mineral density, osteoporosis, and osteoporotic fractures: A genome-wide association study. *Lancet*. 2008;371(9623):1505–12.

207. Rivadeneira F, Styrkársdottir U, Estrada K et al. Twenty bone-mineral-density loci identified by large-scale meta-analysis of genome-wide association studies. *Nat Genet*. 2009;41(11):1199–206.

208. Lee YH, Woo JH, Choi SJ, Ji JD, Song GG. Associations between osteoprotegerin polymorphisms and bone mineral density: A meta-analysis. *Mol Biol Rep*. 2010;37(1):227–34.

209. Wan M, Shi X, Feng X, Cao X. Transcriptional mechanism of bone morphogenetic protein-induced osteoprotegerin gene expression. *J Biol Chem*. 2001;276(13):10119–25.

210. Thirunavukkarasu K, Miles RR, Halladay DL et al. Stimulation of osteoprotegerin (OPG) gene expression by transforming growth factor-β (TGF-β). *J Biol Chem*. 2001;276(39):36241–50.

211. Langdahl BL, Carstens M, Stenkjær L. Polymorphisms in the osteoprotegerin gene and osteoporotic fractures and bone mass. *J Bone Miner Res*. 2000;15(Suppl 1):F159.

212. Rogers A, Hannon RA, Greenfield DM. Polymorphisms of the vitamin D receptor (BsmI, FokI) and osteoprotegerin gene (HincII) and the risk of osteoporosis. *J Bone Miner Res*. 2000;15(Suppl 1):SA158.

213. Xiong DH, Shen H, Zhao LJ et al. Robust and comprehensive analysis of 20 osteoporosis candidate genes by very high-density single-nucleotide polymorphism screen among 405 white nuclear families identified significant association and gene-gene interaction. *J Bone Miner Res*. 2006;21(11):1678–95.

214. Hsu YH, Niu T, Terwedow HA et al. Variation in genes involved in the RANKL/RANK/OPG bone remodeling pathway are associated with bone mineral density at different skeletal sites in men. *Hum Genet*. 2006;118(5):568–77.

215. Mencej-Bedrac S, Prezelj J, Kocjan T et al. The combinations of polymorphisms in vitamin D receptor, osteoprotegerin and tumour necrosis factor superfamily member 11 genes are associated with bone mineral density. *J Mol Endocrinol*. 2009;42(2):239–47.

216. Styrkarsdottir U, Halldorsson BV, Gretarsdottir S et al. Multiple genetic loci for bone mineral density and fractures. *N Engl J Med*. 2008;358(22):2355–65.

217. Koh JM, Park BL, Kim DJ et al. Identification of novel RANK polymorphisms and their putative association with low BMD among postmenopausal women. *Osteoporos Int*. 2007;18(3):323–31.

218. Styrkarsdottir U, Halldorsson BV, Gretarsdottir S et al. New sequence variants associated with bone mineral density. *Nat Genet*. 2009;41(1):15–7.

219. Moon RT, Bowerman B, Boutros M, Perrimon N. The promise and perils of Wnt signaling through beta-catenin. *Science*. 2002;296(5573):1644–6.

220. Nusse R. Wnt signaling in disease and in development. *Cell Res*. 2005;15(1):28–32.

221. Glass DA 2nd, Karsenty G. *In vivo* analysis of Wnt signaling in bone. *Endocrinology*. 2007;148(6):2630–4.

222. Baron R, Rawadi G. Targeting the Wnt/beta-catenin pathway to regulate bone formation in the adult skeleton. *Endocrinology*. 2007;148(6):2635–43.

223. Logan CY, Nusse R. The Wnt signaling pathway in development and disease. *Annu Rev Cell Dev Biol*. 2004;20:781–810.

224. Nusse R, Varmus HE. Wnt genes. *Cell*. 1992;69(7):1073–87.

225. Tuan RS. Cellular signaling in developmental chondrogenesis: N-cadherin, Wnts, and BMP-2. *J Bone Joint Surg Am*. 2003;85(Suppl 2):137–41.

226. Baron R, Rawadi G, Roman-Roman S. Wnt signaling: A key regulator of bone mass. *Curr Top Dev Biol*. 2006;76:103–27.

227. Hu H, Hilton MJ, Tu X, Yu K, Ornitz DM, Long F. Sequential roles of Hedgehog and Wnt signaling in osteoblast development. *Development*. 2005;132(1):49–60.

228. Rodda SJ, McMahon AP. Distinct roles for Hedgehog and canonical Wnt signaling in specification, differentiation and maintenance of osteoblast progenitors. *Development*. 2006;133(16):3231–44.

229. Peifer M, Polakis P. Wnt signaling in oncogenesis and embryogenesis—A look outside the nucleus. *Science*. 2000;287(5458):1606–9.

230. Bienz M, Clevers H. Linking colorectal cancer to Wnt signalling. *Cell*. 2000;103(2):311–20.

231. Slusarski DC, Yang-Snyder J, Busa WB, Moon RT. Modulation of embryonic intracellular Ca^{2+} signaling by Wnt-5A. *Dev Biol*. 1997;182(1):114–20.

232. Kühl M, Sheldahl LC, Malbon CC, Moon RT. Ca^{2+}/calmodulin-dependent protein kinase II is stimulated by Wnt and Frizzled homologs and promotes ventral cell fates in Xenopus. *J Biol Chem*. 2000;275(17):12701–11.

233. Wodarz A, Nusse R. Mechanisms of Wnt signaling in development. *Annu Rev Cell Dev Biol*. 1998;14:59–88.

234. Gong Y, Slee RB, Fukai N et al. LDL receptor-related protein 5 (LRP5) affects bone accrual and eye development. *Cell*. 2001;107(4):513–23.

235. Kalajzic I, Staal A, Yang WP et al. Expression profile of osteoblast lineage at defined stages of differentiation. *J Biol Chem*. 2005;280(26):24618–26.

236. Rawadi G, Vayssière B, Dunn F, Baron R, Roman-Roman S. BMP-2 controls alkaline phosphatase expression and osteoblast mineralization by a Wnt autocrine loop. *J Bone Miner Res*. 2003;18(10):1842–53.

237. Derfoul A, Carlberg AL, Tuan RS, Hall DJ. Differential regulation of osteogenic marker gene expression by Wnt-3a in embryonic mesenchymal multipotential progenitor cells. *Differentiation*. 2004;72(5):209–23.

238. Li X, Zhang Y, Kang H et al. Sclerostin binds to LRP5/6 and antagonizes canonical Wnt signaling. *J Biol Chem*. 2005;280(20):19883–7.

239. Glass DA 2nd, Karsenty G. Molecular bases of the regulation of bone remodeling by the canonical Wnt signaling pathway. *Curr Topics Dev Biol*. 2006;73:43–84.

240. Mao J, Wang J, Liu B et al. Low-density lipoprotein receptor-related protein-5 binds to axin and regulates the canonical Wnt signaling pathway. *Mol Cell*. 2001;7(4):801–9.

241. Tamai K, Zeng X, Liu C et al. A mechanism for Wnt coreceptor activation. *Mol Cell*. 2004;13(1):149–56.

242. Ikeda S, Kishida S, Yamamoto H, Murai H, Koyama S, Kikuchi A. Axin, a negative regulator of the Wnt signaling pathway, forms a complex with GSK-3beta catenin and promotes GSK-3beta-dependent phosphorylation of beta-catenin. *EMBO J*. 1998;17(5):1371–84.

243. Orford K, Crockett C, Jensen JP, Weissman AM, Byers SW. Serine phosphorylation-regulated ubiquitination and degradation of beta-catenin. *J Biol Chem*. 1997;272(40):24735–8.

244. Behrens J, von Kries JP, Kühl M et al. Functional interaction of beta-catenin with the transcription factor LEF-1. *Nature*. 1996;382(6592):638–42.

245. Molenaar M, van de Wetering M, Oosterwegel M et al. XTcf-3 transcription factor mediates beta-catenin-induced axis formation in Xenopus embryos. *Cell*. 1996;86(3):391–9.

246. He TC, Sparks AB, Rago C et al. Identification of c-MYC as a target of the APC pathway. *Science*. 1998;281(5382):1509–12.

247. Tetsu O, McCormick F. Beta-catenin regulates expression of cyclin D1 in colon carcinoma cells. *Nature*. 1999;398(6726):422–6.

248. Kato M, Patel MS, Levasseur R et al. Cbfa1-independent decrease in osteoblast proliferation, osteopenia, and persistent embryonic eye vascularization in mice deficient in Lrp5, a Wnt coreceptor. *J Cell Biol*. 2002;157(2):303–14.

249. Gaur T, Lengner CJ, Hovhannisyan H et al. Canonical Wnt signaling promotes osteogenesis by directly stimulating RUNX2 gene expression. *J Biol Chem*. 2005;280(39):33132–40.

250. Behrens J, Jerchow BA, Würtele M et al. Functional interaction of an axin homolog, conductin, with beta-catenin, APC, and GSK3beta. *Science*. 1998;280(5363):596–9.

251. Aberle H, Bauer A, Stappert J, Kispert A, Kemler R. Beta-catenin is a target for the ubiquitin-proteasome pathway. *EMBO J*. 1997;16(13):3797–804.

252. Jiang J, Struhl G. Regulation of the Hedgehog and Wingless signalling pathways by the F-box/WD40-repeat protein Slimb. *Nature*. 1998;391(6666):493–6.

253. Glinka A, Wu W, Delius H, Monaghan AP, Blumenstock C, Niehrs C. Dickkopf-1 is a member of a new family of secreted proteins and functions in head induction. *Nature*. 1998;391(6665):357–62.

254. Kawano Y, Kypta R. Secreted antagonists of the Wnt signalling pathway. *J Cell Sci*. 2003;116(Pt 13):2627–34.

255. Ladher RK, Church VL, Allen S et al. Cloning and expression of the Wnt antagonists Sfrp-2 and Frzb during chick development. *Dev Biol*. 2000;218(2):183–98.

256. Tamai K, Semenov M, Kato Y et al. LDL-receptor-related proteins in Wnt signal transduction. *Nature*. 2000;407(6803):530–5.

257. Hey PJ, Twells RC, Phillips MS et al. Cloning of a novel member of the low-density lipoprotein receptor family. *Gene*. 1998;216(1):103–11.

258. Mi K, Johnson GV. Role of the intracellular domains of LRP5 and LRP6 in activating the Wnt canonical pathway. *J Cell Biochem*. 2005;95(2):328–38.

259. Little RD, Carulli JP, Del Mastro RG et al. A mutation in the LDL receptor-related protein 5 gene results in the autosomal dominant high-bone-mass trait. *Am J Hum Genet*. 2002;70(1):11–9.

260. Koller DL, Rodriguez LA, Christian JC et al. Linkage of a QTL contributing to normal variation in bone mineral density to chromosome 11q12–13. *J Bone Miner Res*. 1998;13(12):1903–8.

261. Hirschhorn JN, Lindgren CM, Daly MJ et al. Genomewide linkage analysis of stature in multiple populations reveals several regions with evidence of linkage to adult height. *Am J Hum Genet*. 2001;69(1):106–16.

262. Pinson KI, Brennan J, Monkley S, Avery BJ, Skarnes WC. An LDL-receptor-related protein mediates Wnt signalling in mice. *Nature*. 2000;407(6803):535–8.

263. Cheng SL, Lecanda F, Davidson MK et al. Human osteoblasts express a repertoire of cadherins, which are critical for BMP-2-induced osteogenic differentiation. *J Bone Miner Res*. 1998;13(4):633–44.

264. Holmen SL, Zylstra CR, Mukherjee A et al. Essential role of beta-catenin in postnatal bone acquisition. *J Biol Chem*. 2005;280(22):21162–8.

265. Janssens K, van Hul W. Molecular genetics of too much bone. *Hum Mol Genet* 2002;11(20):2385–93.

266. Billin AN, Thirlwell H, Ayer DE. Beta-catenin-histone deacetylase interactions regulate the transition of LEF1 from a transcriptional repressor to an activator. *Mol Cell Biol*. 2000;20(18):6882–90.

267. Brannon M, Brown JD, Bates R, Kimelman D, Moon RT. XCtBP is a XTcf-3 corepressor with roles throughout Xenopus development. *Development*. 1999;126(14):3159–70.

268. Brantjes H, Roose J, van De Wetering M, Clevers H. All Tcf HMG box transcription factors interact with Groucho-related co-repressors. *Nucleic Acids Res*. 2001;29(7):1410–9.

269. Kahler RA, Westendorf JJ. Lymphoid enhancer factor-1 and beta-catenin inhibit Runx2-dependent transcriptional activation of the osteocalcin promoter. *J Biol Chem*. 2003;278(14):11937–44.

270. Qi H, Aguiar DJ, Williams SM, La Pean A, Pan W, Verfaillie CM. Identification of genes responsible for osteoblast differentiation from human mesodermal progenitor cells. *Proc Natl Acad Sci USA*. 2003;100(6):3305–10.

271. de Jong DS, van Zoelen EJ, Bauerschmidt S, Olijve W, Steegenga WT. Microarray analysis of bone morphogenetic protein, transforming growth factor beta, and activin early response genes during osteoblastic cell differentiation. *J Bone Miner Res*. 2002;17(12):2119–29.

272. Hadjiargyrou M, Lombardo F, Zhao S et al. Transcriptional profiling of bone regeneration: Insight into the molecular complexity of wound repair. *J Biol Chem*. 2002;277(33):30177–82.

273. Bennett CN, Longo KA, Wright WS et al. Regulation of osteoblastogenesis and bone mass by Wnt10b. *Proc Natl Acad Sci USA*. 2005;102(9):3324–9.

274. Willert K, Brown JD, Danenberg E et al. Wnt proteins are lipid-modified and can act as stem cell growth factors. *Nature*. 2003;423(6938):448–52.

275. Veeman MT, Axelrod JD, Moon RT. A second canon: Functions and mechanisms of beta-catenin-independent Wnt signaling. *Dev Cell*. 2003;5(3):367–77.

276. Bhanot P, Brink M, Samos CH et al. A new member of the frizzled family from *Drosophila* functions as a Wingless receptor. *Nature*. 1996;382(6588):225–30.

277. Umbhauer M, Djiane A, Goisset C et al. The C-terminal cytoplasmic Lys-thr-X-X-X-Trp motif in frizzled receptors mediates Wnt/beta-catenin signalling. *EMBO J*. 2000;19(18):4944–54.

278. Roman-Roman S, Shi DL, Stiot V et al. Murine Frizzled-1 behaves as an antagonist of the canonical Wnt/beta-catenin signaling. *J Biol Chem*. 2004;279(7):5725–33.

279. Golan T, Yaniv A, Bafico A, Liu G, Gazit A. The human Frizzled 6 (HFz6) acts as a negative regulator of the canonical Wnt. Beta-catenin signaling cascade. *J Biol Chem*. 2004;279(15):14879–88.

280. Kulkarni NH, Halladay DL, Miles RR et al. Effects of parathyroid hormone on Wnt signaling pathway in bone. *J Cell Biochem*. 2005;95(6):1178–90.

281. Bodine PV, Billiard J, Moran RA et al. The Wnt antagonist secreted Frizzled-related protein-1 controls osteoblast and osteocyte apoptosis. *J Cell Biochem*. 2005;96(6):1212–30.

282. Oshima T, Abe M, Asano J et al. Myeloma cells suppress bone formation by secreting a soluble Wnt inhibitor, sFRP-2. *Blood*. 2005;106(9):3160–5.

283. Berndt T, Craig TA, Bowe AE et al. Secreted Frizzled-related protein 4 is a potent tumor-derived phosphaturic agent. *J Clin Invest*. 2003;112(5):785–94.

284. Hsieh JC, Kodjabachian L, Rebbert ML et al. A new secreted protein that binds to Wnt proteins and inhibits their activities. *Nature*. 1999;398(6726):431–6.

285. Vaes BL, Dechering KJ, van Someren EP et al. Microarray analysis reveals expression regulation of Wnt antagonists in differentiating osteoblasts. *Bone*. 2005;36(5):803–11.

286. Bafico A, Liu G, Yaniv A, Gazit A, Aaronson SA. Novel mechanism of Wnt signalling inhibition mediated by Dickkopf-1 interaction with LRP6/Arrow. *Nat Cell Biol*. 2001;3(7):683–6.

287. Zhang Y, Wang Y, Li X et al. The LRP5 high-bone-mass G171V mutation disrupts LRP5 interaction with Mesd. *Mol Cell Biol*. 2004;24(11):4677–84.

288. Boyden LM, Mao J, Belsky J et al. High bone density due to a mutation in LDL-receptor-related protein 5. *N Engl J Med*. 2002;346(20):1513–21.

289. Tian E, Zhan F, Walker R et al. The role of the Wnt-signaling antagonist DKK1 in the development of osteolytic lesions in multiple myeloma. *N Engl J Med*. 2003;349(26):2483–94.

290. Hartmann C, Tabin CJ. Dual roles of Wnt signaling during chondrogenesis in the chicken limb. *Development*. 2000;127(14):3141–59.

291. Gregory CA, Singh H, Perry AS, Prockop DJ. The Wnt signaling inhibitor Dickkopf-1 is required for reentry into the cell cycle of human adult stem cells from bone marrow. *J Biol Chem*. 2003;278(30):28067–78.

292. Mao B, Wu W, Davidson G et al. Kremen proteins are Dickkopf receptors that regulate Wnt/beta-catenin signalling. *Nature*. 2002;417(6889):664–7.

293. Krupnik VE, Sharp JD, Jiang C et al. Functional and structural diversity of the human Dickkopf gene family. *Gene*. 1999;238(2):301–13.

294. Ohnaka K, Tanabe M, Kawate H, Nawata H, Takayanagi R. Glucocorticoid suppresses the canonical Wnt signal in cultured human osteoblasts. *Biochem Biophys Res Commun*. 2005;329(1):177–81.

295. Li X, Liu P, Liu W et al. Dkk2 has a role in terminal osteoblast differentiation and mineralized matrix formation. *Nat Genet*. 2005;37(9):945–52.

296. Semenov M, Tamai K, He X. SOST is a ligand for LRP5/LRP6 and a Wnt signaling inhibitor. *J Biol Chem*. 2005:280(29):26770–5.

297. Winkler DG, Sutherland MS, Ojala E et al. Sclerostin inhibition of Wnt-3a-induced C3H10T1/2 cell differentiation is indirect and mediated by bone morphogenetic proteins. *J Biol Chem*. 2005;280(4):2498–502.

298. Koay MA, Woon PY, Zhang Y et al. Influence of LRP5 polymorphisms on normal variation in BMD. *J Bone Miner Res*. 2004;19(10):1619–27.

299. Gong Y, Vikkula M, Boon L et al. Osteoporosis-pseudoglioma syndrome, a disorder affecting skeletal strength and vision, is assigned to chromosome region 11q12–13. *Am J Hum Genet*. 1996;59(1):146–51.

300. Van Wesenbeeck L, Cleiren E, Gram J et al. Six novel missense mutations in the LDL receptor-related protein 5 (LRP5) gene in different conditions with an increased bone density. *Am J Hum Genet*. 2003;72(3):763–71.

301. Kwee ML, Balemans W, Cleiren E et al. An autosomal dominant high bone mass phenotype in association with craniosynostosis in an extended family is

caused by an LRP5 missense mutation. *J Bone Miner Res.* 2005;20(7):1254–60.

302. Babij P, Zhao W, Small C et al. High bone mass in mice expressing a mutant LRP5 gene. *J Bone Miner Res.* 2003;18(6):960–74.

303. Holmen SL, Giambernardi TA, Zylstra CR et al. Decreased BMD and limb deformities in mice carrying mutations in both Lrp5 and Lrp6. *J Bone Miner Res.* 2004;19(12):2033–40.

304. Fujino T, Asaba H, Kang MJ et al. Low-density lipoprotein receptor-related protein 5 (LRP5) is essential for normal cholesterol metabolism and glucose-induced insulin secretion. *Proc Natl Acad Sci USA.* 2003;100(1):229–34.

305. Ferrari SL, Deutsch S, Choudhury U et al. Polymorphisms in the low-density lipoprotein receptor-related protein 5 (LRP5) gene are associated with variation in vertebral bone mass, vertebral bone size, and stature in whites. *Am J Hum Genet.* 2004;74(5):866–75.

306. Bollerslev J, Wilson SG, Dick IM et al. LRP5 gene polymorphisms predict bone mass and incident fractures in elderly Australian women. *Bone.* 2005;36(4):599–606.

307. van Meurs JB, Rivadeneira F, Jhamai M et al. Common genetic variation of the low-density lipoprotein receptor-related protein 5 and 6 genes determines fracture risk in elderly white men. *J Bone Miner Res.* 2006;21(1):141–50.

308. Agueda L, Bustamante M, Jurado S et al. A haplotype-based analysis of the LRP5 gene in relation to osteoporosis phenotypes in Spanish postmenopausal women. *J Bone Miner Res.* 2008;23(12):1954–63.

309. Giroux S, Elfassihi L, Cole DE, Rousseau F. Replication of associations between LRP5 and ESRRA variants and bone density in premenopausal women. *Osteoporos Int.* 2008;19(12):1769–75.

310. van Meurs JB, Trikalinos TA, Ralston SH et al. Large-scale analysis of association between LRP5 and LRP6 variants and osteoporosis. *JAMA.* 2008;299(11):1277–90.

311. Kiel DP, Ferrari SL, Cupples LA et al. Genetic variation at the low-density lipoprotein receptor-related protein 5 (LRP5) locus modulates Wnt signaling and the relationship of physical activity with bone mineral density in men. *Bone.* 2007;40(3):587–96.

312. Urano T, Shiraki M, Usui T, Sasaki N, Ouchi Y, Inoue S. A1330 V variant of the low-density lipoprotein receptor-related protein 5 (LRP5) gene decreases Wnt signaling and affects the total body bone mineral density in Japanese women. *Endocr J.* 2009;56(4):625–31.

313. Ferrari SL, Deutsch S, Baudoin C et al. LRP5 gene polymorphisms and idiopathic osteoporosis in men. *Bone.* 2005;37(6):770–5.

314. García-Ibarbia C, Pérez-Núñez MI, Olmos JM et al. Missense polymorphisms of the WNT16 gene are associated with bone mass, hip geometry and fractures. *Osteoporos Int.* 2013;24(9):2449–54.

315. Yerges LM, Zhang Y, Cauley JA et al. Functional characterization of genetic variation in the Frizzled 1 (FZD1) promoter and association with bone phenotypes: More to the LRP5 story? *J Bone Miner Res.* 2009;24(1):87–96.

316. Yerges LM, Klei L, Cauley JA et al. A high-density association study of 383 candidate genes for volumetric bone density at the femoral neck and lumbar spine among older men. *J Bone Miner Res.* 2009;24(12):2039–49.

317. Sims AM, Shephard N, Carter K et al. Genetic analyses in a sample of individuals with high or low BMD shows association with multiple Wnt pathway genes. *J Bone Miner Res.* 2008;23(4):499–506.

318. Lee HJ, Koh JM, Hwang JY et al. Association of a RUNX2 promoter polymorphism with bone mineral density in postmenopausal Korean women. *Calcif Tissue Int.* 2009;84(6):439–45.

319. Bustamante M, Nogués X, Agueda L et al. Promoter 2–1025 T/C polymorphism in the RUNX2 gene is associated with femoral neck BMD in Spanish postmenopausal women. *Calcif Tissue Int.* 2007;81(4):327–32.

320. Doecke JD, Day CJ, Stephens AS et al. Association of functionally different RUNX2 P2 promoter alleles with BMD. *J Bone Miner Res.* 2006;21(2):265–73.

321. Vaughan T, Reid DM, Morrison NA, Ralston SH. RUNX2 alleles associated with BMD in Scottish women; interaction of RUNX2 alleles with menopausal status and body mass index. *Bone.* 2004;34(6):1029–36.

322. Vaughan T, Pasco JA, Kotowicz MA, Nicholson GC, Morrison NA. Alleles of RUNX2/CBFA1 gene are associated with differences in bone mineral density and risk of fracture. *J Bone Miner Res.* 2002;17(8):1527–34.

323. Otto F, Thornell AP, Crompton T et al. Cbfa1, a candidate gene for cleidocranial dysplasia syndrome, is essential for osteoblast differentiation and bone development. *Cell.* 1997;89(5):765–71.

324. Hamersma H, Gardner J, Beighton P. The natural history of sclerosteosis. *Clin Genet.* 2003;63(3):192–7.

3

Osteoporosis
Biochemical investigations

IPPOKRATIS POUNTOS and PETER V. GIANNOUDIS

INTRODUCTION

Bone is a dynamic organ that constantly undergoes remodeling. Bone remodeling encapsulates two opposing actions: bone resorption and bone formation. These two processes are combined in time and space at the level of basic multicellular units (BMUs). Bone resorption consists of the actions of osteoclasts and involves the dissolution of bone mineral to its components. In immediate succession, osteoblasts synthesize bone matrix and mineralize the previously created void. Various systemic hormones (e.g., parathyroid hormone, vitamin D, steroid hormones) or locally acting cytokines and growth factors regulate the balance between bone resorption and formation. Under physiologic conditions, this process is completed in a period of 3–6 months. Disturbance of this process, with a preponderance of resorption, can lead to osteoporosis.

Osteoporosis is defined as a systemic disease of the skeleton characterized by low bone mass, deterioration of bone architecture, increased skeletal fragility, and increased fracture risk. It can be diagnosed with the dual-energy x-ray absorptiometry (DEXA) by a simple measurement of the bone mineral density (BMD). This diagnostic modality is currently the gold standard. However, although densitometric techniques can analyze bone mass, bone strength, and architecture *in vivo* are difficult to measure. Furthermore, great variability in DEXA cross-sectional studies exists between "normal" individuals and osteoporosis patients with broad overlapping between the two groups. In this context, the need for alternative biochemical diagnostic tools has been investigated. In recent years, a number of cellular or extracellular components of bone structure have brought to light markers that can specifically reflect on either bone formation or resorption (Figure 3.1).

The aim of this chapter is to describe the available diagnostic bone turnover markers and present their efficacy in diagnosing osteoporosis.

ROUTINE BASELINE BIOCHEMICAL INVESTIGATIONS IN PATIENTS INVESTIGATED FOR OSTEOPOROSIS

Calcium levels

The role of dietary calcium and dairy product intake in the development of osteoporosis has not been fully explored. Nevertheless, it is currently thought that adequate calcium intake improves bone mineral density. Ample calcium intake during childhood and adolescence leads to a higher peak bone mass, which in turn can be considered as an extra deposit for the subsequent years in life (1). In adulthood and especially in postmenopausal women, calcium depletion is associated with increased bone resorption (2). The serum total calcium levels can be within range even in patients with low calcium intake due to compensatory mechanisms; however, the identification and treatment of patients with hypocalcemia could potentially lead to a reduction of bone resorption. Albumin adjustment of total calcium can be useful in correcting total calcium levels skewed by abnormal albumin levels. Ionized calcium measurement can give a more accurate indication of calcium homeostasis.

Vitamin D

Vitamin D is a fat-soluble vitamin that is produced endogenously following sun exposure. Vitamin D promotes intestinal calcium absorption and plays a role in bone growth and remodeling. Vitamin D can be easily determined by measuring the serum 25-hydroxy vitamin D (25[OH]D). The U.S. Institute of Medicine has suggested that 50 nmol/mL should be the lower cutoff limit (3). Some authors suggested that for optimal bone health, the reference value should be increased to 75 nmol/mL (4). Irrespective of which one is considered the lowest reference level,

Bone formation markers

- Total alkaline phosphatase
- Bone-specific alkaline phosphatase
- Ostocalcin (OC)
- C-terminal propeptide of protocolagen type I (PICP)
- N-terminal propeptide of protocolagen type I (P INP)

Bone resorption markers

- Excreted Ca^{++}
- Hidroxyproline
- C-terminal telopeptide of collagen type I
- N-terminal telopeptide of collagen type I
- Tartrate-resistant acid phosphatase (TRAP)
- Deoxypyridinoline
- Pyridinoline
- Bone sialoprotein

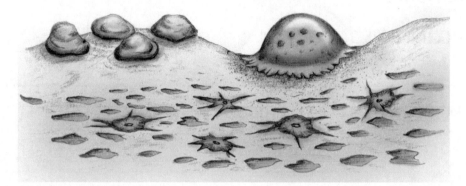

Figure 3.1 Markers of bone formation and resorption.

vitamin D together with calcium levels should be determined as a baseline investigation in every patient investigated for osteoporosis.

Other laboratory investigations

Parathyroid hormone (PTH) analysis is recommended in cases of abnormal serum calcium to investigate the cause of the abnormality. Several centers have introduced PTH measurement in their routine investigation in patients with high clinical suspicion for osteoporosis. A number of laboratory tests can be performed to rule out other causes of osteoporosis. Erythrocyte sedimentation rate can be a useful investigation to rule out inflammatory disease, which can be associated to bone loss. Hypogonadism in men can be screened with serum testosterone. Cortisol and dexamethasone levels should be performed to exclude Cushing syndrome. Serum protein electrophoresis and free light chains could aid in the diagnosis of multiple myeloma. Finally, the measurement of urea and creatinine together with the estimation of the glomerular filtration rates can identify the presence of renal failure, which can inversely affect the skeleton.

DIAGNOSTIC TOOLS: BONE FORMATION MARKERS

Serum total alkaline phosphatase and bone-specific alkaline phosphatase

Alkaline phosphatase (ALP) is a membrane-bound enzyme, which is found attached on glycosyl-phosphatidylinositol moieties present on the outer layer of the cellular membrane of cells (5). The specific function of ALP is currently obscure; however, it seems to play a role in mineralization and osteoid formation (6). The circulating total ALP consists of several dimeric isoforms, which originate in their vast majority from liver and bone; however, spleen, kidney, and placenta contribute with smaller amounts. In healthy adults, bone and liver isoenzymes are present in equal proportions in the circulation. In adolescents and children, bone-ALP prevails to 90% of the total circulating levels because of the skeletal growth. The liver-ALP predominates in patients with abnormal liver function and hepatobiliary pathologies. Once liver disease is ruled out, total ALP activity correlates with the extent of osteoblast activity and represents a simple inexpensive marker of bone metabolism. Caution with result interpretation is recommended as total ALP values are higher in males than in females and rise with age (7,8). The administration of several pharmaceutical agents like, for example, contraceptives, as well as electrolytic disturbances (magnesium, zinc) have been found to reduce its activity (8).

Bone-specific ALP isoform has the advantage of no intergender variation and is not influenced by the circadian rhythm (7). However, cross-reactivity with the liver ALP isoenzyme could be as high as 20% (9). In cases of hepatobiliary pathologies or gestation, bone-specific ALP has higher specificity. In addition, its overall diagnostic value in cases where the total-ALP serum levels significantly exceed the upper normal reference limit can be trivial, as bone-specific ALP can be artificially high, leading to false-positive results (10). From a clinical perspective, the bone-specific ALP isoenzyme measurement has higher specificity compared to total-ALP and can provide an better impression of the level of new bone formation and osteoblast activity (10,11).

Osteocalcin

Osteocalcin (OC) (Gla-protein, glutamic acid) is the most abundant noncollagenous protein of the extracellular bone matrix. Its exact role in the skeleton is obscure, even though it was described 40 years ago. It is a vitamin K–dependent protein that contains three γ-carboxyglutamic residues (12). OC is synthesized by osteoblasts, chondrocytes, and odontoblasts during the formation of extracellular bone matrix (12). It is largely incorporated in bone matrix; however, a small proportion (10%–30%) of the newly synthesized OC is released in the bloodstream (13). In addition to bone formation, it has been shown that small amounts of OC are also released during bone resorption. It is eliminated via the urine; hence, its levels can be artificially raised in patients with renal failure. Data from OC knockout models have shown that osteocalcin-deficient animals had a higher bone mass and bones with improved functional quality (14). In clinical studies, OC has been previously analyzed as a potential marker of bone formation, with findings showing a good correlation between the serum levels of osteocalcin and the level of bone formation but not resorption (15).

The main disadvantage of OC as a marker of osteoporosis is that it is released during both bone formation and resorption. It has a short half-life, it is rapidly degraded *in vivo* and *in vitro*, and substantial interlaboratory variation in the detection technique sensitivity currently exists (16,17,18). Its levels are influenced by vitamin K status, renal function, medications, and circadian rhythm. Long-term bed rest and increased physical activity cause an increase of the OC levels, and its levels vary significantly within the days reaching differences as high as 50%.

Propeptides of procollagen type I

Collagen type I is the most abundant type of collagen seen in the skeletal extracellular matrix. It is formed by the osteoblasts in the form of pre-procollagen. This precursor form of collagen poses two short terminal extension peptides, i.e., the procollagen type 1 C-terminal propeptide (P1CP) and the procollagen type 1 N-terminal propeptide (P1NP) (19). P1CP and P1NP are cleaved during the extracellular metabolism of procollagen and are released to the peripheral circulation, while the central part of the molecule stays incorporated to the bone extracellular matrix (19). P1CP and P1NP circulating levels are not solely the result of bone formation as collagen type I is found in several extraskeletal tissues including skin, tendons, and ligaments. Nonetheless, bone originating P1CP and P1NP has the higher fraction in circulation due to the faster metabolism of bone in comparison to that of the other connective tissues. P1CP is cleared in the liver via the mannose receptor. It has a short half-life of 6–8 minutes and is sensitive to thyroid hormone and insulin growth factor I (20). Diurnal variation of P1CP is significant, with higher values reported in the early hours of the day and lower in the afternoon (21). P1NP is degraded through a scavenger receptor and eliminated through the kidneys, but it is more stable and less affected by the circadian rhythm. Its analysis is expensive, and delayed elimination in cases of renal failure can produce high results (22).

P1CP and P1NP have shown good correlation with the level of bone formation and the levels of the other bone formation markers (23,24). Although their clinical relevance is still questionable, P INP appears to be a more valid method between the two (23,24).

DIAGNOSTIC TOOLS: BONE RESORPTION MARKERS

Urinary-excreted calcium

Urinary-excreted calcium is a historic assessment method to evaluate bone resorption. Bone breakdown releases calcium to the circulation, which in turn, will be excreted through the kidneys. It has been shown that excreted calcium levels are influenced by a number of factors including renal threshold, intestinal absorption, and dietary calcium intake. Therefore, this test is of low sensitivity, and its use is currently abandoned.

Hydroxyproline

Similar to the urinary-excreted calcium, hydroxyproline has poor utility in assessing bone resorption. Significant amounts of urinary hydroxyproline derive from the degradation of newly formed collagen in bone and also other extraskeletal tissues. In addition, its secretion to the urine is tightly dependent on the collagen content in nutrition.

Tartrate-resistant acid phosphatase

Tartrate-resistant acid phosphatase (TRAP) is a lysosomal enzyme and is a member of acid phosphatases. The acid phosphatase is classified as isoenzymes 1–5. They can be inhibited with L+-tartrate, except the band 5; hence, it is termed TRAP. TRAP is found in two isoforms that differ in the presence of sialic acid; TRAP-5a is formed by macrophages, while TRAP-5b is formed by osteoclasts.

Serum TRAP-5b, but not 5a, was found to reflect on the rate of bone resorption (25,26). Serum TRAP-5b activity was shown to be significantly elevated in patients with osteoporosis with a significant negative correlation with bone mineral density (25,26). Serum TRAP-5a activity showed no correlation with serum TRAP-5b activity, with BMD, or with any of the markers of bone turnover (25). Similarly, total serum TRAP was found to be an unsuitable marker of bone resorption (27). TRAP loses approximately 20% of its activity per hour after phlebotomy, which can be prevented by mixing the sample with citrate (28). Patients who have osteoporosis have increased TRAP levels, as do patients with a number of other pathologies, including metastatic carcinoma, Paget disease, hyperthyroidism, multiple myeloma, hairy cell leukemia, and Gaucher disease.

C-terminal and N-terminal telopeptide of collagen type I

The proteolytic degradation of collagen type I results in the release of two fragments of collagen I, the C-terminal and N-terminal telopeptide. These molecules are released to the bloodstream and excreted in the urine. Assays to measure their levels in urine and serum have been developed. Both have shown good correlation with the BMD and are considered satisfactory markers of bone resorption (29,30).

CTX and NTX share the same disadvantages with the propeptides of procollagen type I. The stability of these molecules in serum is linked to the laboratory methodology used. Similar to the P1CP and P1NP, circadian variation is high, and the degradation of extraskeletal collagen type I can affect its levels (31). The menstrual cycle, fasting, diet, exercise, and the administration of medications like contraceptives affect their levels (31).

Pyridinoline and deoxypyridinoline

Pyridinoline (PYD) and deoxypyridinoline (DPD) are trifunctional cross-links that stabilize the mature collagen molecule. During bone resorption, collagen is proteolytically broken down to its components; hence, PYD and DPD are released in the peripheral circulation and excreted in the urine. PYD is found in bone, cartilage, and other extraskeletal tissues, while DPD is mainly found in bone and dentin. Urinary excretion of PYD and DPD is independent to dietary intake as neither is taken up from food. The degradation of newly formed collagen does not influence their levels.

PYD and DPD are considered good markers of bone resorption. Their levels in serum or urine are rather exclusively derived from the skeleton, based on the fact that neither molecules are contained in skin collagen, and bone has higher turnover than cartilage, ligaments, and vessels.

Bone sialoprotein

Bone sialoprotein (BSP) is a phosphorylated glycoprotein that accounts for up to 10% of the noncollagenous proteins of the bone matrix. It is the product of osteoblasts and odontoblasts; hence, it is relatively limited to mineralized tissues. It is believed to be an adhesion molecule of cells to the extracellular matrix and facilitates the organization of the extracellular matrix.

BSP plays a vital role in bone biology. BSP knockout animal studies have defects in skeletogenesis characterized by inhibition of osteoblast clonogenicity, differentiation, and activity (32). BSP has been proposed to be reflected on bone resorption, a finding further strengthened by data showing a sudden drop of BSP in patients treated with intravenous bisphosphonates (33). Furthermore, during antiresorptive treatment, BSP was found to correlate with the levels of other bone resorption markers and the increase of bone mineral density (34).

EMERGING BIOLOGICAL MARKERS OF OSTEOPOROSIS

Novel markers involved in bone cell biology are currently investigated as markers of osteoporosis (Table 3.1). Despite the promising results, their clinical significance is yet to be elucidated. These molecules include a wide variety of proteins, hormones, or microRNAs (miRNAs).

Periostin is a matricellular Gla-containing protein expressed in collagen-rich tissues like bone. It was initially considered to derive specifically from periosteum; however, recent data suggest it is involved in heart morphogenesis and lung and renal diseases, as well as vascular smooth muscle cells. Defects in periostin result in defects in cortical architecture and low mineral density (35). In a recent study, high serum periostin levels were found to be independently associated with increased fracture risk in postmenopausal women (36).

Dickkopf-related protein 1 (Dkk-1) and soluble Frizzled-related protein (sFRP) are Wnt signaling pathway regulatory molecules. Their levels increase in conditions characterized by increased bone resorption (37). A negative association between their levels and BMD has been reported (37). Pathologies like osteoarthritis, rheumatic diseases, and a variety of malignancies influence their circulating levels (38).

Cathepsin K is a catalytic enzyme of collagen type I expressed in osteoclasts. A small amount of cathepsin K is released in the circulation but is degraded quickly by other enzymes like cathepsin S. There is some evidence to suggest that cathepsin K is increased in postmenopausal women with osteoporosis, but its clinical relevance should be further elucidated as this molecule is involved in pathologies like osteoarthritis, atherosclerosis, and cardiovascular diseases (39).

Table 3.1 Emerging circulating markers of bone metabolism in osteoporosis

Proteins/enzymes	Hormone/ growth factors	MicroRNA (miRNA)
Periostin	FGF-23	miRNA-133a
Cathepsin K	Klotho	miRNA-148a
Sclerostin		miRNA-503
Dkk-1		miRNA-21
sFRP		miRNA-23a
Sphingosine-1-phosphate		miRNA-24
RANKL/OPG		miRNA-25
		miRNA-100
		miRNA-125b
		miRNA-214

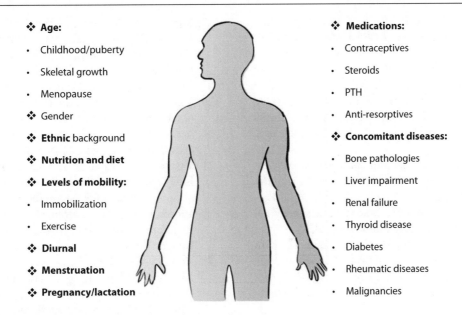

Figure 3.2 Patient-related causes of variability in the levels of biochemical markers.

Sclerostin is an antagonist of the Wnt pathway and is expressed mainly by osteocytes and chondrocytes. Sclerostin was found raised in postmenopausal women, negatively correlated with PTH and estradiol, but its correlation with fracture risk was poor (40,41). In addition, its levels are influenced by a number of pathologies including diabetes, renal insufficiency, atherosclerosis, and others.

Fibroblast growth factor 23 (FGF-23) is a circulating growth factor that regulates the serum levels of inorganic phosphorus and 1,25-dihydroxyvitamin D_3. In a prospective 3-year study including 2868 elderly men, an increase in the baseline levels of FGF-23 was associated with an increased risk of fracture (42). Other similar studies contradict these results, with the role of FGF-23 in depicting low BMD remaining obscure (43).

Finally, a number of single-stranded noncoding RNAs, derived either from the cleavage or translational repression of mRNAs, were investigated as potential markers of osteoporosis. The data are limited; however, mRNA-148a, mRNA-133a, mRNA-503, and others have shown some correlation with either increased osteoclastogenesis or decreased BMD.

CLINICAL UTILITY OF BIOCHEMICAL MARKERS IN DIAGNOSING OSTEOPOROSIS

The aforementioned molecules have shown good correlation to either bone formation or resorption. They have shown some evidence in predicting the presence of bone loss, which correlates with the BMD and the risk of fracture. However, their overall effectiveness in establishing the presence of osteoporosis is poor (44). The marked variability seen can be patient related, but the interlaboratory variability should not be ignored (Figure 3.2). It has been previously shown that this variability can be as high as 30% for the urine-measured markers, while for the serum-measured molecules this figure can be 10%–15% (24). Issues of cross-reactivity and specificity together with numerous exogenous factors that can affect their results limit their clinical significance. Another limitation includes the static nature of these markers and the lack of normal reference values.

In conclusion, the available biochemical molecules can greatly contribute to our understanding of bone physiopathology and provide insight as an assessment tool of a therapeutic response, but their current role as a diagnostic modality is limited. A detailed history and clinical examination that focus on factors related to low bone density together with BMD assessment by DEXA scan are recommended and remain the gold standard. Routine laboratory tests including serum calcium, vitamin D, and thyroid function tests should be the baseline investigations when screening for osteoporosis.

No benefits in any form have been received or will be received from a commercial party related directly or indirectly to the subject of this chapter. No funds were received in support of this study.

REFERENCES

1. Huncharek M, Muscat J, Kupelnick B. Impact of dairy products and dietary calcium on bone-mineral content in children: Results of a meta-analysis. *Bone.* 2008;43(2):312–21.
2. Nakamura K, Saito T, Yoshihara A et al. Low calcium intake is associated with increased bone resorption in postmenopausal Japanese women: Yokogoshi study. *Public Health Nutr.* 2009;12:2366–70.
3. Ross AC, Manson JE, Abrams SA et al. The 2011 report on dietary reference intakes for calcium and

vitamin D from the Institute of Medicine: What clinicians need to know. *J Clin Endocrinol Metab.* 2011;96:53–8.

4. Glendenning P, Taranto M, Noble JM et al. Current assays overestimate 25-hydroxyvitamin D3 and underestimate 25-hydroxyvitamin D2 compared with HPLC: Need for assay-specific decision limits and metabolite-specific assays. *Ann Clin Biochem.* 2006;43:23–30.

5. Harris H. The human alkaline phosphatases: What we know and what we don't know. *Clin Chim Acta.* 1990;186:133–50.

6. Pountos I, Giannoudis PV. Biology of mesenchymal stem cells. *Injury.* 2005;36(Suppl 3):S8–S12.

7. Van Hoof VO, Hoylaerts MF, Geryl H, Van Mullem M, Lepoutre LG, De Broe ME. Age and sex distribution of alkaline phosphatase isoenzymes by agarose electrophoresis. *Clin Chem.* 1990;36: 875–8.

8. Cepelak I, Cvosiscec D. Biochemical markers of bone remodeling. *Biochemia Medica.* 2009;19:17–35.

9. Delmas PD, Eastell R, Garnero P, Seibel MJ, Stepan J, Committee of Scientific Advisors of the International Osteoporosis Foundation. The use of biochemical markers of bone turnover in osteoporosis. *Osteoporos Int.* 2000;11(Suppl 6):S2–17.

10. Martin M, Van Hoof V, Couttenye M, Prove A, Blockx P. Analytical and clinical evaluation of a method to quantify bone alkaline phosphatase, a marker of osteoblastic activity. *Anticancer Res.* 1997;17:3167–70.

11. Woitge HW, Seibel MJ, Ziegler R. Comparison of total and bone-specific alkaline phosphatase in patients with nonskeletal disorder or metabolic bone diseases. *Clin Chem.* 1996;42:1796–804.

12. Ferland G. The vitamin K-dependent proteins: An update. *Nutr Rev.* 1998;56:223–30.

13. Brown JP, Albert C, Nassar BA et al. Bone turnover markers in the management of postmenopausal osteoporosis. *Clin Biochem.* 2009;42:929–42.

14. Ducy P, Desbois C, Boyce B et al. Increased bone formation in osteocalcin-deficient mice. *Nature.* 1996;382:448–52.

15. Delmas PD, Malaval L, Arlot ME, Meunier PJ. Serum bone Gla-protein compared to bone histomorphometry in endocrine diseases. *Bone.* 1985;6:339–41.

16. Blumsohn A, Hannon RA, Eastell R. Apparent instability of osteocalcin in serum as measured with different commercially available immunoassays. *Clin Chem.* 1995;41:318–9.

17. Page AE, Hayman AR, Andersson LM, Chambers TJ, Warburton MJ. Degradation of bone matrix proteins by osteoclast cathepsins. *Int J Biochem.* 1993;25:545–50.

18. Delmas PD, Christiansen C, Mann KG, Price PA. Bone Gla protein (osteocalcin) assay standardization report. *J Bone Miner Res.* 1990;5:5–11.

19. Merry AH, Harwood R, Woolley DE, Grant ME, Jackson DS. Identification and partial characterisation of the non-collagenous amino- and carboxyl-terminal extension peptides of cartilage procollagen. *Biochem Biophys Res Commun.* 1976;71:83–90.

20. Smedsrød B, Melkko J, Risteli L, Risteli J. Circulating C-terminal propeptide of type I procollagen is cleared mainly via the mannose receptor in liver endothelial cells. *Biochem J.* 1990;271:345–50.

21. Vasikaran S, Eastell R, Bruyère O et al., IOF-IFCC Bone Marker Standards Working Group. Markers of bone turnover for the prediction of fracture risk and monitoring of osteoporosis treatment: A need for international reference standards. *Osteoporos Int.* 2011;22:391–420.

22. Koivula MK, Ruotsalainen V, Björkman M et al. Difference between total and intact assays for N-terminal propeptide of type 1 procollagen (P1NP) reflects degradation of pN-collagen rather than denaturation of intact propeptide. *Ann Clin Biochem.* 2010;47:67–71.

23. Ebeling PR, Peterson JM, Riggs BL. Utility of type I procollagen propeptide assays for assessing abnormalities in metabolic bone diseases. *J Bone Miner Res.* 1992;7:1243–50.

24. Charles P, Mosekilde L, Risteli L, Risteli J, Eriksen EF. Assessment of bone remodeling using biochemical indicators of type I collagen synthesis and degradation: Relation to calcium kinetics. *Bone Miner.* 1994;24:81–94.

25. Halleen JM, Ylipahkala H, Alatalo SL et al. Serum tartrate-resistant acid phosphatase 5b, but not 5a, correlates with other markers of bone turnover and bone mineral density. *Calcif Tissue Int.* 2002;71:20–5.

26. Halleen JM, Alatalo SL, Janckila AJ, Woitge HW, Seibel MJ, Väänänen HK. Serum tartrate-resistant acid phosphatase 5b is a specific and sensitive marker of bone resorption. *Clin Chem.* 2001;47:597–600.

27. Halleen JM, Alatalo SL, Suominen H, Cheng S, Janckila AJ, Väänänen HK. Tartrate-resistant acid phosphatase 5b: A novel serum marker of bone resorption. *J Bone Miner Res.* 2000;15:1337–45.

28. Bais R, Edwards JB. An optimized continuous-monitoring procedure for semiautomated determination of serum acid phosphatase activity. *Clin Chem.* 1976;22:2025–8.

29. Sugimoto K, Ikeya K, Iida T et al. An increased serum N-terminal telopeptide of type I collagen, a biochemical marker of increased bone resorption, is associated with infliximab therapy in patients with Crohn's disease. *Dig Dis Sci.* 2016;61:99–106.

30. Garnero P. Biomarkers for osteoporosis management: Utility in diagnosis, fracture risk prediction and therapy monitoring. *Mol Diagn Ther.* 2008;12:157–70.

31. Chubb SA. Measurement of C-terminal telopeptide of type I collagen (CTX) in serum. *Clin Biochem.* 2012;45:928–35.

32. Bouet G, Bouleftour W, Juignet L et al. The impairment of osteogenesis in bone sialoprotein (BSP) knockout calvaria cell cultures is cell density dependent. *PLOS ONE*. 2015;10:e0117402.

33. Seibel MJ, Woitge HW, Pecherstorfer M et al. Serum immunoreactive bone sialoprotein as a new marker of bone turnover in metabolic and malignant bone disease. *J Clin Endocrinol Metab*. 1996;81:3289–94.

34. Shaarawy M, Hasan M. Serum bone sialoprotein: A marker of bone resorption in postmenopausal osteoporosis. *Scand J Clin Lab Invest*. 2001;61:513–21.

35. Bonnet N, Standley KN, Bianchi EN et al. The matricellular protein periostin is required for Sost inhibition and the anabolic response to mechanical loading and physical activity. *J Biol Chem*. 2009;284:35939–50.

36. Rousseau JC, Sornay-Rendu E, Bertholon C, Chapurlat R, Garnero P. Serum periostin is associated with fracture risk in postmenopausal women: A 7-year prospective analysis of the OFELY study. *J Clin Endocrinol Metab*. 2014;99:2533–9.

37. Butler JS, Murray DW, Hurson CJ, O'Brien J, Doran PP, O'Byrne JM. The role of Dkk1 in bone mass regulation: Correlating serum Dkk1 expression with bone mineral density. *J Orthop Res*. 2011;29:414–8.

38. Lane NE, Nevitt MC, Lui LY, de Leon P, Corr M, Study of Osteoporotic Fractures Research Group. Wnt signaling antagonists are potential prognostic biomarkers for the progression of radiographic hip osteoarthritis in elderly Caucasian women. *Arthritis Rheum*. 2007;56:3319–25.

39. Meier C, Meinhardt U, Greenfield JR et al. Serum cathepsin K concentrations reflect osteoclastic activity in women with postmenopausal osteoporosis and patients with Paget's disease. *Clin Lab*. 2006;52:1–10.

40. Mirza FS, Padhi ID, Raisz LG, Lorenzo JA. Serum sclerostin levels negatively correlate with parathyroid hormone levels and free estrogen index in postmenopausal women. *J Clin Endocrinol Metab*. 2010;95:1991–7.

41. Arasu A, Cawthon PM, Lui LY et al., Study of Osteoporotic Fractures Research Group. Serum sclerostin and risk of hip fracture in older Caucasian women. *J Clin Endocrinol Metab*. 2012;97:2027–32.

42. Mirza MA, Karlsson MK, Mellström D et al. Serum fibroblast growth factor-23 (FGF-23) and fracture risk in elderly men. *J Bone Miner Res*. 2011;26:857–64.

43. Lane NE, Parimi N, Corr M et al., Osteoporotic Fractures in Men (MrOS) Study Group. Association of serum fibroblast growth factor 23 (FGF23) and incident fractures in older men: The Osteoporotic Fractures in Men (MrOS) study. *J Bone Miner Res*. 2013;28:2325–32.

44. Miller PD, Baran DT, Bilezikian JP et al. Practical clinical application of biochemical markers of bone turnover: Consensus of an expert panel. *J Clin Densitom*. 1999;2:323–42.

4

Diagnosis
Radiological investigations

DAVID J. HAK and RODRIGO BANEGAS

INTRODUCTION

Radiological methods that can aid in the diagnosis and management of osteoporosis include conventional radiography, dual-energy x-ray absorptiometry (DEXA), quantitative computed tomography (QCT), and high-resolution imaging techniques. Of these, DEXA is currently the most widely used technique for the clinical diagnosis of osteoporosis. Central and peripheral QCT have advantages over DEXA but at present are predominantly used as research tools.

There is much scientific interest in imaging cortical and trabecular bone microstructure *in vivo*, which has become possible with the development of advanced imaging technology. These measurements are typically made at peripheral sites, such as the radius and tibia, using high-resolution computed tomography (CT) and high-resolution magnetic resonance imaging (MRI). While technical issues still need to be addressed to optimize their use, these methods will likely expand our knowledge of the effects of age, disease, and therapy on the skeleton (1).

CONVENTIONAL RADIOGRAPHY

Conventional radiography permits qualitative and semi-quantitative assessment of osteoporosis (2). The main radiographic features of osteoporosis that can be visualized on plain radiographs include increased radiolucency, cortical thinning, altered trabecular patterns, and fragility fractures. The decrease in bone mineral in osteoporosis results in decreased x-ray absorption producing increased radiolucency. Substantial bone loss of at least 30%–50% must be present before increased radiolucency can be observed on conventional radiographs (3). However, the ability to assess radiolucency is limited due to variability in radiographic technique, changes in contrast settings on digital radiographs and picture archiving communication

systems (PACS), and the degree of overlying soft tissues associated with the patient's size.

Cortical thinning results from osseous resorption at endosteal and periosteal sites, along with osseous resorption involving the haversian and Volkmann canals within the intracortical region. With increasing age, there is an imbalance of endosteal bone formation and resorption that leads to a trabeculation of the inner cortical surface and widening of the intramedullary canal.

Cancellous bone, which has a greater surface area, responds faster to metabolic stimuli and thus can demonstrate changes of osteoporosis earlier than cortical bone. The temporal loss of bone mass seen in osteoporosis can be studied by evaluating the trabecular pattern on plain radiographs. The Singh index, reported in 1970, was one of the earliest methods that attempted to stratify trabecular structural changes in the femoral neck with increasing degrees of osteoporosis (4). Changes observed by the Singh index have been shown to correlate with the histomorphometry of iliac crest biopsy. Singh noted that the secondary trabeculae that are not primarily involved in weight bearing disappear first, while the primary trabeculae that are parallel to the axis of weight transmission are preserved until there is advanced osteoporosis (Figure 4.1, Table 4.1).

Morphological evaluation can also be evaluated in the calcaneus. The Jhamaria index closely parallels changes seen with the Singh index and is significantly correlated with age (5). The index ranges from normal bone (grade V) to severe osteoporosis (grade I) and like the Singh index assesses the presence and pattern of compressive and tensile trabeculae (Table 4.2).

Another conventional radiographic finding to suggest the presence of osteoporosis is the demonstration of a low-energy fragility fracture. The most frequent sites for fragility fractures are the spine, hip, wrist, and proximal humerus. Vertebral body compression fractures can be reliably diagnosed with conventional radiographs (Figure 4.2). The presence and number of vertebral compression fractures

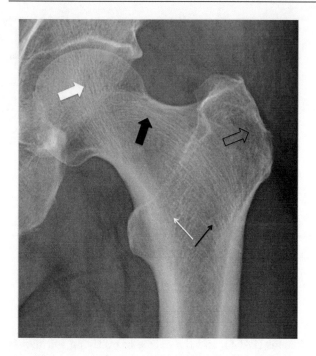

Figure 4.1 Hip radiograph showing the principle tensile (wide black arrow), secondary tensile (thin black arrow), principle compressive (wide white arrow), secondary compressive (thin white arrow), and greater trochanteric (open arrow) trabecular trajectory groups. The Singh classification assesses the progressive loss of these trabecular patterns with increasing bone loss.

are correlated with the degree of osteoporosis. The more severe the osteoporosis, the greater the number of vertebral compression fractures (6).

DUAL-ENERGY X-RAY ABSORPTIOMETRY

DEXA is the most widely used method for measuring bone density. DEXA is a well-standardized and easy to use technique that has a high precision (maximum acceptable precision error, 2%–2.5%) and low radiation dose (1–50 mSv) (7). Central DEXA machines have a large flat table on which the patient lays and a mechanized arm suspended overhead, and they allow measurement of bone density in the hip, spine, and distal radius. These machines are typically used in hospitals and medical offices. Smaller, portable DEXA scanners are available for measuring bone density at peripheral sites such as the distal radius or calcaneus, and they are typically used for osteoporosis screening in drugstores or other community locations.

DEXA scanners produce two x-ray beams that have different peak kilovoltage (30–50 and >70 keV), allowing subtraction of the soft tissue component. The areal bone mineral density (BMD) is typically measured for the lumbar spine, proximal femur, and distal radius. The machine automatically segments the L1–L4 vertebral bodies, femoral neck, and intertrochanteric and trochanteric regions of the proximal femur (Figure 4.3). This segmentation, which is

Table 4.1 Singh index

Grade 6	Grade 5	Grade 4	Grade 3	Grade 2	Grade 1
All trabeculae visible and of normal thickness	Principle tensile and compression trabeculae readily visible with prominence of Ward triangle	Principal tensile trabeculae thinned without loss of continuity	Principle tensile trabeculae thinned and breakage in continuity present	Principle compression trabeculae present, other trabeculae nearly resorbed	Only thin principal compression trabeculae visible

Table 4.2 Jhamari

Grade V	Grade IV	Grade III	Grade II	Grade I
Represents normal healthy bone	Represents normal healthy bone	Represents the borderline between a normal and an osteoporotic bone	Represents osteoporotic bone	Represents advanced stage of osteoporosis
Compression and tensile trabeculae are uniformly present and cross each other. The calcaneus appears to be packed with cancellous bone. The foramen calcanei shows a few thick dense trabeculae comparable in density with those in other parts of the bone	The posterior compression trabeculae are seen as two pillars separated by a well-marked radiolucent area that is due to recession and disappearance of the middle part of the posterior compression trabeculae	There is recession and disappearance of the posterior tensile trabeculae, which stop short at the anterior pillar of the posterior compression trabeculae. This grade represents the borderline between a normal and an osteoporotic bone	Further progression with disappearance of the anterior tensile trabeculae. A thin sheaf of the posterior tensile trabeculae can still be seen which crosses the anterior pillar of the posterior compression trabeculae	Both sets of tensile trabeculae have disappeared completely, and there is also generalized thinning, disappearance, and reduction in the number of compression trabeculae. The bone appears empty and not much denser than the soft tissues

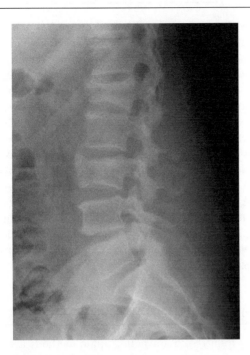

Figure 4.2 Lateral lumbar spine radiograph demonstrating L1 and L3 vertebral compression fractures.

checked and can be corrected by the operator, provides individual BMD measurements in grams per square centimeter.

The raw density information is converted into a patient's T-score and Z-score. The T-score measures the patient's bone density in comparison to a normal population of younger people and is used to estimate the risk of developing a fracture. The World Health Organization (WHO) defined thresholds levels for the diagnosis of osteopenia and osteoporosis. Osteopenia is defined as a T-score of –1 to –2.5 (1–2.5 standard deviations below the mean). Osteoporosis is defined as a T-score less than –2.5 (greater than 2.5 standard deviations below the mean).

The Z-score measures the patient's bone density in comparison to that in people of similar age, sex, and ethnicity. The Z-score is most commonly used in cases of severe osteoporosis to guide further testing for coexisting conditions that may contribute to osteoporosis. Z-scores lower than –2.0 are defined as below the expected range for age.

Although widely used for the measurement of BMD, DEXA has several limitations. DEXA is a two-dimensional measurement and not the volumetric density of the bone or region. The areal BMD measured by DEXA is affected by bone size, overestimating the BMD of larger patients and underestimating the BMD of smaller patients. DEXA also has limitations in measuring BMD in patients with a body mass index greater than 25 kg/m^2. In these obese patients, their soft tissues will elevate BMD measurements due to the x-ray beam attenuation (8). DEXA measurements of the spine and hip can be affected by degenerative changes. Because of the increased bone formation associated with degenerative changes, individuals with substantial degenerative disease will have increased areal density, suggesting a lower fracture risk than is actually present.

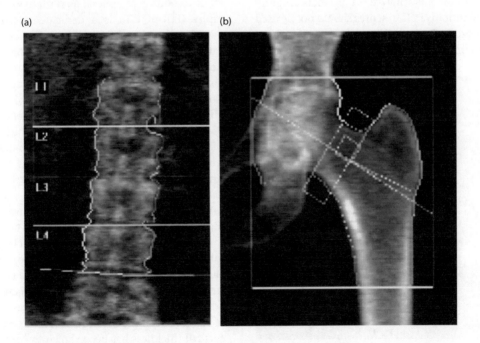

(a)　　　　(b)

Figure 4.3 (a) Posteroanterior dual-energy x-ray absorptiometry (DEXA) image of first through fourth lumbar vertebra. Measurements of the bone mineral content (grams) and area (cm^2) are obtained for each vertebra. These values are compared to an ethnicity- and gender-matched reference database to determine the standard deviation from the mean of either the peak bone mass (T-score) or age-matched bone mineral density (Z-score). (b) DEXA image of the proximal femur showing two defined regions of interest, the femoral neck region (rectangle) and Ward area (square). The areal bone mineral density values of the femoral neck and total hip are used for the World Health Organization definition of osteoporosis (T-score less than –2.5).

Indications for DEXA include women 65 years and older, younger and perimenopausal women with risk factors for fragility fractures, men 70 years and older, and younger men with risk factors for fragility fractures.

QUANTITATIVE COMPUTED TOMOGRAPHY

Quantitative CT is performed using a standard CT scanner with a calibration phantom beneath the patient (Figure 4.4). Standard CT density values measured in Hounsfield units are converted into milligrams hydroxyapatite per cubic centimeter based on the calibration phantom measurements. Quantitative CT scans typically evaluate BMD of the lumbar vertebral bodies and the hip. In comparison to DEXA, quantitative CT provides three-dimensional volumetric measurements of the lumbar spine and proximal femur that are not affected by body size. Quantitative CT offers the ability to separately measure cortical and cancellous bone. This differential measurement is advantageous since high-turnover trabecular bone is more sensitive to changes with disease and therapy. Clinical studies have also shown that quantitative CT BMD of the spine is more sensitive in differentiating patients with osteoporosis from normal individuals without fracture and provides the best capability to discriminate between patients with and without vertebral fractures (9,10).

Disadvantages of quantitative CT are that it requires a higher radiation dose (0.06–2.9 mSv) compared to DEXA. There are only a limited number of longitudinal scientific studies assessing how quantitative CT predicts fragility fractures (7). Quantitative CT T-scores should not be used to define osteoporosis, because these values have not been established for clinical use. Using a T-score threshold of

–2.5 with quantitative CT would define a much higher percentage of patients as having osteoporosis than would be diagnosed with DEXA. However, commonly used clinical criteria using absolute volumetric BMD measurements to characterize fracture risk have been established. Volumetric BMD values of 80–110 mg/cm^3 indicate a mild increase in fracture risk, values 50–80 mg/cm^3 indicate a moderate increase in fracture risk, and values less than 50 mg/cm^3 indicate a severe increase in fracture risk (7).

Indications for the use of quantitative CT instead of DEXA include very small or large individuals in whom DEXA values may not be accurate, older patients with expected advanced degenerative disease of the lumbar spine, and patients requiring high sensitivity to monitor metabolic bone change, such as in patients being treated with parathyroid hormone or corticosteroids (7).

HIGH-RESOLUTION IMAGING TECHNIQUES

Several high-resolution radiographic methods are being developed and optimized to quantify bone architecture, metabolism, and function with the goals of better predicting bone strength and more sensitively monitoring therapeutic interventions.

HIGH-RESOLUTION PERIPHERAL QUANTITATIVE COMPUTED TOMOGRAPHY

High-resolution peripheral quantitative computed tomography (HR-pQCT) is a dedicated extremity imaging machine that provides imaging of trabecular and cortical bone architecture of peripheral sites, such as radius, tibia, and metacarpals. It offers a substantially higher spatial resolution than multidetector CT and MRI (nominal isotropic voxel dimension of 82 mm) (11). Advantages of HR-pQCT are that it allows simultaneous acquisition of BMD, trabecular, and cortical bone architecture. It also has a substantially lower effective radiation dose compared to whole-body multidetector CT and does not include exposure of any radiosensitive organs. Disadvantages are that its use is limited to peripheral skeletal sites and therefore cannot evaluate bone quality in the lumbar spine or hip that are common sites for osteoporotic fragility fractures.

Clinical studies on the usefulness of HR-pQCT for fracture discrimination are limited, and most publications are based on the Strambo or Ofely studies (12,13). For many structural and density HR-pQCT parameters, age-adjusted odds ratios for discriminating fractures are in the range of 1.5–2 (14). In the discrimination of vertebral fractures, cortical thickness has been shown to contribute independently of BMD (12,13). Patients with type 2 diabetes mellitus have a higher incidence of certain fragility fractures despite having normal or increased BMD. A study using HR-pQCT suggests that cortical porosity measurements may be useful to assess increased fracture risk in patients with diabetes (15).

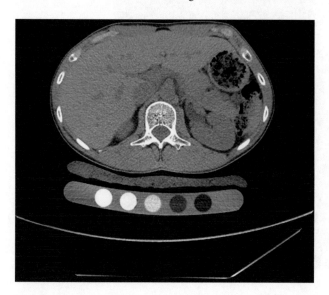

Figure 4.4 Axial computed tomography (CT) scan showing quantitative CT calibration phantom beneath the patient which permits conversion of CT Hounsfield units to milligrams per cubic centimeter of calcium hydroxyapatite. (Image courtesy of Thomas M. Link, MD.)

MULTIDETECTOR COMPUTED TOMOGRAPHY

Multidetector CT is currently in use in clinical practice and offers superior spatial resolution compared with previous spiral CT scanners. However, spatial resolution for imaging of trabecular bone structure is still limited; however, studies have shown that the trabecular bone parameters correlate with those determined on contact radiographs from histologic bone sections and micro-CT (16,17).

Unlike HR-pQCT, multidetector CT can image central regions of the skeleton such as the spine and hip that are common fragility fracture sites. However, substantial radiation exposure is necessary to achieve adequate spatial resolution and image quality, limiting its routine use (18). Multidetector CT measurements of the proximal femur have been shown to improve differentiation between osteoporotic patients with proximal femur fractures and healthy controls (19). Similarly, measurements of the lumbar spine have been shown to improve differentiation between patients with and without osteoporotic spine fractures (20).

MAGNETIC RESONANCE IMAGING

Advances in MRI software and technology have substantially improved the imaging of trabecular bone architecture. While the absence of radiation makes MRI an appealing method to assess bone architecture, at present the technique has been mainly established for peripheral imaging of the distal radius, tibia, and calcaneus (7). Studies have shown that MRI-derived trabecular structure measures correlate well with histology, micro-CT, and biomechanical strength derived from *in vitro* studies (21–23). The spatial resolution with MRI is in the range of trabecular dimensions, which results in substantial partial volume effects, and long acquisition times make imaging susceptible to motion artifacts (7).

REFERENCES

1. Adams JE. Advances in bone imaging for osteoporosis. *Nat Rev Endocrinol.* 2013;9:28–42.
2. Guglielmi G, Muscarella S, Bazzocchi A.Integrated imaging approach to osteoporosis: State-of-the-art review and update. *Radiographics.* 2011;31(5):1343–64.
3. Anil G, Guglielmi G, Peh WC. Radiology of osteoporosis. *Radiol Clin North Am.* 2010;48(3):497–518.
4. Singh M, Nagrath AR, Maini PS. Changes in trabecular pattern of the upper end of the femur as an index of osteoporosis. *J Bone Joint Surg.* 1970;52:457–67.
5. Jhamaria NL, Lal KB, Udawat M, Banerji P, Kabra SG. The trabecular pattern of the calcaneum as an index of osteoporosis. *J Bone Joint Surg Br.* 1983;65(2):195–8.
6. Guglielmi G, Muscarella S, Leone A, Peh WC. Imaging of metabolic bone diseases. *Radiol Clin North Am.* 2008;46(4):735–54.
7. Link TM. Osteoporosis imaging: State of the art and advanced imaging. *Radiology.* 2012;263:3–17.
8. Weigert J, Cann C. DXA in obese patients: Are normal values really normal? *J Womens Imaging.* 1999;1:11–7.
9. Bergot C, Laval-Jeantet AM, Hutchinson K, Dautraix I, Caulin F, Genant HK. A comparison of spinal quantitative computed tomography with dual energy x-ray absorptiometry in European women with vertebral and nonvertebral fractures. *Calcif Tissue Int.* 2001;68(2):74–82.
10. Yu W, Glüer CC, Grampp S et al. Spinal bone mineral assessment in postmenopausal women: A comparison between dual x-ray absorptiometry and quantitative computed tomography. *Osteoporos Int.* 1995;5(6):433–9.
11. Krug R, Burghardt AJ, Majumdar S, Link TM. High-resolution imaging techniques for the assessment of osteoporosis. *Radiol Clin North Am.* 2010;48(3):601–21.
12. Sornay-Rendu E, Boutroy S, Munoz F, Delmas PD. Alterations of cortical and trabecular architecture are associated with fractures in postmenopausal women, partially independent of decreased BMD measured by DXA: The OFELY study. *J Bone Miner Res.* 2007;22(3):425–33.
13. Szulc P, Boutroy S, Vilayphiou N, Chaitou A, Delmas PD, Chapurlat R. Cross-sectional analysis of the association between fragility fractures and bone microarchitecture in older men: the STRAMBO study. *J Bone Miner Res.* 2011;26(6):1358–67.
14. Engelke K, Libanati C, Fuerst T, Zysset P, Genant HK. Advanced CT based *in vivo* methods for the assessment of bone density, structure, and strength. *Curr Osteoporos Rep.* 2013;11(3):246–55.
15. Burghardt AJ, Issever AS, Schwartz AV et al. High-resolution peripheral quantitative computed tomographic imaging of cortical and trabecular bone microarchitecture in patients with type 2 diabetes mellitus. *J Clin Endocrinol Metab.* 2010;95(11): 5045–55.
16. Issever AS, Vieth V, Lotter A et al. Local differences in the trabecular bone structure of the proximal femur depicted with high-spatial-resolution MR imaging and multisection CT. *Acad Radiol.* 2002;9(12):1395–406.
17. Diederichs G, Link TM, Kentenich M et al. Assessment of trabecular bone structure of the calcaneus using multi-detector CT: Correlation with micro-CT and biomechanical testing. *Bone.* 2009;44(5):976–83.
18. Damilakis J, Adams JE, Guglielmi G, Link TM. Radiation exposure in x-ray-based imaging techniques used in osteoporosis. *Eur Radiol.* 2010;20(11):2707–14.
19. Rodríguez-Soto AE, Fritscher KD, Schuler B et al. Texture analysis, bone mineral density, and cortical thickness of the proximal femur: Fracture risk prediction. *J Comput Assist Tomogr.* 2010;34(6): 949–57.

20. Ito M, Ikeda K, Nishiguchi M et al. Multidetector row CT imaging of vertebral microstructure for evaluation of fracture risk. *J Bone Miner Res.* 2005;20(10):1828–36.

21. Link TM, Majumdar S, Lin JC et al. A comparative study of trabecular bone properties in the spine and femur using high resolution MRI and CT. *J Bone Miner Res.* 1998;13(1):122–32.

22. Link TM, Vieth V, Langenberg R et al. Structure analysis of high resolution magnetic resonance imaging of the proximal femur: *In vitro* correlation with biomechanical strength and BMD. *Calcif Tissue Int.* 2003;72(2):156–65.

23. Majumdar S, Kothari M, Augat P et al. High-resolution magnetic resonance imaging: Three-dimensional trabecular bone architecture and biomechanical properties. *Bone.* 1998;22(5):445–54.

5

Development of a fragility liaison service

PAUL ANDRZEJOWSKI and PETER V. GIANNOUDIS

INTRODUCTION

Fragility fractures are defined as those that occur following a low-energy injury that would not usually cause a fracture. In the words of the World Health Organization (WHO), this is equivalent to a low-impact fall from standing height or less (1). They classically encompass neck of femur fractures, lumbar vertebral fractures, and Colles fractures at the wrist, among others. They are by definition "pathologic" and occur in people with reduced bone density for a myriad of reasons. These include medications interfering with the hormonal balance, such as chronic glucocorticoid use or antiandrogen therapy for prostate or breast cancer; medication that inhibits absorption of sufficient vitamin D and calcium; metabolic or endocrine problems; chronic diseases; heavy alcohol intake; family history or genetic defects; and the most common reason, age-related change. These patients often have complicated health-care needs and multiple comorbidities, as well as significant social care needs (2–5). Moreover, they suffer from osteoporosis.

Osteoporosis is a disorder of bone consisting of reduced bone mineral density (BMD) and microarchitectural deterioration of bony tissue. BMD is measured using dual-energy x-ray absorptiometry (DEXA) scanning, usually of lumbar vertebrae and hips. The WHO defines *osteopenia* as a BMD between 1 and 2.5 standard deviations (SDs) below the normal mean for a 30-year-old adult (by which age peak bone mass will usually have been reached) and *osteoporosis* as below 2.5 SDs. These values are referred to as T-scores (2,6). Using these values, it is possible to calculate the 10-year risk of fragility fracture, which can be used to guide therapy.

Loss of estrogen in postmenopausal women leads to increased osteolysis and increases the risk of osteoporosis from 2% at 50 years to over 25% at 80 years; in men there is a 6.6% risk of osteoporosis at 50 years but a 16.6% risk by 80 years, which is usually related to a slower level of new bone turnover as men age (1,3,4,7). In a large, 15-year follow-up study in Australia, after the age of 60, the residual lifetime risk of a fracture for women and men was found to be 44% and 25%, respectively; in patients with osteoporosis, this rose to 65% and 42%, respectively (8). After the age

of 80 years, the risk of hip fracture for both sexes increases exponentially (9). Overall, women remain at a much higher risk, with an approximate 4:1 higher incidence of neck of femur fractures per year than their male counterparts (7).

Osteoporosis is the most common disease of bone and is rising in both incidence and prevalence in the aging population. Interestingly, it has been labeled as the "new epidemic." With increased levels of osteoporosis, a plethora of adverse sequelae naturally follow, including fragility fractures and their potentially fatal outcomes. In 2010, across the European Union's 27 countries, £37 billion (approximately $49.6 billion) were spent annually on osteoporotic fractures, with 1,180,000 quality-adjusted life-years (QALYs) lost. The WHO predicts that the number of people over the age of 65 years will increase by 88% over the next 25 years, and during the period of 2010–2025, the global costs of treating osteoporotic fractures have been predicted to rise by 25% (9–11). In the United Kingdom alone, there are approximately 76,000 hip fractures per year, costing an estimated £2 billion ($2.6 billion) and taking up 1.8 million hospital bed days, with this number set to rise as the elderly population increases (10–13).

Of the estimated 2.7 million hip fractures in the world in 2010, 51% were calculated to be potentially preventable, if we were to define *osteoporosis* as a femoral neck T-score of –2.5 SD or less (7). Fragility fractures, and particularly hip fractures, can have a devastating impact on individuals, with 7% of patients dying within the first month, 30% dying within the first year, and only 30% of patients returning to full function following their injuries (1,11,13).

A pressing need therefore exists for integrated services and systems to cope with the consequences of these fractures and prevent them from occurring in the first place. The care of patients with such injuries should focus on the plurality of issues surrounding their pathogenesis, as well as managing the fracture. This is a multidisciplinary endeavor, including all involved in the care of such patients in order to manage all aspects of care (10,14).

With this in mind, following publication of *The Care of Patients with Fragility Fracture* (the "Blue Book"), a joint publication between the British Orthopaedic Association and the British Geriatrics Society and intense lobbying, and the introduction of the National Hip Fracture Database (NHFD) and Best Practice Tariff, which encourages optimal management in hip fracture patients, increasing emphasis has been made on setting up a fracture liaison service (FLS) (14). They "systematically and proactively" identify patients in either secondary or primary care who sustain fragility fractures, ensure that their risk of a similar event in the future is assessed, and provide appropriate advice or treatment to reduce this risk (15). Patients who have already sustained a fragility fracture are at a two to three times higher risk of a second, with patients sustaining a second hip fracture being 50% more likely to die. It has been shown that an effective FLS can reduce the risk of further fracture by up to 50% (14,16). Numerous national guidelines have been produced that make developing an FLS an absolute priority (1,10,15,16).

FRACTURE LIAISON SERVICE DEVELOPMENT: GUIDELINES AND MODELS

Primary prevention

Current UK National Institute for Health and Care Excellence (NICE) guidance recommends that all patients in at-risk groups be screened and brought in for assessment of fracture risk, with similar guidance by the Royal Osteoporosis Society (Figures 5.1 and 5.2) (1,17).

NICE recommends that risk assessment first take place using a risk stratification tool such as Fracture risk assessment tool (FRAX) or QFracture, which calculates the 10-year risk of fragility fractures based on clinical risk factors. FRAX includes age, sex, weight, height, previous fracture, parental hip fracture, current smoking, glucocorticoids, rheumatoid arthritis, secondary osteoporosis, and alcohol intake of three or more units per day. It can also optionally include BMD T-scores and absolute values. QFracture does not require information on previous fracture, secondary osteoporosis, or BMD but does include several other medical comorbidities and use of tricyclic antidepressants. If the fracture risk falls within the intervention threshold, it is then recommended to go ahead with DEXA scanning, reassess risk when results are back, and consider starting definitive treatment. DEXA scanning should also be considered before initiating any therapy that may have a rapid deleterious effect on bone, such as androgen-inhibiting cancer therapy (1).

This is known as primary prevention and is the ideal situation, with patients being identified at source and before they have the chance to sustain a fragility fracture. Cost analysis suggests that this is the most efficient way to reduce fragility fracture risk and is ideally done using computerized generalized practitioner (GP) records, with patients called in for assessment based on the risks identified on their electronic health record (1). This has been incorporated into the GP QOF (Quality and Outcome Framework), the way GPs in the United Kingdom are remunerated (18).

There have also been large efforts made to establish firm FLS programs in the secondary care setting, which are well placed to identify and seek out patients who may be at higher risk of further fractures, especially those who have already presented to their institution, which are detailed later in this chapter.

FRACTURE LIAISON SERVICE DEVELOPMENT: SETUP

National guidelines from the British Orthopaedic Association and the Royal Osteoporosis Society recommend that every hospital that provides definitive fracture care should have an FLS available. It should be led overall by a designated consultant physician (usually an orthogeriatrician), as well as be fully integrated into the routine orthopedic fracture clinic service, so that there is immediate access to specialist opinion, investigation, and treatment should it be needed. There should also be a linked metabolic bone

---

1. Consider assessment of fracture risk:
   - In all women aged 65 years and over and all men aged 75 years and over
   - In women aged under 65 years and men **aged under 75 years in the presence of risk factors, for example:**
     o Previous fragility fracture
     o Current use or frequent recent use of oral or systemic glucocorticoids
     o History of falls
     o Family history of hip fracture
     o Other causes of secondary osteoporosis
     o Low body mass index (BMI) (less than 18.5 kg/m^2)
     o Smoking
     o Alcohol intake of more than 14 units per week for women and more than 21 units per week for men.

2. Do not routinely assess fracture risk in people aged under 50 years unless they have major risk factors (for example, current or frequent recent use of oral or systemic glucocorticoids, untreated premature menopause or previous fragility fracture), because they are unlikely to be at high risk.

Figure 5.1 Assessing the risk of development fragility fracture. (From National Institute for Health and Care Excellence [NICE]. *Osteoporosis: Assessing the Risk of Fragility Fracture*. Clinical guideline [CG146]. London, UK: NICE, 2012.)

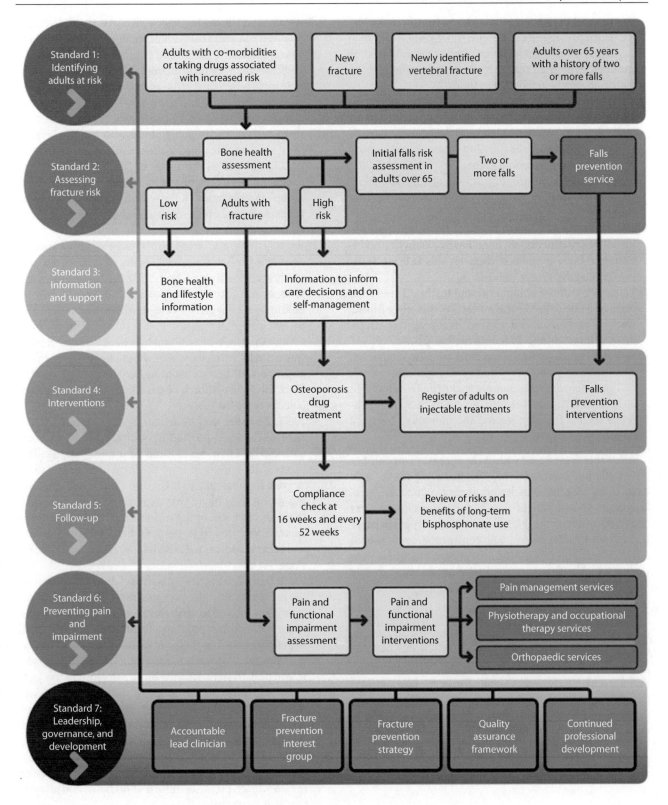

Figure 5.2 Standards of care for osteoporosis and the prevention of fragility fractures (20).

service if required (15). It has been established that central to any FLS is a dedicated clinical practitioner to coordinate all aspects, usually a specially trained nurse, referred to as a fragility prevention practitioner (FPP) (17,19).

They recommend that the "5IQ" model be used when planning and implementing an FLS, as follows:

Identification: All patients aged 50 years and over with a new fragility fracture or vertebral fracture must be "systematically and proactively identified" by the service. This is known as case-finding, and includes all patients who come through accident and emergency with fragility fractures; it is recommended that any fracture with this possibility is reported as such and flagged to the FLS for further review. Patients with other risk factors such as predisposing diseases or medications should also be included. Any such fractures or risks identified by the GP could also be referred into the FLS.

Investigation: Patients require a bone health assessment using FRAX or QFracture and DEXA imaging or blood tests as appropriate, and a comprehensive falls risk assessment if needed, within 3 months of the fracture. A key component is giving the patient sufficient exercises and conditioning following this as well as the pharmacologic intervention, to prevent further fracture.

Information: Patients need to be provided with written information concerning bone health, lifestyle, nutrition, and bone-protection therapy. This is done along the "patient as partner" model.

Intervention: Patients at higher risk of further risk of fractures must be offered bone protection therapy within 5 weeks of assessment and referred for appropriate assessment of interventions to reduce further falls.

Integration: Management plans must be patient centered and integrated between primary and secondary care, and patients who have commenced drug therapy must be reviewed within 4 months to check that an appropriate regime has been started and monitored every 12 months thereafter.

All of this must be set within the context of an emphasis on quality. There must be a database of patients who have been identified as being at risk, which is regularly audited and patient-reported experience measures (PREMs) offered; the FLS team must be appropriately trained and undergo relevant continuing professional development; the FLS should also engage in regular peer review for quality assurance. These have more recently been incorporated into seven overarching standards (Figure 5.2) (16,17).

There is also an emphasis on preventing pain and functional impairment after a fracture, with issues of pain control addressed, and if needed there must be a referral protocol established with the specialist pain service; the FLS must also have access to physiotherapy and occupational therapy and rehabilitation services (17). Ideally, there should also be the facility for referral to services outside the traditional remit, such as podiatry, optometry, smoking and alcohol cessation, and social care services as well as charity organizations (19).

FRACTURE LIAISON SERVICE DEVELOPMENT: PRACTICALITIES

The reality of developing and setting up an FLS requires a number of steps in order to be realized, with the Royal Osteoporosis Society recommending a six-phase approach. The phases are summarized here, but a full set of documents can be obtained from their website (21).

Phase 1: Start out—Initiate a discussion with others involved in caring for patients with osteoporosis, elucidate opinion, and gather and shape ideas. At this stage, a clinical lead or "clinical champion" should be appointed to inspire other clinicians, as well as the hospital management and board, and patient interest groups and ultimately convince them of the merits of an FLS and get them on board with going ahead with setup. A project team must be assembled, a project plan put in place, and a project initiation document or "project brief" created to explain your aims to others. A "stakeholder reference group" that includes all those who may be interested in the project needs to be created and a meeting held with all involved.

Phase 2: Define and scope—This stage is important for developing a better understanding of how things currently are, identifying issues, and generating a thorough process and plan for the project. This should involve holding an engagement event with stakeholders and patient groups, which will fuel enthusiasm for the project and shed light on areas such as what the patient pathway actually involves, which should be mapped; this is an important part of scoping out the current service. Once this information is obtained, you can clearly define objectives for the project.

Phase 3: Measure and understand—The precise level of need of the local population will need to be assessed and analyzed in order to build your business case. This can be done with help from the local information team in your hospital, health board, or clinical commissioning group. It is likely that expert help from people in these departments or organizations will be needed. The capacity required in terms of staffing, imaging, rooms, and other resources will also have to be estimated at this stage.

Phase 4: Design and plan—This should draw together all of the information in the previous three phases and come up with a final plan that can be distributed. A useful way of doing this is holding a facilitated workshop of all relevant parties. Use this information to create a "service specification," which is a document describing the service to be delivered, describe service in terms of the "outputs," and build on this to make your "service model," which describes the components required to detail how it will be delivered in terms of staffing, location, skills, etc. Use the 5IQ model to guide this process. Funding options must be explored and a business case drawn up. Plans to pilot the project must be drawn up considering the workforce, premises, information flows, and integration and communication.

Phase 5: Pilot and implement—Press ahead with what was planned in the previous stage. Ensure to be proactive in capturing and recording data so that the success and utility can be clearly demonstrated or else run the risk of the project being shut down before it can fully begin.

Phase 6: Sustain and share—Aim to implement and sustain the project. Consider linking to formal improvement programs, such as the falls and fragility fracture audit program, continue to train and develop staff, ensure that there is regular audit and measurement of improvement, and maintain your project team and stakeholder reference group with regular and open communication.

FRACTURE LIAISON SERVICE DEVELOPMENT: OUTCOMES AND IMPLICATIONS FOR SERVICE DELIVERY

By 2017 in the United Kingdom, there was a total of 23 established fracture liaison services. Between 2015 and 2017, they covered a population of 5,464,465 patients. A total of 1932 hip fractures were prevented, which translated into £36,608,868 ($49,421,972) saved (19). Significant cost savings have been noted in all countries and regions where a fully integrated FLS has been implemented, making a convincing argument for further widespread rollout, especially for those in charge of local and regional healthcare financing, including public officials and politicians (14). With financial benefits as well as significantly better health-related quality of life for patients, we should hopefully start to see more and more examples of FLSs at local and national levels.

CONCLUSION

This chapter focuses on the pathogenesis and epidemiology of fragility fractures, their importance in the setting of trauma, the importance of an FLS program, and a broad idea of how to implement this in your own hospital. FLSs, if done well, are the future for a modern, integrated fracture care service delivery, particularly for elderly patients, and one that we should embrace with unbridled passion if we want to see the best outcomes for our patients.

REFERENCES

1. National Institute for Health and Care Excellence (NICE). *Osteoporosis: Assessing the Risk of Fragility Fracture. Clinical guideline [CG 146]*. London, UK: NICE, 2012.
2. Christodoulou C, Cooper C. What is osteoporosis? *Postgrad Med J*. 2003;79(929):133–8.
3. Adler RA. Update on osteoporosis in men. Best practice and research. *Clin Endocrinol Metab*. 2018;32(5):759–72.
4. Willson T, Nelson SD, Newbold J, Nelson RE, LaFleur J. The clinical epidemiology of male osteoporosis: A review of the recent literature. *Clin Epidemiol*. 2015;7:65–76.
5. Kanis JA, Cooper C, Rizzoli R, Reginster JY. Executive summary of the European guidance for the diagnosis and management of osteoporosis in postmenopausal women. *Calcif Tissue Int*. 2019;104(3):235–8.
6. Weaver CM, Gordon CM, Janz KF et al. The National Osteoporosis Foundation's position statement on peak bone mass development and lifestyle factors: A systematic review and implementation recommendations. *Osteoporos Int*. 1281;27(4):1281–386.
7. Compston JE, McClung MR, Leslie WD. Osteoporosis. *Lancet*. 2019;393(10169):364–76.
8. Nguyen ND, Ahlborg HG, Center JR, Eisman JA, Nguyen TV. Residual lifetime risk of fractures in women and men. *J Bone Miner Res*. 2007;22(6):781–8.
9. Curtis EM, van der Velde R, Moon RJ et al. Epidemiology of fractures in the United Kingdom 1988–2012: Variation with age, sex, geography, ethnicity and socioeconomic status. *Bone*. 2016;87:19–26.
10. British Orthopaedic Association/British Geriatrics Society. *The Care of Patients with Fragility Fracture ["Blue Book"]*. London, UK: British Orthopaedic Association, 2007, pp. 35–43.
11. Baker PN, Salar O, Ollivere BJ et al. Evolution of the hip fracture population: Time to consider the future? A retrospective observational analysis. *BMJ Open*. 2014;4(4):e004405.
12. Bunning T, Dickinson R, Fagan E et al. *National Hip Fracture Database Annual Report*. London, UK: Royal College of Physicians, Falls and Fragility Fracture Audit Programme, 2018.
13. Healthcare Quality Improvement Partnership. *National Hip Fracture Database Annual Report 2018*. Updated 2019. Available from: https://data.gov.uk/dataset/3a1f3c15-3789-4299-b24b-cd0a5b1f065b/national-hip-fracture-database-annual-report-2018 (accessed July 21, 2019).
14. Pioli G, Bendini C, Pignedoli P, Giusti A, Marsh D. Orthogeriatric co-management—Managing frailty as well as fragility. *Injury*. 2018;49(8):1398–402.
15. British Orthopaedic Association (BOA). British Orthopaedic Association standards for trauma-9 (BOAST 9): Fracture Liaison Services. London, UK: BOA.
16. National Osteoporosis Society (NOS). *Effective Secondary Prevention of Fragility Fractures: Clinical Standards for Fracture Liaison Services*. London, UK: NOS, 2015.
17. National Osteoporosis Society (NOS). *Quality Standards for Osteoporosis and Prevention of Fragility Fractures*. London: NOS, 2017.
18. Mitchell P, Akesson K. How to prevent the next fracture. *Injury*. 2018;49(8):1424–9.
19. Shipman KE, Doyle A, Arden H, Jones T, Gittoes NJ. Development of fracture liaison services: What have we learned? *Injury*. 2017;48(Suppl 7):S4–9.
20. National Osteoporosis Society (NOS). *National Osteoporosis Society—Quality Standards for Osteoporosis and Prevention of Fragility Fractures*. London, UK: NOS, 2017.
21. National Osteoporosis Society (NOS). *Fracture Liaison Service Implementation Toolkit Service Improvement Guide*. London, UK: NOS, 2015.

6

NICE guidelines for medical treatment of osteoporosis
An Update

KATHERINE LOWERY and NIKOLAOS K. KANAKARIS

INTRODUCTION

Since its creation in 1999, as a special health authority, the National Institute for Health and Care Excellence (NICE) aims to improve the quality and reduce the variation of the provided care to patients covered by the National Health Service (NHS) in England. In between its numerous other health- and social care-related initiatives, it has published guidance on a broad spectrum of clinical conditions of high impact and importance. The NICE guidelines are developed by independent multidisciplinary committees that include experts, as well as lay members and represent evidence-based recommendations.

The NICE guidelines for the treatment of osteoporosis were published in conjunction with the guidelines for assessing fragility fractures. These are available from the NICE website and blend with the guidelines from the National Osteoporosis Guideline Group (NOGG). These guidelines were first published in August 2012 and were updated in February 2017 to incorporate the FRAX tool and to follow the cost analysis of bisphosphonates.

This chapter describes the current guidelines for the assessment of fracture risk and the current recommendations for prevention and treatment as advised by NICE for osteoporosis (1).

The guidelines have been developed in order to help the clinician (primary and secondary care providers and hospital specialists) and other health-care professionals to identify those patients at risk and guide treatment. They are also provided to guide service providers and commissioning groups to deliver a service with adequate provisions and systems to ensure patients can be identified and treatment offered appropriately.

ASSESSING THE NEED FOR RISK FRACTURE ASSESSMENT

To ascertain the need for medical treatment, the initial step in the pathway of management advised by NICE is to determine the individual who requires assessment. There are a number of tools to assess the risk. In the United Kingdom, there are two that are in use: FRAX and QFracture. These tools are designed to predict fracture risk, and the primary aim is to identify those individuals who require assessment. These recommendations currently advise assessment of fracture risk in all women aged 65 years and over and all men aged 75 years and over. They also advise to consider assessment of fracture risk in women aged 65 years or less and men aged 75 years or less in the presence of risk factors such as a previous fragility fracture, low bone mass index (BMI less than 18.5 kg/m^2), use of oral or systemic glucocorticoids, smoking, or recurrent fall history (1).

In patients who are younger than 50 years, NICE advises to not routinely assess fracture risk unless there are major risk factors present. These major risk factors include current or frequent recent use of oral or systemic glucocorticoids, untreated premature menopause, or previous fragility fracture (1).

In people aged under 40 years who have a major risk factor, such as history of multiple fragility fracture, major osteoporotic fracture, or current or recent use of high-dose oral or high-dose systemic glucocorticoids (more than 7.5 mg prednisolone or equivalent per day for 3 months or longer), bone mineral density (BMD) should be measured (1).

The recommendations from NICE guide the clinician on whom to assess, and by the presence of clinical risk factors (CRFs), clinicians are alerted to those patients who are at a high risk for fractures.

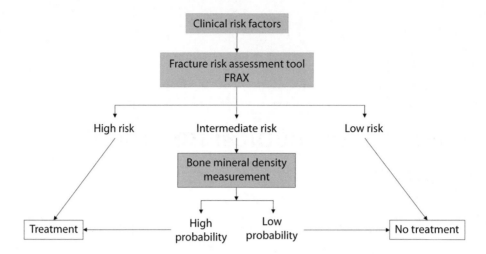

Figure 6.1   A management algorithm for the assessment of patients at risk of fracture.

The tools provided, such as FRAX, are designed to provide thresholds for the use of therapeutic intervention and for the use of BMD scans. The guidelines are there to provide assistance in clinical assessment, but NICE states that the overall decision rests with the individual clinician (1).

Coordinator-based fracture liaison services (FLSs) should be used to systematically identify men and women with fragility fractures.

Fracture risk assessment

Once an individual has been identified as requiring an assessment, the FRAX tool should be utilized and an absolute fracture risk estimated. FRAX algorithms give the 10-year probability of fracture, hip or major osteoporotic fracture (2). In those individuals identified and assessed as having intermediate risk, BMD measurement should be performed and fracture probability reestimated using FRAX.

The National Osteoporosis Guideline Group (NOGG) recommends a management algorithm for the assessment of patients at risk of fracture (Figure 6.1) (2).

The NOGG advises that vertebral assessment should be considered in postmenopausal women and men aged over 50 years if there is a history of more than 4 cm of height loss, kyphosis, recent or current long-term oral glucocorticoid therapy, or a BMD T-score –2.5 SD or less (2).

The NICE advises caution in the interpretation of fracture risk assessment in those patients over the age of 80 years, as fracture risk may be underestimated. Similar advice applies to those patients who have had vertebral fractures or multiple previous fractures, patients who have a high alcohol intake, those who are on high-dose glucocorticoids (greater than 7.5 mg prednisolone or equivalent for 3 months or longer), patients from residential care, and those already prescribed medications that impair bone metabolism.

MEDICAL TREATMENT

The medical treatment of osteoporosis is aimed at both prevention and treatment. The treatment is aimed at providing lifestyle and dietary advice in conjunction with appropriate therapeutic intervention. The guidelines published are in conjunction with the NOGG recommendations (3).

Lifestyle and dietary measures

In those patients who are deemed at increased risk of fracture, a falls risk assessment should be carried out, and regular weight-bearing exercise should be advised.

A recommended daily intake of calcium should be between 700 and 1200 mg. Calcium intake should be assessed and a determination made as to whether this can be achieved through dietary measure alone; if this is not achievable, then supplements should be advised. In those patients who are receiving bone protective therapy, calcium supplementation should be given if dietary intake is below 700 mg daily. Vitamin D supplementation should be considered if the individual has an increased fracture risk or there is evidence of insufficiency. A daily dose of 800 IU cholecalciferol should be advised in postmenopausal women and older men (older than 50 years) at increased risk of fracture.

Therapeutic intervention

There are different therapeutic treatments that can be prescribed to prevent fragility fractures. These include bisphosphonates—alendronate, ibandronate, risedronate, and zoledronic acid. Alternatives to bisphosphonates include raloxifene, denosumab, teriparatide, calcitriol, and hormone replacement therapy. The decision as to which treatment is best lies with the clinician and the patient. The decision should be discussed and tailored to the individual's needs and preferences. The advantages and disadvantages should be discussed. If the patient is unable to comprehend the discussion, this should take place with the responsible carer (4).

Pharmacologic intervention in postmenopausal females

The first-line treatment for postmenopausal women is bisphosphonates, either alendronate or risedronate. In those individuals who cannot tolerate oral bisphosphonates, intravenous bisphosphonate or denosumab is advised. Hormone replacement therapy, raloxifene, or teriparatide can be considered (1,5).

Pharmacologic intervention for osteoporosis in males

Alendronate and risedronate are the first-line treatments in men. Zoledronic acid or denosumab are alternatives, but if the patient cannot tolerate those or they are contraindicated, teriparatide can also be considered. In males, the femoral neck BMD T-scores should be based on the National Health and Nutrition Examination Survey (NHANES) female reference database (2).

Glucocorticoid-induced osteoporosis

The recommendations for both males and females who are greater than 70 years of age taking high doses of glucocorticoids (greater than 7.5 mg/day prednisolone) should be considered for bone protective therapy. In premenopausal females and younger males who are taking high-dose glucocorticoids, bone protective therapy should also be considered. In these patients who are at high risk of fracture, treatment should begin at the onset of glucocorticoid therapy. First-line treatment is alendronate and risedronate. Zoledronate or teriparatide are alternative options if these are contraindicated or patients are intolerant of first-line options.

Duration of treatment

Once treatment with bone protective medication has commenced, a review of the patient should occur. This should include an assessment of potential adverse effects and compliance with the treatment. Potential adverse effects include dyspepsia-type symptoms, and these often occur within the first month. Patients should also be questioned on potential symptoms of atypical fractures, such as thigh or groin pain.

The NICE advised that patients who are commenced on bisphosphonates should have an assessment for the continuing need for treatment at 3–5 years. For those individuals who are at high risk of fracture, alendronate can be continued for up to 10 years and risedronate up to 7 years. These durations are in line with the Scottish (5) and the NOGG (3) guidelines. Continuation of bisphosphonate treatment beyond 3–5 years can generally be recommended in individuals over 75 years old, those with a history of hip or vertebral fracture, those who sustain a fracture while on treatment, and those taking oral glucocorticoids (1). If the bone-sparing treatment is discontinued, then fracture risk should be reassessed after any new fracture, regardless of when this occurs. If no new fracture occurs, assessment of fracture risk should be performed again after 18 months to 3 years. Discussion of stopping bisphosphonate treatment after 3–5 years should include patient choice, fracture risk, and life expectancy.

Guidelines for review and recommendations to continue treatment after 5 years in those individuals at high risk are taken from the National Osteoporosis Guideline Group. Their recommendation to discontinue treatment in those patients who are not at increased risk following an assessment of BMD is based on reducing potential adverse effects on the skeleton, such as atypical fractures (3). "Drug holidays" have not shown that adverse effects on the skeleton have been reduced (5).

If a patient sustains a fracture while on bone-sparing treatment, the clinician must assess the patient for adherence to treatment, and an assessment must be made to exclude secondary causes of osteoporosis (1).

SUMMARY

The guidelines from the NICE and the NOGG are published to help the clinician determine those at an increased fracture risk and guide the assessment and treatment process. Universally, these individuals are identified using tools such as FRAX and arranging for appropriate further investigations if risk is intermediate. Following determination, the patient can be provided appropriate education and pharmacologic treatment.

REFERENCES

1. National Institute for Health and Care Excellence (NICE). *Osteoporosis: Assessing the Risk of Fragility Fracture. Clinical guideline [CG 146].* London, UK: NICE, 2012. Available from https://pathways.nice.org.uk/pathways/osteoporosis
2. University of Sheffield. FRAX. Fracture Risk Assessment Tool. Available from: https://www.sheffield.ac.uk/FRAX/
3. National Osteoporosis Guideline Group. Assessment of fracture risk. Available from: https://www.sheffield.ac.uk/NOGG/mainrecommendations.html
4. National Institute for Health and Care Excellence (NICE). *Biphosphonates for treating osteoporosis.* Technology appraisal guidance [TA464]. London, UK: NICE, 2017. Available from: https://www.nice.org.uk/guidance/ta464/chapter/1-Recommendations
5. https://www.sign.ac.uk/sign-142-management-of-osteoporosis-and-the-prevention-of-fragility-fractures, accessed 28 February 2020

7

Role of bisphosphonates and denosumab

BLOSSOM SAMUELS, YI LIU, and JOSEPH LANE

INTRODUCTION

Bisphosphonate

Osteoporosis is an extremely common disease, expected to increase to a prevalence of approximately 200 million individuals worldwide. In the United States alone, it has been estimated that about 54 million men and women have osteoporosis, or its precursor, osteopenia. Osteoporosis is characterized by decreasing bone mass and diminishing microarchitecture, resulting in increased bone fragility and fractures. This disease poses a major social problem due to high rates of morbidity and mortality following fractures. Hip fractures in elderly patients carry an extremely high mortality rate of approximately 10% at 1 month and 30% at 1 year. The mortality impact is greater for men than women, and in older patients (1). After a hip fracture, many older individuals fail to fully recover. It has been reported that among hip fracture patients who were independent in self-care prior to their fractures, 20%–60% will need assistance with daily activities for 1 and 2 years after fracture due to functional disability (2).

As individuals age, their bone density and muscle mass both decline, resulting in increased risk for falls and associated injuries. It has been reported that 95% of hip fractures are due to falls. Economically, osteoporosis carries a large cost, estimated to be $25.3 billion by 2025. Each year over 300,000 individuals ages 65 and older are hospitalized for hip fractures. The estimated annual prevalence of hip fractures globally is expected to reach 4.5 million by 2050 (3).

Pharmacotherapy and fall prevention interventions are the main tools to prevent hip fractures. The medications currently used to treat osteoporosis include bisphosphonates, denosumab, estrogen or combined estrogen and progesterone therapy, raloxifene, combined estrogen and bazedoxifene, teriparatide, abaloparatide, and romosozumab. The discussion in this chapter focuses on the major antiresorptive agents, drugs known to reduce osteoclastic bone resorption and lower bone turnover, which include bisphosphonates and denosumab (4,5).

MECHANISM

Bisphosphonates are a class of agents that have been widely used as the first-line treatment of osteoporosis and a number of other conditions involving excessive bone resorption, including skeletal complications of malignancy, osteogenesis imperfecta, and Paget disease. Etidronate, the first bisphosphonate approved in the United States, was used in 1968 to treat a young patient with myositis ossificans progressive. Etidronate was considered to also have several other potential benefits, including the capacity to prevent heterotopic ossification after total hip replacement and spinal cord injury. Then, in the 1970s, with more bisphosphonates available, these medications were employed to treat a number of conditions such as Paget disease and hypercalcemia of malignancy. In the 1990s, after bone densitometry use widened, bisphosphonates became standard treatment for patients diagnosed with osteoporosis. For more than 40 years, bisphosphonates have been used worldwide for the treatment of osteoporosis (6).

Bisphosphonates decrease osteoclastic activity and have been shown to decrease the risk of osteoporotic fractures. Bones are constantly undergoing remodeling in a lifelong process to ensure that mature bone is broken down by osteoclasts (resorption) and new bone is built by osteoblasts (bone formation). Bisphosphonates intervene to slow the process of bone loss. These drugs concentrate in trabecular bone, an area of high bone turnover, where they are selectively internalized by osteoclasts, accumulate intracellularly, and ultimately inhibit bone resorption. Over several years of research, the mechanisms by which bisphosphonates inhibit bone resorption have been investigated, resulting in the classification of these drugs into distinct categories (7).

Bisphosphonates are chemically stable analogues of inorganic pyrophosphate (PPi) (6). They can be divided into two main categories, either non-nitrogen-containing or nitrogen-containing bisphosphonates. The non-nitrogen-containing bisphosphonates include clodronate, etidronate, and tiludronate. These drugs function by causing the incorporation of a nonhydrolyzable analogue of adenosine triphosphate (ATP), thereby disrupting cellular metabolism and causing apoptosis of osteoclasts. Nitrogen-containing bisphosphonates, which include pamidronate, neridronate, olpadronate, alendronate, ibandronate, risedronate, and zoledronate, work by inhibiting farnesyl pyrophosphate (FPP) synthase in the mevalonate pathway. By inhibiting lipid synthesis within osteoclasts, these drugs disrupt plasma membrane targeting, causing an accumulation of toxic metabolites that ultimately diminish osteoclastic activity and survival (7).

CLINICAL DATA

Increased bone mineral density

Bisphosphonates have been used to increase bone mineral density (BMD) and reduce fracture risk in women with postmenopausal osteopenia and osteoporosis, men with osteoporosis, patients receiving glucocorticoids, and a number of other conditions. By causing a reduction in osteoclastic activity, bone resorption diminishes, and bone turnover markers (BTMs) rapidly decrease. In general, the maximum effect is achieved in 3–6 months after initiating treatment. This effect will persist while on bisphosphonate therapy, and the new steady state is maintained for 10 years or longer. Bisphosphonates differ in their binding affinity and antiresorptive potency (8). Nitrogen-containing bisphosphonates are generally considered more potent than non-nitrogen-containing bisphosphonates. The reported potency for nitrogen-containing bisphosphonates is zoledronate > risedronate ≫ ibandronate > alendronate (9).

With treatment, patients can achieve a moderate increase in their BMD (8). Zoledronate, a potent bisphosphonate with high affinity for mineralized bone and sites of high bone turnover, is administered annually through a 5 mg intravenous infusion. The HORIZON-Pivotal Fracture Trial (HORIZON-PFT) randomized postmenopausal women with osteoporosis to receive either zoledronate ($n = 3889$) or placebo ($n = 3876$) at baseline, 12 months, and 24 months. After being followed for 3 years, results showed that patients who received zoledronate achieved a statistically significant increase in their BMD at the total hip (6.0%), lumbar spine (6.7%), and femoral neck (5.1%) (10). In order to avoid renal injury, it is recommended to only use intravenous zoledronate in patients with CrCl greater than 30–35 mL/min (11). Of note, most clinical trials utilizing bisphosphonates also provided calcium and vitamin D supplementation to participants. It is recommended that clinicians carefully dose these supplements in order to ensure calcium and vitamin D levels remain within recommended ranges, avoiding complications related to hypercalcemia or vitamin D toxicity (4).

Vertebral and nonvertebral fractures

Bisphosphonates have been shown to reduce the risk of both vertebral and nonvertebral fractures. The American College of Physicians (ACP) issued a clinical practice update in 2017 recommending that clinicians offer antiresorptive therapy with either bisphosphonates or denosumab to treat patients with a diagnosis of osteoporosis. The ACP's recommendation for bisphosphonates is based on high-quality evidence that demonstrated a reduction in vertebral, nonvertebral, and hip fractures when postmenopausal women were treated with bisphosphonates, specifically alendronate, risedronate, and zoledronic acid, or denosumab. There was evidence that ibandronate reduced risk of vertebral fractures; however, there was insufficient evidence to show that it reduced risk of hip and other nonvertebral fractures (4). Bisphosphonates generally cause a greater reduction in risk of vertebral fractures than nonvertebral fractures. Nonetheless, alendronate, risedronate, and zoledronate have demonstrated the remarkable ability to reduce hip fracture risk by up to 40% (6). The ACP recommends that treatment for osteoporosis be continued for 5 years to reduce the risk for fractures involving the hips and spine (4).

A review combining data from 24 randomized controlled trials (RCTs) was recently published investigating the impact of bisphosphonates on fracture risk. This included 21,335 in the bisphosphonate group and 17,862 in the placebo group across trials using alendronate (six studies), risedronate (five studies), etidronate (four studies), zoledronic acid (four studies), clodronate (two studies), ibandronate (one study), minodronate (one study), and pamidronate (one study). Results showed that bisphosphonate use contributed to a reduction in the risk of overall osteoporotic fractures, vertebral fractures, and nonvertebral fractures. There was insufficient evidence to demonstrate overall osteoporotic fracture risk reduction with etidronate (12).

Adherence

Compliance with bisphosphonate use remains a very important factor in the efficacy of these drugs. Adherence to oral bisphosphonates has been a major problem, with reports showing that less than 50% of individuals starting oral bisphosphonates continue them for more than 1 year (11). In a cohort of 664 women with a mean follow-up period of about 27 months, patients had taken their bisphosphonate for an average of 14.4 months associated with an adherence rate of only 57%. Comparing pretreatment to 6 months or more follow-up bone density results, this study found a continuous relationship between adherence and changes in BMD (13). Another study of 171,063 individuals followed for 1–2.5 years revealed a 46% increased fracture risk in noncompliant patients compared to those who were compliant (11).

Poor adherence has been associated with several factors, including concern about drug side effects, inconvenience of taking medications, comorbid conditions, use of multiple medications, poor understanding of benefits, absence of symptoms for underlying disease, age, socioeconomic status, and health plan costs (4,11). Various administration options are available for oral bisphosphonates, including daily, weekly, and monthly formulation. An enteric-coated risedronate has been introduced that, compared to the traditional daily formulation, has demonstrated efficacy and safety in a 2-year randomized, controlled, noninferiority study. This delayed release risedronate may be a favorable option for patients who have difficulty complying with a daily dosing schedule. Intravenous zoledronate administered yearly also offers a convenient option for delivering a defined dose and avoiding gastrointestinal intolerance (14).

Change in bone turnover markers

Bisphosphonates diminish bone resorption, thereby causing a reduction in BTMs. Conversely, high BTM levels are associated with low BMD and increased fracture risk in untreated postmenopausal women. Many clinicians use BTMs to identify patients with high bone turnover and monitor osteoporosis treatment. After discontinuing long-term bisphosphonates, the persistence of low BTM levels may suggest continued antiresorptive benefit (11).

BTMs should be monitored to assess patients' response to bisphosphonates. In fact, the International Osteoporosis Foundation has proposed defining failure to respond to treatment as "two or more incident fragility fractures or by lack of BTM response and a significant decrease in BMD" (15). In studies using bone markers to monitor response to treatment, alendronate and ibandronate were shown to result in greater reductions in BTMs than risedronate. Patients who experience the largest reduction in their BTMs demonstrated higher BTMs at baseline and high levels of adherence to taking their bisphosphonate medication (16).

Some have suggested that BTMs should be used to predict fracture risk. This is supported by a post hoc analysis of the Fracture Intervention Trial that reported an association between fewer vertebral fractures and greater suppression of serum procollagen type 1 N-terminal propeptide (P1NP), bone-specific alkaline phosphatase (BSAP), and C-terminal cross-linking telopeptide (CTX) in alendronate-treated patients. Other studies investigating the relationship between BTMs and fracture risk have not always demonstrated this association, which may be due in part to variability in BTM tests. With evidence suggesting that lower BTM levels may convey reduced fracture risk, many clinicians choose to restart bisphosphonate therapy once BTM levels begin to rise and exceed the lower half of the premenopausal range (11).

Glucocorticoid-induced osteoporosis

Although steroids are used to treat many inflammatory conditions, these drugs carry a significant risk of contributing to bone loss and the development of glucocorticoid-induced osteoporosis (GIOP). The use of bisphosphonates to prevent and treat GIOP has been investigated in several studies. Results were analyzed in a recent systematic review of 27 RCTs involving 3075 adults with inflammatory bowel disease treated with steroids for at least 1 year who were randomized to receive either bisphosphonates or placebo. There was moderate-certainty evidence supporting bisphosphonates for prevention and treatment of GIOP in the spine and hips, high-certainty evidence that bisphosphonates decrease the risk of vertebral fractures, and low-certainty evidence that bisphosphonates make little or no impact on fracture risk at nonverbal sites. This review overall supported the use of bisphosphonates in patients receiving long-term treatment with glucocorticoids (17). Other sources have cited evidence supporting the use of alendronate, risedronate, as well as teriparatide to reduce fracture risk in patients being treated with glucocorticoids (4).

Fracture healing

The effect of bisphosphonates on fracture healing has been an area of study for several years. It has been proposed that bisphosphonates, by inhibiting bone resorption, may contribute to a significant delay in this key stage of fracture healing. The majority of clinical reports involving acute fracture healing after treatment with bisphosphonates demonstrate that healing is not impaired. However, there are reports that suggest that upper limb fractures may have some delay in healing time (18). Ng et al. reported that patients who received bisphosphonates prior to their fracture had a 6-day delay in average healing time compared to those who did not receive bisphosphonates. There was no increased risk of nonunion (19). In another study involving a systematic review of the literature, distal radius fractures had significantly prolonged union time among patients being treated with bisphosphonates (20). In regard to the atypical femoral fractures (AFFs) that may occur in patients with histories of long-term bisphosphonate use, studies show a delay in union time in an estimated 26% of published cases (21).

Studies have also investigated the impact of initiating bisphosphonates (less than 3 months) following acute fracture. Several studies show no significant delay in healing time in either upper or lower limb fractures when bisphosphonates are initiated early after fracture (18). Seo et al. reported that early initiation of bisphosphonates after surgery did not impact fracture union in osteoporotic patients who had undergone fixation of proximal humerus fractures (22). Similarly, Li et al. reported in a review of 10 randomized controlled studies with 2888 patients who received early initiation of bisphosphonates after surgery that there was no delay in fracture healing time either radiologically or clinically (23).

SIDE EFFECTS

Atypical fracture

First reported in 2008, bisphosphonate use has been associated with the occurrence of AFFs (11). The risk of AFFs with bisphosphonates appears to be related to the duration of treatment. For postmenopausal women taking bisphosphonates for less than 2 years, the reported rate of atypical fractures was 1.78 per 100,000. This rate increased to more than 100 per 100,000 once women remained on bisphosphonates for 8 years or longer (4).

AFFs occur in the subtrochanteric region and diaphysis of the femur. The fractures also tend to occur in healthy, active individuals who were younger than patients who sustain typical femoral fractures. AFFs are associated with minimal or no trauma and prodromal pain. These fractures have characteristic findings that include bilateral or unilateral cortical thickening (hypertrophy) in the lateral side of the subtrochanteric region, transverse orientation (although they may become oblique as they progress medially), and noncomminuted or minimally comminuted appearance. These fractures may be incomplete (involving only the lateral cortex) or complete (extending through both the lateral and medial cortices of the femur with an associated medial cortical spike). These findings distinguish AFFs from typical fractures and suggest that they undergo a different pathogenesis (24).

For management, patients found to have a cortical lesion should undergo further evaluation with magnetic resonance imaging (MRI) or computed tomography (CT) if MRI is not available. MRI will be able to detect a fracture line and bone edema or hyperemia to suggest stress fracture, while CT can detect a fracture line and any associated bone formation. Radionucleotide bone scans are helpful for detecting areas of hyperemia; however, these scans lack the specificity of an MRI or CT for detecting fractures. Bisphosphonates and any other antiresorptive agents should be discontinued immediately. Calcium and vitamin D levels should be supplemented appropriately. Prophylactic nail fixation is recommended in cases of incomplete fracture when there is a visible fracture line and symptoms of pain; however, if the pain is minimal, patients may participate in a 2- to 3-month trial period of limited weight-bearing on the affected side using assistive devices (i.e., cane or walker) for ambulation and transfers. If symptoms fail to improve with this trial, then it is recommended to proceed with prophylactic nail fixation. Limited weight-bearing is recommended for patients with cortical thickening and no evidence of a fracture line and with incomplete fractures with no pain. There are several reports that support the use of an anabolic agent such as teriparatide to heal these AFFs (24).

Osteonecrosis of jaw

Osteonecrosis of the jaw (ONJ) is a rare condition that occurs in a minority of patients treated with bisphosphonates and denosumab. It was initially reported in 2003 in patients with metastatic cancer who were being treated with high-dose intravenous bisphosphonates (11). ONJ incidence remains greatest in the oncology patient populations, ranging from 1% to 15%, since this population undergoes frequent treatments with oncology-dose bisphosphonates and denosumab. Patients receiving these antiresorptive agents for osteoporosis typically receive lower doses at a less frequent rate than cancer patients, and their incidence of ONJ is much lower at an estimated 0.001%–0.1% (25). Of note, ONJ also occurs individuals who are not exposed to antiresorptive agents at an incidence of 1/3000 patients per year according to a single study (11).

ONJ has specific characteristics that include evidence of "(a) exposed necrotic bone in the maxillofacial region that has been present for at least 8 weeks of appropriate therapy; (b) exposure to potent anti-resorptive agents (BPs or denosumab) or anti-angiogenic agents; (c) no history of radiation therapy to the jaw" (11). The pathophysiology of ONJ remains unclear. Proposed factors include local bacterial infection, immune dysfunction, role of inflammation, soft tissue toxicity, oversuppression of bone remodeling by antiresorptive agents, inhibition of angiogenesis, effects of bisphosphonates on $\gamma\delta$ T cells and on monocyte and macrophage function. Several risk factors for developing ONJ have been identified, including invasive dental procedures (extractions or implants), smoking, diabetes mellitus, poor oral hygiene, chronic inflammation, ill-fitting dentures, and use of certain drugs such as glucocorticoids, chemotherapy, and anti-angiogenic agents. Asian populations appear to have a higher incidence of ONJ (11,25).

Preventative strategies to reduce the incidence of ONJ include good oral hygiene, addressing any active oral disease before beginning antiresorptive drugs, and avoiding invasive dental procedures. The American Dental Association and the American Association of Oral and Maxillofacial Surgeons do not advise that patients taking bisphosphonates for osteoporosis discontinue treatment for their invasive dental procedures given the long half-life of bisphosphonates (11). However, some experts suggest that patients at high risk for ONJ, such as those with cancer undergoing oncology-dose antiresorptive therapy, may consider holding therapy after invasive dental procedures until the surgical sites heal (25).

Management depends on several factors, including the stage of the disease, size of the lesions, and presence of contributing drug therapy and comorbidity. Treatment includes conservative options, such as topical antibiotic oral rinses and systemic antibiotic therapy, and surgical debridement if needed. There is early evidence supporting using teriparatide to enhance healing. Several experimental management strategies for ONJ include bone marrow stem cell intralesional transplantation, low-level laser therapy, local platelet-derived growth factor application, hyperbaric oxygen, and tissue grafting (25).

Cardiovascular

There is some controversial literature about the risk of cardiovascular events with bisphosphonates; however, the majority of studies show no increased risk of cardiovascular events, stroke, myocardial infarction, or cardiovascular death (4). In fact, several studies have demonstrated that bisphosphonate use is associated with reduced mortality in men and women with osteoporotic fractures after 18 months to 2 years of treatment. This mortality reduction is only partially related to the reduced risk of fractures.

The mechanism for this mortality benefit is unclear; however, the immunomodulatory effects that bisphosphonates exert on the development of vascular disease have been proposed as a possible mechanism. To investigate, a longitudinal study of a rheumatoid arthritis population with a high prevalence of bisphosphonate use and vascular disease was conducted in the United States, enrolling patients in the National Data Bank for Rheumatic Diseases. Results demonstrated that the risk of myocardial infarction, after adjusting for several confounders, was significantly reduced while on bisphosphonates compared to when not on bisphosphonates. This study suggested that bisphosphonates may offer a significant mortality reduction in older patients, as they often have both cardiovascular disease and osteoporosis. Future studies are needed to further define the mechanism by which bisphosphonates may reduce cardiovascular events (26).

Other adverse events

There is an association between the use of oral bisphosphonates and the occurrence of mild upper gastrointestinal symptoms, which does not appear to be linked to the use of any particular bisphosphonate. Studies have reported various adverse events associated with zoledronic acid use including hypocalcemia, influenza-like symptoms, uveitis, arthritis, arthralgias, and headaches. Several of these symptoms with zoledronic acid are associated with an acute phase reaction that is typically observed after some patients receive intravenous bisphosphonate for the first time. Ibandronate use has been associated with myalgias, cramps, and limb pain. Bisphosphonates have not been linked to any increased risk of cancer (4,11).

ANTIRESORPTIVE DENOSUMAB

Mechanism

In contradistinction to bisphosphonates, denosumab is a full human monoclonal antibody that targets the receptor activator of nuclear factor–κB ligand (RANKL) with high affinity and specificity, preventing it from binding to its receptor activator of nuclear factor–κB (RANK) in the extracellular milieu. This inhibition prevents bone resorption by impairing the development, activation, and survival of osteoclasts (27).

Pharmacokinetics

The bioavailability of denosumab 60–120 mg administered subcutaneously was reported to be 61%–64%. The baseline RANKL level, quasi-steady-state constant, and RANKL degradation rate were 614 ng/mL, 138 ng/mL, and 0.00148 h^{-1}. After administration of denosumab 60 mg, the mean maximum denosumab concentration was 6.75 mcg/mL with a median time to maximum concentration of 10 days. The mean half-life was 25.4 days (28). Unlike bisphosphonates, denosumab is not excreted by the kidney (29). Therefore, dosage adjustment is not required in patients with renal impairment (29). In contrast to bisphosphonates, denosumab does not incorporate into bone.

Clinical data

INCREASED BONE MINERAL DENSITY

In the Fracture Reduction Evaluation of Denosumab in Osteoporosis (FREEDOM) trial that involved 7808 postmenopausal women, denosumab was associated with an increase in BMD of 9.2% at the lumbar spine (LS) and 6.0% at the total hip (TH) as compared with placebo at 36 months' follow-up (30). The FREEDOM extension trial is a 7-year open-label extension study following the 3-year FREEDOM trial in which all patients were given denosumab in the extension period (31). The study was completed by 2626 patients. In the long-term group, patients receiving 10 years of denosumab continued to have an increase in BMD from FREEDOM baseline by 21.7% at the LS, 9.2% at TH, 9.0% at FN, and 2.7% at the one-third radius at 10-year follow-up. In the crossover group where women received 7 years of denosumab after 3 years of placebo, BMD increased from extension baseline by 16.5% at the LS, 7.4% at TH, 7.1% at FN, and 2.3% at one-third radius (31). The FREEDOM extension trial confirmed long-term efficacy of denosumab.

Compared with bisphosphonates, denosumab showed more significant BMD increase in postmenopausal women with osteoporosis (32–34). In one study, patients were given either denosumab subcutaneous every 6 months or oral alendronate every week after 1 year of alendronate. In subjects switching to denosumab, greater BMD gain was found at all anatomic sites in the denosumab group compared with subjects continuing alendronate ($P < 0.0125$ at all sites) (32). In another randomized open-label study, 1 year of denosumab significantly increased BMD compared with oral risedronate at LS (3.4% versus 1.1%), TH (2.0% versus 0.5%), and FN (1.4% versus 0%, $P < 0.0001$ at all sites) (33). Likewise, denosumab was superior to ibandronate in increasing BMD at all sites in a randomized open-label study that involved 833 postmenopausal women ($P < 0.001$ at all sites) (34). This was further confirmed by a RCT of 643 postmenopausal women previously treated with oral bisphosphonates. Subjects were assigned to either denosumab biannually or zoledronic acid once a year. At 12 months, denosumab had a significantly greater increase compared with zoledronic acid at LS (3.2% versus 1.1%), TH (1.9% versus 0.6%), and FN (1.2% versus −0.1%, $P < 0.001$ at all sites) (35).

An anabolic agent like teriparatide, a parathyroid hormone analogue, directly stimulates osteoblasts to improve bone mass and volume as well as decreases fracture risk (36). The denosumab and teriparatide administration study (DATA) is a RCT involving 94 postmenopausal osteoporotic women to evaluate the effect of teriparatide, denosumab, or combination therapy (37). At 24 months, LS BMD increased more in the combination group (12.9%) than in the teriparatide group (9.5%) alone or in the denosumab group (8.3%, $P < 0.01$). A similar difference was detected at the FN (6.8% in the combination group versus 2.8% in the teriparatide group and 4.1% in the denosumab group, $P < 0.01$) and TH (6.3% in the combination group, 2.0% in the teriparatide group, and 3.2% in the denosumab group, $P < 0.001$) (38). The authors further investigated the sequencing of denosumab and teriparatide by conducting the DATA-Switch study. In DATA-Switch, women originally assigned to teriparatide received denosumab (teriparatide to denosumab group), those originally assigned to denosumab received teriparatide (denosumab to teriparatide group), and those originally assigned to both received an additional 24 months of denosumab alone (combination to denosumab group) (39). At 48 months, LS BMD had the greatest increase in the teriparatide to denosumab group (18.3%), compared with 14% in denosumab to teriparatide group and 16% in combination to denosumab group, although such difference was not statistically significant. The combination to denosumab group was associated with the largest BMD increase at both FN (9.1% versus 8.3% in teriparatide to denosumab and 4.9% in denosumab to teriparatide group, $P < 0.05$) and TH (8.6% versus 6.6% in teriparatide to denosumab and 2.8% in denosumab to teriparatide group, $P < 0.05$) (38). The results of the DATA-Switch study suggested the importance of the orders of antiosteoporotic agent.

In addition to bone protective benefits in postmenopausal women with osteoporosis, the previous study also demonstrated increased BMD with denosumab in men with low BMD (39). Of the 228 subjects completing 1 year of follow-up, denosumab increased BMD by 5.7% at LS, 2.4% at TH, and 2.1% at FN ($P < 0.015$ at all sites compared with placebo) (39). In addition, a recently published study revealed that denosumab was both noninferior and superior to risedronate in patients receiving glucocorticoids treatment with regard to BMD gain in LS (4.4% versus 2.3% in glucocorticoid-continuing, $P < 0.0001$ and 3.8% versus 0.8% in glucocorticoid-initiating group, $P < 0.0001$) (40).

CHANGE IN BONE TURNOVER MARKER

The pharmacodynamic effect of denosumab is best evaluated through bone turnover markers. In the FREEDOM extension trial, denosumab resulted in a decrease of bone resorption marker, serum C-telopeptide (CTX), by 59% in 36 months compared with a mild increase by 2% in placebo group. The suppression of CTX continues in the extension group for 84 months and remains statistically different when compared with the crossover group in 84 months' follow-up (31). Similarly, bone formation marker, P1NP, was significantly decreased in the extension group in 84 months' follow-up, whereas there was no change in P1NP in the crossover group (31). The reduction in bone turnover marker was related to persistent BMD gain and reduction of fracture risk in the FREEDOM extension trial.

FRACTURE DATA

Fracture

In addition to BMD increase, denosumab was associated with fracture risk reduction in osteoporotic patients. In the FREEDOM trial, denosumab decreased vertebral fracture by 68% as well as lowered hip fracture by 40% and nonvertebral fracture by 20% compared with the placebo group in postmenopausal osteoporotic women (30). The incidence of new vertebral fracture (range 0.90%–1.86%) and nonvertebral fracture (range 0.84%–2.55%) remained low in the FREEDOM extension trial in a 10-year follow-up (31). Very few studies were not designed or statistically designed to evaluate the reduction of fractures as the endpoint due to the relatively low incidence rate of fracture. However, most of the clinical trials showed that patients in the denosumab group had lower accumulative fracture risk. In men with osteoporosis, two subjects sustained clinical fractures in the placebo group, and one subject was found to have cal fracture in the denosumab-treated group (39).

Fracture healing

With regard to fracture healing status, post hoc analysis of the FREEDOM trial failed to detect any delayed healing or nonunion in patients receiving denosumab for 3 years. In addition, the administration of denosumab was not associated with an increased risk of surgical complication after surgery (41). This study suggested that denosumab could be a safe option for those patients who required surgery to manage underlying fractures. In contradistinction to teriparatide, there is no enhancement of fracture healing or spinal fusion.

Safety, tolerability, and long-term monitoring

LONG-TERM USE CONCERNS/BETTER COMPLIANCE

Adherence and compliance of medication is always of great importance to medical illness, especially for chronic diseases like osteoporosis. In a multicenter randomized clinical trial, the adherence (risk ratio [RR] 0.58), compliance (RR 0.48), and persistence (RR 0.54) of denosumab were significantly higher than weekly alendronate (all $P < 0.05$). In addition, subjects involved in this study demonstrated a preference and satisfaction of denosumab over alendronate (42).

INFECTIONS/IMMUNE EFFECT

RANKL/RANK not only has an essential role in osteoclastogenesis but was also involved in immune system functions. As a result, denosumab may have a theoretical side effect of immune suppression and thus increased infection risk. However, the infectious or immune complications of denosumab remain conflicting. In the original FREEDOM trial, increased incidence of hospitalization for cellulitis was found in the denosumab group (30). In the FREEDOM extension trial, the infection rate was similar in the long-term group and crossover group. The overall incidence of infection in the FREEDOM extension trial has remained low over the 10-year follow-up (31).

SEVERE HYPOCALCEMIA

Denosumab can cause severe hypocalcemia, especially in those patients with underlying chronic kidney disease, hypoparathyroidism, or malabsorption. In the FREEDOM extension trial, the incidence of hypocalcemia is about 0.1 per 100 participant years and remained similar throughout the time course (31). In a postmarket report of denosumab, eight cases of severe hypocalcemia were reported. Severe hypocalcemia usually happens within 30 days after denosumab administration. Concurrent calcium supplementation is necessary to prevent hypocalcemia. It is recommended that calcium levels be monitored in patients taking denosumab, especially in those with chronic kidney deficiency.

ATYPICAL FRACTURE

Atypical fracture located in the subtrochanteric area has been reported to be associated with antiresorptive agent exposure (43). In the FREEDOM extension trial, each group reported one case of atypical fracture, and the overall cumulative incidence remained very low (0.8 per 10000 participant-years) (31).

OSTEONECROSIS OF JAW

ONJ is a rare complication of antiresorptive agents. Although the pathophysiology of ONJ is yet to be elucidated, oversuppression of bone turnover from antiresorptive agents may play an important role. The overall frequency of ONJ related to antiresorptive agent in osteoporotic patients was estimated at 0.001%–0.01% (44). The incidence of ONJ in patients receiving denosumab varied from 0 to 30.2 per 100,000 patient-years (45). Although there was no study directly comparing the incidence of ONJ between bisphosphonates and denosumab, the incidence rate of ONJ in theory would be lower in denosumab, as denosumab does not incorporate and lacks an antiangiogenic effect.

In the FREEDOM extension trial, 13 ONJ cases were identified: 7 in the long-term group and 6 in the crossover group (31). A recent meta-analysis identified the risk factors of developing denosumab-related ONJ including previous bisphosphonates treatment, diabetes, and advanced age (46). However, the authors failed to find the relationship between the duration and dosage of denosumab use and ONJ occurrence (46).

REBOUND EFFECT

Although limited data are available, current studies and case series have linked the discontinuation of denosumab with a rebound response of BMD, BTMs, and vertebral fragility risk (47).

Bone and colleagues conducted a randomized, blinded, placebo-controlled study where they followed postmenopausal women with osteopenia who received denosumab every 6 months for 2 years (48). After denosumab discontinuation, BMD returned to baseline at all measured sites over 2 years but remained higher than previously treated placebo (48). An increase in bone resorption markers was also observed with cessation of therapy. There was no increase in clinical fracture risk observed after discontinuation of denosumab (48). However, vertebral fractures have been observed within 2–10 months after denosumab discontinuation. In a recent systematic review by Anastasilakis and colleagues, 24 patients were found to have vertebral fractures after denosumab discontinuation, with the majority (92%) having multiple vertebral compression fractures (49). Patients who received denosumab for more than 2 years had more fractures than patients who received denosumab for less than 2 years (49). This is consistent with a recent post hoc analysis of the FREEDOM trial that demonstrated the vertebral fracture rate quickly increased upon denosumab discontinuation to the level observed in untreated participants (50). In this study, participants with previous history of vertebral fractures or who sustained vertebral fractures during denosumab treatment were at the highest risk of getting new vertebral fracture after denosumab discontinuation (odds ratio 3.9 95%, confidence interval 2.1–7.2) (50).

Additionally, a strategy to prevent bone loss after denosumab cessation is in need of further investigation. Limited data suggest that posttreatment with bisphosphonates could prevent BMD loss after denosumab discontinuation and may theoretically decrease fracture risk (51). A recent prospective clinical trial was conducted to investigate whether a single dose of zoledronate could prevent the decrease in BMD and increase in BTMs after discontinuation of denosumab. The study included 57 female participants with osteoporosis who were treated with denosumab and then randomized to either receive zoledronate ($n = 27$) or two additional monthly 60 mg denosumab injections ($n = 30$) beginning 6 months after the last denosumab treatment. At 24 months from randomization, lumbar BMD in the zoledronate group was unchanged from baseline, while the denosumab group experienced a decrease from the 12-month value by 4.82% $\pm$ 0.7% ($P < 0.001$). Femoral neck BMD results demonstrated similar changes. There was no correlation between BMD and BTMs at baseline or

12 months. Vertebral fractures occurred in 3 patients from the denosumab group and 1 patient from the zoledronate group. Altogether the results indicated that zoledronate, independent of BTMs, helped to prevent bone loss at 24 months. However, clinical follow up is recommended since this effect varies among individuals (52).

SUMMARY

Both bisphosphonate and denosumab provide protection from low-energy fracture. Bisphosphonates bind to bone with prolonged half-life (greater than 30 years). Denosumab has a 2-month duration and does not bind to bone. Denosumab can be used in patients with renal dysfunction. Neither agent enhances fracture healing.

REFERENCES

1. Haentjens P. Meta-analysis: Excess mortality after hip fracture among older women and men. *Ann Intern Med.* 2010;152(6):380.
2. Dyer SM, Crotty M, Fairhall N et al. A critical review of the long-term disability outcomes following hip fracture. *BMC Geriatr.* 2016;16:158.
3. Marks R. Hip fracture epidemiological trends, outcomes, and risk factors, 1970–2009. *Int J Gen Med.* 2010;3:1–17.
4. Qaseem A, Forciea MA, McLean RM, Denberg TD; Clinical Guidelines Committee of the American College of Physicians. Treatment of low bone density or osteoporosis to prevent fractures in men and women: A clinical practice guideline update from the American College of Physicians. *Ann Intern Med.* 2017;166(11):818–39.
5. Yusuf AA, Cummings SR, Watts NB et al. Real-world effectiveness of osteoporosis therapies for fracture reduction in post-menopausal women. *Arch Osteoporos.* 2018;13(1):33.
6. Russell RG. Bisphosphonates: The first 40 years. *Bone.* 2011;49(1):2–19.
7. Rogers MJ, Crockett JC, Coxon FP, Mönkkönen J. Biochemical and molecular mechanisms of action of bisphosphonates. *Bone.* 2011;49(1):34–41.
8. Watts NB, Diab DL. Long-term use of bisphosphonates in osteoporosis. *J Clin Endocrinol Metab.* 2010;95(4):1555–65.
9. Lewiecki EM. Bisphosphonates for the treatment of osteoporosis: Insights for clinicians. *Ther Adv Chronic Dis.* 2010;1(3):115–28.
10. Sunyecz J. Zoledronic acid infusion for prevention and treatment of osteoporosis. *Int J Womens Health.* 2010;2:353–360.
11. Adler RA, El-Hajj Fuleihan G, Bauer DC et al. Managing osteoporosis in patients on long-term bisphosphonate treatment: Report of a task force of the American Society for Bone and Mineral Research. *J Bone Miner Res.* 2016;31(10):1910.
12. Byun JH, Jang S., Lee S et al. The efficacy of bisphosphonates for prevention of osteoporotic fracture: An update meta-analysis. *J Bone Metab.* 2017;24(1):37.
13. Weycker D, Lamerato L, Schooley S et al. Adherence with bisphosphonate therapy and change in bone mineral density among women with osteoporosis or osteopenia in clinical practice. *Osteoporos Int.* 2012;24(4):1483–9.
14. McClung MR, Balske A, Burgio DE, Wenderoth D, Recker RR. Treatment of postmenopausal osteoporosis with delayed-release risedronate 35 mg weekly for 2 years. *Osteoporos Int.* 2013;24(1):301–10.
15. Diez-Perez A, Adachi JD, Agnusdei D et al. Treatment failure in osteoporosis. *Osteoporos Int.* 2012;23(12):2769–74.
16. Naylor KE, Jacques RM, Paggiosi M et al. Response of bone turnover markers to three oral bisphosphonate therapies in postmenopausal osteoporosis: The TRIO study. *Osteoporos Int.* 2016;27(1):21–31.
17. Allen CS, Yeung JH, Vandermeer B, Homik J. Bisphosphonates for steroid-induced osteoporosis. *Cochrane Database Syst Rev.* 2016;10:CD001347.
18. Kates SL, Ackert-Bicknell CL. How do bisphosphonates affect fracture healing? *Injury.* 2016;47. doi: 10.1016/s0020-1383(16)30015-8.
19. Ng AJ, Yue B, Joseph S, Richardson M. Delayed/nonunion of upper limb fractures with bisphosphonates: Systematic review and recommendations. *ANZ J Surg.* 2014;84(4):218–24.
20. Molvik H, Khan W. Bisphosphonates and their influence on fracture healing: A systematic review. *Osteoporos Int.* 2015;26(4):1251–60.
21. Edwards BJ, Bunta AD, Lane J et al. Bisphosphonates and nonhealing femoral fractures: Analysis of the FDA Adverse Event Reporting System (FAERS) and international safety efforts. *J Bone Joint Surg Am.* 2013;95(4):297–307.
22. Seo JB, Yoo JS, Ryu JW, Yu KW. Influence of early bisphosphonate administration for fracture healing in patients with osteoporotic proximal humerus fractures. *Clin Orthop Surg.* 2016;8(4):437–43.
23. Li YT, Cai HF, Zhang ZL. Timing of the initiation of bisphosphonates after surgery for fracture healing: A systematic review and meta-analysis of randomized controlled trials. *Osteoporos Int.* 2015;26(2):431–41.
24. Shane E, Burr D, Abrahamsen B et al. Atypical subtrochanteric and diaphyseal femoral fractures: Second report of a task force of the American Society for Bone and Mineral Research. *J Bone Miner Res.* 2014;29(1):1–23.
25. Khan AA, Morrison A, Hanley DA et al. Diagnosis and management of osteonecrosis of the jaw: A systematic review and international consensus. *J Bone Miner Res.* 2015;30(1):3–23.
26. Wolfe F, Bolster MB, O'Connor CM, Michaud K, Lyles KW, Colón-Emeric CS. Bisphosphonate use is associated with reduced risk of myocardial infarction in patients with rheumatoid arthritis. *J Bone Miner Res.* 2013;28:984–91.

27. Baron R, Ferrari S, Russell RG. Denosumab and bisphosphonates: Different mechanisms of action and effects. *Bone*. 2011;48(4):677–92.

28. Sutjandra L, Rodriguez RD, Doshi S et al. Population pharmacokinetic meta-analysis of denosumab in healthy subjects and postmenopausal women with osteopenia or osteoporosis. *Clin Pharmacokinet*. 2011;50(12):793–807.

29. Block GA, Bone HG, Fang L, Lee E, Padhi D. A single-dose study of denosumab in patients with various degrees of renal impairment. *J Bone Miner Res*. 2012;27(7):1471–9.

30. Cummings SR, San Martin J, McClung MR et al. Denosumab for prevention of fractures in postmenopausal women with osteoporosis. *N Engl J Med*. 2009;361(8):756–65.

31. Bone HG, Wagman RB, Brandi ML et al. 10 years of denosumab treatment in postmenopausal women with osteoporosis: Results from the phase 3 randomised FREEDOM trial and open-label extension. *Lancet Diabetes Endocrinol*. 2017;5(7):513–23.

32. Kendler DL, Roux C, Benhamou CL et al. Effects of denosumab on bone mineral density and bone turnover in postmenopausal women transitioning from alendronate therapy. *J Bone Miner Res*. 2010;25(1):72–81.

33. Roux C, Hofbauer LC, Ho PR et al. Denosumab compared with risedronate in postmenopausal women suboptimally adherent to alendronate therapy: Efficacy and safety results from a randomized open-label study. *Bone*. 2014;58:48–54.

34. Recknor C, Czerwinski E, Bone HG et al. Denosumab compared with ibandronate in postmenopausal women previously treated with bisphosphonate therapy: A randomized open-label trial. *Obstet Gynecol*. 2013;121(6):1291–9.

35. Miller PD, Pannacciulli N, Brown JP et al. Denosumab or zoledronic acid in postmenopausal women with osteoporosis previously treated with oral bisphosphonates. *J Clin Endocrinol Metab*. 2016;101(8):3163–70.

36. Ensrud KE, Crandall CJ. Osteoporosis. *Ann Intern Med*. 2017;167(3):ITC17–32.

37. Tsai JN, Uihlein AV, Lee H et al. Teriparatide and denosumab, alone or combined, in women with postmenopausal osteoporosis: The DATA study randomised trial. *Lancet*. 2013;382(9886):50–6.

38. Leder BZ, Tsai JN, Uihlein AV et al. Denosumab and teriparatide transitions in postmenopausal osteoporosis (the DATA-Switch study): Extension of a randomised controlled trial. *Lancet*. 2015;386(9999):1147–55.

39. Orwoll E, Teglbjaerg CS, Langdahl BL et al. A randomized, placebo-controlled study of the effects of denosumab for the treatment of men with low bone mineral density. *J Clin Endocrinol Metab*. 2012;97(9):3161–9.

40. Saag KG, Wagman RB, Geusens P et al. Denosumab versus risedronate in glucocorticoid-induced osteoporosis: A multicentre, randomised, double-blind, active-controlled, double-dummy, non-inferiority study. *Lancet Diabetes Endocrinol*. 2018;6:445–54.

41. Adami S, Libanati C, Boonen S et al. Denosumab treatment in postmenopausal women with osteoporosis does not interfere with fracture-healing: Results from the FREEDOM trial. *J Bone Joint Surg Am*. 2012;94(23):2113–9.

42. Kendler DL, McClung MR, Freemantle N et al. Adherence, preference, and satisfaction of postmenopausal women taking denosumab or alendronate. *Osteoporos Int*. 2011;22(6):1725–35.

43. Shane E, Burr D, Abrahamsen B et al. Atypical subtrochanteric and diaphyseal femoral fractures: Second report of a task force of the American Society for Bone and Mineral Research. *J Bone Miner Res*. 2014;29(1):1–23.

44. Khan AA, Morrison A, Kendler DL et al. Case-based review of osteonecrosis of the jaw (ONJ) and application of the international recommendations for management from the International Task Force on ONJ. *J Clin Densitom*. 2017;20(1):8–24.

45. Khan AA, Morrison A, Hanley DA et al. Diagnosis and management of osteonecrosis of the jaw: A systematic review and international consensus. *J Bone Miner Res*. 2015;30(1):3–23.

46. de Oliveira CC, Brizeno LA, de Sousa FB, Mota MR, Alves AP. Osteonecrosis of the jaw induced by receptor activator of nuclear factor-kappa B ligand (Denosumab): Review. *Med Oral Patol Oral Cir Bucal*. 2016;21(4):e431–9.

47. Lamy O, Gonzalez-Rodriguez E, Stoll D, Hans D, Aubry-Rozier B. Severe rebound-associated vertebral fractures after denosumab discontinuation: Nine clinical cases report. *J Clin Endocrinol Metab*. 2017;102(2):354–8.

48. Bone HG, Bolognese MA, Yuen CK et al. Effects of denosumab treatment and discontinuation on bone mineral density and bone turnover markers in postmenopausal women with low bone mass. *J Clin Endocrinol Metab*. 2011;96(4):972–80.

49. Anastasilakis AD, Polyzos SA, Makras P, Aubry-Rozier B, Kaouri S, Lamy O. Clinical features of 24 patients with rebound-associated vertebral fractures after denosumab discontinuation: Systematic review and additional cases. *J Bone Miner Res*. 2017;32(6):1291–6.

50. Cummings SR, Ferrari S, Eastell R et al. Vertebral fractures after discontinuation of denosumab: A post hoc analysis of the randomized placebo-controlled FREEDOM trial and its extension. *J Bone Miner Res*. 2017. Epub 2017/11/07.

51. Reid IR, Horne AM, Mihov B, Gamble GD. Bone loss after denosumab: Only partial protection with zoledronate. *Calcif Tissue Int*. 2017. Epub 2017/05/14.

52. Anastasilakis AD, Papapoulos SE, Polyzos SA, Appelman-Dijkstra NM, Makras P. Zoledronate for the prevention of bone loss in women discontinuing denosumab treatment. A prospective 2-Year clinical Trial. *J Bone Miner Res*. 2019;34(12):2220–8.

8

The role of anabolic agents

NIFON K. GKEKAS, EUSTATHIOS KENANIDIS, PANAGIOTIS ANAGNOSTIS, MICHAEL POTOUPNIS, DIMITRIOS G. GOULIS, and ELEFTHERIOS TSIRIDIS

INTRODUCTION

Osteoporosis is a systemic skeletal disease affecting millions of people worldwide. It is characterized by low bone mineral density (BMD) and microarchitectural deterioration of bone tissue, predisposing to increased risk of fracture (1). The clinical significance of osteoporosis is on the fractures that arise. In the United Kingdom, approximately 536,000 new fragility fractures occur each year (2).

The primary goal of osteoporosis management is the prevention of fractures. Antiresorptive and osteoanabolic agents are the two major classes of antiosteoporotic medication. The former is the first-line and most commonly used drug category, which acts by suppressing the osteoclastic-mediated bone resorption and bone turnover (3). Osteoanabolic compounds stimulate and promote bone formation by activation of osteoblasts and bone remodeling. They are usually used as a second-line treatment with proven antifracture efficacy, mainly retained for patients with severe osteoporosis and high fracture risk, who are unresponsive to antiresorptive therapy. There is still inconsistency concerning the optimal sequence of administration of anabolic agents. As they can be used only for a limited period, the patients require an antiresorptive therapy afterward to consolidate BMD gains (4).

The only approved anabolic agents for the treatment of osteoporosis in the United States are teriparatide, a parathyroid hormone (PTH) synthetic analogue, and abaloparatide, a PTH-related peptide (PTHrP) synthetic analogue (3). Both of them reduce the incidence of vertebral and nonvertebral fractures and have been approved by the U.S. Food and Drug Administration (FDA). Abaloparatide has not yet been approved by the European Medicines Agency (EMA). A third agent with a dual mechanism of action characterized both by suppressing osteoclastic and inducing osteoblastic activity has also emerged. This refers to romosozumab, which is a humanized monoclonal antibody against sclerostin (one of the main inhibitors of the Wnt pathway) and shows efficacy in reducing vertebral, nonvertebral, and hip fracture risk. However, its approval remains under consideration by the FDA, given concerns regarding increased cardiovascular events (5,6).

The purpose of this chapter is to present the current evidence on the efficacy and safety of the new anabolic antiosteoporotic agents.

MECHANISM OF ACTION OF TERIPARATIDE AND ABALOPARATIDE

Teriparatide is a peptide composed of the first 34 amino acids of the N-terminal end of PTH. Abaloparatide is a 34 amino acid recombinant, synthetic analogue of PTHrP that is identical to human PTHrP at amino acids 1–22 but differs in amino acids 23–34 to maximize its stability and anabolic activity (7,8).

PTH is an 84 and PTHrP a 36 amino acid polypeptide encoded by interrelated genes that bind to the same PTH 1 receptor (PTH1R). PTH is secreted by the parathyroid glands and plays a crucial role in the regulation of calcium and phosphate metabolism. PTH increases serum calcium concentrations via promotion of an osteoclast-mediated calcium release from the bone, proximal renal tubular calcium reabsorption, and indirectly, by intestinal calcium and phosphorus absorption via an increase in calcitriol formation in the kidney (9).

PTHrP is produced by many different tissues and exerts its effects via paracrine actions. It also increases bone resorption and renal tubular calcium reabsorption, without playing any role in intestinal calcium absorption (8). PTHrP can modulate chondrocyte differentiation and osteoblast function, mammary gland formation, calcium transport through the placenta, vascular smooth muscle differentiation, tooth development, and pancreatic β-cell proliferation (8). Experimental studies have shown that selective deletion of the PTHrP gene leads to decreased bone formation and bone mass. PTHrP loss of function has also been associated with skeletal deformities in humans, such as in Blomstrand chondrodysplasia (8).

Notably, the osteoanabolic influence of PTH and PTHrP analogues has been demonstrated only at a low dosage and by intermittent administration, whereas continuous stimulation of PTH1R (such as in primary hyperparathyroidism) enhances bone turnover and consequently results in bone resorption (10). To date, it is not entirely understood why the continuous versus intermittent exposure to PTH/PTHrP causes different effects on the bone (11).

CLINICAL USE OF TERIPARATIDE AND ABALOPARATIDE

Osteoanabolic agents are mostly advocated as a second-line antiosteoporotic treatment, given their substantial cost. They should be considered in specific groups, such as in patients with severe osteoporosis or high risk of fracture, failure of alternative antiosteoporotic agents, intolerability or contraindications to them, glucocorticoid-induced osteoporosis, chronic obstructive lung disease, transplant bone disease, or any type of illness with an "inherent" requirement to build new bone (12).

Treatment with PTH/PTHrP analogues should be avoided in individuals with a history of renal stones and is contraindicated in patients with hypercalcemic disorders, primary or secondary hyperparathyroidism, or anyone at increased risk for osteosarcoma (e.g., history of Paget disease, radiation involving the skeleton, bone metastases) (13).

Teriparatide

Teriparatide is administered subcutaneously at a daily dose of 20 μg, for a total of 24 months. The suggested underlying mechanisms for teriparatide's anabolic effect, although not fully elucidated, may include Wnt 10b signaling stimulation, sclerostin inhibition, and increased insulin-like growth factor-1 and osteocalcin production (14).

Teriparatide has proven efficacy in reducing vertebral and nonvertebral fracture risk in postmenopausal women with osteoporosis (15). It has also shown greater antifracture efficacy compared with alendronate in patients with glucocorticoid-induced osteoporosis (16). Furthermore, teriparatide is effective in male osteoporosis, by increasing BMD, even 30 months after its cessation, and reducing vertebral fracture risk (17). There is also evidence for higher resolution of osseous defects of the oral cavity compared with placebo (18), which is important in cases of jaw osteonecrosis (19). Moreover, in a recent comparative study in postmenopausal women with severe osteoporosis, teriparatide was more effective in decreasing the risk of new vertebral and clinical fractures when compared with weekly risedronate, after 24 months of therapy (no difference in nonvertebral fracture risk was observed) (20).

Abaloparatide

Abaloparatide is administered subcutaneously and has a higher selectivity for the RG and a lower affinity for the R0 conformation of the PTH1R compared with teriparatide, yielding a more potent osteoanabolic effect (21). It induces bone formation, avoiding the coupling with bone resorption (22). Animal and human studies have shown that abaloparatide can significantly increase both cortical thickness and trabecular bone mass (23–25).

In connection with clinically translatable outcomes, the Abaloparatide Comparator Trial in Vertebral Endpoints (ACTIVE) showed the superiority of abaloparatide and teriparatide against placebo concerning morphometric vertebral fracture risk in postmenopausal women at high risk of fracture (mean age 69 years) (26). In detail, abaloparatide reduced the risk of new morphometric vertebral fractures and nonvertebral fractures compared with placebo. It also demonstrated a higher risk reduction for major osteoporotic fractures (upper arm, wrist, hip, or clinical spine) compared with placebo or teriparatide (26). Furthermore, it was tolerated well with a very low risk of adverse events, including nausea, dizziness, and headaches. Additionally, the incidence of hypercalcamia was lower with abaloparatide compared with teriparatide (26).

Both teriparatide administration and abaloparatide administration should be followed by an antiresorptive agent to keep up the gain in BMD (27). Following the initial treatment with abaloparatide, sequential therapy with alendronate not only maintained but also increased the BMD gain and reduced new radiographic vertebral fractures (28).

The treatment duration of both teriparatide and abaloparatide is limited to 24 months, based on trials that were terminated by the risk of osteosarcoma in rodent models, which, however, has not been reproduced in human studies (13).

ROMOSOZUMAB

The discovery of the Wnt signaling pathway was crucial for the understanding of osteoblastic differentiation. Major extracellular inhibitors of this pathway are sclerostin and Dickkopf-1, which are secreted by the osteocytes that bind to lipoprotein receptor-related proteins 5 and 6, eventually suppressing osteoblastic activity, differentiation, and survival (29). The inhibition of sclerostin also suppresses the osteoclastic activity, since sclerostin upregulates the synthesis of the receptor activator of nuclear factor–κB ligand (RANKL), which is the primary determinant of osteoclastic differentiation (29).

Romosozumab is a humanized monoclonal antibody against sclerostin that demonstrated an increase in bone formation combined with a decrease in bone resorption in both animal and human studies. This dual action changes bone architecture by rapidly increasing both trabecular and cortical bone mass, as well as bone stiffness (30).

In two hallmark clinical studies (6,31), romosozumab was associated with a significant reduction of vertebral and clinical fractures at 12 and 24 months. However, the reduction in nonvertebral and hip fractures was noticed only when romosozumab and alendronate were evaluated together at 24 months (6). Patients randomized to romosozumab/alendronate achieved higher BMD values at all skeletal sites compared with alendronate alone (6). It must be emphasized that the discontinuation of romosozumab was followed by bone loss and the return of BMD to pretreatment levels, whereas the sequential administration of denosumab further increased BMD (32). Higher risk in severe adjudicated cardiovascular disease (CVD) events, however, was observed with romosozumab compared with alendronate (6). The exact pathogenetic mechanisms of this observation have not been elucidated, but these concerns have suspended romosozumab's approval by the FDA.

SEQUENTIAL THERAPY

The sequence of administration of anabolic and antiresorptive agents determines the impact of skeletal response. In general, the ideal therapeutic strategy after discontinuation of an osteoanabolic therapy has not been established. Several studies have demonstrated that administration of antiresorptive therapy after an anabolic agent consolidates the BMD gain induced by the latter (28). In the absence of sequential antiresorptive therapy, BMD benefits will eventually be reduced, as bone loss declines at a rate of up to 4% per year (33). Anabolic therapy should always be followed by administration of an antiresorptive agent, with denosumab providing the greatest benefit, especially after its prior combination with teriparatide (34).

CONCLUSIONS

Osteoanabolic agents are used as second-line drugs for the treatment of osteoporosis in patients with severe osteoporosis and high fracture risk, unresponsive to antiresorptive compounds. PTH synthetic analogue teriparatide, PTHrP synthetic analogue abaloparatide, and the sclerostin-inhibitor romosozumab, by stimulating bone formation appear to be effective in increasing BMD in all skeletal sites and in reducing vertebral and nonvertebral fracture risk. Romosozumab is still under approval by the FDA because an increased cardiovascular risk remains under investigation. In general, osteoanabolic agents should always be followed by administration of an antiresorptive agent, such as bisphosphonates or denosumab, the latter having a greater effect.

REFERENCES

1. Vestergaard P, Rejnmark L, Mosekilde L. Increased mortality in patients with a hip fracture-effect of premorbid conditions and post-fracture complications. *Osteoporos Int.* 2007;18(12):1583–93.

2. Svedbom A, Hernlund E, Ivergard M et al. Osteoporosis in the European Union: A compendium of country-specific reports. *Arch Osteoporos.* 2013;8:137.

3. Black DM, Rosen CJ. Clinical practice. Postmenopausal osteoporosis. *N Engl J Med.* 2016;374(3):254–62.

4. Anagnostis P, Gkekas NK, Potoupnis M et al. New therapeutic targets for osteoporosis. *Maturitas* 2019;120:1–6.

5. Cosman F, Crittenden DB, Ferrari S et al. FRAME Study: The foundation effect of building bone with 1 year of romosozumab leads to continued lower fracture risk after transition to denosumab. *J Bone Miner Res.* 2018;33(7):1219–26.

6. Saag KG, Petersen J, Brandi ML et al. Romosozumab or alendronate for fracture prevention in women with osteoporosis. *N Engl J Med.* 2017;377(15):1417–27.

7. Makino A, Takagi H, Takahashi Y et al. Abaloparatide exerts bone anabolic effects with less stimulation of bone resorption-related factors: A comparison with teriparatide. *Calcif Tissue Int.* 2018;103(3):289–97.

8. Wysolmerski JJ. Parathyroid hormone-related protein: An update. *J Clin Endocrinol Metab.* 2012;97(9):2947–56.

9. Akerstrom G, Hellman P, Hessman O et al. Parathyroid glands in calcium regulation and human disease. *Ann N Y Acad Sci.* 2005;1040:53–8.

10. Lewiecki EM, Miller PD. Skeletal effects of primary hyperparathyroidism: Bone mineral density and fracture risk. *J Clin Densitom.* 2013;16(1):28–32.

11. Tsiridis E, Morgan EF, Bancroft JM et al. Effects of OP-1 and PTH in a new experimental model for the study of metaphyseal bone healing. *J Orthop Res.* 2007;25(9):1193–203.

12. Diez-Perez A, Adachi JD, Agnusdei D et al. Treatment failure in osteoporosis. *Osteoporos Int.* 2012;23(12):2769–74.

13. Cipriani C, Irani D, Bilezikian JP. Safety of osteoanabolic therapy: A decade of experience. *J Bone Miner Res.* 2012;27(12):2419–28.

14. Cusano NE, Costa AG, Silva BC et al. Therapy of osteoporosis in men with teriparatide. *J Osteoporos.* 2011;2011:463675.

15. Neer RM, Arnaud CD, Zanchetta JR et al. Effect of parathyroid hormone (1-34) on fractures and bone mineral density in postmenopausal women with osteoporosis. *N Engl J Med.* 2001;344(19):1434–41.

16. Saag KG, Shane E, Boonen S et al. Teriparatide or alendronate in glucocorticoid-induced osteoporosis. *N Engl J Med.* 2007;357(20):2028–39.

17. Kaufman JM, Orwoll E, Goemaere S et al. Teriparatide effects on vertebral fractures and bone mineral density in men with osteoporosis: Treatment and discontinuation of therapy. *Osteoporos Int.* 2005;16(5):510–6.

18. Bashutski JD, Eber RM, Kinney JS et al. Teriparatide and osseous regeneration in the oral cavity. *N Engl J Med.* 2010;363(25):2396–405.

19. Cheung A, Seeman E. Teriparatide therapy for alendronate-associated osteonecrosis of the jaw. *N Engl J Med*. 2010;363(25):2473–4.
20. Kendler DL, Marin F, Zerbini CAF et al. Effects of teriparatide and risedronate on new fractures in post-menopausal women with severe osteoporosis (VERO): A multicentre, double-blind, double-dummy, randomised controlled trial. *Lancet* 2018;391(10117):230–40.
21. Hattersley G, Dean T, Corbin BA et al. Binding selectivity of abaloparatide for PTH-type-1-receptor conformations and effects on downstream signaling. *Endocrinology*. 2016;157(1):141–9.
22. Doyle N, Varela A, Haile S et al. Abaloparatide, a novel PTH receptor agonist, increased bone mass and strength in ovariectomized cynomolgus monkeys by increasing bone formation without increasing bone resorption. *Osteoporos Int*. 2018;29(3):685–97.
23. Chandler H, Lanske B, Varela A et al. Abaloparatide, a novel osteoanabolic PTHrP analog, increases cortical and trabecular bone mass and architecture in orchiectomized rats by increasing bone formation without increasing bone resorption. *Bone*. 2018;120:148–155.
24. Bilezikian JP, Hattersley G, Fitzpatrick LA et al. Abaloparatide-SC improves trabecular microarchitecture as assessed by trabecular bone score (TBS): A 24-week randomized clinical trial. *Osteoporos Int*. 2018;29(2):323–8.
25. Chew CK, Clarke BL. Abaloparatide: Recombinant human PTHrP (1-34) anabolic therapy for osteoporosis. *Maturitas* 2017;97:53–60.
26. Miller PD, Hattersley G, Riis BJ et al. Effect of abaloparatide vs placebo on new vertebral fractures in postmenopausal women with osteoporosis: A randomized clinical trial. *JAMA* 2016;316(7):722–33.
27. Leder BZ, Tsai JN, Jiang LA et al. Importance of prompt antiresorptive therapy in postmenopausal women discontinuing teriparatide or denosumab: The Denosumab and Teriparatide Follow-up study (DATA-Follow-up). *Bone* 2017;98:54–8.
28. Bone HG, Cosman F, Miller PD et al. ACTIVExtend: 24 months of alendronate after 18 months of abaloparatide or placebo for postmenopausal osteoporosis. *J Clin Endocrinol Metab*. 2018;103(8):2949–57.
29. Suen PK, Qin L. Sclerostin, an emerging therapeutic target for treating osteoporosis and osteoporotic fracture: A general review. *J Orthop Translat*. 2016;4:1–13.
30. Graeff C, Campbell GM, Pena J et al. Administration of romosozumab improves vertebral trabecular and cortical bone as assessed with quantitative computed tomography and finite element analysis. *Bone*. 2015;81:364–9.
31. Cosman F, Crittenden DB, Adachi JD et al. Romosozumab treatment in postmenopausal women with osteoporosis. *N Engl J Med*. 2016;375(16):1532–43.
32. McClung MR, Brown JP, Diez-Perez A et al. Effects of 24 months of treatment with romosozumab followed by 12 months of denosumab or placebo in postmenopausal women with low bone mineral density: A randomized, double-blind, phase 2, parallel group study. *J Bone Miner Res*. 2018;33(8):1397–406.
33. Eastell R, Nickelsen T, Marin F et al. Sequential treatment of severe postmenopausal osteoporosis after teriparatide: Final results of the randomized, controlled European Study of Forsteo (EUROFORS). *J Bone Miner Res*. 2009;24(4):726–36.
34. Tsai JN, Uihlein AV, Lee H et al. Teriparatide and denosumab, alone or combined, in women with postmenopausal osteoporosis: The DATA study randomised trial. *Lancet* 2013;382(9886):50–6.

Current and emerging pharmacological agents in the treatment of osteoporosis

JAMES X. LIU and THOMAS A. EINHORN

INTRODUCTION

Over the past 15 years, there have been significant strides in the advancement of new pharmacologic agents in the treatment of osteoporosis. Current treatment options include drugs that reduce both bone resorption and formation and strengthen trabecular bone to prevent stress risers (concentrated points of stress that lead to acute fractures). The most effective drugs that are currently available to treat osteoporosis include the antiresorptives agents such as the bisphosphonates, and the receptor activator of nuclear factor–κB ligand (RANKL) inhibitor, denosumab. Bone-building agents that stimulate bone formation and resorption, also known as the anabolic class of drugs, are parathyroid hormone (PTH) analogues. Collectively, these agents have established efficacy that is supported in the literature. Denosumab has been shown to reduce the risk of vertebral fracture by 70%, hip fractures by 40%–50%, and nonvertebral fractures by 20%–30% (1), while PTH analogues reduce the risk of vertebral fractures by 60%–65% (2).

However, there are limitations to the current treatment regimen. Bisphosphonates require inconvenient and complex dosing regimens that result in poor compliance. Many PTH drugs require daily injections that many patients find objectionable. It has been shown that more than 50% of patients discontinue their treatment plan within 12 months of initial osteoporosis therapy (3). Long-term treatment with these drugs causes concerns over patient safety. Because of these major issues, there is an urgent need for new therapies that reduce the risk of nonvertebral fractures, have reliable safety profiles, and can be conveniently dosed.

This chapter gives an overview of raloxifene, which belongs to the class of selective estrogen receptor modulators (SERMs), as well as the emerging osteoporotic drugs romosozumab, which is an inhibitor of sclerostin, and abaloparatide, which belongs to the PTH-related peptide class of drugs (Table 9.1).

RALOXIFENE

Raloxifene is a benzothiophene nonsteroidal derivative that binds to estrogen receptors. It is a second-generation SERM that acts as an estrogen receptor agonist or antagonist depending on the target tissue. The ideal SERM acts as estrogen receptor agonist by exerting a protective effect on bone, while maintaining breast and uterine safety via its estrogen receptor antagonist activity (4). Raloxifene was initially approved by the U.S. Food and Drug Administration for the treatment and prevention of osteoporosis in postmenopausal women. In 2007, the indications were extended to reduce invasive breast cancer risk in postmenopausal women with osteoporosis (5). Raloxifene is currently the only drug in its class that is approved for long-term treatment in the prevention of fragility fractures.

Mechanism of action

Raloxifene exerts its action as either an estrogen agonist or antagonist depending on the specific tissue that it targets. There are two primary isoforms of estrogen receptors: estrogen receptor alpha (ERα), which is primarily an activating receptor, and estrogen receptor beta (ERβ), which is primarily an inhibiting receptor (6). ERβ exerts its inhibitory action on ERα by forming a heterodimer. Thus, the levels of expression that are unique to a particular tissue type have different levels of isoforms that will direct cellular responsiveness to estrogens. In general, raloxifene functions as an estrogen agonist in bone and lipid metabolism and functions as an estrogen antagonist in breast and uterine tissue.

The estradiol and estrogen receptor interaction induces a cellular cascade that ends with interaction with the estrogen-responding element in DNA. Estrogen receptors do not have a single binding site, rather they have two domains: one domain for estrogen-type ligands and another domain for antiestrogen-type ligands such as SERM (5).

Table 9.1 Summary of the effects of osteoporotic drugs observed in clinical trials on bone mineral density (BMD) and fracture risk reduction

Drug	Drug class	Mechanism of action	Mode of delivery	Study phase	Pivotal trials	Increase in BMD	Fracture risk reduction
Raloxifene	SERM	Binds to estrogen receptor α and β –> estrogen agonist in bone, estrogen antagonist in breast and uterine tissue	Oral	Launched	(15–17)	LS 4.3%[a] FN 1.9%[a]	Vertebral fractures 39%[b]
Romosozumab	Anabolic	Sclerostin monoclonal antibody that affects the Wnt/β-catenin pathway	SC or IM injection	III	(26,30,31,42,43)	LS 11.3%[c] TH 4.1%[c]	N/A
Abaloparatide	Anabolic	Synthetic PTH analog –> intermittent activation of PTH type I receptor	SC injection	III	(38–40)	LS 6.7%[d] TH 2.6%[d]	Major osteoporotic 67%[e]

Abbreviations: FN, femoral neck; IM, intramuscular; LS, lumbar spine; SC, subcutaneous; SERM, selective estrogen receptor modulator; TH, total hip.

[a] Raloxifene 60 mg/day for 7 years (16).

[b] Raloxifene 60 mg/day for 4 years (15).

[c] Romosozumab 210 mg monthly for 12 months (31).

[d] Abaloparatide 80 μg daily for 24 weeks (38).

[e] Abaloparatide 80 μg daily for 18 months (40).

The differential pharmacologic effects of SERMs are due to the three primary mechanisms: differential expression of estrogen receptors depending on the target tissue, differential conformation of the estrogen receptor itself, and differential estrogen receptor binding to coregulator proteins, of which more than 20 have been previously described (7). Coregulator proteins primarily function as activating or repressing transcriptional regulators that modulate receptor activity. The action of SERMs is related to the ligand binding domain of the estrogen receptor; the presence of coactivating or corepressing interaction on the receptor surface determines whether the estrogen receptor ultimately activates the DNA estrogen-responding element or promotes proteasomal release (8). Over the past 10 years, there has been an expansion in the number of coregulator families of estrogen receptors being defined. The intracellular mechanisms are also likely to be influenced by other tissue-related proteins that alter gene transcription and translation through phosphorylation. Although the mechanism of SERMs on bone, breast, and endometrial tissue has been described, many of the exact subcellular processes are still being evaluated (8).

EFFECTS ON BONE

On bone tissue specifically, raloxifene binds to estrogen receptors and induces an activating response, analogous to the response of estrogens. There are two simultaneous actions that are downstream from the SERM-estrogen-receptor interaction: osteoclast activity inhibition and osteoblast activity induction (9). Osteoclast activity inhibition is mediated by raloxifene's effect on interleukin-6

(IL-6) and tumor necrosis factor α (TNF-α) levels in the osseous microenvironment, which mirrors the action that is seen with estrogen replacement therapy in postmenopausal women. Other cytokines that are modulated by the estronergic effect include IL-1β, RANK, RANKL, and osteoprotegerin. Osteoprotegerin, which is an inhibitor of bone resorption, suppresses osteoclast activity and also suppresses the production of the bone-resorbing cytokine IL-6. Osteoclasts respond with a faster rate of apoptosis and slower differentiation rate partly induced by the higher rates of osteoblast maturation and differentiation that result from the osteoprotegerin/RANK/RANKL system. Consequentially, there is a reduction of bone resorption and an increase in bone mineral density (10).

EFFECTS ON OTHER TISSUES

Unlike its effects on bone, raloxifene exerts an estrogen antagonist effect in breast tissue by blocking coactivator binding. Not only does this block the transcription of the estrogen receptor regulated gene, it may also exert additional effects on estrogen bioavailability, estrogen-induced collagen synthesis, or effects on insulin-like growth factors (IGFs). Because of these interactions, raloxifene has been shown to inhibit breast cancer cell growth via two mechanisms: by reducing human telomerase reverse transcriptase expression (Htert) and reducing vascular endothelial growth factor expression in estrogen receptor positive breast carcinomas. Estrogen receptor negative breast carcinomas are also affected by raloxifene due to the SERM's downregulation of glutathione and induction of apoptosis in breast cells.

There is evidence that raloxifene increases the risk of thromboembolic events in postmenopausal women. Recent studies have shown that raloxifene therapy increases the activities of factors VIII, XI, and XII, as well as significantly reduces the APC sensitivity ratio (11). This results in significant increases in prothrombin fragments 1 and 2 and significant decreases in the activities of antithrombin and protein C with continued raloxifene administration. Data demonstrate that raloxifene therapy results in a procoagulant state (5).

Clinical efficacy

Numerous studies have shown that raloxifene is a safe and effective medication to be used in the treatment of osteoporosis (12,13). Phase I studies show that raloxifene is a safe drug to take at doses up to 200–600 mg per day. Phase II studies show that raloxifene is as effective as estrogen for short-term suppression of bone turnover, significantly lowers low-density lipoprotein (LDL) and total serum cholesterol, and increases high-density lipoprotein (HDL) cholesterol without effects on the uterus (14).

Measurement of bone mineral density is the most common test used to diagnose and monitor osteoporosis and response to treatment. Johnston et al. (13) conducted a prospective trial on 1145 healthy postmenopausal women 45–60 years of age to randomly receive daily raloxifene versus placebo. Bone mineral density was measured and increased from baseline 36 months in the raloxifene group in a dose-dependent manner.

The often-cited MORE (Multiple Outcomes of Raloxifene Evaluation) trial examined 7705 postmenopausal women with osteoporosis and randomized patients to placebo ver1sus raloxifene 60 or 120 mg/day. Patients were from 25 countries and had been postmenopausal for at least 2 years and had osteoporosis. Over the course of 4 years, cumulative relative risks (RRs) for one or more new vertebral fractures were 0.64 with raloxifene 60 mg/day and 0.57 for raloxifene 120 mg/day. There was a 50% fracture risk reduction in the treatment arm, with the reduction slightly higher in patients receiving 120 mg per day. The study also demonstrated a significant reduction in ankle fractures. The data confirmed that raloxifene was efficacious in reducing the risk for fragility fractures in postmenopausal women with osteoporosis (15). All types of breast cancer were reduced with raloxifene by 62%. Estrogen receptor positive breast cancer incidence was decreased with raloxifene but had no effect on estrogen receptor negative breast cancers.

The CORE (Continuing Outcomes Relevant to Evista) study was a multicenter, double-blind, placebo-controlled clinical trial that investigated the incidence of invasive breast cancer in the same women enrolled in the MORE trial. After examining 4011 women with a mean age of 65.8 years, it was determined that after 7 years of raloxifene therapy, lumbar spine and femoral neck bone mineral density significantly increased 4.3% and 1.9%, respectively.

Patients in the trial experienced a 50% reduction in the raloxifene group in the overall incidence of breast cancer (16).

The RUTH (Raloxifene Use for the Heart) trial was a multicenter, double-blind, randomized, placebo-controlled trial assessing the effect of raloxifene on cardiovascular events. The trial examined 10,101 postmenopausal women with a mean age of 67.5 years with a mean treatment duration of 5.6 years and concluded that raloxifene has a hazard ratio of 0.65 and risk reduction of 0.13% for the risk of developing vertebral fractures (17). This study also demonstrated a 44% high incidence of venous thromboembolic events, with a 1.2 per 1000 woman-years absolute risk increase for the raloxifene group versus the placebo group (17).

Safety profile

The MORE (14) and CORE (12) studies demonstrated significant increased incidences of deep venous thrombosis (DVT) and pulmonary embolism (PE) for patients in the raloxifene group. The greatest risk for DVT and PE occurred in the initial 4 months of treatment. Increases in the absolute risk of venous thromboembolism (VTE) in the raloxifene group was 1.8 per 100 persons in the MORE trial and 1.2 per 100 persons in the RUTH study. Due to raloxifene's accelerating effect on blood coagulation and reduction in anticoagulation, raloxifene is contraindicated in women with a complication or history of VTE, as well as in patients who are considered high risk, such as long-term immobile patients and patients with hypercoagulation disorders.

The RUTH trial (17) showed that raloxifene did not significantly affect the risk of coronary artery disease. However, while there was no difference in the incidence of stroke in the raloxifene group, the incidence of specifically fatal stroke was 2.2/1000 person-years in the raloxifene group versus 1.5/1000 person-years in the placebo group.

The most frequently reported adverse events for patients taking raloxifene are reported to be peripheral edema (0.65%) and VTE (0.16%). The vasomotor instability syndrome, also known as "hot flashes," has been associated with raloxifene use. This entity can be characterized by peripheral vasodilation with cutaneous flushing, sweating, chills, anxiety, and rapid heart rate. While raloxifene slightly increases the incidence of hot flashes relative to placebo (28% versus 21%) (18), it does not alter its natural history and does not affect the total duration of symptoms until symptom resolution (19).

ROMOSOZUMAB

Romosozumab is a humanized monoclonal antibody to sclerostin. Sclerostin is an inhibitor of the Wnt signaling pathway that modulates its bone anabolic effects. Romosozumab allows the Wnt signaling pathway to function without the inhibition of sclerostin, thus promoting osteoanabolic effects. The drug is currently undergoing phase III clinical trials for the treatment of osteoporosis and is primarily used in the subcutaneous injection form (20). Similar to PTH and PTH-related peptides, romosozumab is classified as an anabolic agent. The discovery of the Wnt signaling pathway in bone metabolism and studies of disorders of high bone mass in which sclerostin is not usually expressed, namely sclerosteosis and van Buchem disease, identified the Wnt pathway inhibitor sclerostin as a new pharmacologic target in the treatment of osteoporosis.

Mechanism of action

Sclerostin, produced primarily by osteocytes, is a monomeric glycoprotein that is a product of the SOST gene. SOST mRNA expression has been shown in bone marrow, cartilage, kidney, heart, and pancreatic tissue. The antagonist effects of sclerostin on the Wnt signaling pathway have been well established (21). The Wnt/β-catenin pathway has major effects on osteoblast differentiation and proliferation. Activation of the pathway involves binding of the Wnt ligand to LDL receptor-related proteins 5 and 6 (LRP5/LRP6 complex), which results in the inactivation of GSK-3β, which functions to target β-catenin. β-Catenin accumulates in the cytoplasm and is translocated into the nucleus where it upregulates the transcription of numerous target genes that stimulate differentiation of mesenchymal stem cells in the skeletal cells, which includes differentiation of osteoblasts and chondrocytes (22). Sclerostin inhibits the activity of the LRP5/LRP6 complex, preventing the binding of Wnt and stopping the Wnt/β-catenin signaling, thus inhibiting the osteoblast proliferation and differentiation.

SCLEROSTIN DEFICIENCY

Two well-studied rare autosomal recessive sclerosing bone disorders that are characterized by abnormally high bone mass are sclerosteosis and van Buchem disease. Both diseases have the common etiology of deficient SOST gene function, which leads to impaired synthesis of the secreted glycoprotein sclerostin. Sclerostin has two primary functions that ultimately lead to catabolic effects in bone: it binds to the first propeller of LRP5/6 receptor and directly antagonizes the Wnt/β-catenin pathway in osteoblasts, and also acts on neighboring osteocytes to increase the RANKL expression and the RANKL/osteoprotegerin ratio, thus stimulating osteoclastic bone resorption (23). As a result, patients with sclerostin deficiency have thickened skulls, facial and jawbone enlargement, mandibular prognathism, and frontal bone prominence (24).

Targeted deletion of the SOST gene in mice significantly increased bone mineral density as well as thickness of the distal femur and cortical area of the femoral shaft. Compared with wild-type mice, the surface mineralization rate, mineral appositional rate, and bone formation rate increased by 249%, 143%, and 396%, respectively (25). Because sclerostin-deficient humans and animals lacked

complications in organs other than the skeleton, sclerostin became an attractive target for the development of a new anabolic agent.

PRECLINICAL STUDIES

There were several important preclinical studies to investigate the effect of sclerostin inhibition on bone metabolism. In a study by Li et al. (26), sclerostin antibodies were given subcutaneously twice per week for 5 weeks in a rodent model of osteoporosis. The 5-week treatment resulted in significant increase in bone mineral density and skeletal strength. The treatment reversed the bone loss associated with the osteoporotic rodent model and restored the bone mass to levels greater than sham-operated control animals. The histological results showed increased bone formation, increased cortical thickness, and decreased central porosity. This effect was reversible with discontinuation of the treatment.

A study done in cynomolgus monkeys who were exposed to once-monthly subcutaneous sclerostin antibody injections demonstrated dose-dependent increases in bone formation, cortical thickness, and bone mineral density. Biomechanical studies showed significantly increased strength of the vertebrae in the animals treated with two injections of the antibody compared to control animals. The study showed even short-term exposure of animals to sclerostin antibody resulted in dramatic improvements in bone mass and strength (27).

To further characterize the mechanism of sclerostin antibodies, a study examined bone biopsies in a rodent model of osteoporosis and male cynomolgus monkeys after treatment with antibody for 5 and 10 weeks, respectively. The results demonstrated that the new bone formation occurred even at quiescent surfaces. The treatment increased the rate of activation of bone modeling and extended the formation period of existing remodeling sites (28). These data support the targeting of sclerostin as agents that stimulate bone formation.

Clinical efficacy

There are currently three human monoclonal sclerostin inhibitors in the public domain: romosozumab (Amgen and UCB), blosozumab (Elli Lilly), and BPS804 (Norvartis) (29).

The first human trial included 72 healthy men and postmenopausal women who were given once-monthly romosozumab injections or placebo. Results showed that with a high dose (10 mg/kg subcutaneous), bone formation markers of procollagen type 1 N-terminal propeptide (P1NP), bone alkaline phosphatase (BAP), and osteocalcin reached levels of 184%, 126%, and 176% above baseline after 30 days. The bone resorption marker carboxy-terminal collagen cross-links (CTX) decreased by 54% at 14 days. These same values returned to baseline 2 months after injection. The bone mineral density of the lumbar spine and hip significantly increased by 5.3% and 2.8%, respectively, on day 85 (30). Computed tomography (CT) analysis of a subset of these patients revealed improvement in trabecular and cortical bone mass as well increased whole bone stiffness. The benefits were maintained for 3 months following the last dose of romosozumab.

A phase II study to assess the safety and tolerability of romosozumab was conducted in 419 postmenopausal women who were aged 55–85 years and had bone mineral density T-scores between −2.0 and greater than −3.5 (31). Different doses and dosing intervals were compared with placebo, oral alendronate 70 mg weekly, and subcutaneous teriparatide 20 μg daily. Placebo versus romosozumab injections were randomly assigned at a frequency of once-monthly or once every 3 months, with the primary endpoint being spine bone marrow density measurement after 12 months of therapy. After 383 participants completed the protocol, the study demonstrated that all doses of romosozumab induced significant increases in bone mineral density. The highest dose of romosozumab, 210 mg once-monthly, increased bone mineral density of the spine, hip, and femoral neck by 11.3%, 4.1%, and 3.7%, respectively, after 1 year. More importantly, the increases in bone mineral density were greater than that with either alendronate or teriparatide.

Continuation of romosozumab treatment of 210 mg once-monthly for a second year further increased spine and hip bone mineral density to 15.2% and 5.5%, respectively. During the second year of treatment, serum levels of P1NP and CTX remained below baseline, indicating continuous and stable decrease in bone turnover with prolonged romosozumab treatment. For patients who discontinued treatment, serum P1NP and CTX gradually returned to baseline values (29). These studies indicated that romosozumab has a significant antiresorptive effect that is exerted by a RANKL-dependent mechanism.

The results of the preclinical and early clinical studies are promising. The efficacy of these agents to reduce fracture risk and long-term tolerability will be assessed in the ongoing phase III clinical study being performed with romosozumab. It is currently unknown whether long-term treatment will yield a sustained anabolic effect. The safety profile of the drug has yet to be completely elucidated, including a phase I study of patients with chronic kidney disease.

ABALOPARATIDE

Abaloparatide (PTHrP[1–34]) is a 34 amino acid synthetic analog of PTH-related peptide (PTHrP). PTH is the primary hormone that maintains calcium and phosphate homeostasis. The effect of PTH heavily depends on the pattern of PTH release: chronically elevated PTH levels, as seen with hyperparathyroidism, exert a dramatic catabolic effect on bone metabolism. Intermittent PTH administration increases bone mass and exerts an anabolic effect on bone. However, the anabolic effect of PTH analogs is followed by an increase in bone resorption due to the coupling effect,

which limits the overall increase in bone mass that can be achieved with this therapy (32). Uncoupling of bone formation with resorption would maximize the anabolic effect that can be achieved with PTH and PTHrP.

Mechanism of action

PTH primarily targets bone and kidney. Cellular activity requires the binding of PTH/PTHrP type 1 receptor (PTH1R), which is found on the surface of osteoblasts and stromal cells of bone and apical membranes of renal tubules (33). When PTH binds to PTH1R, multiple signaling pathways are activated, the most important of which is the receptor-mediated activation of Gs protein α subunit. This results in the production of cyclic AMP, activation of phospholipase C, and activation of protein kinase A (PKA). The PKA pathway is responsible for the catabolic and anabolic effects of PTH and its related compounds. The expression of RANKL on bone cells is induced by the PKA pathway via PTH.

Monocyte chemoattractant protein-1 (MCP-1) and IL-18 are both regulated by PTH and exert their effects through the PKA pathway. However, the two cytokines serve opposite functions: MCP-1 promotes osteoclastogenesis, while IL-18 inhibits osteoclast formation. Thus, PTH can regulate bone metabolism through the specific cytokines that are upregulated; anabolic pathways are initiated from transient cytokine regulation, while catabolic pathways result from constant expression and continuous activation of osteoclasts (34).

Furthermore, it has been reported that PTH1R activation can directly modulate the Wnt signaling pathway. β-Catenin can be modulated by LRP6 or Disheveled protein, which are downstream components of the Wnt pathway. It was recently demonstrated that phosphorylation of β-catenin by PKA may lead to divergent outcomes in gene expression, which include both promotion and inhibition of osteoclastogenesis, depending on the cytokine environment (35). Intermittent PTH administration causes phosphorylation of LRP6, stabilizing β-catenin, which leads to anabolic pathways, while continuous PTH exposure did not have these downstream effects (36). Thus, via multiple signaling cascade systems, the microenvironment surrounding the PTH/PTHrP receptor interaction can ultimately lead to competing pathways in bone metabolism.

PRECLINICAL STUDIES

In ovariectomized (OVX) rat models of osteoporosis, subcutaneous injection of PTHrP (1–34) was given daily to study the effects of bone mineral density, bone histomorphometrics, and biomechanical parameters. The results showed increased lumbar and femoral bone mineral density following peptide administration. There was also significantly improved bone biomechanical properties, enhanced bone strength, and increased bone formation. The study concluded that once daily or every other day injection of PTHrP (1–34) significantly improved bone strength and bone mineral density of the rats without a significant change in serum calcium and phosphate levels in treated rats (37).

Clinical efficacy

Abaloparatide has similar or even greater potency relative to PTHrP. It has demonstrated promising results in preclinical studies while exerting a limited hypercalcemic effect (37). Currently, it is given as a daily injection, which acts on the type 1 PTH receptor to stimulate bone formation. Studies have demonstrated good clinical tolerance and marked bone formation with dissociation of resorption markers at doses up to 80 μg per day, over a 7-day exposure period (35). There are several key clinical studies that demonstrate good clinical efficacy of abaloparatide.

A phase II clinical trial has shown promising effects of abaloparatide on bone mineral density of the lumbar spine, hip, and femoral neck in postmenopausal women with osteoporosis. Designed as a multicenter, multinational, double-blind, placebo-controlled trial, 222 women were randomly assigned to receive 24 weeks of treatment with daily subcutaneous injections of placebo, abaloparatide, or teriparatide. At the end of the 24-week period, bone mineral density increased by 2.9%, 5.2%, and 6.7% in the abaloparatide 20, 40, and 80 μg groups, respectively. The teriparatide group yielded a 5.5% increase in lumbar spine bone mineral density. Femoral neck and hip bone mineral density improved by 3.1% and 2.6% with abaloparatide 80 μg. The study demonstrated that abaloparatide not only significantly improved bone mineral density of the hip and spine in a dose-dependent fashion but did so at a greater efficacy than the currently marketed dose of teriparatide (38).

The ACTIVE (Abaloparatide Comparator Trial in Vertebral Endpoints) trial was a phase III double-blinded, randomized controlled trial conducted in 10 different countries (39). To assess the prevention of fracture in postmenopausal women, 2463 women were randomized to abaloparatide 80 μg daily, teriparatide 20 μg daily, or placebo for 18 months. Abaloparatide and teriparatide both reduced the risk of major osteoporotic fractures by 67% and 30%, respectively. The effect of abaloparatide was significantly improved from placebo, but treatment with teriparatide was not significantly different (40). The risk of wrist fracture was 1.2% in the placebo group and 0.5% in the abaloparatide group. The teriparatide group was significantly higher at 1.8% risk (41). The incidence of hypercalcemia was lower with abaloparatide (3.4%) versus teriparatide (6.4%) ($P = 0.006$). The ACTIVE trial concluded that the use of subcutaneous abaloparatide significantly reduced the risk of new vertebral and nonvertebral fractures over the 18-month course of administration.

Early studies have shown significant improvement in bone marrow density that is a result of the anabolic activity of abaloparatide. Furthermore, results seem to show superior efficacy of abaloparatide over teriparatide. This new anabolic option is promising, and numerous studies are currently being conducted to identify the exact indications and safety profile of this anabolic agent.

CONCLUSION

There are a wide variety of drug classes that are used to treat osteoporosis and prevent fragility fractures. Some classes of drugs, such as SERMs, although clinically established, are still being rigorously studied to improve their efficacy and safety profile. Although there are several effective modalities and drug classes for the treatment of osteoporosis, continuous efforts are being made to develop sophisticated, convenient agents that increase clinical efficacy while minimizing the risk of adverse events. Progress in this emerging field of medicine is rapid, particularly at the speed to which novel targets become effective pharmacologic agents. Among the most promising new agents, the sclerostin inhibitor romosozumab and the PTHrP analog abaloparatide are the nearest to becoming available for clinical use. The challenge will be to most appropriately use these new medications to effectively treat osteoporotic patients.

REFERENCES

1. Black DM, Delmas PD, Eastell R et al. Once-yearly zoledronic acid for treatment of postmenopausal osteoporosis. *N Engl J Med*. 2007;356(18):1809–22.
2. Neer RM, Arnaud CD, Zanchetta JR et al. Effect of parathyroid hormone (1-34) on fractures and bone mineral density in postmenopausal women with osteoporosis. *N Engl J Med*. 2001;344(19):1434–41.
3. McClung MR. Emerging therapies for osteoporosis. *Endocrinol Metab*. 2015;30(4):429–35.
4. D'Amelio P, Isaia GC. The use of raloxifene in osteoporosis treatment. *Expert Opin Pharmacother*. 2013;14(7):949–56.
5. Gizzo S, Saccardi C, Patrelli TS et al. Update on raloxifene: Mechanism of action, clinical efficacy, adverse effects, and contraindications. *Obstet Gynecol Surv*. 2013;68(6):467–81.
6. Rey JR, Cervino EV, Rentero ML, Crespo EC, Alvaro AO, Casillas M. Raloxifene: Mechanism of action, effects on bone tissue, and applicability in clinical traumatology practice. *Open Orthop J*. 2009;3:14–21.
7. Riggs BL, Hartmann LC. Selective estrogen-receptor modulators—Mechanisms of action and application to clinical practice. *N Engl J Med*. 2003;348(7):618–29.
8. Jordan VC. Selective estrogen receptor modulation: Concept and consequences in cancer. *Cancer Cell*. 2004;5(3):207–13.
9. Taranta A, Brama M, Teti A et al. The selective estrogen receptor modulator raloxifene regulates osteoclast and osteoblast activity *in vitro*. *Bone*. 2002;30(2):368–76.

10. Messalli EM, Mainini G, Scaffa C et al. Raloxifene therapy interacts with serum osteoprotegerin in post-menopausal women. *Maturitas*. 2007;56(1):38–44.

11. Azevedo GD, Franco RF, Baggio MS, Maranhao TM, Sa MF. Procoagulant state after raloxifene therapy in postmenopausal women. *Fertil Steril*. 2005;84(6):1680–4.

12. Martino S, Cauley JA, Barrett-Connor E et al. Continuing outcomes relevant to Evista: Breast cancer incidence in postmenopausal osteoporotic women in a randomized trial of raloxifene. *J Natl Cancer Inst*. 2004;96(23):1751–61.

13. Johnston CC, Jr., Bjarnason NH, Cohen FJ et al. Long-term effects of raloxifene on bone mineral density, bone turnover, and serum lipid levels in early postmenopausal women: Three-year data from 2 double-blind, randomized, placebo-controlled trials. *Arch Intern Med*. 2000;160(22):3444–50.

14. Ettinger B, Black DM, Mitlak BH et al. Reduction of vertebral fracture risk in postmenopausal women with osteoporosis treated with raloxifene: Results from a 3-year randomized clinical trial. Multiple Outcomes of Raloxifene Evaluation (MORE) Investigators. *JAMA*. 1999;282(7):637–45.

15. Delmas PD, Ensrud KE, Adachi JD et al. Efficacy of raloxifene on vertebral fracture risk reduction in postmenopausal women with osteoporosis: Four-year results from a randomized clinical trial. *J Clin Endocrinol Metab*. 2002;87(8):3609–17.

16. Siris ES, Harris ST, Eastell R et al. Skeletal effects of raloxifene after 8 years: Results from the continuing outcomes relevant to Evista (CORE) study. *J Bone Miner Res*. 2005;20(9):1514–24.

17. Barrett-Connor E, Mosca L, Collins P et al. Effects of raloxifene on cardiovascular events and breast cancer in postmenopausal women. *N Engl J Med*. 2006;355(2):125–37.

18. Cohen FJ, Lu Y. Characterization of hot flashes reported by healthy postmenopausal women receiving raloxifene or placebo during osteoporosis prevention trials. *Maturitas*. 2000;34(1):65–73.

19. Goldstein SR, Duvernoy CS, Calaf J et al. Raloxifene use in clinical practice: Efficacy and safety. *Menopause*. 2009;16(2):413–21.

20. Costa AG, Bilezikian JP, Lewiecki EM. Update on romosozumab: A humanized monoclonal antibody to sclerostin. *Expert Opin Biol Ther*. 2014;14(5):697–707.

21. Krause C, Korchynskyi O, de Rooij K et al. Distinct modes of inhibition by sclerostin on bone morphogenetic protein and Wnt signaling pathways. *J Biol Chem*. 2010;285(53):41614–26.

22. Krishnan V, Bryant HU, Macdougald OA. Regulation of bone mass by Wnt signaling. *J Clin Invest*. 2006;116(5):1202–9.

23. Tu X, Delgado-Calle J, Condon KW et al. Osteocytes mediate the anabolic actions of canonical Wnt/β-catenin signaling in bone. *Proc Natl Acad Sci USA*. 2015;112(5):E478–86.

24. Beighton P, Barnard A, Hamersma H, van der Wouden A. The syndromic status of sclerosteosis and van Buchem disease. *Clin Genet*. 1984;25(2):175–81.

25. Li X, Ominsky MS, Niu QT et al. Targeted deletion of the sclerostin gene in mice results in increased bone formation and bone strength. *J Bone Miner Res*. 2008;23(6):860–9.

26. Li X, Ominsky MS, Warmington KS et al. Sclerostin antibody treatment increases bone formation, bone mass, and bone strength in a rat model of postmenopausal osteoporosis. *J Bone Miner Res*. 2009;24(4):578–88.

27. Ominsky MS, Vlasseros F, Jolette J et al. Two doses of sclerostin antibody in cynomolgus monkeys increases bone formation, bone mineral density, and bone strength. *J Bone Miner Res*. 2010;25(5):948–59.

28. Ominsky MS, Niu QT, Li C, Li X, Ke HZ. Tissue-level mechanisms responsible for the increase in bone formation and bone volume by sclerostin antibody. *J Bone Miner Res*. 2014;29(6):1424–30.

29. Appelman-Dijkstra NM, Papapoulos SE. Sclerostin inhibition in the management of osteoporosis. *Calcif Tissue Int*. 2016;98(4):370–80.

30. Padhi D, Jang G, Stouch B, Fang L, Posvar E. Single-dose, placebo-controlled, randomized study of AMG 785, a sclerostin monoclonal antibody. *J Bone Miner Res*. 2011;26(1):19–26.

31. McClung MR, Grauer A, Boonen S et al. Romosozumab in postmenopausal women with low bone mineral density. *N Engl J Med*. 2014;370(5):412–20.

32. McClung MR, San Martin J, Miller PD et al. Opposite bone remodeling effects of teriparatide and alendronate in increasing bone mass. *Arch Intern Med*. 2005;165(15):1762–8.

33. Lee K, Brown D, Urena P et al. Localization of parathyroid hormone/parathyroid hormone-related peptide receptor mRNA in kidney. *Am J Physiol*. 1996;270(1 Pt 2):F186–91.

34. Lee M, Partridge NC. Parathyroid hormone signaling in bone and kidney. *Curr Opin Nephrol Hypertens*. 2009;18(4):298–302.

35. Polyzos SA, Makras P, Efstathiadou Z, Anastasilakis AD. Investigational parathyroid hormone receptor analogs for the treatment of osteoporosis. *Expert Opin Investig Drugs*. 2015;24(2):145–57.

36. Taurin S, Sandbo N, Qin Y, Browning D, Dulin NO. Phosphorylation of β-catenin by cyclic AMP-dependent protein kinase. *J Biol Chem*. 2006;281(15):9971–6.

37. Xu J, Rong H, Ji H et al. Effects of different dosages of parathyroid hormone-related protein 1-34 on the bone metabolism of the ovariectomized rat model of osteoporosis. *Calcif Tissue Int*. 2013;93(3):276–87.

38. Leder BZ, O'Dea LS, Zanchetta JR et al. Effects of abaloparatide, a human parathyroid hormone-related peptide analog, on bone mineral density in postmenopausal women with osteoporosis. *J Clin Endocrinol Metab*. 2015;100(2):697–706.

39. Miller PD, Hattersley G, Riis BJ et al. Effect of abaloparatide versus placebo on new vertebral fractures in postmenopausal women with osteoporosis: A randomized clinical trial. *JAMA*. 2016;316(7):722–33.

40. Cosman F, Hattersley G, Hu MY, Williams GC, Fitzpatrick LA, Black DM. Effects of abaloparatide-SC on fractures and bone mineral density in subgroups of postmenopausal women with osteoporosis and varying baseline risk factors. *J Bone Miner Res*. 2017;32(1):17–23.

41. Harslof T, Langdahl BL. New horizons in osteoporosis therapies. *Curr Opin Pharmacol*. 2016;28:38–42.

42. Padhi D, Allison M, Kivitz AJ et al. Multiple doses of sclerostin antibody romosozumab in healthy men and postmenopausal women with low bone mass: A randomized, double-blind, placebo-controlled study. *J Clin Pharmacol*. 2014;54(2):168–78.

43. McColm J, Hu L, Womack T, Tang CC, Chiang AY. Single- and multiple-dose randomized studies of blosozumab, a monoclonal antibody against sclerostin, in healthy postmenopausal women. *J Bone Miner Res*. 2014;29(4):935–43.

10

Monitoring/surveillance of medical treatment

KONSTANTINOS D. STATHOPOULOS and ANDREAS F. MAVROGENIS

INTRODUCTION

Osteoporosis constitutes a major public health problem worldwide, as it is associated with significant morbidity, mortality, and costs resulting from fractures of the central and peripheral skeleton. In 2006, all osteoporotic fractures accounted for 2.7 million in men and women in Europe at a direct cost of €36 billion (39.6 billion US dollars) (1); a 2010 estimate elevated these costs to €38.7 or $42.57 billion in 27 European countries (2,3). In the United States, osteoporotic fractures account for more than 432,000 hospital admissions, almost 2.5 million medical office visits, and about 180,000 nursing home admissions annually; the respective estimated cost to the U.S. health-care system for 2005 was $17 billion (4). To cope with the significant burden of this disease, it is important that clinicians identify those patients who are at a higher risk for fracture and treat them appropriately. Treatment consists of modification of personal habits such as smoking andl alcohol consumption, increased physical activity with specific exercise programs to preserve or increase muscle strength, implementation of strategies to reduce falls in the elderly, proper nutrition with regard to protein as well as calcium and vitamin D intake, and pharmacologic agents including per os or intravenous bisphosphonates, selective estrogen receptor modulators (SERMs), receptor activator of nuclear factor–κB ligand RANKL inhibitor denosumab, 1–34 PTH analogue teriparatide hormone replacement therap and strontium ranelate (3,4). Newer FDA approved agents for the pharmacological treatment of postmenopausal osteoporosis include PTHrP analogue abaloparatide, and sclerostin antibody romosozumab.

Since the clinical significance of osteoporosis lies in the fractures that arise and clinicians are advised to treat patients with a high risk of fracture (3,4), it would seem that the ideal method of monitoring drug therapy with regard to efficacy would be to compare the individual's pretreatment fracture risk with the fracture risk after one or more years of pharmacological therapy and then decide whether therapy with that specific agent was successful, and if it should be continued or not. However, as recently shown in the study of Wang, Bolland, and Grey (5), even when numerous clinical guideline recommendations (developed either by professional societies, government organizations, or other sources) are considered, only 3% of them recommend estimation of fracture risk for monitoring of drug therapy. There are probably numerous etiologies that could explain this finding, perhaps the most obvious being that there is no single technique available to actually measure the fracture risk of an individual. Even when specific fracture risk calculators (algorithms) are considered, such as FRAX, which is a widely available and easy to use validated tool for the estimation of the 10-year probability of fracture of an individual, they can only be used to estimate fracture risk before the commencement of therapy and are not approved for the monitoring of therapy. When failure of therapy is considered, there also seems to be agreement among clinicians and researchers that the occurrence of a single fragility fracture in a patient receiving pharmacologic therapy does not necessarily demonstrate that the treatment has failed (6). This notion is supported by clinical findings demonstrating that pharmacologic agents reduce osteoporotic fracture rates by 30%–70% but not 100%, meaning that even when patients use potent drugs, fractures still occur under therapy, and fracture risk is not eliminated. As a consequence, most authors suggest that monitoring of therapy should target the pre- and posttreatment evaluation of parameters of bone strength that are usually easily accessible in the clinical setting. It has been suggested that the best available of these parameters is the bone mineral density (BMD) as measured by dual-energy x-ray absorptiometry (DEXA) (2–5,7). To assess response to treatment, some authors also recommend the use of bone turnover markers (BTMs) (2–5,7). It is our understanding that both of these approaches are helpful, since BMD can be considered a surrogate of bone strength, while BTMs can signal an individual's response to therapy; however, we believe that monitoring of therapy should incorporate more information that would capture more elements of fracture risk. This chapter reviews these two approaches to monitor the efficacy of osteoporosis therapy

Table 10.1 Methods and their validation for the monitoring of osteoporosis

Methods	Validation
Dual-energy x-ray absorptiometry	+
Bone turnover markers	+/−
Quantitative computed tomography (FEMUR)	+
FRAX	−
Peripheral quantitative computed tomography	−
Quantitative ultrasound	−

of an individual in the clinical setting and provide some insight into other techniques or strategies that might be useful in achieving this goal (Table 10.1).

MONITORING BONE MINERAL DENSITY (DUAL-ENERGY X-RAY ABSORPTIOMETRY)

BMD as a surrogate of bone strength

Osteoporosis was defined in the 1990s as a disease characterized by low bone mass and deterioration of bone micro-architecture, leading to enhanced bone fragility and increased fracture risk (8,9). To give a more complete definition, a National Institutes of Health Consensus Conference in 2000 further described osteoporosis as a skeletal disorder characterized by compromised bone strength predisposing to an increased risk for fracture (10,11). The term *bone strength* is a key element in our understanding of what osteoporosis really signifies. From a biomechanical perspective, bone strength is defined as a bone's maximal resistance to loading (12). To determine whether a bone will fail under loading, one should consider the loads or forces applied to the bone and its structural strength or resistance to these loads. Since it is impossible to measure in real time the forces generated during a traumatic event in an individual, it is important to recognize that the ultimate strength of a bone in vivo can only be assessed indirectly. Moreover, during the last 15 years, we have come to appreciate that bone strength relies not only on the quantity of bone—estimated by measuring bone mineral mass and/or "density"—but also on another set of properties, usually referred to as "bone quality" (12–14). These properties include bone geometry, macro- and microarchitectural elements of both types of bone tissue that comprise all of our bones (i.e., trabecular and cortical), as well as the material properties of bone tissue itself including its organic (mostly collagen) and inorganic (hydroxyapatite) components, and also on the levels of tissue damage accumulation and repair (13,14). Finally, in effect, both mass and structure depend essentially on bone turnover (12–14). Bone mineral mass can be assessed *in vivo* with the use of quantitative densitometric techniques such as DEXA or quantitative computed tomography (QCT).

DEXA is a two-dimensional technique that provides measurements of bone mineral mass (BMC, mg) per projected total area (cm^2), thus referred to as areal BMD (mg/cm^2) (3,4,8–10). It is currently used for the diagnosis of osteoporosis, the diagnostic criterion being a BMD measurement equal to or more than 2.5 standard deviations below the young female reference mean (T-score $\leqq$ −2.5 standard deviation), at the lumbar spine, total proximal femur, and femoral neck (3,4,15,16). Areal BMD has been acknowledged to correlate fairly well to bone strength, as it accounts for approximately two-thirds of the variance of bone strength *in vitro* of isolated bones, such as the vertebral body or proximal femur, based on experimental studies (3). Moreover, areal BMD at the osteoporotic level has been recognized as an important risk factor for fragility fractures, as there is evidence from cross-sectional and prospective studies that the risk for fracture substantially increases up to threefold for each standard deviation decrease in BMD (3,17). Consequently, it only seems logical that monitoring areal BMD in patients who receive pharmacologic therapy for osteoporosis would be an excellent method in the clinical setting. However, several issues need to be considered.

What does an increase in areal BMD really mean?

Monitoring BMD could be ideal in patients who are treated with bone-forming agents; since formation of new bone is anticipated, BMD increase is expected to reflect the patient's response to treatment. In that context, if a patient presents with a higher BMD after 1 year of therapy, it could well be concluded that this patient is responsive to treatment; in contrast, if BMD declines during that period, this may be a sign of nonresponsiveness. The critical question when serial measurements are considered is whether the results obtained are to be trusted. As with all quantitative tests, with DEXA BMD measurement, the main sources of variability are factors related to the patient, the technologist, and the apparatus (densitometer) (18). Knowledge of the magnitude of this variability is essential to determine when a BMD change is real. Patient-related factors may include the existence of spinal deformities such as scoliosis or spondylosis at the lumbar spine, extraosseous ossifications, osteoarthritis of the hip, and others. In these cases, it is recommended that BMD differences should be taken under clinical consideration only after appropriate selection of the radiological site that offers the most trustworthy reading (usually the femoral neck in most cases). Also, given the variety of DEXA apparatus available, it is important that serial measurements are performed with the same apparatus so that differences of BMD are accurately compared, as there is significant interapparatus variance (19). Additionally, the accuracy of measurements depends highly upon the DEXA technologist who needs to check system calibration and make adjustments as necessary, and who is also responsible for patient positioning, data acquisition, and analysis. According to the International Society for Clinical Densitometry (ISCD), it is mandatory that at least one practicing DEXA technologist in a facility has a valid certification in bone densitometry (18). Accurate detection of BMD changes during treatment requires that the change is greater than the precision error of the measurement. BMD precision (i.e., reproducibility of the measurement) is the ability of the same densitometer and technologist to obtain the same result when measuring a patient multiple times over a short period. In clinical practice, the method most widely used to categorize changes in BMD during therapy is to estimate the least significant change (LSC), which is derived from the standard deviation of the precision error of the measurement. With a confidence interval of 95%, the LSC is calculated as $2.77 \times CV$ (coefficient of variation). As a result, for serial measurements, only changes greater than the LSC can be attributed to the pharmacologic treatment, while smaller changes may be related to measurement error (18). According to the latest ISCD position statement, LSC should be expressed as an absolute value in gram per square centimeter (g/cm^2). This is preferable to using %CV as it is less affected by the baseline BMD value. The LSC for each DEXA technologist should not exceed 5.3% for the lumbar spine, 5.0% for the total hip, and 6.9% for the femoral neck (18). When all of these are considered, changes of BMD with bone-forming agents may offer valuable information as to whether response to treatment has been achieved and if the patient should continue the therapy with the same agent. It must be noted, however, that in patients who had previously used antiresorptive agents, response to treatment in terms of BMD after switching to bone-forming agents may be of a smaller magnitude than observed with treatment-naive patients (20).

When antiresorptive agents are considered, it would be logical to expect that BMD changes of an individual patient would be considerably smaller than those observed with bone-forming agents. Moreover, since antiresorptives primarily prevent bone loss, potential increases of bone mass need to be explained within the context of their individual mechanism of action in order to be credible. For instance, increases of BMD with bisphosphonates as previously discussed by Ego Seeman (21) result from the (partial) filling of already excavated resorption cavities, as these agents do not promote further bone formation. Since net bone mass gain is expected to be moderate (possibly in the magnitude of 3%–4% per year for the first 18–24 months of treatment for most oral bisphosphonates), especially in patients without a previously high remodeling rate, further gains of BMC after that time are thought to be a result of secondary mineralization rather than more filling of resorption cavities (21). As a result, adequate response to treatment within the same patient might be inferred if such gains of BMD are achieved, or at least if bone loss is prevented, and BMD remains stable within LSC limits. Treatment failure with antiresorptives, as expected, would entail bone mass to decrease substantially in serial measurements, possibly at the magnitude of 4% per year or more (6).

These considerations are in line with a previous ISCD position statement (22) that states that serial BMD testing can monitor response to therapy by finding an increase or stability of bone density, while nonresponse could be inferred by finding loss of bone density, bearing in mind that the expected change in BMD should exceed the LSC.

Associations between changes in areal BMD and fracture risk

Given that areal BMD is a significant parameter of bone strength, it would be safe to preclude that increases of BMD result in increases of bone strength, and thus could be associated with decreases of fracture incidence. It is important to bear in mind that while the positive association between BMD and bone strength has been validated for isolated bones *in vitro*, and has been shown to be linear, the same relation does not necessarily apply *in vivo*, and there is no readily accessible method that can be used in order to provide proof of concept as far as risk of fracture is concerned. Since fractures are stochastic events and multiple factors are implicated, we have no way of knowing how much of a difference in BMD, if any, would be needed in order to prevent a certain fracture from happening in a single osteoporotic individual. Moreover, with the use of more advanced techniques, we have come to appreciate that the architectural elements of a bone structure may contribute substantially to its strength, rather than BMD alone. Other considerations with BMD entail that while the absolute value of BMD may have a high specificity for fracture at the threshold for osteoporosis, nevertheless, it has a low sensitivity, i.e., many fractures are documented in individuals with sometimes normal BMD or T-scores in the range of osteopenia (3,4). Furthermore, it has been shown that for a certain value of BMD, the risk for fracture increases substantially with ageing, so that older individuals have greater risk of fracture even if they have the same BMD as younger individuals (3).

To explore the relation between areal BMD and fracture risk for populations, we rely on data provided by randomized controlled trials (RCTs) where the effects of a pharmacologic agent versus placebo are considered. In such cases, it has been shown that the relationship (negative association) between increases in BMD and decreases in fracture risk is not linear, while in other instances results have been contradictory (7,23–26). Most studies have been performed with antiresorptive agents, since only one bone-forming agent was marketed worldwide until recently ; therefore, we must be careful when attempting to compare results from different studies, as each one has a unique design, population of patients, inclusion and exclusion criteria, etc., and such comparisons are of limited value. Although increases in BMD from various pharmacologic treatments may differ substantially, reported reductions in vertebral fracture risk have been found in many cases to be similar. For example, risedronate and raloxifene, based on the results of their clinical trials, were found to produce approximately the same decrease of relative risk for vertebral fractures, despite the fact that risedronate was shown to increase BMD at the spine more than raloxifene (27–31). Moreover, changes of BMD at the femoral neck explained only 7% of the reduction of nonvertebral fracture risk with risedronate, and changes of BMD at the lumbar spine explained only 4% of the reduction of vertebral fracture risk with raloxifene (3,27,32). Comparisons between patients with greater BMD gains as opposed to those with smaller gains after therapy with risedronate have also suggested that greater increases in BMD did not translate into greater decreases of fracture risk (31,32). Although a significant association has been shown between increases of areal BMD with teriparatide resulting in decreases of vertebral fracture risk (33), comparisons between risedronate and teriparatide based on RCTs have previously suggested that even if teriparatide results in far larger increases of areal BMD at the spine after 12 months of treatment (approximately 7% as opposed to 4% with risedronate), the relative risk reduction for vertebral fractures was found to be almost identical to that of both of these agents (29–34). Moreover, in the case of alendronate, one study showed that fracture risk was decreased even in patients who had decreases in BMD (35). In the case of raloxifene, patients with reductions in BMD during treatment had similar incident vertebral fracture rates to those with increases of BMD (27). However, with other agents such as strontium ranelate, and denosumab, a strong association has been found between increases in BMD and reduction of fracture risk (36–38).

Such observations suggest that for some agents such as teriparatide, denosumab, or strontium ranelate, their antifracture efficacy can be explained in terms of increases of areal BMD, while for others such as raloxifene, alendronate, or risedronate, fracture risk reduction cannot be explained by changes in areal BMD. Some studies have also suggested that even smaller gains or small decreases of BMD with some agents may be associated with significant decreases of fracture risk in patients under medication as compared to those receiving placebo. As a result, it might be advisable to rely on areal BMD changes in terms of fracture risk reduction not for all, but for selected pharmaceutical agents where evidence from RCTs exists, and after ensuring that comparisons of serial measurements actually present real differences if changes exceed LSC.

Authors' considerations

It is our understanding that the use of serial BMD measurements by DEXA may be useful when estimating response to treatment of an individual. Osteoporosis has been characterized as a "silent disease," and there is strong evidence to support that patients fail to adhere to treatments for long periods of time, since, among other reasons, they are unable to comprehend and measure the benefit of continuing treatment. Repeat DEXA scans every 1–2 years might be helpful in this regard, in encouraging patients to continue taking their medication, provided that their

physicians explain to them the context in which their results should be interpreted. Moreover, in cases where significant reductions (i.e., greater than 4% per year) of BMD under treatment are encountered, secondary causes for bone loss might be sought after and discovered or different treatment regimens can be applied.

MONITORING BONE TURNOVER MARKERS

BTMs measured in blood and/or urine were introduced in the early 1990s as surrogates of the rate of bone turnover of an individual at any given time. The most commonly used markers of bone formation measured in blood include bone-specific alkaline phosphatase (BALP), procollagen type 1 amino-terminal propeptide (P1NP), and osteocalcin, while markers of bone resorption include carboxy-terminal telopeptide cross-linked type 1 collagen (CTX) and type 1 collagen amino-terminal telopeptide (NTX) (39,40). Most of these can be detected with immunoassays using antibodies that recognize specifically a component of bone matrix released either during bone formation (P1NP) or resorption (CTX), while other assays recognize an enzymatic activity associated with the osteoblast (BALP). The use of such markers has multiple advantages since they are easily obtainable, a variety of assays is available, most are quite inexpensive (although not reimbursed from several national social security systems worldwide), and measurements provide information beyond the scope of BMD (3,40). In a current position paper, Vasicaran et al. suggested that serum CTX should be used as the reference standard for bone resorption and serum P1NP for bone formation (41).

One of the major applications of BTMs after their introduction in clinical practice has been to detect patients with high bone turnover before commencement of therapy. In such cases, evidence of elevated markers above the normal reference range signifies that these patients are rapidly losing bone mass, and thus the microarchitecture of both trabecular and cortical bone is rapidly deteriorating. As a result, inhibition of further bone loss with the use of antiresorptive agents might be advisable in those with already low BMD, so as to minimize the risk of subsequent fractures. However, BTMs do not provide any information concerning the diagnosis of osteoporosis, and their utility for decision-making, as well as their routine clinical application, has been debated, based on a number of issues mainly regarding the accuracy of measurements (41). Namely, of concern are both the biological (preanalytical) variability that most of these markers exhibit, as well as the multiple methodologies applied by different laboratories for some of them. Preanalytical variability as previously discussed by Hannon and Eastell includes sex, age, menopausal status, fasting status, time of day of sample collection (circadian), pregnancy/lactation, exercise, fractures, comorbidities (thyroid and parathyroid disease, renal disease, etc.), and use of drugs (glucocorticoids, anticonvulsants, and others) (42). Analytical variability refers to the methodology used to process the specimen after collection. It must be noted that the lack of consensus as to which assays and methods should be used for each marker poses difficulties, as it is problematic to compare values obtained by different methods in different laboratories. Standardization of measurements so that they are universally comparable is a demanding task that entails that the marker is clearly defined by molecular structure and weight and then reference standard materials as well as calibrators for the clinical laboratories are produced (42).

Theoretical considerations suggest that a high rate of bone turnover above the normal range in patients with already compromised bone strength (as in osteoporosis) would signify increased risk of fracture; rapid and increased bone resorption counterbalanced by slow and partial filling of resorption cavities with bone formation would result in net loss of bone mass and structural decay, thereby increasing the propensity to fracture. As a result, it could be postulated that the use of BTMs could be linked and potentially provide further information concerning fracture risk. A number of previously published prospective studies in treatment-naive postmenopausal women of the general population suggested that increase of a marker of bone resorption or formation was associated with increased fracture risk (42–50). However, due to the lack of an adequate number of relevant studies or studies addressing specifically patients with osteoporosis, the heterogeneity of the markers used as well as the multiple predicted outcomes in terms of fracture types in previously published studies, lack of consistency concerning assays and methods used by researchers, and other methodological issues, there is no consensus in the literature, and most researchers suggest that further research is needed in order to deduct safer conclusions.

Monitoring efficacy

The use of BTMs for monitoring osteoporosis treatment has been previously included in the guidelines of numerous scientific societies throughout the world (3,4,7,51). BTMs exhibit larger and more rapid responses to pharmacologic agents than BMD, and their measurements are indicative of the agents' mechanism of action; while changes of BMD are estimated not earlier than after 12 months of therapy, changes of BTMs (especially with antiresorptive agents) are usually detected within days or weeks of starting treatment (41). The direction of the response and its magnitude and time course differ by treatment and by BTM, and the nature of their response is determined by the mechanism of action of the drug. For instance, with antiresorptive agents such as bisphosphonates, markers of bone resorption decrease significantly within usually 4 weeks of treatment, followed by a decrease in bone formation markers after that time (41). However, the actual amount of decrease of bone resorption has been shown to be different even for agents of the same class such as bisphosphonates; alendronate has been shown to decrease bone resorption markers

more than risedronate in clinical trials (29,52). For all per os bisphosphonates, reduction of bone turnover has been shown to reach a plateau after approximately 6–9 months of therapy, and BTMs may remain almost at the same lower levels for many years if therapy is continued. However, with denosumab, which has a different mechanism of action and is administered subcutaneously every 6 months, bone resorption markers have been shown to decrease at about 90% 1 month after the injection and then slowly rise 10% or more until the completion of the 6-month period (53). The route of administration of a drug is another determinant of the BTM response; more rapid decrease in bone resorption is seen with intravenous alendronate than with the oral formulation. Zoledronic acid, which is only administered intravenously, also reduces bone resorption more rapidly than alendronate by mouth (53–55). Teriparatide, on the other hand, as a bone-forming agent induces a different pattern of response with regard to BTMs; bone formation markers significantly increase after 1 month of treatment, and increases continue for another 5 months until they reach a plateau, while bone resorption markers start to increase significantly after about 3 months of treatment (56).

In an individual basis, the use of BTMs for the monitoring of treatment requires a baseline measurement, and a repeat measurement at some defined point during treatment. The ability to detect change between the two values with confidence depends on the reproducibility of the measurements, which is expressed as a coefficient of variation (CV). As for BMD, to be trustworthy ($P < 0.05$), the change in measured value must also exceed the least significant change (LSC), which is calculated according to the formula $2.77 \times CV$ (4,7,41,42). To improve accuracy even further, biological variability can be reduced by obtaining samples in the early morning after an overnight fast, and serial measurements should be made at the same time of day and at the same laboratory (4,7). Therapy-induced changes in BTMs provide evidence that the patient responds to the treatment and may also reveal patients with low compliance and/or persistence in some cases. If no decrease in bone resorption and bone formation markers is detected after 12 months of therapy with a potent bisphosphonate in a previously untreated patient, then it could be postulated that the patient did not receive the medication as instructed. However, in patients who transition from one per os bisphosphonate to another, further decrease of bone resorption markers might not be detected after the transition even with good compliance and persistence, and the same applies when transitioning from a more to a less potent antiresorptive agent (39). Delay in the onset of increases of bone formation markers can also be encountered in patients who transition to teriparatide after the use of bisphosphonates (3,39).

Changes in BTMs with treatment are often associated with changes in BMD, both for antiresorptive agents and for anabolic therapy (57–59). Especially for antiresorptives, however, clinical results have been inconsistent for the different agents, and changes in BMD were not found to be closely related to the reported fracture risk reduction. More specifically, percent change of BMD at the lumbar spine explained 18% of the reduction of vertebral fracture risk with risedronate and 11% with alendronate (31,60). The effect of antiresorptive therapy on BMD, however, has been shown to be greater in women with higher BTMs at baseline. For example, the increase in spine BMD in response to hormone replacement therapy was found to be greater in those patients with higher u-NTX at baseline (61). The relationship between decrease of BTMs with antiresorptives and decrease of fracture risk has also been assessed by previously published studies (26–29,61–63). These studies suggest that there is a positive association between changes in BTMs and fracture risk: the larger the decrease in BTMs, the larger is the reduction in fracture risk. In the VERT study, the change in u-CTX and u-NTX at 3–6 months explained 54%–77% of the fracture risk reduction with risedronate (64). In the MORE study, the change in PINP and OC explained 28% and 34%, respectively, of the vertebral fracture risk reduction with raloxifene (28).

Monitoring adherence and persistence

Adherence to treatment is poor in all chronic diseases, and osteoporosis is no exception. Also, there is evidence to suggest that the response to treatment is suboptimal in those who adhere poorly (41,65,66). Various strategies have been developed to improve adherence, but there is limited evidence to suggest that the use of BTMs may actually help in that direction. In a randomized open study of postmenopausal women treated with raloxifene (67), patients have been shown to benefit by interviews performed regularly by a nurse as opposed to patients who performed no visits, but information concerning the results of measurements of urinary NTX did not seem to improve patients' adherence any further. In another study with patients receiving risedronate for 1 year (68), those who were informed for measurements of urinary NTX at two different time intervals (10th and 22nd weeks of treatment) were not shown to have any benefit concerning persistence as opposed to patients who did not receive such feedback. Of interest also is the finding that patients who were informed that they responded well to therapy had better persistence, while in those who were informed that they were not responding, persistence was worse. Another study assessing the utility of monitoring BTMs on adherence to bisphosphonate treatment suggested that a positive impact in patients who were informed they were good responders was only seen when the decrease in BTMs levels was marked (greater than 30%) (69).

Authors' considerations

It is our understanding that the use of BTMs may certainly be helpful in monitoring osteoporosis therapy. Our experience obtained from our clinical practice suggests that while

preanalytical and analytical variability cannot be ruled out, a baseline measurement of both P1NP and CTX before, and a new measurement of both of these markers at a selected time (i.e., 3 months) after the initiation of therapy provide fairly accurate insight concerning the response to treatment. We advise our patients to provide morning specimens after overnight fasting and ask for measurements to be made with the same assays and methods at the same clinical laboratory. We have found that detailed history with regard to previous medication may also be helpful for further assessment of the results of BTM measurements. A decrease of BTMs with the use of an antiresorptive agent is indicative in our view that the patient actually responds to therapy, even if areal BMD with DEXA remains stable within LSC limits. That is because DEXA cannot provide information at the microarchitectural level of either the trabecular or cortical bone where most of the changes produced by antiresorptives could be detected, and only captures differences of "total" (integral) BMD that is more prone to projectional or position errors. In cases where no significant change in BTMs is detected, we feel that other possibilities such as nonresponse, problematic adherence/persistence, or secondary causes of bone loss need to be explored. Response to treatment with BTMs may also signify, in our opinion, that a particular patient may also have decreased risk of fracture in terms of improved or retained microarchitecture of the vertebrae or the hip, for instance, but since fractures are stochastic events and each patient represents a different entity and has a unique musculoskeletal system at the time of presentation, we do not see how a safe correlation between change in BTMs and fracture risk can be achieved.

NOVEL METHODS FOR MONITORING TREATMENT

Imaging techniques other than DEXA currently used for research include quantitative ultrasound (QUS), quantitative computed tomography (QCT) performed either at the central (spine, hip) or peripheral (radius, tibia) skeleton (pQCT), high-resolution peripheral QCT (HR-pQCT), and high-resolution magnetic resonance imaging (HR-MRI). By consensus, none of these techniques can be used for the diagnosis of osteoporosis; however, there are data to suggest that some of them could be used for estimation of fracture risk, and in some cases possibly for monitoring of therapy. QUS measures the speed of sound (SOS) and broadband ultrasound attenuation (BUA) at peripheral skeletal sites such as the heel, but there is no clear evidence that these parameters are clinically useful in monitoring therapy (7). QCT provides measurements of bone mineral mass and volumetric (mg/cm^3) BMD of the trabecular and cortical compartment separately, while peripheral QCT enables the study of long bones such as the radius and tibia by capturing geometrical and structural properties such as bone cross-sectional areas (CSAs), bone perimeters at the periosteal and endosteal surfaces, and mean cortical thickness. According to the ISCD 2015 executive summary, total femur trabecular

BMD measured by QCT predicts hip fractures and hip BMD measured by DEXA in postmenopausal women and older men (grade: fair-B-W). Integral and trabecular BMD of the proximal femur measured by QCT can be used to monitor age- and treatment-related BMD changes (grade: fair-B-W) (70). This position has been based on a significant number of prospective studies with three-dimensional QCT of the hip in women treated with alendronate, zolendronic acid, ibandronate, raloxifene, teriparatide, and denosumab (71–81). However, it must be noted that radiation exposure is significantly higher with QCT (by a factor of 50–100) than with DEXA, and it is less available than DEXA in most countries (71). Previous position statements for the use of pQCT for monitoring of treatment were not in favor of the technique due to lack of relevant information from large prospective clinical trials; HR-pQCT is a fairly new technique that is still not widely available, so again there are no conclusions to be drawn yet concerning its utility for monitoring of treatment.

REFERENCES

1. Johnell O, Kanis JA. An estimate of the worldwide prevalence and disability associated with osteoporotic fractures. *Osteoporos Int.* 2006;17:1726–33.
2. Strom O, Borgstrom F, Kanis JA et al. Osteoporosis: Burden, health care provision and opportunities in the EU. A report prepared in collaboration with the International Osteoporosis Foundation (IOF) and the European Federation of Pharmaceutical Industry Associations (EFPIA). *Arch Osteoporos.* 2011;6(1–2):59–155.
3. Kanis JA, Compston J, Cooper C et al. European Guidance. *Osteoporos Int.* 2013;24(1):23–57.
4. Cosman F, de Beur SJ, LeBOff MS et al. *Osteoporos Int* 2014; 25(10): 2359–81.
5. Wang M, Bolland M, Grey A. Management recommendations for osteoporosis in clinical guidelines. *Clin Endocrinol.* 2016;84:687–92.
6. Diez-Perez A, Adachi JD, Agnusdei D et al. Treatment failure in osteoporosis. *Osteoporos Int.* 2012;23(12):2769–74.
7. Bruyere O, Reginster JY. Monitoring of osteoporosis therapy. *Best Practice Res Clin Endocrinol Metabol.* 2014;28:835–41.
8. Consensus development conference: Prophylaxis and treatment of osteoporosis. *Osteoporos Int.* 1991;1:114–7.
9. Consensus Development Conference. Diagnosis, prophylaxis, and treatment of osteoporosis. *Am J Med.* 1993;94:646–50.
10. Kanis JA, Gluer CC, for the Committee of Scientific Advisors, International Osteoporosis Foundation. An update on the diagnosis and assessment of osteoporosis with densitometry. *Osteoporos Int.* 2000;11:192–202.
11. Klibanski A, Adams-Campbell L, Bassford T et al. NIH consensus development panel on osteoporosis prevention, diagnosis and treatment. Osteoporosis prevention, diagnosis, and therapy. *JAMA* 2001;285:785–95.
12. Cole JH, van der Meulen MCH. Whole bone mechanics and bone quality. *Clin Orthop Relat Res.* 2011;469:2139–49.
13. Seeman E, Delmas PD. Bone quality: The material and structural basis of bone strength and fragility. *N Engl J Med.* 2006;354:2250–61.
14. Seaman E. Bone quality: The material and structural basis of bone strength. *J Bone Miner Metab.* 2008;26:1–8.
15. World Health Organization (WHO). *Assessment of fracture risk and its application to screening for postmenopausal osteoporosis.* Technical report series 843. Geneva, Switzerland: WHO, 1994.
16. Kanis JA. Assessment of fracture risk and its application to screening for postmenopausal osteoporosis: Synopsis of a WHO report. WHO Study Group. *Osteoporos Int.* 1994;4:368–81.
17. Marshall D, Johnell O, Wedel H. Meta-analysis of how well measures of bone mineral density predict occurrence of osteoporotic fractures. *BMJ* 1996;312:1254–9.
18. Lewiecki EM, Binkley N, Morgan SL et al. on behalf of the International Society for Clinical Densitometry. Best practices for dual-energy x-ray absorptiometry measurement and reporting: International Society for Clinical Densitometry Guidance. *J Clin Densitom.* 2016;19(2):127–40.
19. Kolta S, Ravaud P, Fechtenbaum J et al. Follow-up of individual patients on two DXA scanners of the same manufacturer. *Osteoporos Int.* 2000;11:709–13.
20. Obermayer-Pietsch BM, Marin F, McCloskey EV et al. Effects of two years of daily teriparatide treatment on BMD in postmenopausal women with severe osteoporosis with and without prior antiresorptive treatment. *J Bone Miner Res.* 2008;23:1591–600.
21. Seeman E. Is a change in bone mineral density a sensitive and specific surrogate of anti-fracture efficacy? *Bone* 2007;41(2007):308–17.
22. Baim S, Wilson CR, Lewiecki EM et al. Precision assessment and radiation safety for dual-energy x-ray absorptiometry: Position paper of the International Society for Clinical Densitometry. *J Clin Densitom.* 2005;8:371–8.
23. Cummings SR, Karpf DB, Harris F et al. Improvement in spine bone density and reduction in risk of vertebral fractures during treatment with antiresorptive drugs. *Am J Med.* 2002;112:281–9.
24. Delmas PD, Seeman E. Changes in bone mineral density explain little of the reduction in vertebral or nonvertebral fracture risk with anti-resorptive therapy. *Bone* 2004;34:599–604.
25. Hochberg MC, Greenspan S, Wasnich RD et al. Changes in bone density and turnover explain the reductions in incidence of nonvertebral fractures that occur during treatment with antiresorptive agents. *J Clin Endocrinol Metab.* 2002;87:1586–92.

26. Delmas PD, Li Z, Cooper C. Relationship between changes in bone mineral density and fracture risk reduction with antiresorptive drugs: Some issues with meta-analyses. *J Bone Mineral Res.* 2004;19: 330–7.

27. Sarkar S, Mitlak BH, Wong M et al. Relationships between bone mineral density and incident vertebral fracture risk with raloxifene therapy. *J Bone Mineral Res.* 2002;17:1–10.

28. Ettinger B, Black DM, Mitlak BH. Reduction of vertebral fracture risk in postmenopausal women with osteoporosis treated with raloxifene: Results from a 3-year randomized clinical trial. Multiple outcomes of raloxifene evaluation (MORE) investigators. *JAMA* 1999;282(7):637–45.

29. Harris, ST, Watts NB, Genant HK. Effects of risedronate treatment on vertebral and nonvertebral fractures in women with postmenopausal osteoporosis. *JAMA* 1999;282:1344–52.

30. Reginster J, Minne HW, Sorensen OH et al. Randomized trial of the effects of risedronate on vertebral fractures in women with established postmenopausal osteoporosis. Vertebral Efficacy with Risedronate Therapy (VERT) Study Group. *Osteoporos Int.* 2000;11:83–91.

31. Watts NB, Cooper C, Lindsay R et al. Relationship between changes in bone mineral density and vertebral fracture risk associated with risedronate: Greater increases in bone mineral density do not relate to greater decreases in fracture risk. *J Clin Densitom.* 2004;7:255–61.

32. Watts NB, Geusens P, Barton IP, Felsenberg D. Relationship between changes in BMD and nonvertebral fracture incidence associated with risedronate: Reduction in risk of nonvertebral fracture is not related to change in BMD. *J Bone Mineral Res.* 2005;20:2097–104.

33. Chen P, Miller PD, Delmas PD et al. Change in lumbar spine BMD and vertebral fracture risk reduction in teriparatide-treated postmenopausal women with osteoporosis. *J Bone Mineral Res.* 2006;21:1785–90.

34. Neer RM, Arnaud CD, Zanchetta JR, Prince R. Effect of parathyroid hormone (1–34) on fractures and bone mineral density in postmenopausal women with osteoporosis. *N Engl J Med.* 2001;344(19):1434–41.

35. Chapurlat RD, Palermo L, Ramsay P et al. Risk of fracture among women who lose bone density during treatment with alendronate. The fracture intervention trial. *Osteoporos Int.* 2005;16:842–8.

36. Bruyere O, Roux C, Detilleux J et al. Relationship between bone mineral density changes and fracture risk reduction in patients treated with strontium ranelate. *J Clin Endocrinol Metabolism.* 2007;92:3076–81.

37. Bruyere O, Roux C, Badurski J et al. Relationship between change in femoral neck bone mineral density and hip fracture incidence during treatment with strontium ranelate. *Curr Med Res Opin.* 2007;23:3041–5.

38. Austin M, Yang YC, Vittinghoff E et al. Relationship between bone mineral density changes with denosumab treatment and risk reduction for vertebral and nonvertebral fractures. *J Bone Mineral Res Official J Am Soc Bone Mineral Res.* 2012;27:687–93.

39. Burch J, Rice S, Yang H et al. Systematic review of the use of bone turnover markers for monitoring the response to osteoporosis treatment: The secondary prevention of fractures, and primary prevention of fractures in high-risk groups. *Health Technol Assess.* 2014;18(11):1–180.

40. Seibel MJ. Biochemical markers of bone turnover: Part I: Biochemistry and variability. *Clin Biochem Rev.* 2005;26:97–122.

41. Vasikaran S, Eastell R, Bruyère O et al. Markers of bone turnover for the prediction of fracture risk and monitoring of osteoporosis treatment: A need for international reference standards. *Osteoporos Int.* 2011;22:391–420.

42. Hannon R, Eastell R. Preanalytical variability of biochemical markers of bone turnover. *Osteoporos Int.* 2000;11:S30–S44.

43. Akesson K, Ljunghall S, Jonsson B et al. Assessment of biochemical markers of bone metabolism in relation to the occurrence of fracture: A retrospective and prospective population-based study of women. *J Bone Miner Res.* 1995;10:1823–9.

44. Garnero P, Hausherr E, Chapuy M-C et al. Markers of bone resorption predict hip fracture in elderly women: The EPIDOS prospective study. *J Bone Miner Res.* 1996;11:1531–8.

45. Gerdhem P, Ivaska KK, Alatalo SL et al. Biochemical markers of bone metabolism and prediction of fracture in elderly women. *J Bone Miner Res.* 2004;19:386–93.

46. Ross PD, Kress BC, Parson RE et al. Serum bone alkaline phosphatase and calcaneus bone density predict fractures: A prospective study. *Osteoporos Int.* 2000;11:76–82.

47. Sornay-Rendu E, Munoz F, Garnero P, Duboeuf F, Delmas PD. Identification of osteopenic women at high risk of fracture: The OFELY study. *J Bone Miner Res.* 2005;20:1813–9.

48. van Daele PL, Seibel MJ, Burger H et al. Case–control analysis of bone resorption markers, disability, and hip fracture risk: The Rotterdam study. *BMJ* 1996;312:482–3.

49. Vergnaud P, Garnero P, Meunier PJ et al. Undercarboxylated osteocalcin measured with a specific immunoassay predicts hip fracture in elderly women: The EPIDOS study. *J Clin Endocrinol Metab.* 1997;82:719–24.

50. Szulc P, Chapuy MC, Meunier PJ, Delmas PD. Serum undercarboxylated osteocalcin is a marker of the risk of hip fracture in elderly women. *J Clin Invest.* 1993;91:1769–74.

51. Eisman J, Ebeling P, Ewald D et al. *Clinical Guideline for the Prevention and Treatment of Osteoporosis in Postmenopausal Women and Older Men.* The Royal

Australian College of General Practitioners, 2010. Available from: https:// www.racgp.org.au.

52. Black DM, Cummings SR, Karpf DB et al. Randomised trial of effect of alendronate on risk of fracture in women with existing vertebral fractures. Fracture Intervention Trial Research Group. *Lancet* 1996;348(9041):1535–41.

53. Vasikaran SD, Khan S, McCloskey EV, Kanis JA. Sustained response to intravenous alendronate in postmenopausal osteoporosis. *Bone Miner.* 1995;17:517–20.

54. Saag K, Lindsay R, Kriegman A, Beamer E, Zhou W. A single zoledronic acid infusion reduces bone resorption markers more rapidly than weekly oral alendronate in postmenopausal women with low bone mineral density. *Bone* 2007;40:1238–43.

55. McClung M, Lewiecki E, Cohen S et al. Denosumab in postmenopausal women with low bone mineral density. *N Engl J Med.* 2006;354:821–31.

56. Arlot M, Meunier PJ, Boivin G et al. Differential effects of teriparatide and alendronate on bone remodeling in postmenopausal women assessed by histo-morphometric parameters. *J Bone Miner Res.* 2005;20:1244–53.

57. Greenspan SL, Resnick NM, Parker RA. Early changes in biochemical markers of bone turnover are associated with long-term changes in bone mineral density in elderly women on alendronate, hormone replacement therapy, or combination therapy: A three-year, double-blind, placebo-controlled, randomized clinical trial. *J Clin Endocrinol Metab.* 2005;90:2762–7.

58. Chen P, Satterwhite JH, Licata AA et al. Early changes in biochemical markers of bone formation predict BMD response to teriparatide in postmenopausal women with osteoporosis. *J Bone Mineral Res.* 2005;20:962–70.

59. Munck-Brentano T, Biver E, Chopin F et al. Clinical utility of serum bone turnover markers in postmenopausal osteoporosis therapy monitoring: A systematic review. *Semin Arthritis Rheum.* 2011;41:157–69.

60. Cummings SR, Karpf DB, Harris F et al. Improvement in spine bone density and reduction in risk of vertebral fractures during treatment with antiresorptive drugs. *Am J Med.* 2002;112:281–9.

61. Chesnut CH, Bell NH, Clark GS et al. Hormone replacement therapy in postmenopausal women: Urinary N-telopeptide of type I collagen monitors therapeutic effect and predicts response of bone mineral density. *Am J Med.* 1997;102:29–37.

62. Reginster J-Y, Sarkar S, Zegels B et al. Reduction in PINP, a marker of bone metabolism, with raloxifene treatment and its relationship with vertebral fracture risk. *Bone* 2004;34:344–51.

63. Sarkar S, Reginster J-Y, Crans GG et al. Relationship between changes in biochemical markers of bone turnover and BMD to predict vertebral fracture risk. *J Bone Miner Res.* 2004;19:394–401.

64. Bauer DC, Black DM, Garnero P et al. Change in bone turnover and hip, non-spine, and vertebral fracture in alendronate-treated women: The fracture intervention trial. *J Bone Miner Res.* 2004;19:1250–8.

65. Siris ES, Harris ST, Rosen CJ et al. Adherence to bisphosphonate therapy and fracture rates in osteoporotic women: Relationship to vertebral and nonvertebral fractures from two US claims databases. *Mayo Clin Proc.* 2006;81:1013–22.

66. Blouin J, Dragomir A, Moride Y et al. Impact of noncompliance with alendronate and risedronate on the incidence of nonvertebral osteoporotic fractures in elderly women. *Br J Clin Pharmacol.* 2008;66:117–27.

67. Reginster J-Y, Sarkar S, Zegels B et al. Reduction in PINP, a marker of bone metabolism, with raloxifene treatment and its relationship with vertebral fracture risk. *Bone* 2004;34:344–51.

68. Eastell R, Barton I, Hannon RA et al. Relationship of early changes in bone resorption to the reduction in fracture risk with risedronate. *J Bone Miner Res.* 2003;18:1051–6.

69. Clowes JA, Peel NFA, Eastell R. The impact of monitoring on adherence and persistence with antiresorptive treatment for post-menopausal osteoporosis: A randomized controlled trial. *J Clin Endocrinol Metab.* 2004;89:1117–23.

70. Shepherd J, Schousboe JT, Broy SB, Engelke K, Leslie WD. Executive Summary of the 2015 ISCD Position Development Conference on Advanced Measures from DXA and QCT: Fracture Prediction Beyond BMD. *J Clin Densitom.* 2015;18(3):274–85.

71. Engelke K, Lang T, Khosla S et al. Clinical use of quantitative computed tomography (QCT) of the hip in the management of osteoporosis in adults: The 2015 ISCD Official Positions Part I. *J Clin Densitom.* 2015;18(3):338–58.

72. Keaveny TM, Hoffmann PF, Singh M et al. Femoral bone strength and its relation to cortical and trabecular changes after treatment with PTH, alendronate, and their combination as assessed by finite element analysis of quantitative CT scans. *J Bone Miner Res.* 2008;23(12):1974–82.

73. Black DM, Greenspan SL, Ensrud KE et al. The effects of parathyroid hormone and alendronate alone or in combination in postmenopausal osteoporosis. *N Engl J Med.* 2003;349(13):1207–15.

74. Lewiecki EM, Keaveny TM, Kopperdahl DL et al. Once-monthly oral ibandronate improves biomechanical determinants of bone strength in women with postmenopausal osteoporosis. *J Clin Endocrinol Metab.* 2009;94(1):171–80.

75. Engelke K, Fuerst T, Dasic G et al. Regional distribution of spine and hip QCT BMD responses after one year of once-monthly ibandronate in postmenopausal osteoporosis. *Bone* 2010;46(6):1626–32.

76. Eastell R, Lang T, Boonen S et al. Effect of once-yearly zoledronic acid on the spine and hip as measured by quantitative computed tomography: Results of the HORIZON Pivotal Fracture Trial. *Osteoporos Int.* 2010;21(7):1277–85.

77. Miller PD, Delmas PD, Lindsay R et al. Early responsiveness of women with osteoporosis to teriparatide after therapy with alendronate or risedronate. *J Clin Endocrinol Metab.* 2008;93(10):3785–93.

78. Yang L, Sycheva AV, Black DM, Eastell R. Site-specific differential effects of once-yearly zoledronic acid on the hip assessed with quantitative computed tomography: Results from the HORIZON Pivotal Fracture Trial. *Osteoporos Int.* 2013;24(1):329–38.

79. Poole KE, Treece GM, Gee AH et al. Denosumab rapidly increases cortical bone in key locations of the femur: A 3D bone mapping study in women with osteoporosis. *J Bone Miner Res.* 2015;30(1):46–54.

80. Borggrefe J, Graeff C, Nickelsen TN et al. Quantitative computed tomographic assessment of the effects of 24 months of teriparatide treatment on 3D femoral neck bone distribution, geometry, and bone strength: Results from the EUROFORS study. *J Bone Miner Res.* 2010;25(3):472–81.

81. Genant HK, Libanati C, Engelke K et al. Improvements in hip trabecular, subcortical, and cortical density and mass in postmenopausal women with osteoporosis treated with denosumab. *Bone* 2013;56(2):482–8.

11

Systemic complications of osteoporosis medical treatment

KONSTANTINOS G. MAKRIDIS and STAMATINA-EMMANOUELA ZOURNTOU

INTRODUCTION

In the osteoporotic bone, there is a great disruption of its microarchitectural structure, characterized by a decrease of its density, a "porous" (as a sponge) composition, and a disturbance of the trabecular skeleton. The combination of these factors leads to a reduction in bone resistance, mainly to compression forces, increasing the risk of bone fractures.

Bone mass is increased at the beginning of the embryonic and infant ages, and then the rate of growth decreases until the age of puberty. The increase is almost completed during the 18th–20th years of life, and from that age onward, a small amount of bone is formed up to the age of 28–30 years. This bone mass represents the peak bone mass and begins to decline with age progress in both women and men. The onset of loss develops much earlier in women than men as a result of menopause.

Bone is a living tissue, and its metabolism aims to both restore and maintain the anatomical and functional integrity as well as the maximum bone mass. Thus, within a decade, the entire bone tissue has been completely replaced. This process is called *remodeling*. Remodeling is under the control of several hormones, consisting of (a) the fragmentation and absorption of the minimal bone products of the bone loss, leaving finally a "bump" to the bone, and then (b) repairing the damage, filling the hole, with new healthy bone. The first process is called *absorption* and is performed by cells present on the inner surface of the bone, the osteoclasts. The second process is called *bone reshaping* and is performed by osteoblasts, which are in close proximity to osteoclasts. Among these cells, there is cooperation and interaction so that osteoblasts are activated by osteoclasts to correct the damage caused by the latter (1).

Substances produced by these two types of cells (osteoclasts, osteoblasts), as well as bone tissue degradation products, are called bone remodeling or metabolism markers. These indicators are tools in both investigating osteoporosis and monitoring the effectiveness of antiosteoporotic treatment (2).

Currently existing medicines, which are clearly only given by experts, are divided into three categories: (a) antiabsorption drugs, which are substances that reduce the absorption capacity of osteoclasts, thus limiting bone loss and giving osteoblasts time to repair the damage; (b) anabolic agents, which act by increasing the activity of osteoblasts to produce new bone; and (c) dual action agents (Table 11.1).

While the efficacy of these drugs on osteoporosis has been proven, there are many reported systemic complications that may affect the treatment and should be analyzed in detail.

SYSTEMIC COMPLICATIONS OF BISPHOSPHONATES

Bisphosphonates are structurally similar to pyrophosphate and act by inhibiting activation of enzymes that utilize pyrophosphate. Presenting high affinity with calcium, they stick to the bone where calcium ions are abundant, forming a chemical complex there. Osteoclasts digest these complexes, and their apoptosis begins due to inhibition of specific metabolic pathways.

Oral bisphosphonates can cause adverse events from the gastrointestinal tract, like dyspepsia, gastritis, stomach pain, and erosions of the esophagus. This can be prevented by remaining seated upright for 30–60 minutes after taking the medication (3).

Intravenous bisphosphonates can give fever and flu-like symptoms after the first infusion, which are thought to occur because of their potential to activate human T cells (3). Many patients report that at the first intravenous dose of zoledronate or monthly oral dose of ibandronate or risedronate they experience one or more symptoms of acute-phase reactions such as fever, muscle aches, and arthritis-like symptoms. These symptoms occur within

Table 11.1 Antiosteoporotic drugs

Class and drug	Brand name	Form	Frequency	Gender
Antiresorptive Agents				
Bisphosphonates				
Alendronate	Fosamax	Oral	Daily/weekly	Women + men
Alendronate	Binosto	Oral	Weekly	Women + men
Ibandronate	Boniva, Bonviva	Oral	Monthly	Women
Ibandronate	Boniva	Intravenous	Every 3 months	Women
Risedronate	Actonel	Oral	Daily/weekly/monthly	Women + men
Risedronate	Atelvia	Oral	Weekly	Women
Zoledronic acid	Reclast, Aclasta	Intravenous	Yearly	Women + men
Receptor Activator of Nuclear Factor–κB Ligand (RANKL) Inhibitor				
Denosumab	Prolia	Injection	Every 6 months	Women + men
Calcitonin				
Calcitonin	Fortical, Miacalcin	Nasal spray	Daily	Women
Calcitonin	Miacalcin	Injection	Varies	Women
Estrogen (Hormone Therapy)				
Estrogen	Multiple brands	Oral	Daily	Women
Estrogen	Multiple brands	Transdermal	Weekly	Women
Selective Estrogen Receptor Modulators (SERMs)				
Raloxifene	Evista	Oral	Daily	Women
Tissue Selective Estrogen Complex (TSEC)				
Estrogen/bazedoxifene	Duavee	Oral	Daily	Women
Anabolic Agents				
Parathyroid Hormone (PTH) Analogue				
Teriparatide	Forteo, Forsteo	Injection	Daily	Women + men
Parathyroid Hormone-Related Protein (PTHrp) Analogue				
Abaloparatide	Tymlos	Injection	Daily	Women
Dual Action Bone Agent				
Strontium ranelate	Protelos	Oral	Daily	Women + men

24–36 hours and last up to 3–5 days. They can successfully be reduced with acetaminophen at doses of 500–1000 mg before and after infusion (3).

Mild hypocalcemia may occur without any clinical significance. Iritis is a rare adverse effect caused more likely by intravenous bisphosphonates.

Renal failure is another reported adverse event with the use of these drugs, although its frequency is very low. This happens because approximately 50%–60% of administered bisphosphonate is excreted unchanged by the kidneys, with the remainder taken up by bone. Considering that many patients also use other agents that are nephrotoxic, such as nonsteroidal anti-inflammatory drugs or diuretics, the presence of preexisting renal impairment and dehydration at the time of bisphosphonate infusion increases the risk for renal toxicity.

In any case, serum creatinine levels and glomerular filtration rate should be calculated before administration of bisphosphonates, especially of intravenous ones (4).

One study reported a case report with systemic inflammatory response after intravenous administration of zoledronic acid. He was a pediatric patient with complex medical problems, and he developed tachycardia, fever, hypotension, moderate acute respiratory distress syndrome, and pulmonary hemorrhage beginning 3 hours after completion of the infusion and resolving the third day (5).

Kesikburun et al. reported a case of aggravation of myasthenia gravis after taking alendronate for corticoid-induced osteoporosis. Stopping the administration and turning to intravenous ibandronate improved the symptoms (6).

Cutaneous adverse reactions to bisphosphonates have been recorded, although their incidence is rare, estimated to be 1 per 10,000. Rash, pruritus, urticaria, angioedema, Stevens-Johnson syndrome, and toxic epidermal necrolysis are the systemic complications occurring after administration of bisphosphonates (7).

Herrera reported another rare complication after zoledronic acid infusion. Orbital inflammation occurred in a chronic immunosuppressive patient, but it was rapidly resolved with oral prednisone (8).

Recent studies have reported bisphosphonate use (specifically zoledronate and alendronate) as a risk factor for atrial fibrillation relating to fluctuations in calcium blood levels. An association between the timing of the infusion or the acute phase reaction following the infusion has not yet been proven. Moreover, no increase in the rate of atrial fibrillation has been recorded even in oncologic patients who receive 10-times-higher doses of bisphosphonates. Definitely, the evidence is not clear and more studies are necessary to prove this complication (9).

Several studies have evaluated whether bisphosphonate use is associated with an increased risk of esophageal cancer. Most of them do not provide any strong evidence regarding the association between bisphosphonates administration and this serious complication, and definitely more data are necessary to prove it (10).

SYSTEMIC COMPLICATIONS OF DENOSUMAB

Denosumab is a human monoclonal antibody for the treatment of osteoporosis, metastases to bone, and giant cell tumor of bone. It is a receptor activator of nuclear factor–κB ligand (RANKL) inhibitor preventing the development of osteoclasts.

Denosumab may lower the calcium levels in the blood causing spasms or cramps in the muscles and numbness and tingling in the fingers, toes, or around the mouth. The majority of reported cases were patients with chronic kidney disease or patients with heart or lung transplantation (11–15). A blood test of calcium levels must be advised to every patient prior to therapy with denosumab, and 1000 mg of calcium and 400 IU of vitamin D daily must be given. Moreover, monitoring of calcium, magnesium, and phosphorus in patients with chronic kidney disease is highly recommended (16).

Several infections such as pneumonia, diverticulitis, appendicitis, sepsis, pyelonephritis, urinary tract infection, and cellulitis have been reported in patients taking denosumab. The mechanism of action might be connected to the role of RANKL in the immune system. RANKL is expressed by T-helper cells and is thought to be involved in dendritic cell maturation (17). However, it seems that their relative risk was not statistically significant compared to placebo (16,18).

Anaphylaxis and skin-related rashes especially in the mouth, groin, and thigh have been mentioned, but no fatal outcomes occurred from these complications (16). In any case, the existence of such lesions should be reported to health-care providers, and patients should practice good dental care during treatment.

SYSTEMIC COMPLICATIONS OF CALCITONIN

Calcitonin is a 32 amino acid linear polypeptide hormone that is produced in humans primarily by the parafollicular cells (also known as C-cells) of the thyroid gland. It acts to reduce blood calcium by inhibiting osteoclast activity in bones and renal tubular cell reabsorption of Ca^{2+} and phosphate, thus opposing the effects of parathyroid hormone (PTH).

Common side effects with nasal calcitonin are a runny nose, headache, back pain, and nosebleed (epistaxis) (17).

Side effects in patients receiving intramuscular or subcutaneous calcitonin are dose related and can occur in up to 80% of patients on high doses. Generally, they are not serious, and the most common are gastrointestinal consisting of anorexia, nausea, vomiting, a metallic taste, or rarely, diarrhea. Vascular phenomena, such as flushing or shivering, are the next most common, followed by dermatologic changes, including a local rash at the injection site, a generalized rash, and pruritus. These skin changes are usually not immunologic in origin. True allergic reactions consisting of urticaria and anaphylaxis are rare. Because most side effects are dose related and decrease in severity with duration of use, the calcitonin dose may be reduced and gradually increased as tolerated (19–22).

The use of calcitonin has been implicated in liver and breast cancers. Although the data do not definitively support the discontinuation of calcitonin in these cases, use of this medication should be reviewed from time to time with the health-care provider (23).

SYSTEMIC COMPLICATIONS OF ESTROGEN, SELECTIVE ESTROGEN RECEPTOR MODULATORS, AND TISSUE SELECTIVE ESTROGEN COMPLEX

The estrogen receptors α and β affect osteoclast apoptosis and the use of estrogens, estrogen modulators, and the tissue selective estrogen complex (TSEC) as antiosteoporotic agents have been extensively analyzed.

When used alone, estrogens have a potential increased risk for venous thromboembolic disorders, breast cancer, cardiac events, stroke, and endometrial cancer. To reduce this risk, it is important to be prescribed the hormone progesterone in combination with estrogen (hormone therapy [HT]) for those women who have a uterus. Estrogen therapy (ET) is prescribed for women who have had hysterectomies. Side effects may include vaginal bleeding in women with a uterus on HT, breast tenderness, and gallbladder disease (24).

Selective estrogen receptor modulators are nonsteroidal synthetic drugs with similar effects on bone as estrogen, but without any of the adverse events on breast and endometrium tissues.

Tamoxifen is useful in the treatment of osteoporosis, but the adverse effects such as hot flushes and the increased risk of developing endometrial cancer can limit its use.

Raloxifene is associated with an acceptable endometrial profile and has not demonstrated tamoxifen-like effects in the uterus but has been associated with adverse effects such as venous thromboembolism and vasomotor symptoms (25).

Bazedoxifene is relatively safe and well tolerated without exhibiting breast or endometrial stimulation and having a lower risk for venous thromboembolism. Its advantage over raloxifene is that it increases endothelial nitric oxide synthase activity and does not antagonize the effect of 17β-estradiol on vasomotor symptoms (26).

The first TSEC combines conjugated estrogens and the selective estrogen receptor modulator (SERM) bazedoxifene for a positive synergistic action. This combination allows for the benefits of estrogen with regard to relief of vasomotor symptoms without estrogenic stimulation of the endometrium (26).

SYSTEMIC COMPLICATIONS OF PARATHYROID HORMONE AND PARATHYROID HORMONE-RELATED PROTEIN ANALOGUES

Teriparatide is a recombinant protein form of PTH consisting of the first (N-terminus) 34 amino acids, which is the bioactive portion of the hormone (27).

Common adverse effects of teriparatide include nausea, headache, dizziness, leg cramps, and limb pain. Sometimes, a slight elevation in serum and urine calcium levels can occur, but the risk of kidney stones is minimal (28).

In animal studies performed in immature rats, very high doses of teriparatide that were given for a long period of time increased the incidence of osteosarcoma; however, there is no evidence that this risk is similar to that in humans (28).

In patients with Paget disease, with undiagnosed high levels of alkaline phosphatase or calcium, and those who have received bone radiotherapy, teriparatide should not be given (28).

Abaloparatide is 34 amino acid synthetic analogue of parathyroid hormone-related protein (PTHrP). It has 41% homology to PTH (1–34) and 76% homology to PTHrP (1–34) C.

Common adverse effects include hypercalciuria, dizziness, nausea, headache, fatigue, abdominal pain, and vertigo. The risk of developing osteosarcoma is similar to teriparatide in humans; however, the use of both must not last over 2 years (27).

SYSTEMIC COMPLICATIONS OF STRONTIUM RANELATE

Strontium ranelate is a strontium salt of ranelic acid having similar nuclear size as calcium and acting as a dual-action bone agent. The most common side effects include nausea, diarrhea, headache, and eczema, but severe effects are rare. Occasionally, severe allergic reactions are reported including rash with eosinophilia and systemic symptoms (DRESS syndrome) (29,30).

DRESS syndrome is a severe adverse drug-induced reaction presenting as a diffuse maculopapular skin rash with fever, hematologic abnormalities (leukocytosis, eosinophilia, and/or atypical lymphocytosis), and multiorgan involvement. In such cases, even more severe reactions may occur like systemic reactivation of human herpesviruses (HHV-6 and HHV-7), Epstein-Barr virus, and cytomegalovirus (31).

In general, the use of strontium has been restricted due to the increased risk of venous thromboembolism, pulmonary embolism, and serious cardiovascular disorders, including myocardial infarction (32). Regarding this complication, no clear data exist about the exact mechanism of action, and it seems that is mediated by several factors apart from strontium ranelate (33).

REFERENCES

1. Akkawi I, Zmerly H. Osteoporosis: Current concepts. *Joints.* 2018;6(2):122–7.
2. Lorentzon M. Treating osteoporosis to prevent fractures: Current concepts and future developments. *J Intern Med.* 2019;285(4):381–94.
3. Khan M, Cheung AM, Khan AA. Drug-related adverse events of osteoporosis therapy. *Endocrinol Metab Clin North Am.* 2017;46(1):181–92.
4. Pazianas M, Abrahamsen B. Osteoporosis treatment: Bisphosphonates reign to continue for a few more years, at least? *Ann N Y Acad Sci.* 2016;1376(1):5–13.
5. Trivedi S, Al-Nofal A, Kumar S, Tripathi S, Kahoud RJ, Tebben PJ. Severe non-infective systemic inflammatory response syndrome, shock, and end-organ dysfunction after zoledronic acid administration in a child. *Osteoporos Int.* 2016;27(7):2379–82.
6. Kesikburun S, Güzelküçük U, Alay S, Yavuz F, Tan AK. Exacerbation of myasthenia gravis by alendronate. *Osteoporos Int.* 2014;25(9):2319–20.
7. Musette P, Kaufman JM, Rizzoli R, Cacoub P, Brandi ML, Reginster JY. Cutaneous side effects of antiosteoporosis treatments. *Ther Adv Musculoskelet Dis.* 2011;3(1):31–41.
8. Herrera I, Kam Y, Whittaker TJ, Champion M, Ajlan RS. Bisphosphonate-induced orbital inflammation in a patient on chronic immunosuppressive therapy. *BMC Ophthalmol.* 2019;19(1):51.
9. Barrett-Connor E, Swern AS, Hustad CM et al. Alendronate and atrial fibrillation: A meta-analysis of randomized placebo-controlled clinical trials. *Osteoporos Int.* 2012;23(1):233–45.
10. Brown JP, Morin S, Leslie W et al. Bisphosphonates for treatment of osteoporosis: Expected benefits, potential harms, and drug holidays. *Can Fam Physician.* 2014;60(4):324–33.
11. Saleem S, Patel S, Ahmed A, Saleem N. Denosumab causing severe, refractory hypocalcaemia in a patient with chronic kidney disease. *BMJ Case Rep.* 2018;2018.

12. De Muynck B, Leys M, Cuypers J, Vanderschueren D, Delcroix M, Belge C. Hypocalcemia after denosumab in a pulmonary hypertension patient receiving epoprostenol. *Respiration.* 2018;95(2):139–42.

13. Shrosbree JE, Elder GJ, Eisman JA, Center JR. Acute hypocalcaemia following denosumab in heart and lung transplant patients with osteoporosis. *Intern Med J.* 2018;48(6):681–7.

14. Huynh AL, Baker ST, Stewardson AJ, Johnson DF. Denosumab-associated hypocalcaemia: Incidence, severity and patient characteristics in a tertiary hospital setting. *Pharmacoepidemiol Drug Saf.* 2016;25(11):1274–8.

15. Laskowski LK, Goldfarb DS, Howland MA, Kavcsak K, Lugassy DM, Smith SW. A RANKL wrinkle: Denosumab-induced hypocalcemia. *J Med Toxicol.* 2016;12(3):305–8.

16. Zaheer S, LeBoff M, Lewiecki EM. Denosumab for the treatment of osteoporosis. *Expert Opin Drug Metab Toxicol.* 2015;11(3):461–70.

17. Khosla S. Increasing options for the treatment of osteoporosis. *N Engl J Med.* 2009;361(8):818–20.

18. Watts NB, Roux C, Modlin JF et al. Infections in postmenopausal women with osteoporosis treated with denosumab or placebo: Coincidence or causal association? *Osteoporos Int.* 2012;23(1):327–37.

19. Henriksen K, Byrjalsen I, Andersen JR et al. SMC021 investigators. A randomized, double-blind, multicenter, placebo-controlled study to evaluate the efficacy and safety of oral salmon calcitonin in the treatment of osteoporosis in postmenopausal women taking calcium and vitamin D. *Bone.* 2016;91:122–9.

20. Rossini M, Adami G, Adami S, Viapiana O, Gatti D. Safety issues and adverse reactions with osteoporosis management. *Expert Opin Drug Saf.* 2016;15(3):321–32.

21. Chung SY, Chen TH, Lai SL, Huang CH, Chen WH. Hypercalcemia and status epilepticus relates to salmon calcitonin administration in breast cancer. *Breast.* 2005;14(5):399–402.

22. Siminoski K, Josse RG. Prevention and management of osteoporosis: Consensus statements from the Scientific Advisory Board of the Osteoporosis Society of Canada. 9. Calcitonin in the treatment of osteoporosis. *CMAJ.* 1996;155(7):962–5.

23. Sun LM, Lin MC, Muo CH, Liang JA, Kao CH. Calcitonin nasal spray and increased cancer risk: A population-based nested case-control study. *J Clin Endocrinol Metab.* 2014;99(11):4259–64.

24. Cartwright B, Robinson J, Seed PT, Fogelman I, Rymer J. Hormone replacement therapy versus the combined oral contraceptive pill in premature ovarian failure: A randomized controlled trial of the effects on bone mineral density. *J Clin Endocrinol Metab.* 2016;101(9):3497–505.

25. Qaseem A, Forciea MA, McLean RM, Denberg TD, Clinical Guidelines Committee of the American College of Physicians. Treatment of low bone density or osteoporosis to prevent fractures in men and women: A clinical practice guideline update from the American College of Physicians. *Ann Intern Med.* 2017;166(11):818–39.

26. Pickar JH, Komm BS. Selective estrogen receptor modulators and the combination therapy conjugated estrogens/bazedoxifene: A review of effects on the breast. *Post Reprod Health.* 2015;21(3):112–21.

27. Pioszak AA, Parker NR, Gardella TJ, Xu HE. Structural basis for parathyroid hormone-related protein binding to the parathyroid hormone receptor and design of conformation-selective peptides. *J Biol Chem.* 2009;284(41):28382–91.

28. Verhaar HJ, Lems WF. PTH analogues and osteoporotic fractures. *Expert Opin Biol Ther.* 2010;10(9):1387–94.

29. Moreno-Higueras M, Callejas-Rubio JL, Gallo-Padilla L. Dress syndrome and bilateral panuveitis caused by strontium ranelate. *Med Clin.* 2017;149(7):317–8.

30. Adwan MH. Drug Reaction with Eosinophilia and Systemic Symptoms (DRESS) syndrome and the rheumatologist. *Curr Rheumatol Rep.* 2017;19(1):3.

31. Drago F, Cogorno L, Broccolo F, Ciccarese G, Parodi A. A fatal case of DRESS induced by strontium ranelate associated with HHV-7 reactivation. *Osteoporos Int.* 2016;27(3):1261–4.

32. Bolland MJ, Grey A. Ten years too long: Strontium ranelate, cardiac events, and the European Medicines Agency. *BMJ.* 2016;354:i5109.

33. Atteritano M, Catalano A, Santoro D, Lasco A, Benvenga S. Effects of strontium ranelate on markers of cardiovascular risk in postmenopausal osteoporotic women. *Endocrine.* 2016;53(1):305–12.

12

Complications of medical treatment
Atypical fractures

OWEN DIAMOND, NATALIE C. ROLLICK, and DAVID L. HELFET

INCIDENCE OF ATYPICAL FRACTURES

With the ensuing "Silver Tsunami" and increasing recognition of the incidence of osteoporosis, bisphosphonates have become one of the most widely utilized drugs. Bisphosphonates have established a role in the primary and secondary prevention of fragility fractures (1). There is, however, a paradoxical effect with the use of bisphosphonates for some patients. Numerous case reports and case series have shown an increase in the presentation of atypical femoral fractures (AFFs) (Figure 12.1a) in patients exposed to long-term bisphosphonate therapy (2–6).

Bisphosphonates work by suppressing bone resorption and hence slow the loss of bone mass. They have been shown to successfully reduce the incidence of fragility fractures (7). However, this interference in bone turnover has a consequence for normal bone homeostasis.

It is well recognized that AFFs are a complication associated with the prolonged use of bisphosphonates (8). Medical and public concerns related to bisphosphonate side effects have led to a considerable decrease in their extended use and interest in the possible benefits of a "bisphosphonate holiday" (9–11).

It has been estimated that the relative risk of patients experiencing an AFF while taking bisphosphonates is high; however, the absolute risk of these fractures in patients on bisphosphonates is low, ranging from 3.2 to 50 cases per 100,000 person-years. Long-term use may be associated with higher risk of about 100 per 100,000 person-years (4). In a study from two large trauma centers in the United Kingdom, which reviewed 3515 consecutive patients with a fracture of the proximal femur, there was 156 fractures in the subtrochanteric region and 251 femoral shaft fractures. The atypical fracture pattern was seen in 27 patients (7%; 29 femoral shaft or subtrochanteric fractures). Twenty-two patients with 24 atypical fractures were receiving bisphosphonate treatment at the time of fracture for a mean of 4.6 years (2).

ETIOPATHOLOGY

Normal bone undergoes constant turnover, with osteoclasts and osteoblasts working in tandem. Osteoclast cells have a role of "chomping away" along the length of long bones in a formation called *cutting cones*. Homeostasis is completed when the osteoclasts' cutting cones are followed behind by osteoblasts laying down new bone, which can then be mineralized. It is a combination of osteoclasts "eating or engulfing" small disruptions in the normal architecture of the bone followed by the laying down of new bone by osteoblasts that prevents crack propagation and ensures normal homeostasis of the bone superstructure. Bisphosphonates act by preventing the normal function of osteoclasts, thereby reducing bone resorption with the aim of having a net gain in bone density. Although this has proven successful in reducing the risk of some fragility-type fractures, it unfortunately compromises the normal osteoclast homeostatic function, normal bone remodeling and repair capacity. In the femur, the reduction in the osteoclast function of "mopping up" subclinical microfractures eventually leads to accumulation of microdamage (Figure 12.1b). These microfractures can propagate and ultimately clinically present as an AFF (12,13).

Clinical presentation and radiological findings

Most patients with an AFF present following a low-energy fall, or they may not have experienced any associated trauma whatsoever, presenting similarly to a pathologic fracture (i.e., an abnormal bone fracturing under a normal physiologic load). It is estimated that 25%–45% of patients will have prodromal symptoms such as thigh pain (2,14). Clinical workup of every patient includes a detailed history, inquiring about any preceding pain in the injured limb and also any symptoms in the nonfractured

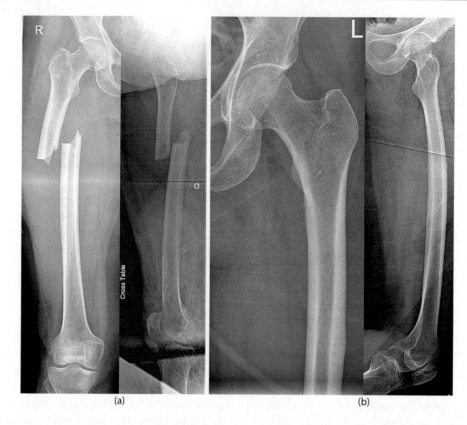

(a)   (b)

Figure 12.1 (a) Anteroposterior (AP) and lateral radiographs (left images) demonstrate a displaced right-sided subtrochanteric atypical femur fracture. (b) Contralateral left femur AP and lateral radiographs at the time of injury demonstrate endosteal changes, lateral bowing, and a transverse line extending from the lateral cortex.

contralateral limb because both femurs have been exposed to the same bisphosphonate risk for an AFF. The contralateral limb should be x-rayed when there is any suspicion that the femur fracture being treated is related to bisphosphonate use. It is important to inquire about the duration of any bisphosphonate therapy or other bone metabolizing medications.

CRITERIA FOR AN ATYPICAL FRACTURE

The American Society for Bone and Mineral Research (ASBMR) task force developed an initial (2010) and then a revised (2014) case definition of AFFs (4,8). Its definition for an AFF is that of a fracture located along the femoral diaphysis from just distal to the lesser trochanter to just proximal to the supracondylar flare. At least four of the five major features should be present (see Figure 12.1a) (4,15).

Major features

1. Fracture is located anywhere along the femur from just distal to the lesser trochanter to just proximal to the supracondylar flare.
2. Associated with no trauma or minimal trauma, as in a fall from a standing height or less.
3. Transverse or short oblique configuration.

4. Noncomminuted.
5. Complete fractures extend through both cortices and may be associated with a medial spike; incomplete fractures involve only the lateral cortex.

Minor features

1. Localized periosteal reaction of the lateral cortex
2. Generalized increase in cortical thickness of the diaphysis
3. Prodromal symptoms such as dull or aching pain in the groin or thigh
4. Bilateral fractures and symptoms
5. Delayed healing
6. Comorbid conditions (e.g., vitamin D deficiency, rheumatoid arthritis, hypophosphatasia)
7. Use of pharmaceutical agents (e.g., bisphosphonates, glucocorticoids, proton pump inhibitors)

TREATMENT OPTIONS

Complete fractures

A complete fracture requires surgery, and the patient must be optimized for the procedure. Pre-op workup should include full-length femur radiographs, laboratory investigations (including bone profile), and Orthogeriatric/Internal Medicine review. First presentation of subtrochanteric or diaphyseal AFF can be treated with a cephalomedullary nail in most cases. This is dependent on adequate reduction, bone contact, and alignment (Figure 12.2a). Patients on long-term bisphosphonate who have fractures may have both increased anterior and increased lateral bowing of the femur. It is imperative to focus on the correct entry point for antegrade nailing. Ensure that the entry point is at the junction of the anterior and middle third of the trochanter on the lateral intraoperative fluoroscopic view. This is important to allow adequate reduction of the fracture and also to prevent anterior cortex perforation distally (16). In a trochanteric entry nail, the entry point on the anteroposterior (AP) intraoperative fluoroscopic view needs to be at the highest point and most medial point on the trochanter. Allowing the entry point to inadvertently drift laterally on the trochanter will create a varus deformity in the proximal femur, which is associated with an increased risk of failure (Figure 12.3a) (17).

Evidence suggests that although time to healing is increased for bisphosphonate fractures, intramedullary nailing should remain the mainstay of treatment on primary presentation (18). Experience has shown us that these AFFs occur after the femur has developed a varus deformity proximally. If the varus deformity of the proximal femur is not adequately corrected and reduced at the time of initial antegrade nailing, then there is a high risk of failure (see Figure 12.3a,b) (19–21).

Impending fracture

Patients on long-term bisphosphonate therapy may present with symptoms of pain without a history of injury. Radiographs may show an incomplete or impending fracture (see Figure 12.1b). An impending fracture can often be described as the dreaded black line on x-rays. It is advised that any patient who has an atypical fracture on one side

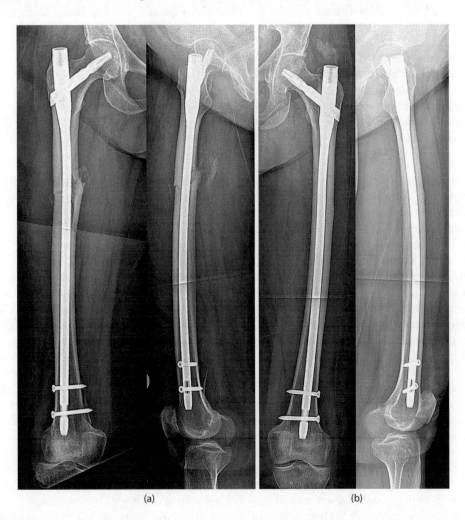

(a)　　　　　　　　　　　　　(b)

Figure 12.2 (a) Anteroposterior (AP) and lateral radiographs following treatment of a right atypical femur fracture from patient in Figure 12.1a. A cephalomedullary (trochanteric femoral nail) was inserted along with debridement of the femoral stress fracture using an osteotome through a small incision. Bone graft and Bone Morphogenic Protein was placed along with reamer bone graft biological augmentation. X-ray is at 26 months and shows complete union of the fracture. Note the correct entry point on the AP and lateral x-rays. (b) Left femoral AP and lateral radiographs 26 months following surgery illustrate healed atypical fracture in the patient from Figure 12.1b. Patient symptoms have settled, and black line has disappeared.

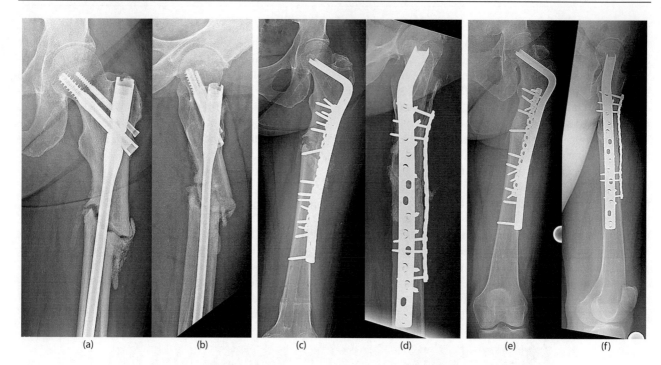

(a) (b) (c) (d) (e) (f)

Figure 12.3 (a) Femoral nail in varus malreduction. (Note that the lateral entry point for the nail and the profile of the lesser trochanter is suspicious for a rotational malalignment.) (b) Lateral x-ray showing malreduction of the fracture. The proximal segment remains flexed. The nail diameter is also too small for this medullary canal. (c) Post-op anteroposterior (AP) radiograph of salvage surgery with orthogonal plating technique. (Note the effort needed with the blade plate to take the fracture out of varus.) (d) Post-op lateral radiograph showing reduction of the previously flexed proximal segment. This is done using the anterior plate initially before application of the blade plate. (e) One-year post-op AP radiograph. (f) One-year post-op lateral radiograph.

and a history of prolonged bisphosphonate exposure has radiographic imaging performed on the contralateral side with AP and lateral images of the femur. Radiological signs include endosteal thickening of the lateral cortex, transverse black lines that usually appear to start at the lateral cortex (see Figure 12.1b). It is estimated that up to 40% of patients who present with a bisphosphonate AFF on one side will have the contralateral femur affected (22). If there is doubt about the contralateral side, then advanced imaging including computed tomography (CT) and magnetic resonance imaging (MRI) have been advocated to confirm the effect on the femur. MRI can also be utilized for follow-up to evaluate the success of conservative treatment.

The ASBMR recommends that patients with incomplete fractures and no pain, or those with periosteal thickening but no cortical lucency, should limit weight-bearing and avoid vigorous activity. Reduced activity should be continued until there is no bone edema detected on an MRI or no increased activity detected on a bone scan (4). Patients who have pain and radiological signs of impending fracture should be treated surgically to reduce symptoms and prevent progression to complete fracture. It has been suggested that up to 30% of patients with radiographic changes go on to a complete fracture within 6 months (4). It is our preference to treat these patients with a cephalomedullary nail to protect the femoral neck as well as address the impending fracture (Figure 12.2b). This prophylactic procedure can be done during the same admission to hospital but in a

separate surgical session. It would be our preference that the surgery is staged approximately 7–10 days apart.

Nonunion of atypical fractures

In our experience, each patient presenting with a nonunion will have individual nuances that need to be appreciated, but general principles can be applied in all cases. Although it is well recognized that these patients with AFF have a high need for revision surgery, the underlying diagnosis of infection must always be considered. History and examination should identify any suggestion of infection. Red flags to look out for are a history of wound-healing problems, continued ooze following the index procedure, previous courses of antibiotics, or even previous washouts. Preoperative workup involves checking the white cell count, C-reactive protein, and erythrocyte sedimentation rate. If indicated, an aspiration can be performed and a staged procedure utilized with both local and systemic delivery of antibiotics between stages.

When the nonunion surgery is to be undertaken, it is vital to never underestimate the importance of preoperative planning. It must be established what exactly the previous fixation method was and the reason for failure. What exact metalwork/hardware will have to be removed (which manufacturer and specific implants), and if the hardware is broken, how will this complicate extraction?

After many years of experience with different techniques, our preference for definitive reconstruction for these failed AFF cases is an orthogonal plating method, involving a 95° blade plate (4.5 mm) in combination with an anterior 3.5 mm plate (23). We have achieved good results with this technique and find it allows excellent fracture reduction and, importantly, adequate compression. The method of using the blade plate reliably takes the fracture, which has usually failed in varus into a more physiologic valgus alignment allowing forces to work with the hardware to optimize the chances of osseous union. Preoperative AP and lateral radiographs and CT scan imaging are carefully scrutinized for angular and rotational deformity. It is crucial to template blade insertion angle to adequately correct varus angulation. This often means inserting the blade at less than 95° in relation to the femoral shaft.

For the procedure, the patient is positioned supine on a radiolucent Jackson table with a bump placed under the affected hip. Previous incisions are extended to accommodate a lateral subvastus approach to the proximal femur and facilitate implant removal.

The guidewire for a 95° angled blade plate (Synthes, Paoli, Pennsylvania) is placed at the previously templated angle relative to the femoral shaft in the coronal plane and centrally through the femoral neck on the sagittal plane in order to restore appropriate proximal femoral valgus angulation. The seating chisel is then inserted and used to gain control of the proximal fragment.

The nonunion is then debrided back to bleeding bone. All fibrous tissue and callous are meticulously removed from the nonunion, and cultures are sent to rule out indolent infection. The healthy bone edges are freshened with osteotomes and a 2.0 mm drill. Reduction is then obtained with standard reduction clamps. A 3.5 mm reconstruction plate (Synthes) is contoured and provisionally applied to the anteromedial surface of the femur in order to control sagittal plane forces and act as an additional clamp for the blade placement.

The chisel is then removed, and the blade plate is inserted. Care is taken to obtain anatomical alignment in both the coronal and sagittal planes on fluoroscopy. The defect within the head and neck secondary to the removed cephalomedullary screw is generally beneath the blade plate and should be filled with allograft chips or demineralized bone matrix prior to plate application. With the 3.5 mm reconstruction plate offering malleable bony support and preventing a flexion deformity, an articulated tensioning device is then used to compress the fracture through the blade plate. Both plates are then completely secured to the femur with cortical screw fixation, and when possible, interfragmentary fixation (either through the blade or through the 3.5 mm plate) is placed after the fracture has been appropriately tensioned. The wounds are irrigated, and biological augmentation is added as per surgeon preference. The wounds are closed in a layered fashion over a drain (23).

Case example 1 shown in Figure 12.3a,b presents an AFF that was initially treated with a reconstruction nail, but the reduction was suboptimal. Note on the AP x-ray (Figure 12.3a) the fracture has been left in varus malalignment. On the lateral x-ray (Figure 12.3b), the proximal fragment is flexed relative to the distal fragment. In this example, the diameter of the femoral nail is also too small for the femoral canal and therefore not giving enough stability at the fracture site. This patient had ongoing pain because the fracture was not uniting. Figure 12.3c,d show the postoperative x-ray films following removal of the nail and treatment with the orthogonal plating technique (NB correction of the flexion and varus deformity). One year following surgery the patient's pain had resolved, and x-rays (Figure 12.3e,f) show complete bony union.

Case example 2 illustrates an example where the wrong device was selected for the presenting fracture type. Figure 12.4a–c show the sequential failure of an AFF fixed initially with a two-hole sliding hip screw (SHS). Progressive varus at the fracture site was noted as the construct gradually failed. This case was treated by removing the SHS and using the orthogonal plating technique to reduce the deformity (i.e., flexion and varus) and compress the fracture. (Figure 12.4d,e are the postoperative x-rays, and Figure 12.4f shows the radiographs at 1 year illustrating fracture union.)

Case example 3 demonstrates an AFF initially treated with a cephalomedullary nail (Figure 12.5a,b) that failed to progress to osseous union in an expected time frame (Figure 12.5c,d). Hence, the hardware underwent fatigue failure (Figure 12.5e). This was initially revised with a single blade plate (Figure 12.5f). This represents our learning curve with the technique and shows how even with the blade plate it is essential to get adequate bone contact and compression so as to encourage healing. Good bone contact also improves load sharing between the bone and the hardware device, so giving sufficient time for union prior to fatigue of the hardware. In this example, the fracture was slow to unite (Figure 12.5g); hence, the blade plate fatigued (Figure 12.5h). All is not lost and this case was salvaged with our orthogonal plating technique (Figure 12.5i,j) and shows how it can be used in such challenging cases to ultimately achieve osseous union (Figure 12.5k).

We employ the "diamond concept" described by Giannoudis et al. in treating patients with nonunions. The diamond concept has five different factors that must be present for therapy to work:

1. Osteogenic cells
2. Osteoconductive scaffold
3. Osteoinductive growth factors
4. Adequate vascularity
5. Favorable mechanical environment

For our patients, this entails biological supplementation of nonunions with growth factors, mesenchymal cells, and scaffolding (24). Patients who have presented as a nonunion in our unit are assessed for a metabolic bone work through a specialist in our institution's metabolic bone service. This involves assessing parathormone, 25-hydroxyvitamin D, calcium, and bone-specific alkaline phosphatase.

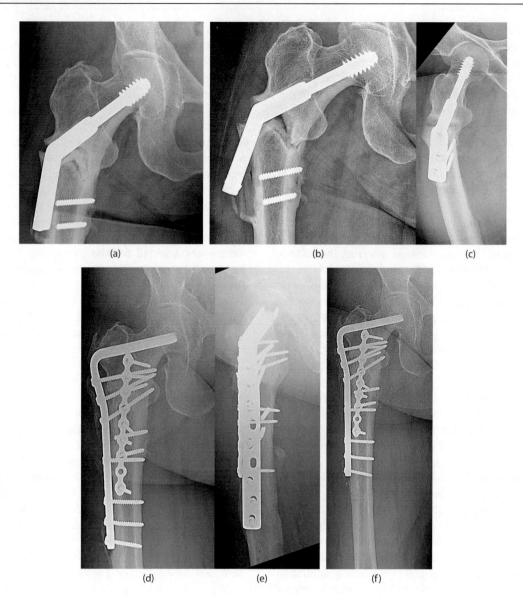

Figure 12.4 (a) Atypical femoral fracture fixed with a sliding hip screw. (Note the residual varus at the level of the fracture.) (b) Failing sliding hip screw fixation (anteroposterior [AP] radiograph). (c) Failing sliding hip screw fixation (lateral radiograph). (d) Salvage surgery with orthogonal plating technique using a blade plate (AP radiograph). (e) Post-op salvage surgery (lateral radiograph). (f) One year after salvage surgery (AP radiograph).

The majority of patients receive supplementation of vitamin D and calcium. Recent publications have suggested that there may be a role for teriparatide in reducing the time to union for patients undergoing revision surgery for previous failed fixation of an AFF (25).

Method of mobilization

It has been our preference to treat patients postoperatively with early mobilization, with toe-touch weight-bearing to a maximum of 20 pounds for the first 4 weeks and then to gradually progress to full weight-bearing under the supervision of a physiotherapist. This has been our postoperative protocol for patients treated with a cephalomedullary nail for a first presentation and for those revision patients treated

with our dual-plating technique. The protocol allows patients to regain confidence mobilizing, allow the soft tissues to settle, and then introduce full weight-bearing and more active rehabilitation exercises once the wound is healed, quads function has returned, and postoperative pain has resolved.

Patients with AFFs are often elderly, poly-comorbid and have poor tolerance for prolonged immobility. Recent research has highlighted the dangers of immobility in the elderly and the inability of elderly patients to comply with protected weight-bearing instructions(26). Therefore, we work closely with our physiotherapists and rehabilitation physicians to ensure that patients are not exposed to the high risks of immobility if they fail with protected weight-bearing. In these instances, we ask the patients to mobilize weight-bearing as tolerated but with the support of a walker frame for 6 weeks.

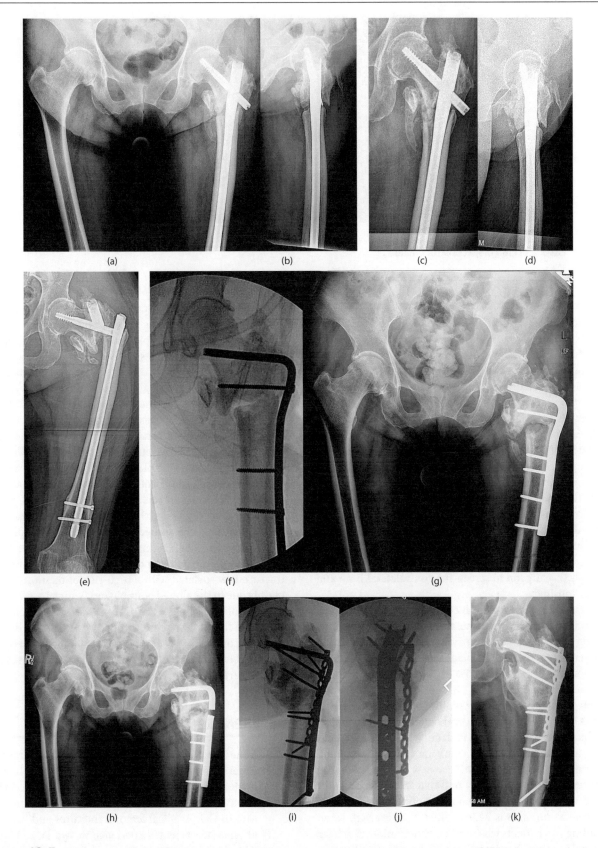

Figure 12.5 (a) Anteroposterior radiograph of atypical femoral fracture (AFF) treated with cephalomedullary nail. (b) Lateral radiograph of AFF treated with cephalomedullary nail. (c) AFF slow to unite. (d) Lateral x-ray showing no evidence of union. (e) Ultimate fatigue failure of the device due to nonunion. (f) Fluoroscopy showing correction of varus but not enough bone contact or compression of the fracture. (g) Fracture not healing. Insufficient reduction or bone contact. Not enough load sharing with the plate. (h) Ultimate fatigue failure of the blade plate. (i) Revision to orthogonal plating with good bone contact and compression. (j) Second plate placed anteriorly. (k) Fracture went on to unite after orthogonal plating.

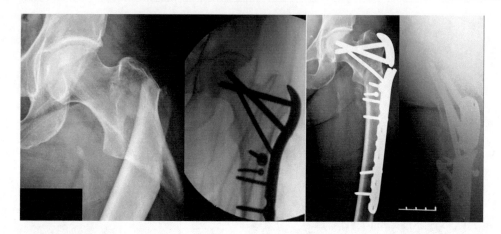

Figure 12.6 Locking plate construct failure.

EXPECTED OUTCOMES

It is expected that the majority of patients on long-term bisphosphonate therapy will not experience the complication of an AFF. However, it is recognized that there is a definite increased relative risk to the normal population, and it is estimated that long-term bisphosphonate use is associated with a 100 per 100,000 person-years risk (4). Research is ongoing into why certain people develop AFFs while others do not given the same exposure to bisphosphonates. The role of a bisphosphonate holiday and how this might reduce the AFF incidence further is another area of important research (27,28).

For those who do experience an AFF, recognition of the fracture pattern is vital to patient outcome. Recognition alerts the surgeon of the high risk of failure associated with this fracture type compared to other more common fractures in this area. Recognition is also important so as to direct the surgeon to screen the contralateral limb and treat accordingly.

A systematic review by Koh et al. suggested with respect to overall results in all treatments (intramedullary nailing, locking compression plating, dynamic hip screw, dynamic condylar screw, and angled blade plate) that fracture healing should be expected in 85% of patients after the index procedure (15).

Antegrade intramedullary nailing on first presentation of an AFF is associated with good outcomes for the majority of patients, with attention to detail with fastidious technique, and should be the surgeon's mainstay of treatment. Lee et al. found in a retrospective review of 75 AFFs treated by antegrade intramedullary nail that 29 (63%) fractures healed within 6 months without complications. The average time to union was 24.9 weeks (11–48 weeks), when excluding two patients who went on to nonunion. A greater percentage of AFFs primarily treated with plate fixation require revision surgery (31.3%) than fractures treated with intramedullary nailing (12.9%) (15).

Our experience with single plating of AFF demonstrated mixed results. When using locking plates, there can be failure in up to 30% of cases (29). Even well-reduced constructs can

fail (Figure 12.6). This may be due to the increased time to union for AFFs on bisphosphonates, meaning the construct is exposed to strain for longer; hence, there is greater risk of hardware fatigue. Locking plate constructs may be especially vulnerable due to the stiffness of the construct and the length of time that there is stress concentration on the plate at the point where it fatigued (Figure 12.6). Our theory is that an orthogonal plate reconstruction gives more balance to the fixation. Excellent compression of the bone means there is good bone contact and hence improved load sharing. Also, the strength of the blade plate is more resistant to failure. We have experience of blade plate fracture when used without the supplemental plate, adequate bone contact, and load sharing. Ultimately this case was addressed with our dual-plating technique and progressed to ultimate osseous union.

In summary, AFF related to prolonged bisphosphonate usage presents a challenging problem for today's orthopedic surgeons. The patient population is often frail, and the fracture is associated with a high risk of fixation failure, mainly due to the altered bone biology, which increases the time to union and hence the time that hardware is exposed to fatigue failure. We presented our experience in dealing with the complications of this fracture along with a robust and reliable technique that can be used in those cases that require revision.

REFERENCES

1. Bone HG, Hosking D, Devogelaer JP et al. Ten years' experience with alendronate for osteoporosis in postmenopausal women. *N Engl J Med*. 2004;350(12):1189.
2. Thompson RN, Phillips JR, McCauley SH, Elliott JR, Moran CG. Atypical femoral fractures and bisphosphonate treatment: Experience in two large United Kingdom teaching hospitals. *J Bone Joint Surg Br*. 2012;94(3):385.
3. Warren C, Gilchrist N, Coates M, Frampton C, Helmore J, McKie J, Hooper G. Atypical subtrochanteric fractures, bisphosphonates, blinded radiological review. *ANZ J Surg*. 2012;82(12):908.

4. Shane E, Burr D, Abrahamsen B et al. Atypical sub-trochanteric and diaphyseal femoral fractures: Second report of a task force of the American Society for Bone and Mineral Research. *J Bone Miner Res.* 2014;29(1):1.

5. Phillips HK, Harrison SJ, Akrawi H, Sidhom SA. Retrospective review of patients with atypical bisphosphonate related proximal femoral fractures. *Injury* 2017;48(6):1159.

6. Nieves JW, Cosman F. Atypical subtrochanteric and femoral shaft fractures and possible association with bisphosphonates. *Curr Osteoporos Rep.* 2010;8(1):34.

7. Wells GA, Cranney A, Peterson J et al. Alendronate for the primary and secondary prevention of osteoporotic fractures in postmenopausal women. *Cochrane Database Syst Rev.* 2008;23(1):CD001155.

8. Shane E, Burr D, Ebeling PR et al. Atypical subtrochanteric and diaphyseal femoral fractures: Report of a task force of the American Society for Bone and Mineral Research. *J Bone Miner Res.* 2010;25(11):2267.

9. Adams AL, Adams JL, Raebel MA et al. Bisphosphonate drug holiday and fracture risk: A population-based cohort study. *J Bone Miner Res.* 2018;33(7):1252.

10. Lovy AJ, Koehler SM, Keswani A, Joseph D, Hasija R, Ghillani R. Atypical femur fracture during bisphosphonate drug holiday: A case series. *Osteoporos Int.* 2015;26(6):1755.

11. Kong SY, Kim DY, Han EJ et al. Effects of a "drug holiday" on bone mineral density and bone turnover marker during bisphosphonate therapy. *J Bone Metab.* 2013;20(1):31.

12. Ettinger B, Burr DB, Ritchie RO. Proposed pathogenesis for atypical femoral fractures: Lessons from materials research. *Bone.* 2013;55(2):495.

13. Geissler JR, Bajaj D, Fritton JC. American Society of Biomechanics Journal of Biomechanics Award 2013: Cortical bone tissue mechanical quality and biological mechanisms possibly underlying atypical fractures. *J Biomech.* 2015;48(6):883.

14. Kang JS, Won YY, Kim JO et al. Atypical femoral fractures after anti-osteoporotic medication: A Korean multicenter study. *Inte Orthop.* 2014;38(6):1247.

15. Koh A, Guerado E, Giannoudis PV. Atypical femoral fractures related to bisphosphonate treatment: Issues and controversies related to their surgical management. *Bone Joint J.* 2017;99-B(3):295.

16. Park JH, Lee Y, Shon OJ, Shon HC, Kim JW. Surgical tips of intramedullary nailing in severely bowed femurs in atypical femur fractures: Simulation with 3D printed model. *Injury* 2016;47(6):1318.

17. Yoon RS, Donegan DJ, Liporace FA. Reducing subtrochanteric femur fractures: Tips and tricks, do's and don'ts. *J Orthop Trauma.* 2015;29(Suppl 4):S28.

18. Egol KA, Park JH, Rosenberg ZS, Peck V, Tejwani NC. Healing delayed but generally reliable after bisphosphonate-associated complete femur fractures treated with IM nails. *Clin Orthop Relat Res.* 2014;472(9):2728.

19. Lee KJ, Yoo JJ, Oh KJ et al. Surgical outcome of intramedullary nailing in patients with complete atypical femoral fracture: A multicenter retrospective study. *Injury.* 2017;48(4):941.

20. Jiang L, Zheng Q, Pan Z. What is the fracture displacement influence to fracture non-union in intramedullary nail treatment in subtrochanteric fracture? *J Clin Orthop Trauma.* 2018;9(4):317.

21. Ruecker AH, Rueger JM. Pertrochanteric fractures: Tips and tricks in nail osteosynthesis. *Eur J Trauma Emerg Surg.* 2014;40(3):249.

22. Schilcher J, Aspenberg P. Incidence of stress fractures of the femoral shaft in women treated with bisphosphonate. *Acta Orthop.* 2009;80(4):413.

23. Rollick NC, Bear J, Diamond O, Wellman DS, Helfet DL. Orthogonal plating with a 95° blade plate for salvage of unsuccessful cephalomedullary nailing of atypic femur fractures: A technical trick. *J Orthop Trauma.* 2019;33(6):e246–e250.

24. Giannoudis PV, Ahmad MA, Mineo GV, Tosounidis TI, Calori GM, Kanakaris NK. Subtrochanteric fracture non-unions with implant failure managed with the "Diamond" concept. *Injury.* 2013;44(Suppl 1):S76.

25. Mastaglia SR, Aguilar G, Oliveri B. Teriparatide for the rapid resolution of delayed healing of atypical fractures associated with long-term bisphosphonate use. *Eur J Rheumatol.* 2016;3(2):87.

26. Kammerlander C, Pfeufer D, Lisitano LA, Mehaffey S, Bocker W, Neuerburg C. Inability of older adult patients with hip fracture to maintain postoperative weight-bearing restrictions. *J Bone Joint Surg Am.* 2018;100(11):936.

27. McClung MR. Bisphosphonate therapy: How long is long enough? *Osteoporos Int.* 2015;26(5):1455.

28. McClung M, Harris ST, Miller PD et al. Bisphosphonate therapy for osteoporosis: Benefits, risks, and drug holiday. *Am J Med.* 2013;126(1):13.

29. Prasarn ML, Ahn J, Helfet DL, Lane JM, Lorich DG. Bisphosphonate-associated femur fractures have high complication rates with operative fixation. *Clin Orthop Relat Res.* 2012;470(8):2295.

13

Biomechanical considerations for fixation of osteoporotic bone

PETER AUGAT and CHRISTIAN VON RÜDEN

MECHANICAL PROPERTIES OF BONE

Bone's main physical function is to provide the skeletal support for the body and enable movement and load transfer between joints. Bone has the unique feature to adapt itself to a changing mechanical environment by bone remodeling. In young and healthy bone, its composition and functional competence are maintained by a well-balanced osteoclastic bone resorption and osteoblastic bone formation. This functional adaptation is achieved by an orchestrated remodeling process resulting in adaptation of bone structure and of intrinsic material properties. Later in life, age and osteoporosis lead to bone loss caused by an imbalanced and excessive bone remodeling (1). The loss of bone mineral becomes apparent by a reduction in bone mineral density as measured by computed tomography (CT) or dual-energy x-ray absorptiometry (DEXA) and at later stages is visible on plain x-ray images. Associated with the loss of bone mineral and change in material properties is also a dramatic change in bone mechanical competence. The mechanical competence of bone determines its resistance to fracture and response to external loads. During aging and osteoporosis, the amount of bone is reduced, the microarchitecture destabilized, and the intrinsic material properties deteriorated, leading to enhanced bone fragility and increased fracture risk. This becomes clinically manifested with an age- and osteoporosis-related increase of bone fractures (2). Age-related degradation of mechanical competence of bone appears to be more pronounced for mechanical properties associated with bone failure than for those associated with bone stiffness. While elastic moduli in tension or compression, which describe the stiffness of bone, degrade by only about 2% per decade, failure properties like toughness or ultimate strain show an age-related decrease of about 5%–10% per decade (3).

While the role of the inorganic components on bone's mechanical competence is reasonably well understood, much less is known about the effect of collagenous and noncollagenous proteins. Ninety percent of bone's organic matrix is composed of type I collagen, a structural protein composed of three polypeptide chains with a defined amino acid sequence. There is increasing evidence suggesting that changes in protein content and structure play important roles in age- and disease-related changes in bone (4). In particular, the organic matrix is considered to be responsible for bone's ductility and its ability to absorb energy prior to fracturing (5,6). Collagen undergoes numerous posttranslational modifications with aging and disease, including both enzymatic and nonenzymatic cross-linking. Enzymatic cross-linking of collagen is generally considered to have a positive effect on bone's mechanical properties, while nonenzymatic cross-linking can lead to deteriorated bone mechanical properties with aging and disease. Noncollagenous proteins (e.g., osteopontin, osteocalcin), which compose 10% of bone's organic matrix, may act as the glue that holds mineralized collagen fibers together and thus may play a role in the prevention of harmful microdamage formation.

The age- and osteoporosis-related changes in bone mass, bone architecture, and bone material properties lead to a dramatic decline in bone's mechanical competence. At the age of 80 years, bone strength of the proximal femur is reduced by more than 50% from its strength at a young age (7). Even more pronounced is the loss of mechanical competence at the spine where the strength reduction during lifetime has been reported to amount to up to 70% (8). These dramatic age-related changes in the material properties indicate that the factor of risk for fracture is increased, and traumatic events that are benign at a young age will become enormously hazardous in the elderly. With aging, not only the strength of bone decreases but also the loads acting on the skeleton change. Muscle performance and coordination deteriorate and lead to an increased risk of falling. Elderly individuals also have a decreased ability to support falls. The energy generated during a fall largely exceeds the energy required to cause a fracture of the

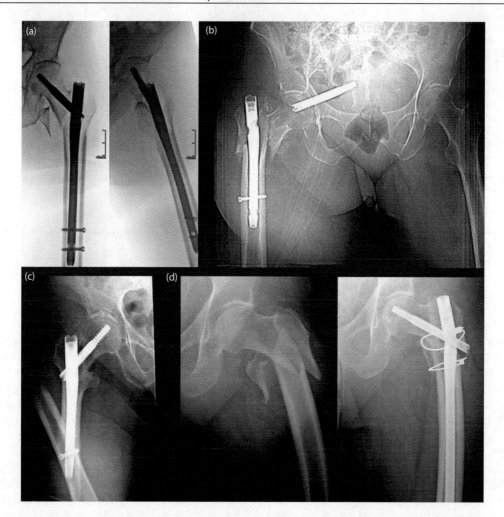

Figure 13.1 Complications in fractures of the femur due to adequate trauma in patients with advanced age and/or osteoporosis. (a) Unstable fixation due to lack of lateral support of the lag screw in an AO/OTA type A3.3 fracture. (b) Loosening and migration of the lag screw in a cephalomedullary nail. (c) Inadequate length of intramedullary implant after femoral shaft fracture. (d) Failure of intramedullary nail after fixation of unstable AO/OTA type A3.3 fracture.

femur. Thus, without any energy absorption by soft tissue dampening, muscle contraction, or compensatory movement, the load acting on the femur during falling would inevitably lead to hip fracture (9).

Finally, fractures in individuals with advanced age and osteoporosis also occur during high-energy traumatic events (10). Due to changes in lifestyle, the activity level of elderly individuals is continuously increasing. Accordingly, the risk of accidents with adequate trauma that will lead to fracture also increases. These fractures related to adequate traumatic events often do not present at those locations typical for fractures due to osteoporosis but require similar attention (Figure 13.1).

FRACTURE FIXATION IN OSTEOPOROTIC BONE

The reduction of bone's mechanical competence with age and osteoporosis not only leads to an increased risk for fractures but also aggravates their operative treatment.

The outcome of fracture treatment in frail patients often is unpredictable and often results in catastrophic failure of internal fracture fixation. In these situations, fixation often fails from failure of bone rather than breakage of the metallic implant (11). The consequences of failure of the bone around metallic implants are multifaceted but typically include loss of fracture reduction, malalignment, and penetration of metallic implants into joints or other places were implants do not belong. (Figure 13.1 shows a screw cut out after trochanteric fracture fixation in osteoporotic bone.) Often these bone failures occur gradually rather than during a singular catastrophic event. The friction between the metallic implant and the bone causes complete destruction of the already rarified bone and typically leaves empty cavities behind, a situation that is only to be solved by joint replacement.

Age and osteoporosis reduce the fixation strength for internal fracture fixation implants and constitute a challenge for stable and enduring fracture fixation (12). The fixation strength of osteosynthesis implants is reduced by up to 70% in osteoporotic and aged bone compared to normal healthy bone (13). Typically, the strength reduction is more pronounced for implants in trabecular bone compared to implants for long bones and shaft fractures. Implants for long bone and shaft fractures typically rely on implant fixation in cortical bone. Osteoporosis and aging affect cortical bone primarily by thinning of the cortex; thus, the reduction of implant fixation strength is associated with loss of cortical thickness. Compared to thick cortices, the holding force decreases by 1000 N (or 50%) per 1 mm loss of cortical thickness. This might generate differences in the holding power of bone screws of up to 2000 N within an individual bone and highlights the importance of placing bone screws in the bone with thick cortices wherever possible (14).

PRINCIPLES OF FRACTURE FIXATION IN OSTEOPOROTIC BONE

Implants that are employed for open reduction and internal fixation (ORIF) have commonly been developed for normal, healthy bone. Recently, more and more implants provide optional features addressing typical complications occurring in elderly and osteoporotic bone. Successful fracture treatment still relies on accurate and stable fixation of the fracture. Moreover, fracture fixation in osteoporotic bone needs to be stable enough to allow for immediate weight-bearing, as the elderly can typically not cope with reduced weight-bearing recommendations.

In osteoporotic bone, it is paramount to consequently and thoughtfully apply the techniques for stable fracture fixation. Often it might be necessary to modify these techniques in order to improve and optimize the fixation and achieve satisfactory healing results (15).

Fracture treatment by ORIF has the following aims:

a. Primary stability of the fracture in order to initiate fracture healing under functional movement
b. Correct alignment and adequate fracture reduction in order to avoid malalignment and inadequate joint loading
c. Secondary stability in order to enable bony consolidation
d. Promotion of bone formation and prevention of delayed union or nonunion

Primary stability

Primary stability of the fracture after ORIF is a prerequisite for successful fracture healing under functional movement, partial or full weight-bearing. Achieving sufficient primary stability in osteoporotic bone requires consequent application of basic biomechanical principles. The most critical point in fracture fixation of osteoporotic bone constitutes the interface between osteosynthesis implant and bone. Thus, one important goal should be to minimize stress at the bone and implant interface. This can be successfully achieved by choosing internal fixation devices that allow

load sharing with the host bone. The most intuitive way to maximize load sharing is obtained by fixation devices providing a large contact area between implant and bone. Plates should be long, providing many locking options, and should be broad, providing larger surface areas and more possibilities for screw placement. Plates with a larger contact area effectively reduce the local compressional strain on the bone. Similarly, more thinner screws generate smaller local strain in cortical as well as trabecular bone compared to fewer thicker screws (16). Thinner screws have the additional advantage of providing more flexibility and thus the ability to distribute the load within a larger volume of bone, thus reducing local stress on bone tissue. But using more screws for fracture fixation increases construct stiffness and dynamic stability, while at the same time, screw penetration becomes more likely due to elevated strain in the bone around the screws (17). Thus, an improvement in primary stability does not necessarily lead to improved secondary stability, and vice versa (see later in chapter).

Intramedullary implants achieve load sharing by intramedullary contact of the nail and by interlocking of the screws. Longer nails having multiple locking options are ideally suited to minimize stress within bone areas that are in contact with the screws. Increased bone contact of the nail in the intramedullary canal has shown to considerably improve fixation stability (18). Increased bone contact can be achieved by purchase of the nail tip in subchondral bone, which has shown to increase fixation stability and decrease stress around locking screws (18). Also, longer nails, larger nail thickness, and adequate reaming of the intramedullary canal can all increase nail bone contact and thus lead to better stability of long bone fractures (Figure 13.2) (19). Not only the nail itself but also the locking screws provide possibilities to improve fixation stability in intramedullary nailing. Modern intramedullary nails provide a multitude of locking options, particularly at the metaphyseal site of the nail. The design (20) of the locking screws and their number (21,22) both have shown to improve primary fixation stability. Interestingly, by locking the nail in a freehand technique, which is often required for distal locking in longer nails, the locking screws get jammed by their imperfect alignment and this improves fixation stability, in particular the torsional and shear stability in long bone fractures (Figure 13.3) (23).

Correct alignment and accurate fracture reduction

Correct alignment and accurate fracture reduction are essential to obtain good functional outcome and an adequate healing response. Only with correct functional alignment can the load transfer through the fracture and through the adjacent joints be reconstituted. The first and most important step in fracture fixation is thus the correct alignment of the load axes. Fractures involving the joint require in addition anatomical reduction to restore the bony anatomy and joint surfaces. As reduced weight-bearing or

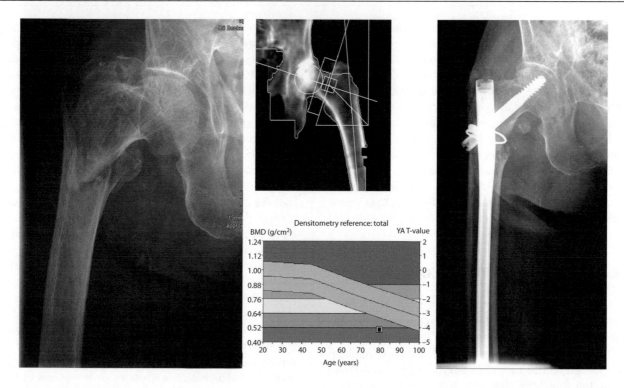

Figure 13.2 Trochanteric fracture in an 80-year-old man with severe osteoporosis (T: −4.1) fixed with a long Gamma nail (Stryker, Mahwah, New Jersey) and one additional cerclage providing axial and bending stiffness.

unloading of the fracture is often impossible for elderly and fragile individuals, maintenance of fracture reduction typically requires osteosynthesis of the fracture.

Whenever possible, ligamentotaxis should be employed to initiate the reduction of the fracture. If necessary, the reduction needs to be performed by open reduction of the fracture fragments. Prior to the application of the osteosynthesis, the alignment of the correct load axes and the correct rotation of the anatomical axes need to be verified. Care has to be taken to maintain these axes during the application of the osteosynthesis. Precontoured anatomical locked plates have the inherent risk to readjust fracture

fragments if reduction is not maintained during their application. In contrast to conventional plates, locked plates cannot be employed for fracture reduction but need to be applied to an already reduced fracture. Angle variability of the locking screws may additionally impede reduction maintenance, as those screws may deflect at the end of the screw insertion process. Thus, for contoured locking plates, the correct and careful placement of the first screws in the joint block is paramount. In the shaft area, temporary conventional screws may assist the alignment of the plate by pulling the plate toward the prealigned fracture. Care has to be taken so as not to lose correct alignment by pulling

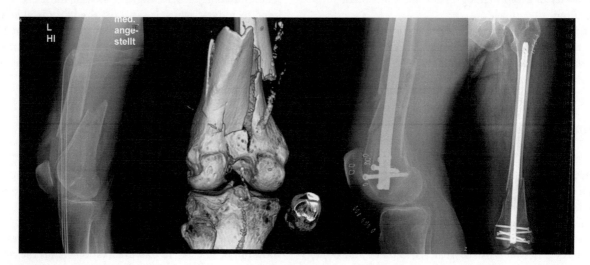

Figure 13.3 Distal femur AO/OTA type C3 fracture in an 86-year-old woman after slipping in the bathroom. Fixation with long retrograde femur nail using multiple locking screw options.

the fracture fragments toward the plate. Depending on the fixation principle, the conventional screw should be removed or replaced by a locking screw in order to avoid a stress rising effect at the plate.

If the aim of the fracture fixation is to rigidly fix the fracture and promote direct bone healing, compressional techniques can be employed to perfect the reduction maneuver. Lag screws are frequently employed to readjust bone blocks in metaphyseal fractures. These lag screws can also be employed to readjust diaphyseal fractures. In any case, lag screw fixations need to be secured by buttress plates in the metaphyseal area and neutralization plates in the diaphyseal area. Fracture compression can also be achieved by mechanisms inherent to the fixation implant. In extramedullary as well as in intramedullary implants, compression techniques allow for a well-controlled adaptation of fracture fragments and effective fracture reduction but may be technically demanding (24–26). In addition to improving the fracture reduction, compression provides increased primary and secondary stability by load sharing between implant and bone (27). The biomechanical principle of intramedullary compression osteosynthesis is based on the implantation of a movable intramedullary nail that is statically interlocked in distal round holes and dynamically interlocked in a proximal oblong hole. Distraction of the nail against the proximal interlocking screw by means of a compression screw leads to a relative movement of the proximal fragment directed distally against the nail (27). In simple fractures, nonunions, and osteotomies, this results in direct contact of the main fragments under increasing compression. In humerus fractures, compression interlocking has been shown to reduce the fracture gap and increase the biomechanical stiffness (28). However, it included the risk of bending or loosening of the locking screw in the dynamic oblong holes. Thus, it has been recommended to add an additional static locking screw and provide more axial stability of the construct (28). Also, fractures of the tibial shaft have been shown to benefit from compression nailing if the fractures are mostly transverse and have sufficient surface contact among the main fragments (29). Through better fracture reduction, increased mechanical stability, and decreased shear movement (19), the time to bony union and the rate of delayed unions can be significantly reduced by compression (29,30). It should be mentioned that the forces generated by compression of the fracture fragments can easily exceed 1000 N (29); therefore, compression should be applied with caution and gently in osteoporotic bone to avoid iatrogenic fractures.

Finally, bone transplants (autologous spongiosa), bone grafts, or bone cements play an important role in obtaining adequate and sustaining fracture reduction. These materials support the restoration of joint surfaces and enable their correct alignment (31). Residual voids and gaps can be filled even if they are quite irregular by injectable material. If joint surfaces can be accurately reconstructed with sufficient stability, functional movement and joint loading can be initiated earlier and complications associated with prolonged joint immobilization can be avoided.

Secondary stability

Secondary stability of fracture fixation is required to enable bony consolidation and maintain anatomical alignment. It first relies on sufficient primary stability. Secondary stability under weight-bearing and functional movement cannot be achieved without primary stability of the fracture fixation construct. In addition, bone fatigue by brittle failure, creep, or trabecular crushing has to be prevented. In osteoporotic bone, the limiting factor for secondary stability is its diminished fatigue strength. Bone fatigue occurs at locations at which the strain of bone tissue exceeds its yield strain. Thus, for secondary stability, it is essential to avoid excessive strain and strain concentrations. As discussed for achievement of primary stability, implants that distribute the strain over a larger area by large surfaces or by more screws or bolts may prevent bone from early fatigue.

The design of implants such as screws and blades has shown to determine its secondary stability. Lag screws for the fixation of hip fractures have frequently been tested biomechanically in order to identify the design with the largest secondary stability and the smallest risk for screw migration and cut-out through the femoral head. Due to their larger contact surface, lag screws with a screw design in which each turn of the thread contributes to the contact surface exhibit a higher migration resistance as compared to lag screws with blade designs (32). Implants with additional features such as antirotation or antigliding mechanisms divert loads from the bone to the implant, thereby reducing excessive shear or tensile loads (32). Examples are additional antirotation screws in dynamic hip screw systems (Figure 13.4); struts on screws, which prevent screw rotation (33); or supporting plates for femoral neck pins (Figure 13.5) (34). For these implants, it is essential that the added feature does not negatively affect the strength of the implant itself and that their application does not require modification of the surgical procedure. The aim of these add-on implant features should be to only strengthen the bone implant interface without adding any risk of technical or surgical complication.

In order to maximize the secondary stability of osteosynthesis constructs, loading scenarios that would generate excessive strains locally must be avoided. Thus, it is always beneficial to place screws at positions that provide stable anchorage, such as regions with dense trabecular bone or subcortical regions. For example, the placement of dynamic hip screws has been shown to benefit from subcortical placement of the lag screw within the femoral head (35). Even if the optimal placement for lag screws in cephalomedullary implants appears to be slightly different than for extramedullary implants (36,37), the concept of placing screws in more stable bone regions remains valid. Nevertheless, it is critical to determine those regions for each type of implant separately, as for different types of screws, the optimal region for placement appears to be different (38,39).

One frequently employed technique to improve secondary stability and prevent bone failure is the augmentation

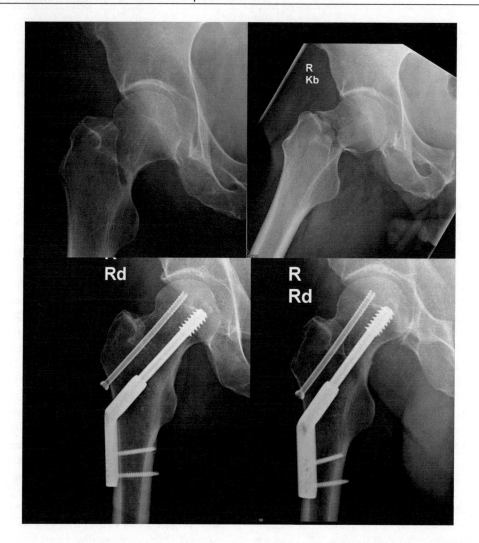

Figure 13.4 Femoral neck fracture, Garden type 3 in a 72-year-old male fixed with dynamic hip screw (DePuy Synthes, Oberdorf, Switzerland) and antirotational screw.

of bone with bone cements, autologous bone material, allografts, or bone grafts. All of these materials can be employed to fill voids, stabilize implants, and provide mechanical support. In addition, some of these materials also enhance the biological repair of the fracture or the fracture defect (40). In particular, for the stabilization of osteoporotic fractures in trabecular regions including the spine, the wrist, the tibial plateau, and the hip, injectable materials that harden *in situ* have become very popular. For stabilization of osteoporotic vertebral fractures, kyphoplasty and vertebroplasty have become a standard procedure (41). While the most frequent artificial augmentation material remains polymethyl methacrylate (PMMA), some more biologically active materials such as hydroxyapatite, calcium sulfate, or calcium phosphate find increased applications. The main advantages of PMMA include biological inertness, absence of inflammatory reaction, and most importantly, immediate multidirectional mechanical stability with stiffness ranging between cortical and trabecular bone (42). Calcium phosphate and calcium sulfate cements, although being biologically active and osteoconductive,

have the disadvantage of lower mechanical stiffness and earlier failure compared to PMMA cements, primarily in loading situations that include shear. For primarily axial loading situations, these cements have obtained satisfactory clinical results (43).

Augmentation of bone around implants has been most effective for the augmentation of screws with bone cement. This technique effectively transmits load from the metallic implant to the bone and distributes the stress over a larger amount of bone tissue (44,45).

Promotion of bone formation and prevention of delayed union or nonunion

It has long been known that the mechanical environment is one of the most important factors affecting the progression of bone healing (46). Recent experimental studies confirmed clinical experience that diaphyseal fractures respond differently to mechanical loading compared to metaphyseal fractures (47,48). In fractures involving

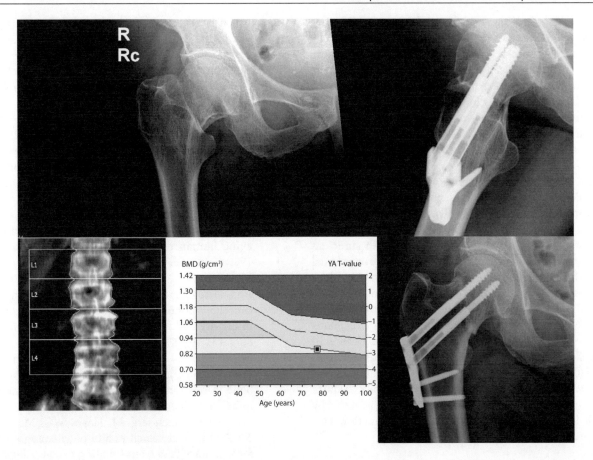

Figure 13.5 Medial femoral neck fracture, Pauwels type 3 in a 78-year-old woman with osteoporosis (T: −2.7) stabilized by TargonFN plate construct (Aesculap, Tuttlingen, Germany) combining parallel pins with telescoping technique and with angular stability provided by a buttress plate.

the shaft, the principle of elastic fixation that stimulates periosteal callus formation by interfragmentary movement (secondary healing response) should be employed (49). Although the optimal amount of interfragmentary movement is not exactly known, numerous preclinical studies have been able to identify a range of motion parameters shown to be favorable for diaphyseal fracture healing (15,50,51). In essence, initial strain values within the fracture that were below 15% were consistently found to be compatible with bone healing. The strongest positive responses in terms of callus stimulation were found for strains between 2% and 10% (50). Furthermore, the direction of strain plays an important part in the success of the healing process. Mechanical stimulation inducing axial strain has shown to stimulate the healing response predominantly by periosteal callus formation. In contrast, shear strain, in particular within the fracture gap, appears to be less stimulatory or may even inhibit bone formation in the fracture gap (52,53).

Modern implants for the treatment of long bone diaphyseal fractures include intramedullary nails with various locking options and a variety of locking plate constructs. Intramedullary nails provide a maximum of axial stabilization due to their placement in the load axis of the bone. Rotational and bending stability has to be provided by

sufficient nail thickness and the generous use of the nail's locking options (19). Thus, in the central diaphysis, a long intramedullary nail with intramedullary reaming and a maximum of locking distally and proximally should be the primary choice. Locking plate constructs may be a valid alternative for certain fracture situations. Locking plates rely on a stable interlock between the plate and the screws. Deformation under load bearing in diaphyseal fractures mainly occurs by bending of the plate. The amount of interfragmentary movement depends largely on the working length of the plate (distance between the two locking screws opposite the fracture gap). This provides the surgeon with the option to manipulate the amount of strain in the fracture gap and thus to stimulate the secondary healing response. Another possibility to influence the mechanical stability is provided by using different plate materials. Titanium plates are preferable to steel plates because they provide more elastic deformation. Recent developments in locking plate constructs aimed for the further option to increase interfragmentary motion in diaphyseal fractures fixed with locking plates. Increased axial deformation at the fracture site can be achieved by targeted manipulation of the locking screws or the plate itself. Using special locking screw designs (far cortical locking [54], dynamic locking screw [55]), the fracture can be dynamized, and the secondary healing response can be successfully stimulated (56). Alternatively, the dynamization can also be introduced by special plate design that allows the locking screws to be dynamically locked into the plate (57,58). The clinical benefit of these dynamization features has yet to be demonstrated, especially for the treatment of osteoporotic fractures. Finally, for stable plate constructs that heal by a primary healing response, it is essential to avoid fracture gaps and achieve accurate fracture reduction and alignment (49).

Fractures in the metaphyseal area affect mainly cancellous bone that heals by membranous healing: osteoid is formed by mesenchymal cells within the hematoma region and is then sequentially replaced by woven bone and remodeled into lamellar bone (47). With sufficient mechanical stability, there is rarely any cartilage or external callus formation (59). The healing response in cancellous bone is closely localized to the injured region and rarely extends beyond a few millimeters from the traumatized area (60). The healing of gaps or defects in cancellous bone is rather slow or incomplete. Therefore, defects in cancellous bone should be avoided by accurate reduction or by filling any remaining defect with bone graft material. In particular, C-type fractures involving the joints require a maximum of mechanical stability that can be achieved by stable locking plate constructs often in combination with compression screws.

SUMMARY

In elderly patients and patients with osteoporosis, the amount of bone and its mechanical quality are drastically reduced leading to a deterioration of bones mechanical competence. This not only results in the well-known phenomenon of fragility fractures but also in an increased difficulty in the stable and persisting fixation of these fractures. Fixation of fracture in fragile bone requires consequent application of accepted techniques for stable fracture fixation aiming at primary stability of the fracture, correct alignment and adequate fracture reduction, secondary stability, and promotion of bone formation. Specially adapted techniques such as compression or augmentation can support the basic techniques. In addition, specially designed implants for osteoporotic fracture fixation or the combination of multiple implants provide powerful options to enhance the stability of fracture fixation. Although internal fixation and successful healing of fractures in fragile bone will remain a challenge, consequent application of fixation techniques in combination with new techniques to improve fixation will avoid failure of fixation and healing.

REFERENCES

1. Seeman E, Delmas PD. Bone quality—The material and structural basis of bone strength and fragility. *N Engl J Med*. 2006;354:2250–61.

2. Augat P, Schorlemmer S. The role of cortical bone and its microstructure in bone strength. *Age Ageing*. 2006;35(Suppl 2):ii27–31.

3. Burstein AH, Reilly DT, Martens M. Aging of bone tissue: Mechanical properties. *J Bone Joint Surg Am*. 1976;58:82–6.

4. Garnero P. The role of collagen organization on the properties of bone. *Calcif Tissue Int*. 2015;97:229–40.

5. Osterhoff G, Morgan EF, Shefelbine SJ, Karim L, McNamara LM, Augat P. Bone mechanical properties and changes with osteoporosis. *Injury*. 2016;47(Suppl 2):S11–20.

6. Zioupos P, Currey JD, Hamer AJ. The role of collagen in the declining mechanical properties of aging human cortical bone. *J Biomed Mater Res*. 1999;45:108–16.

7. McCalden RW, McGeough JA, Court-Brown CM. Age-related changes in the compressive strength of cancellous bone. The relative importance of changes in density and trabecular architecture. *J Bone Joint Surg Am*. 1997;79:421–7.

8. Mosekilde L, Mosekilde L, Danielsen CC. Biomechanical competence of vertebral trabecular bone in relation to ash density and age in normal individuals. *Bone*. 1987;8:79–85.

9. van den Kroonenberg AJ, Hayes WC, McMahon TA. Hip impact velocities and body configurations for voluntary falls from standing height. *J Biomech*. 1996;29:807–11.

10. Augat P, Weyand D, Panzer S, Klier T. Osteoporosis prevalence and fracture characteristics in elderly female patients with fractures. *Arch Orthop Trauma Surg*. 2010;130:1405–10.

11. Cornell CN, Ayalon O. Evidence for success with locking plates for fragility fractures. *HSS J*. 2011;7:164–9.

12. Goldhahn J, Suhm N, Goldhahn S, Blauth M, Hanson B. Influence of osteoporosis on fracture fixation—A systematic literature review. *Osteoporos Int*. 2008;19:761–72.

13. von Rüden C, Augat P. Failure of fracture fixation in osteoporotic bone. *Injury*. 2016;47:3–10.

14. Seebeck J, Goldhahn J, Stadele H, Messmer P, Morlock MM, Schneider E. Effect of cortical thickness and cancellous bone density on the holding strength of internal fixator screws. *J Orthop Res*. 2004;22:1237–42.

15. Augat P, Simon U, Liedert A, Claes L. Mechanics and mechano-biology of fracture healing in normal and osteoporotic bone. *Osteoporos Int*. 2005;16(Suppl 2):S36–43.

16. Hungerer S, Eberle S, Lochner S et al. Biomechanical evaluation of subtalar fusion: The influence of screw configuration and placement. *J Foot Ankle Surg*. 2013;52:177–83.

17. Mair S, Weninger P, Hogel F, Panzer S, Augat P. [Stability of volar fixed-angle plating for distal radius fractures. Failure modes in osteoporotic bone]. *Unfallchirurg*. 2013;116:338–44.

18. Huang SC, Lin CC, Lin J. Increasing nail-cortical contact to increase fixation stability and decrease implant strain in antegrade locked nailing of distal femoral fractures: A biomechanical study. *J Trauma*. 2009;66:436–42.

19. Augat P, Penzkofer R, Nolte A et al. Interfragmentary movement in diaphyseal tibia fractures fixed with locked intramedullary nails. *J Orthop Trauma*. 2008;22:30–6.

20. Holper B, Tschegg EK, Stanzl-Tschegg S, Gabler C. [Possibilities for improving fatigue properties of interlocking screws of solid tibial nails. A mathematical model with practical conclusions]. *Unfallchirurg*. 2002;105:140–6.

21. Freeman AL, Craig MR, Schmidt AH. Biomechanical comparison of tibial nail stability in a proximal third fracture: Do screw quantity and locked, interlocking screws make a difference? *J Orthop Trauma*. 2011;25:333–9.

22. Chan DS, Nayak AN, Blaisdell G et al. Effect of distal interlocking screw number and position after intramedullary nailing of distal tibial fractures: A biomechanical study simulating immediate weight-bearing. *J Orthop Trauma*. 2015;29:98–104.

23. Augat P, Buehren V. Intramedullary nailing of the distal tibia. Does angular stable locking make a difference? *Unfallchirurg*. 2015;118:311–7.

24. Schmidt-Rohlfing B, Heussen N, Knobe M, Pfeifer R, Kaneshige JR, Pape HC. Reoperation rate after internal fixation of intertrochanteric femur fractures with the percutaneous compression plate: What are the risk factors? *J Orthop Trauma*. 2013;27:312–7.

25. Hoffmann S, Paetzold R, Stephan D, Puschel K, Buehren V, Augat P. Biomechanical evaluation of interlocking lag screw design in intramedullary nailing of unstable pertrochanteric fractures. *J Orthop Trauma*. 2013;27:483–90.

26. Ruecker AH, Rupprecht M, Gruber M et al. The treatment of intertrochanteric fractures: Results using an intramedullary nail with integrated cephalocervical screws and linear compression. *J Orthop Trauma*. 2009;23:22–30.

27. Buhren V. [Intramedullary compression nailing of long tubular bones]. *Unfallchirurg*. 2000;103:708–20.

28. Muckley T, Diefenbeck M, Sorkin AT, Beimel C, Goebel M, Buhren V. Results of the T2 humeral nailing system with special focus on compression interlocking. *Injury*. 2008;39:299–305.

29. Hogel F, Gerber C, Buhren V, Augat P. Reamed intramedullary nailing of diaphyseal tibial fractures: Comparison of compression and non-compression nailing. *Eur J Trauma Emerg Surg*. 2013;39:73–7.

30. Gonschorek O, Hofmann GO, Buhren V. Interlocking compression nailing: A report on 402 applications. *Arch Orthop Trauma Surg*. 1998;117:430–7.

31. Iundusi R, Gasbarra E, D'Arienzo M, Piccioli A, Tarantino U. Augmentation of tibial plateau fractures with an injectable bone substitute: CERAMENT. Three year follow-up from a prospective study. *BMC Musculoskelet Disord*. 2015;16:115.

32. Born CT, Karich B, Bauer C, von Oldenburg G, Augat P. Hip screw migration testing: First results for hip screws and helical blades utilizing a new oscillating test method. *J Orthop Res*. 2011;29:760–6.

33. Koller H, Zenner J, Hitzl W et al. The impact of a distal expansion mechanism added to a standard pedicle screw on pullout resistance. A biomechanical study. *Spine J*. 2013;13:532–41.

34. Eschler A, Brandt S, Gierer P, Mittlmeier T, Gradl G. Angular stable multiple screw fixation (Targon FN) versus standard SHS for the fixation of femoral neck fractures. *Injury*. 2014;45(Suppl 1):S76–80.

35. Baumgaertner MR, Curtin SL, Lindskog DM, Keggi JM. The value of the tip-apex distance in predicting failure of fixation of peritrochanteric fractures of the hip. *J Bone Joint Surg Am*. 1995;77:1058–64.

36. Kane P, Vopat B, Heard W et al. Is tip apex distance as important as we think? A biomechanical study examining optimal lag screw placement. *Clin Orthop Relat Res*. 2014;472:2492–8.

37. Kuzyk PR, Zdero R, Shah S, Olsen M, Waddell JP, Schemitsch EH. Femoral head lag screw position for cephalomedullary nails: A biomechanical analysis. *J Orthop Trauma*. 2012;26:414–21.

38. Nikoloski AN, Osbrough AL, Yates PJ. Should the tip-apex distance (TAD) rule be modified for the proximal femoral nail antirotation (PFNA)? A retrospective study. *J Orthop Surg Res*. 2013;8:35.

39. Kouvidis GK, Sommers MB, Giannoudis PV, Katonis PG, Bottlang M. Comparison of migration behavior between single and dual lag screw implants for intertrochanteric fracture fixation. *J Orthop Surg Res*. 2009;4:16.

40. Van Lieshout EM, Alt V. Bone graft substitutes and bone morphogenetic proteins for osteoporotic fractures: What is the evidence? *Injury*. 2016;47(Suppl 1):S43–6.

41. Savage JW, Schroeder GD, Anderson PA. Vertebroplasty and kyphoplasty for the treatment of osteoporotic vertebral compression fractures. *J Am Acad Orthop Surg*. 2014;22:653–64.

42. Kammerlander C, Neuerburg C, Verlaan JJ, Schmoelz W, Miclau T, Larsson S. The use of augmentation techniques in osteoporotic fracture fixation. *Injury*. 2016;47(Suppl 2):S36–43.

43. Bajammal SS, Zlowodzki M, Lelwica A et al. The use of calcium phosphate bone cement in fracture treatment. A meta-analysis of randomized trials. *J Bone Joint Surg Am*. 2008;90:1186–96.

44. Kammerlander C, Erhart S, Doshi H, Gosch M, Blauth M. Principles of osteoporotic fracture treatment. *Best Pract Res Clin Rheumatol*. 2013;27:757–69.

45. Schliemann B, Wahnert D, Theisen C et al. How to enhance the stability of locking plate fixation of proximal humerus fractures? An overview of current biomechanical and clinical data. *Injury*. 2015;46:1207–14.

46. Goodship AE, Kenwright J. The influence of induced micromovement upon the healing of experimental tibial fractures. *J Bone Joint Surg Br*. 1985;67:650–5.

47. Sandberg OH, Aspenberg P. Inter-trabecular bone formation: A specific mechanism for healing of cancellous bone. *Acta Orthop*. 2016;87:459–65.

48. Sandberg O, Bernhardsson M, Aspenberg P. Earlier effect of alendronate in mouse metaphyseal versus diaphyseal bone healing. *J Orthop Res*. 2017;35(4):793–799.

49. Claes L, Recknagel S, Ignatius A. Fracture healing under healthy and inflammatory conditions. *Nat Rev Rheumatol*. 2012;8:133–43.

50. Claes LE, Heigele CA, Neidlinger-Wilke C et al. Effects of mechanical factors on the fracture healing process. *Clin Orthop Relat Res*. 1998;(355 Suppl):S132–47.

51. Simon U, Augat P, Utz M, Claes L. A numerical model of the fracture healing process that describes tissue development and revascularisation. *Comput Methods Biomech Biomed Engin*. 2011;14:79–93.

52. Augat P, Burger J, Schorlemmer S, Henke T, Peraus M, Claes L. Shear movement at the fracture site delays healing in a diaphyseal fracture model. *J Orthop Res*. 2003;21:1011–7.

53. Steiner M, Claes L, Ignatius A, Simon U, Wehner T. Disadvantages of interfragmentary shear on fracture healing—Mechanical insights through numerical simulation. *J Orthop Res*. 2014;32:865–72.

54. Bottlang M, Feist F. Biomechanics of far cortical locking. *J Orthop Trauma*. 2011;25(Suppl 1):S21–8.

55. Plecko M, Lagerpusch N, Andermatt D et al. The dynamisation of locking plate osteosynthesis by means of dynamic locking screws (DLS)—An experimental study in sheep. *Injury*. 2013;44:1346–57.

56. Bottlang M, Lesser M, Koerber J et al. Far cortical locking can improve healing of fractures stabilized with locking plates. *J Bone Joint Surg Am*. 2010;92:1652–60.

57. Bottlang M, Tsai S, Bliven EK et al. Dynamic stabilization of simple fractures with active plates delivers stronger healing than conventional compression plating. *J Orthop Trauma*. 2017;31(2):71–77.

58. Bottlang M, Tsai S, Bliven EK et al. Dynamic stabilization with active locking plates delivers faster, stronger, and more symmetric fracture-healing. *J Bone Joint Surg Am*. 2016;98:466–74.

59. Han D, Han N, Chen Y, Zhang P, Jiang B. Healing of cancellous fracture in a novel mouse model. *Am J Transl Res*. 2015;7:2279–90.

60. Charnley J, Baker SL. Compression arthrodesis of the knee; A clinical and histological study. *J Bone Joint Surg Br*. 1952;34-B:187–99.

14

The fix and treat principle
An update

VASILEIOS P. GIANNOUDIS and PETER V. GIANNOUDIS

INTRODUCTION

Osteoporosis is a disease affecting the bones, characterized by low bone mass and disruption of bone microarchitecture, leading to compromised bone strength and an increase in the risk of fractures. The incidence of this disease (fragile bones) increases after the age of 50 years. It has been estimated that worldwide, one in three women over age 50 years will experience osteoporotic fractures, as will one in five men aged over 50 years (1). Moreover, Kanis and Johnell reported that in women over 45 years of age, osteoporosis accounts for more days spent in hospital than many other diseases such as diabetes, myocardial infarction, and breast cancer (2).

Osteoporosis is associated with a great cost burden to the health-care system. In Europe, the disability due to osteoporosis is greater than that caused by cancers (with the exception of lung cancer) and is equivalent if not greater than that lost to a number of protracted conditions such as rheumatoid arthritis, asthma, and hypertension.

Over 200 million women are affected annually from osteoporosis (10% of women aged 60 years, 20% of women aged 70 years, 40% of women aged 80 years, and greater than two-thirds of women aged 90 years) (3). In the United States, approximately 2 million osteoporotic fractures occur annually, with 800,000 emergency room attendances and half a million hospitalizations (4). Worldwide, osteoporosis causes more than 8.9 million fractures per year, resulting in an osteoporotic fracture every 3 seconds, of which 1.6 million were at the hip, 1.7 million were at the forearm, and 1.4 million were clinical vertebral fractures. Europe and the Americas accounted for 51% of all these fractures, while most of the remainder occurred in the Western Pacific region and Southeast Asia (5). Gullberg et al. estimated that by 2050, the worldwide incidence of hip fracture in men is projected to increase by 310% and 240% in women, compared to rates in 1990 (6).

Noteworthy, these numbers quantifying the degree of the osteoporosis impact to the society are only estimates and as such are more likely than not underestimating the significance of the problem. Interestingly, osteoporosis has been characterized as a silent disease until fractures happen, which can lead then to significant secondary health problems and even mortality. Not surprisingly, a survey that was carried out by the International Osteoporosis Foundation (IOF) demonstrated denial of personal risk by postmenopausal women, absence of conversation about osteoporosis with their general practitioner, and limited access to diagnosis and treatment before the occurrence of the first fracture, highlighting the problem of underdiagnosis and undertreatment of the disease (7).

Accordingly, several organizations have taken the initiative to increase the awareness of the problem so that all the patients that require treatment would receive the appropriate medication. For instance, recently, the IOF recommended specific aims in order to foresee good bone health throughout the life span of an individual: (a) attainment of potential peak bone mass during childhood and adulthood periods; (b) control of environmental factors and personal health-related factors to prevent early bone loss; and (c) prevention and treatment of osteoporosis in the elderly (8).

With regard to fracture prevention, several educational and screening programs have been developed to contribute to the increased awareness of the disease, identification of patients, and implementation of treatment. However, in order to introduce more effective prevention programs, specific initiatives were introduced such as orthogeriatric services and fracture liaison services (FLSs) (9). This was based on the argument that assessment of patients via the clinical setting, which would allow the acquisition of all the necessary investigations, referrals to appropriate specialists, and prescription of treatment along with longer follow-up, would safeguard more robust engagement of patients and higher success rates.

Remarkably, the vast majority of individuals at high risk who already had at least one osteoporotic fracture are neither identified nor treated (7). Kanis et al. reported that a prior fracture is associated with an 86% increased risk of any fracture (10).

Dang et al. investigated the risks and characteristics of recurrent osteoporotic/fragile fractures. The Medicare Standard Analytical Files database was used to identify patients over a 5-year period older than 65 years of age who had osteoporosis or osteopenia and sustained a fragility fracture of the proximal humerus, distal radius, hip, ankle, and vertebral column. The incidence and type of recurrent fracture were investigated over a 3-year period. Out of 1,059,212 patients who had an initial fragility fracture, 5.8% had a subsequent fracture within 1 year from their initial fracture, 8.8% within 2 years, and 11.35% within 3 years. At 3-year follow-up, hip fractures were the most frequent type of subsequent fracture regardless of the initial fracture type (6.5%, $P < 0.05$). The authors concluded that patients who have any type of fragility fracture have a notable risk of subsequent fractures within 3 years, especially hip fractures. These patients should be evaluated and treated for underlying risks factors, including osteoporosis and/or osteopenia (11). Interestingly, other studies have reported similar findings.

Warriner et al. found that initial hip fracture increased the risk of contralateral fracture by 3.7 times and the risk of vertebral fracture by 3.6 times (12). Sobolev et al. (13) reported that a prior fracture at any site increases the risk of hip fracture by 2.4 times. The authors went on to state that a second hip fracture has more than 50% higher mortality than the index event. A meta-analysis has demonstrated that a history of fracture at any skeletal site is associated with approximately a doubling of future fracture risk (10).

More interestingly, Edwards et al. highlighted that half of patients presenting with a hip fracture were noted to have sustained a previous non-hip fragility fracture. This finding suggests that those patients admitted to hospital with an incident fragility fracture epitomize a highrisk-patient cohort where interventions including medical bone protection treatment and falls preventions are justified (14). In addition, it would make sense that if patients are offered appropriate advice at the time of the hospital stay, where they are in bed, immobilized, and appreciating the implications of fracture treatment, they may be more agreeable to starting therapy to lessen the risk of further fractures.

Consequently, such an opportunity at the time of hospital stay is defined as the *fix and treat principle*. This approach represents one model where effective initiation of treatment can reduce future fracture risk.

FIX AND TREAT PRINCIPLE

The fix and treat principle is heavily reliant on a preestablished FLS. The objective of an FLS is to ensure that all patients older than 50 years presenting to acute care services with a fragility fracture at any skeletal site, undergo fracture risk assessment and receive treatment in accordance with relevant national clinical guidelines for osteoporosis. The FLS also safeguards that falls risk is addressed among older patients by being referred to appropriate local services focusing on falls prevention.

Van Geel et al. presented a prospective cohort study on their experiences of the Glasgow FLS—the first established in the United Kingdom in 1999 (15). Between 1999 and 2007, 5011 patients were reviewed in the FLS, with all of these patients being recommended calcium and vitamin D supplementation, with approximately 50% of them also being recommended bisphosphonates if they met preset criteria. Note that in order to receive a bisphosphonate recommendation, patients did not need to have an osteoporotic T-score (-2.5 or less). Despite FLS being recommended worldwide as a treatment strategy, these services are yet to be implemented. Consequently, there is limited high-quality literature investigating the use of osteoporotic medications while adhering to an FLS model.

Aguado-Maestro et al. (16) investigated whether such an opportunity of initiation of treatment in patients presenting with a proximal femoral fragility fracture is used successfully in elderly patients over an 18-month period. Included into the study were 1004 patients (278 male) who met the inclusion criteria. The mean age was 82.01 years and mean length of stay (LOS) was 19.54 days. Three hundred and six patients (30.5%) had at least another fragility fracture before the index episode (mean 1.40 fractures; standard deviation [SD]: 0.71 fractures; range: 1–6 fractures). Only 16.4% were under complete osteoporosis treatment on admission, defined as receiving calcium with vitamin D and a bisphosphonate or an alternative agent. When we compared patients without a history of a previous fragility fracture (group A) and patients with at least another previous fragility fracture (group B), we found that patients in group B had a significantly lower abbreviated mental test score (AMTS), lower bone mineral density (BMD) as evident on the dual-energy x-ray absorptiometry (DEXA) scan, an inferior mobility before admission, and a higher incidence of extracapsular fractures ($P < 0.05$). On discharge, patients in group B had a higher chance of receiving complete bone protection compared to group A (27.9% versus 41.7%; $P < 0.01$). This was attributed to the observation that patients in group B were more likely to be reviewed by orthogeriatricians following discharge than those in group A.

The authors highlighted that there was still room for improvement in terms of ensuring that more patients can be educated and be discharged on bone protection medication.

Huntjens et al. compared outcomes for fracture patients who were admitted to a university hospital with a FLS with those for fracture patients who presented to a general hospital without a FLS (17). The results were analyzed according to the intention-to-treat principle. After 15 months, the FLS patients had a 28% lower risk of sustaining refractures (hazard ratio [HR] 0.72%, 95% confidence interval [CI] 0.52–0.98), which increased to 56% by 24 months (HR 0.44%, 95% CI 0.25–0.79). After correction for age, sex, and baseline fracture location, during 2 years of follow-up, 35% fewer patients died in the FLS group as compared to those not managed by a FLS.

Nakayama et al. investigated refracture rates for patients managed by a hospital with a FLS and compared them with those for a hospital without a FLS (18). During 3 years of follow-up, observed rates of refracture were lower at the FLS hospital by 33% (HR 0.67%, 95% CI 0.47–0.95) and 41% (HR 0.59%, 95% CI 0.39–0.90) for refracture and major refractures, respectively. The number needed to treat (NNT) to prevent one new fracture during 3 years was 20.

Overall the usefulness of FLS has been confirmed in several countries. For instance, audit data gathered by the West Glasgow FLS estimated that for a hypothetical cohort of 1000 fragility fracture patients managed by FLS, 18 fractures may be prevented, providing an overall savings of £21,000 ($26,250 USD) (19). Similarly, cost-effectiveness has been validated in Canada (20).

Of interest in addition to the implementation of the FLS being used as a vehicle for secondary bone prevention, national initiatives have further contributed to this goal. In the United Kingdom in 2007, the British Orthopaedic Association (BOA) and British Geriatrics Society (BGS) announced consensus guidance on the care of fragility fracture patients (21), where the importance of establishing an orthogeriatric service and an FLS was highlighted, while at the same time the launch of the National Hip Fracture Database (NHFD) was publicized (22). The NHFD has become the largest continuous audit of acute hip fracture care and post-hip fracture secondary prevention globally, having more than half a million cases documented up to February 2018. Moreover, the UK Royal Osteoporosis Society (formerly the National Osteoporosis Society) announced a strategy that recognized the importance of implementation of an FLS in every hospital. In addition, Royal Osteoporosis Society established a Service Development Team that is collaborating with hospitals throughout the United Kingdom to improve access to FLS. The Fracture Liaison Service Database (FLS-DB) was commissioned by the Healthcare Quality Improvement Partnership (HQIP) as a new national audit as part of the Falls and Fragility Fracture Audit Programme (FFFAP) delivered by the Royal College of Physicians (23). The FLS-DB involves two national audit components: a facilities audit and a patient audit. At the same time, the Department of Health (DH) published guidelines for preventing falls and fractures and effective interventions in health and social care (i.e., respond to the first fracture, prevent the second through FLSs in acute and primary care; early intervention to restore independence).

All of these coordinated national UK initiatives have contributed to improvement in the management of elderly patients with fragility fractures.

In addition to the aforementioned National Initiative, a global organization, the Fragility Fracture Network (FFN) has been contributing to the implementation of strategies for secondary prevention of fragility fractures. It has successfully created a multidisciplinary network of experts expressing one voice supporting the view that policy change in relation to the management of fragility fractures can only happen at a national level, and development and implementation of multidisciplinary national coalitions are the most effective way to achieve this.

A recent systematic review and meta-analysis of orthogeriatric care models concluded that collaboration between orthopedic surgeons and geriatricians can improve outcomes after hip fracture (24).

Despite all of these developments that appear to be successful in some nations like the United Kingdom, the IOF recently summarized the usefulness of the most commonly used osteoporosis treatments specifically in the context of secondary fracture prevention (25). The authors concluded, "In light of the diverse array of effective osteoporosis treatments which are available to reduce future fracture risk, it is of great concern that a pervasive and persistent secondary prevention care gap is evident throughout the world (14)".

This is evidenced by a decreasing number of bisphosphonate prescriptions in patients who are at high risk of developing osteoporotic fractures and those who should be commenced on medications postoperatively following the sustainment of fragility fractures.

Ongoing efforts, therefore, are essential to publicize the findings of studies supporting the effectiveness and cost savings produced in health-care models where the fix and treat principle among other initiatives are applied successfully.

REFERENCES

1. Kanis JA, Johnell O, Oden A et al. Long-term risk of osteoporotic fracture in Malmo. *Osteoporos Int.* 2000;11:669.
2. Kanis JA, Johnell O, Oden A et al. Epidemiology of osteoporosis and fracture in men. *Calcif Tissue Int.* 2004;75:90.
3. Johnell O, Kanis JA. An estimate of the worldwide prevalence and disability associated with osteoporotic fractures. *Osteoporos Int.* 2006;17:1726.
4. Singer A, Exuzides A, Spangler L et al. Burden of illness for osteoporotic fractures compared with other serious diseases among postmenopausal women in the United States. *Mayo Clin Proc.* 2015;90(1):53–62.
5. Kanis JA. WHO Technical Report, University of Sheffield, UK, 2007, 66.
6. Gullberg B, Johnell O, Kanis JA. World-wide projections for hip fracture. *Osteoporos Int.* 1997;7:407.
7. International Osteoporosis Foundation. How fragile is her future? 2000.
8. Cooper C, Dawson-Hughes B, Gordon CM, Rizzoli R. Healthy nutrition, healthy bones: How nutritional factors affect musculoskeletal health throughout life. In Jagait CK, Misteli L, eds. *World Osteoporosis Day Thematic Report.* Nyon, Switzerland: International Osteoporosis Foundation, 2015.
9. Perreault S, Dragomir A, Desgagné A et al. Trends and determinants of antiresorptive drug use for osteoporosis among elderly women. *Pharmacoepidemiol Drug Saf.* 2005;14(10):685–95.

10. Kanis JA, Johnell O, De Laet C et al. A meta-analysis of previous fracture and subsequent fracture risk. *Bone*. 2004;35:375.

11. Dang DY, Zetumer S, Zhang AL. Recurrent fragility fractures: A cross-sectional analysis. *J Am Acad Orthop Surg*. 2019;27(2):e85–91.

12. Warriner AH, Patkar NM, Yun H, Delzell E. Minor, major, low-trauma, and high-trauma fractures: What are the subsequent fracture risks and how do they vary? *Curr Osteoporos Rep*. 2011;9(3):122–8.

13. Sobolev B, Sheehan KJ, Kuramoto L, Guy P. Excess mortality associated with second hip fracture. *Osteoporos Int*. 2015;26(7):1903–10.

14. Edwards BJ, Bunta AD, Simonelli C, Bolander M, Fitzpatrick LA. Prior fractures are common in patients with subsequent hip fractures. *Clin Orthop Relat Res*. 2007;461:226–30.

15. van Geel TACM, Bliuc D, Geusens PPM et al. Reduced mortality and subsequent fracture risk associated with oral bisphosphonate recommendation in a fracture liaison service setting: A prospective cohort study. *PLOS ONE* 2018;13(6):e0198006.

16. Aguado-Maestro I, Panteli M, García-Alonso M, Bañuelos-Díaz A, Giannoudis PV. Incidence of bone protection and associated fragility injuries in patients with proximal femur fractures. *Injury*. 2017;48(Suppl 7):S27–33.

17. Huntjens KM, van Geel TA, van den Bergh JP et al. Fracture liaison service: Impact on subsequent non-vertebral fracture incidence and mortality. *J Bone Jt Surg Am*. 2014;96:e29.

18. Nakayama A, Major G, Holliday E, Attia J, Bogduk N. Evidence of effectiveness of a fracture liaison service to reduce the re-fracture rate. *Osteoporos Int*. 2016;27:873–9.

19. McLellan AR, Wolowacz SE, Zimovetz EA et al. Fracture liaison services for the evaluation and management of patients with osteoporotic fracture: A cost-effectiveness evaluation based on data collected over 8 years of service provision. *Osteoporos Int*. 2011;22(7):2083–98.

20. Yong JH, Masucci L, Hoch JS, Sujic R, Beaton D. Cost-effectiveness of a fracture liaison service—A real-world evaluation after 6 years of service provision. *Osteoporos Int*. 2016;27(1):231–40.

21. British Orthopaedic Association/British Geriatrics Society. *The Care of Patients with Fragility Fracture ["Blue Book"]*. 2nd ed. London, UK: British Orthopaedic Association, 2007.

22. Royal College of Physicians. The national hip fracture database. London. 2018.

23. Royal College of Physicians. Fracture liaison service database (FLS-DB). London. 2018.

24. Grigoryan KV, Javedan H, Rudolph JL. Orthogeriatric care models and outcomes in hip fracture patients: A systematic review and meta-analysis. *J Orthop Trauma*. 2014;28(3):e49–55.

25. Harvey NC, McCloskey EV, Mitchell PJ et al. Mind the (treatment) gap: A global perspective on current and future strategies for prevention of fragility fractures. *Osteoporos Int*. 2017;28:1507–29.

15

Principles of management of osteoporotic fractures

SETH M. TARRANT and ZSOLT J. BALOGH

INTRODUCTION

The prevalence of osteoporotic fractures is a major health burden (1). As the population ages and has increased functional expectations, surgical optimization of function within finite health budgets is a challenge. Classical fixation principles need to be modified to a new osteoporotic paradigm. Decreased bone healing potential in osteoporosis (2), impaired stem cell function (3), the pro-inflammatory environments (4), and increased implant failure highlight the difficulties faced in the oncoming epidemic.

The first principle of management is choosing the correct indication for the right patient to potentially operate on. The AO principles of early return to function and mobility apply to osteoporotic fracture (5). In this fragile population, extended immobility leads to increased morbidity (6) and mortality (7), as best evidenced in osteoporotic hip fracture care. The converse is that surgery is inherently risky, expensive, and may have little benefit functionally in low-demand patients, such as geriatric distal radius fractures (8). The limited functional reserve and the reduced propensity to compensate through adjacent joints necessitates the restoration of the residual function for maintenance of mobility and independence.

A potentially fragile physiologic status must next be taken into account. Geriatric patients sustaining osteoporotic fractures are immunosuppressed (9), sarcopenic (10) and often anticoagulated. The soft tissue compromise from expanding hematoma, the stress from blood loss and the direct skin impact from the initial trauma must be considered with surgical approach. The likelihood of ongoing bleeding and the chance of revision can also affect the approach and fixation used. Gaythorne Girdlestone's analogy of the surgeon to the gardener, as opposed to the carpenter (11), is critical in a patient cohort that has inherently frail soft tissue planes in addition to a fragile skeleton.

Cognitive status, age, residential status, and comorbidity influence surgical decision in the osteoporotic patient as they are independent predictors of the outcome. Due to impaired physiologic reserve and the increased energy expenditure needed with impaired mobility, rehabilitation may be integral to recovery. A patient who cannot follow instructions should not undergo a surgical procedure that needs significant cooperation in the success of the management plan. A patient who is wheelchair- or bedbound may not warrant an extensive operation that has a significant complication profile, such as revision arthroplasty (Figure 15.1).

Once patient factors are accounted for, the fracture pattern, the element classically focused on as dictating treatment, can be considered. Despite being generally low-energy trauma incidents, fracture of osteoporotic bone can lead to patterns that are comminuted, complex, and more challenging than younger bone (12). Obtaining secure fixation of orthopedic implants to osteoporotic bone is challenging (13), and there is known failure from both implant pullout and nonunion. Failed operative management without viable revision options puts the patient into higher risk than the nonoperative treatment. Equivalence has been shown between operative and nonoperative treatment, but within nonoperative groups a subset of malunion may have a worse result. Hence deciding which patient may benefit from surgical intervention and tailoring treatment to individual physiology and functional goals must rely on clinical experience and surgical acumen (14).

FIXATION PRINCIPLES

Healthy bone can be considered as a stiff spring, deforming under load and regaining form upon release (15). The fragility of osteoporotic bone is a consequence of mineral and protein content depletion that changes the bone's structural properties. Rigidity (the opposition of deformation), resistance (the ability to absorb energy), fatigue resistance (the adaption to repetitive loads), and resistance to fracture

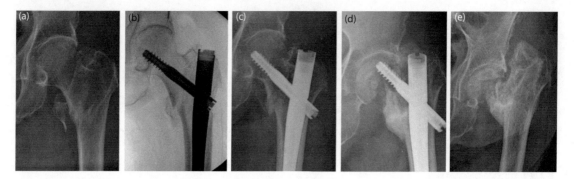

Figure 15.1 An intertrochanteric proximal femur fracture in a nursing home patient with chronic renal failure and diabetes (a) had a technically acceptable closed reduction and percutaneous femoral nail fixation (b). At the 1-month mark, the fracture had compressed (c); however, it developed aseptic nonunion and screw cut-out over the course of a year (d). The patient was cognitively impaired, the nail was removed, and salvage arthroplasty was not offered (e).

(progression of a defect) are all reduced. Anisotropy is amplified: the increasing trabecular alignment allows for greater strength in the axis of principal load. However, this reorganization of depleting resources increases fracture risk when atypical force is applied across the bone, as seen in low-energy falls (16).

An understanding of absolute and relative stability is critical in fixation of osteoporotic bone, which is more brittle and fractures more easily than normal bone. As the diaphyseal cortex thins, the diameter of the bone increases in order to maintain the bones' structural stiffness to bending and torsion (17). Conventional plating technique refined by the AO consisted of generating compression across the fracture site with rigid internal fixation, with absolute stability and primary bone healing being the main objectives (5). This often needs extensive soft tissue dissection, and focus in the last two decades has been toward incorporating biological fixation, relying on relative stability constructs with minimally invasive techniques (18). At the cortical level in osteoporosis, a thinner cortex allows for less purchase of screw thread, so more cortices and threads may be needed (Figure 15.2). As bone mineral density decreases, so does a screw's holding ability, and a large volume of research has been dedicated to designing an implant more suitable to osteoporotic bone (19). Decreasing bone mineral density is a predictor for fixation failure (20), but determining the quantitative extent of osteoporosis is difficult for the clinician. At the bone-implant interface, load can exceed strain tolerance rendering rigid constructs undesirable. Life expectancy has increased over the last six decades since the AO was established, and osteoporotic fractures increasing in turn. No one principle is absolutely applicable, and the injury pattern, anatomical location, and patient goals must be considered.

PLATING

Traditional plating osteosynthesis relies on friction between the plate and the cortical surface of the bone, which are compressed to each other. This friction is generated by the hold of the screws in cortical bone, and in osteoporosis, it is challenging to generate the torque needed to hold a plate against bone using cortical screws. High stresses at the bone-implant interface and poor screw holding power result in a high possibility of failure. Relative stability constructs, such as intramedullary nails and minimally invasive bridge plating, are desirable; however, they are not always feasible. The advent of the locking screw-plate interface has broadened osteosynthesis options, with increased stability and reliable fixation compared with conventional plates in osteoporotic bone (21). Locking screws started as "Schuhli" nuts, a device that locked the head onto the outside of the standard LCP plate (22). Modern locking screws have a threaded hole in the plate. This creates a fixed-angle device that will only fail if all screws on one side of the fracture fail at the individual screw-bone interface, if the implant cuts out of bone, or if the implant breaks (13). Locking screws inserted in bicortical, and even unicortical, constructs show less displacement from axial loading than bicortical nonlocking screw constructs. However, when cantilever forces are applied after axial loading, disrupting the bone-plate interface, bicortical locking screws are far superior (23). When nonlocking cortical screws are needed, hybrid constructs offer greater stiffness and also increase the pullout torque of the nonlocking screw (24).

The metaphyseal-diaphyseal junction and periarticular regions are commonly injured in osteoporotic fractures. Periarticular locking plates provide options to provide rigid fixation around articular surfaces where needed and maintain overall mechanical alignment. Modern plating systems have lengths where a bridging construct to a comminuted junctional fracture can be applied, providing adequate working length for a relative stability construct if needed.

The use of minimally invasive plates, with external radiolucent insertion devices, has extended plating indications and limited surgical exposure. The optimal length for a minimally invasive plate osteosynthesis for bridging comminuted metaphyseal or diaphyseal segments is the longest plate that will not jeopardize joint structure or neurovascular bundles. Plate length is one of the few controllable

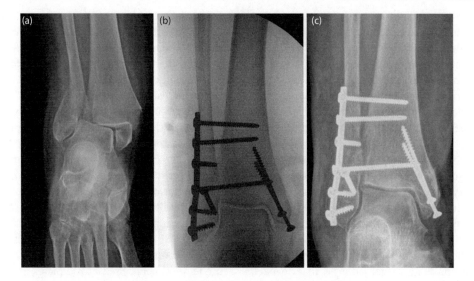

Figure 15.2 An osteoporotic fracture of the ankle (a) requires more cortical purchase to achieve rigid articular fixation (b). Subtle lucencies around the top two tricortical screws and a fracture through the bottom syndesmotic screw are observed, but the patient has achieved the primary goal of maintenance of reduction and union (c).

variables. When plating the distal femur, short plates are a risk factor for failure (25). It is recommended to have a plate that extends proximal to the lesser trochanter to avoid a stress riser and allow a working length to avoid nonunion. Plates extending to the greater trochanter, requiring proximal contouring, have shown excellent results with 95% union rates when coupled with unrestricted weight-bearing. Plates below the lesser trochanter in united fractures are at risk of late, secondary periorthotic fracture (26).

Some anatomical areas benefit from multiple plate constructs. The distal humerus is a common area where rigid fixation and early ranging are optimal, as the joint poorly tolerates immobility. Dual plates are biomechanically stronger (27). Whether the plates are "parallel" or "orthogonal" ("90-90") has been shown to make no difference in clinical outcomes in the adult upper limb (28), despite biomechanical studies showing increased torsional strength with orthogonal plating (29). Bicolumnar 90-90 plating, using multiple mini-fragment plates (at least four), in osteoporotic patients has had encouraging results in reaching high union rates (30). This concept can be applied to other long bone fracture sites: double plating for the distal femur has been advocated in osteoporotic bone to avoid varus collapse and hardware failure (31). However, soft tissue dissection must be taken into account when gaining the exposure to apply multiple plates.

Even with relative stability concept plating applied for the metaphysis and diaphysis, the associated articular fracture requires absolute stability fixation, typically with interfragmentary compression screws outside of the plate. The distal condylar femur fracture in the geriatric population is a challenging, exponentially increasing anatomical location that often has intra-articular involvement (26). As a consequence, plating has become the standard modality of treatment. More complex intra-articular patterns have a tendency to have plate fixation, which may skew

outcomes, suggesting intramedullary nailing is superior in comparative trials (32). The downside to plate fixation is the extra-axial nature of implant positioning: patients are often not allowed to weight-bear due to surgical concerns regarding implant failure and hence loss of reduction with a non-load-sharing implant, with nonunion traditionally high approaching 20% (33). On the contrary, single-center reviews for distal femoral plating have demonstrated that early weight-bearing achieves union rates of 95% when a long construct is utilized (13 holes or greater) with a large working distance (5 holes on average) (26). The quality of evidence looking at the optimal solution for distal femoral osteosynthesis is traditionally poor (34), with multicenter randomized control trials (RCTs) looking at early weight-bearing with plate fixation (NCT02475941) and plating versus nailing (SOLVED; NCT00429663) aiming to better define the role of plating.

Buttress plating is advantageous for metaphyseal fractures. The proximal tibia can have complex fracture patterns in osteoporotic bone. The principles of articular restoration are paramount, whether through a plate of separate interfragmentary screws. Comminution and impaction of osteoporotic bone mean anatomical restoration of the metaphysis cannot always be achieved. One or more plates per plateau is recommended (35). Buttressing can be performed through both open and minimally invasive methods with similar results, complications, and reoperation rates in a younger population (36). There is a paucity of high-quality evidence looking at the tibial buttress in geriatric populations (37). Minimally invasive buttress techniques are attractive options in the osteoporotic patient to respect the soft tissue envelope.

Despite plating being a satisfying tool for anatomical reduction, there is controversy in its use compared with nonoperative options, particularly in the upper limb that does not bear weight. In low-demand patients, nonanatomical union can still produce reasonable functional outcomes with avoidance of operative complications.

The osteoporotic distal radius fracture has had good functional outcomes from fixation with plating after loss of closed reduction (38). Over the last two decades, there has been a steady rise in the plating of geriatric wrist fractures (39,40). Functional outcomes, however, have been shown to be no better than closed reduction in unstable distal radius fractures in patients over 65 years (8). A later multicenter RCT had a conversion rate of 41% in the nonoperative group to plate fixation, demonstrating the trauma community sentiment that complex intra-articular fracture patterns are best served by plating osteosynthesis (41). Despite this, functional and quality life scores do not significantly differ.

The proximal humerus is commonly fractured in the geriatric population. Plate osteosynthesis in two-part fractures has slightly better function than intramedullary nailing in the short term (42); however, this diminishes by 3 years, and when fixation is randomized against sling immobilization for displaced fracture, there are no medium-term differences in functional outcomes (43). High rates of complication from plate fixation in osteoporotic proximal humerus fractures may be related to the lack of differentiation between which cohorts benefit from operative and nonoperative management. Malunion, malreduction, avascular necrosis, and screw cut-out have been reported in over 50% of patients (44). Anatomical reduction with fixation is a predictor of better function irrespective of the severity of preoperative displacement (45). Overall the quality of evidence for proximal humerus fixations is poor (46).

The olecranon is another classically injured bone in elderly falls. Traditionally, simple fractures were fixed with tension band wiring (TBW) constructs, but as anatomical plates and locking screws have been developed, a shift toward their use has been witnessed without high-quality evidence (47). Meta-analysis shows no difference between functional outcomes between TBW and plating, but plating shows less complications in the adult population (48). With TBW constructs, it is vital to direct in a longitudinal transcortical orientation, not intramedullary, to prevent excessive back-out (49). Cancellous bone in osteoporosis cannot be expected to hold any form of reduction. Nonoperative management in the elderly cohort performs well functionally in retrospective studies (50). Whether fixation is needed at all was explored through an RCT looking at the role of operative (fixation via TBW or plate) versus nonoperative management. The study was terminated due to the complication rate in the operative group (81.8%) (51). A similarly designed RCT comparing intervention versus nonoperative management is currently recruiting (52). An RCT comparing plates versus TBW in an adult population (TBW mean age: 43 ± 16, Plate: 52 ± 17) demonstrated comparable patient- and surgeon-reported outcome measures. A subset of this study would have been osteoporotic; however, this was not explored (53).

In osteoporotic bone, the use of hybrid plating is a powerful technique. Cortical screws allow reduction of the fracture, and locking screws augment the pullout strength of fixation. Biomechanical models demonstrate that locking screws placed between cortical screws and the fracture increase the torque needed to remove the cortical screws. Additionally, ensuring that there are at least three bicortical locking screws are present on either side or within the fracture improves fatigue strength of hybrid constructs (24).

Despite the attraction of locking plates for fragility fractures, they are not always suitable for implantation. Acetabular fractures are common examples of this, with careful anatomical contouring of plates needed in addition to trajectories of screws that are not amenable to engaging in traditional locking holes. Ultimately, anatomical reduction is paramount to a good result (54). In the elderly, fractures of the anterior column hemitransverse pattern are common, with a tendency of central subluxation of the femoral head. Specialized plates made to buttress the quadrilateral plate are available but are not superior to having rigid anterior column plating with long screws into the ischium (55). Despite anatomical plates being readily available for nearly every part of the body, "traditional plates" could achieve similar outcomes as long as reduction and fixation principles are adhered to.

IMPACTION CONSTRUCTS

Impaction methods of fixation promote controlled collapse of the fracture. Fracture patterns that have already impacted themselves, such as valgus femoral neck fractures, lend themselves to this fixation principle. A greater degree of initial displacement leads to worse outcomes, including avascular necrosis, and is a predictor of impaction device failure, so the fracture pattern must be carefully examined (56). The two major fixation devices for this pattern are cannulated screws and sliding hip screw (SHS), which is often augmented with a cannulated screw for rotational control. Minimally invasive plating techniques can also be employed with impaction devices and have been shown to have equivalent results to cephalomedullary devices in unstable pertrochanteric fractures (57).

The SHS has been shown to be a stable device with the ability to compress the fracture intraoperatively. Having a tip-apex distance of less than 25 mm on both views prevents failure (58). Careful use of image intensifiers should avoid penetration through the joint surface when properly implanted. Helical blades are a modification of the conventional sliding screw used in impaction implants. Upon insertion, impaction of cancellous bone occurs around the flanges of the blade, allowing for improved purchase in the femoral head. Biomechanical studies have shown the blade to be superior to a screw in both rotational control and resistance to collapse (59). Clinically, the blade has mixed results, with some studies resulting in less loss of fixation and implant migration than the dynamic screw (60) and others showing a high cut-out rate with a blade (15%) compared to a screw (3%) (61). Within blade failures, atypical medial cut-out has been reported (62).

Cannulated screws are generally suitable for nondisplaced or valgus impacted fractures of the femoral head. Care must be taken to examine preoperative and intraoperative lateral radiographs to make sure there is no displacement of the head. Greater than 15° of valgus angulation or posterior tilt is predictive of treatment failure, and arthroplasty should be considered so the patient endures only one operation (63). Impaction-type constructs for hip fracture have a reoperation rate of approximately 20% over the course of 2 years (64). Loss of femoral offset has been of concern, with the hypothesis of poorer function in the impaction device. Initial displacement is a predictor of femoral neck impaction collapse, as is age of the patient. Impaction of 11–15 mm is the threshold of worsening pain and mobility (56).

Cannulated screws can be inserted through a smaller incision or even percutaneously. Despite being a construct relying on impaction, initial intraoperative compression in a controlled setting is desirable with cannulated screws. A configuration of three screws in an inverted triangle is superior to a standard triangle (65), with care needed to ensure the lowest screw is not inserted distal to the lesser trochanter, which can precipitate subtrochanteric fracture in osteoporotic bone (66). The ability to control the rate of fracture collapse is desirable and is reduced in biomechanical models when a fully threaded posterior screw is inserted (67). *In vivo*, use of two or three fully threaded screws in an inverted triangle is associated with decreased neck shortening, with a partially threaded screw used per surgeon discretion to reduce inferior head ptosis or achieve calcar compression (68). The use of washers is often incorporated into cannulated screw constructs. In case series where adequate reduction is achieved, washers prevent fixation failure. The greater surface area is useful in the metaphyseal lateral cortical bone to generate compressive force on screw insertion (69).

Despite implantation into stable femoral neck fracture configurations, failure does occur (70). An ever-present surgical principle is to only perform one, definitive operation in the osteoporotic patient. Novel screw configurations focusing on medial calcar support and differing planes of screw orientation have theoretical advantages and biomechanical evidence of better tolerating dynamic forces and moments through gait than the classic inverted triangle (71). Compelling clinical data are needed before wide acceptance. Fortunately, arthroplasty salvage has excellent 5-year survival rates (72).

Regional variation exists in choice between implants, and surgeons within an institution will often have a preference between SHS and cannulated screws. The multinational FAITH study (Fixation using Alternative Implants for the Treatment of Hip fractures) demonstrated that the reoperation rate was similar between the two groups. SHS implants had a higher rate of avascular necrosis (9% versus 5%). Furthermore, of those implants revised, SHS had more reoperations for conversion to total hip, as opposed to change of fixation implants (64). The authors performed subgroup analyses demonstrating an advantage of the SHS in both displaced and basicervical fractures, by having lower reoperation rates, which makes biomechanical sense.

NAILING

Intramedullary nailing (IMN) is an attractive fixation option for osteoporotic fracture and is being increasingly utilized (73). The bone-implant interface strain can be reduced by having the implant within the load-bearing axis. Relative stability constructs can hence reduce nonunion and implant failure, with the construct being allowed to deform without jeopardizing interlocking screws. IMNs are load-sharing, minimally invasive, and often time-efficient compared with achieving the same fixation goals of plating. As fracture complexity increases, the ability to achieve satisfactory reduction with plating can become difficult and require extensile surgical approaches.

Intramedullary nails for the treatment of proximal femur fractures have been shown to be biomechanically advantageous to SHS constructs when the fracture extends out the lateral cortex, with less mechanical failure *in vivo* (74). Likewise, a fracture pattern with a detached greater trochanter benefits from nail fixation compared to SHS (75), as do transverse/reverse oblique or subtrochanteric proximal femur fractures (76). Other extramedullary devices such as 95° blade plate have fallen out of common use, and attempts to incorporate angular-stable fixation principles, which are theoretically advantageous in osteoporotic bones, have been unsuccessful. Proximal femur locking plates have demonstrated high failure rates and should not be routinely used when a load-sharing nail can be employed (77).

Despite the mechanical advantages, early nail designs showed greater complications (78). Modern nail designs may have lessened this, and a well-randomized comparison to SHS is needed (79). IMN randomized against SHS for "unstable" (AO31A2) fracture patterns has shown equivalent failure rates and functional outcomes; however, fixation with SHS is prone to 1 cm more of femoral neck shortening (80). In the subset of patients able to walk over 150 m premorbidly, IMN have better functional outcomes compared to SHS, likely due to IMN prevention of neck shortening. It can be recommended that high-functioning patients receive IMN from a functional perspective (81).

Short femoral nails for proximal femur fractures offer the advantage of being less invasive, avoiding anterior cortical penetration in the osteoporotic patient with a short arc of radius femoral bow, and having distal locking performed through the targeting device. Short nails have shown equivalent results for stable and unstable pertrochanteric fractures without subtrochanteric extension (82). Classifications have tried to define stability, and an unstable fracture is usually accepted as when the medial calcar is comminuted and provides insufficient structural support (57). In a fall-prone population, shorter nails have been hypothesized to have an increased rate of secondary periorthotic fracture (83). This is not borne out in

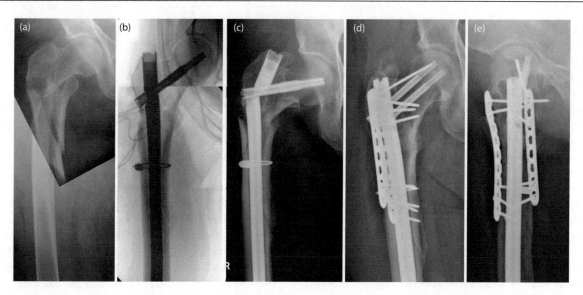

Figure 15.3 Comminuted proximal femur (a) underwent reduction with cerclage and long femoral nail (b). Despite excellent reduction, implant failure occurred at the 3-month mark (c). This was revised with nail exchange and augmented with bone graft from intramedullary reamings. Two small fragment locking compression plates were applied to provide rotational control (d and e) (x-ray at 1-year postrevision).

meta-analysis (84), and if a patient is at high fall risk, it may be rational to span the entire femur. This has to be weighed up with the increased blood loss and surgical time in inserting long nails (84). Short nails have to be performed with care: occult intraoperative peri-implant fracture does occur due to a combination of tight femoral canals, limited nail diameter options, and impaction. It is advised in osteoporotic bone to avoid impacting the nail down a tight femoral canal with force, and ream to an appropriate diameter if needed.

Mechanical failure can be reduced in both long and short femoral nailing by aiming for "three-point" proximal fixation. Having a lag screw that does not engage the lateral cortex and a tip-apex distance of greater than 25 mm are the greatest predictors of failure (85). Excessive shortening of the femoral neck during recovery and healing leads to an inability to retain ambulatory capacity and failure of the construct. It has been shown to not be associated with the "stability" of the fracture pattern (86). A screw within the center of the femoral head is traditionally the aim of fixation, and having the screw placed in the inferior neck on anteroposterior (AP) radiographs and central on the lateral leads to higher stiffness and load-to-failure in biomechanical models (87). Inferior neck screw positioning has also clinically been shown to reduce cut-out in unstable fracture patterns (88). Consequently, a tip-apex distance referenced off the inferior calcar, "CalTAD$_{AP}$," has been proposed as a better predictor of nail failure (89). Nailing in a varus position has also been shown to lead to failure (57). All attempts should be made to properly reduce the fracture pattern to avoid varus neck-shaft angle. A slightly medial entry point in relation to the greater trochanter will aid this, particularly in subtrochanteric fractures. In the event of nail failure, revision nailing with a focus on compression and rotational control at the fracture site is

advocated to achieve excellent clinical outcomes for the patient (Figure 15.3).

Intramedullary nailing ideally uses minimally invasive techniques. If the fracture pattern does not align in a satisfactory position, open reduction may be needed. Subtrochanteric femur fractures are a common scenario for this. This is a group that has a high nonunion and implant failure rate (90). Biomechanically, the restoration of the medial buttress (compression side of the femur) by indirect or soft tissue preserving direct-reduction techniques is critical to minimize the risk of failure (91). Cerclage wires to hold the reduced cortical fragments in reduced position around the intramedullary nail have had good clinical results and afford stability to gain optimal nail entry point (92). This can be done in a percutaneous method, avoiding extensive subvastus exposure (93). Other options providing anatomical reduction before nail insertion may include unicortical plating of the lateral cortex. Reducing the fracture during nailing and leaving no device to maintain reduction has also been shown to have good results with preserved soft tissues and periosteal blood supply (94).

Fractures in the periarticular regions fall into the extended indication of nailing and require careful preoperative planning. Nailing techniques provide advantages for soft tissue preservation and reduced morbidity from dissection, but limitations exist. Multiplanar locking options exist in many nailing systems, allowing for greater biomechanical stability in periarticular osteoporotic bone with capacious medullary canal. Furthermore, the advent of "screw-in-screw" fixation allows for further fragment-specific targeting. In proximal humerus biomechanical models, screw-in-screw configurations prevent fracture collapse (95). Retrograde femoral nail constructs hold similar problems. They are an attractive option for distal femur fractures

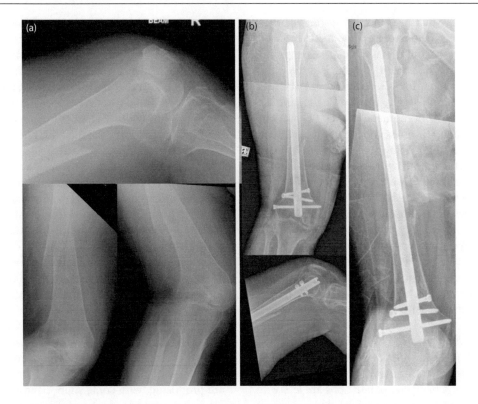

Figure 15.4 A severely osteoporotic, nonambulatory nursing home patient with cognitive impairment sustained a distal femoral spiral fracture, complicated by preexisting fixed flexion and valgus deformity of the knee (a). Primary goals of care are pain relief and to allow for easier nursing care. A minimally invasive retrograde nail can achieve reduction without disturbance of the fracture biology (post-op x-rays [b]) with callus formation displayed at the 3-month mark (c).

(Figure 15.4), with better patient-reported outcomes when compared to plating on the surface (96). However, heterogeneity in fracture patterns exists, particularly in relation to the level of articular involvement (32). Better-designed studies accounting for complex intra-articular fracture patterns not suitable for pure relative stability constructs (AO 33C2 and C3) need to be conducted to determine whether plates or nails show any clinical advantage.

Several IMN design features have been engineered specifically for osteoporotic bone. The proximal portion of the nail tends to be of greater diameter than standard trochanteric nails, allowing for greater implant contact. Singular lag screw constructs are favored, with a set screw that inserts from the proximal nail and engages into grooves on the lag screw, preventing rotation of the head on the shaft and controlling axial compression. The importance of engaging the set screw and controlling rotational moments has been highlighted in cases where lag screw migration into the pelvis has occurred (97).

The helical blade construct has been utilized with nail devices. In similar fashion to SHS constructs, it is hypothesized to give superior hold in the femoral head (98). Clinically, however, the blade has equivalent performance to screws in unstable fracture patterns (61). Perforations in helical blade designs allow for cement to be infiltrated, increasing the bone-implant interface, stiffness, and implant stability in biomechanical studies (99). In the clinical setting, cement augmentation of helical blade

is well tolerated with few complications (100). For retrograde femoral nails, distal spiral blades are used and hold the advantage of compacting cancellous bone, avoiding deformation on loading, and are both stiffer and stronger than conventional screws (101). Another strategy for osteoporotic bone is the use of distal "screw and nut" systems. These allow a retrograde nail to be used in a distal femur fracture with a condylar split, with the wide surface area of the nut generating compression across the articular surface via the screw threaded through the nail (102).

In the older patient, the radius of curvature (ROC) of the chosen nailing system is important. As humans age, the femur shortens, and the anterior bow of the femur increases. Race, sex, and height all affect femoral bow (103). This is seen more so in females, with the anterior femoral bow constantly increasing with age (104). Larger nail curvatures in a bowed femur will end in the anterior portion of the distal femur (105), and maintaining an anterior entry point can aid in preventing perforation of the anterior cortex (106). Most modern nails have a shorter radius of curvatures, with an ROC of 150 cm matching a geriatric femoral bow more closely than 200 cm ROC nails, leading to less cortical perforation and fracture (107). In the Asian population, a further reduction in ROC to 100 cm leads to better central positioning than 150 cm ROC nails (108).

IMN designs for the osteoporotic shoulder fracture have attempted to address the overall poor results with plate fixation (109). Traditionally considered a non-weight-bearing joint, it can often have increased forces transmitted across it with mobility aids. The humeral nail is attractive, from its minimally invasive nature and load-sharing philosophy, but accounts for a small percentage of proximal humeral internal fixation (109). Helical blades can be used to better suit osteoporotic bone. Humeral nails have less complications than proximal humeral plating (42), but complications are common, and osteoporotic cohorts have worse functional outcomes than younger cohorts with humeral nails (110). Reoperation rates have been cited as 13% for Neer type 2, 17% for type 3, and 63% for type 4 humeral fractures in systematic review (111). The nature of the shoulder joint may preclude the patient from gaining significant functional benefit from fixation, and the reoperation rate and risk and cost of further surgery must be considered.

The minimally invasive nature of the nail is important in patients with multiple comorbidities and a reduced quality of soft tissue and bone. Lateral malleolus fractures, despite being low-energy mechanisms and with union rates of 99% with plating (112), have a relatively high rate of complications associated with more invasive plating fixation: 30% in a young population (113) and 40% in the elderly population (114). Fibular nails are a minimally invasive option, and wound complications in elderly populations are less with nails than with plates (114). A study of distal fibular fractures (with a mean age of 65 years and 75% having significant systemic comorbidities) demonstrated complications of 20%, including a 5% revision rate for failure (115). The role of fibular nails has been further explored by randomizing with open plate fixation in a cohort over 65 years, demonstrating lower infection rates in nailing compared with ORIF, with reoperation and union rates similar. The overall cost of the nail, when taking into account complications, is cheaper on cost-benefit analysis (116).

AUGMENTATION

Osteoporotic fractures often occur in metaphyseal areas, with preexisting alterations to trabecular architecture.

Fracture and subsequent reduction can result in large cancellous bone defects that can benefit from augmentation. Osteosynthesis in osteoporotic bones is less successful with decreasing mineralization (117). The general principle of augmentation is that the material must provide structural support to fill a void and be of low morbidity. Stimulation of union through osteogenicity, osteoinductivity, and/or osteoconductivity is desirable, but not all augments hold these properties.

Autograft has traditionally been accepted as the gold standard. It is biocompatible, osteoinductive, osteoconductive, and osteogenic. Autologous cancellous bone is usually harvested from the anterior iliac crest, with other sites including the distal femur or proximal tibia. There is a general lack of availability in the osteoporotic patient. There has additionally been a high complication rate associated with the donor site. These include iatrogenic fracture, bleeding, infection, and local pain up to the 12-month mark (118).

Allograft can be in the form of processed bone crunch, struts, or graft. Intramedullary fibular grafts have been incorporated in proximal humeral fractures to address medial column loss and varus fracture collapse in combination with plate osteosynthesis. Biomechanical studies are promising, with some supporting clinical data (119). The same principle can be applied to the distal humerus (120). Most literature surrounding cortical onlay strut grafting is involved in periprosthetic fractures of the hip, which performs well with cerclage cables in conjunction with plate and screws (121). In unstable fracture and osteoporotic fracture patterns, this can be incorporated to provide stability if rigid fixation is needed.

Synthetic bone grafts are attractive solutions. They include porous materials, bioactive glasses, glass–ceramics, synthetic polymers, and calcium phosphates and sulfates. They lack autograft donor-site morbidity, the possibility of disease transmission, and histoincompatibility risk of allograft. However, many of these augments are expensive with limited evidence (17).

Calcium phosphate bone cement injection into metaphyseal bone defects shows promise for preventing fracture

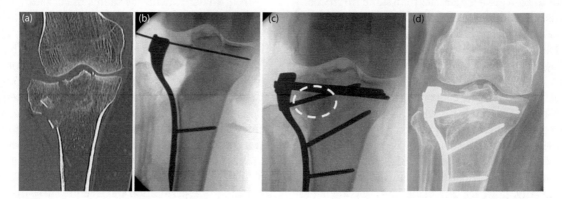

Figure 15.5 (a) A comminuted osteoporotic lateral tibial plateau fracture that had significant compression of the metaphyseal bone; (b) Rigid buttress fixation and augmentation were applied; (c) Radiopaque calcium phosphate implanted is shown within the oval; (d) At the 1-year mark union was achieved with a painless, functional range.

collapse (Figure 15.5). Calcium phosphate has the ability to osseointegrate and provides an osseoconductive scaffold (122). It increases screw pullout strength in osteoporotic bones models when infiltrated into cortical screw holes (123). It is an attractive option compared to traditional polymethyl methacrylate (PMMA) cement that can cause exothermic-related bone necrosis in the vulnerable fracture environment in addition to being difficult to remove in revision settings. PMMA is additionally not authorized as a weight-bearing construct (123). Calcium sulfate cement has been utilized in maintaining fracture reduction in proximal humeral fracture settings (124). It does however dissolve within 8 weeks, which may prematurely withdraw augmenting benefits, as seen in early collapse of tibial plateau fixation (125).

Augmenting constructs with PMMA cement has had many varied applications in osteoporotic bone. The concern for bone necrosis from the exothermic reactions can be obviated when limited amounts are employed (126). Cement that has a predictable viscosity, allowing for controlled injection and uniform distribution, should be used with care so that is does not perforate through articular surfaces. Radiopaque contrast material can be injected prior to cement application to prevent this complication (127). Cement augmentation is used in proximal femur fractures through perforations in the lag device that sits in the femoral head. This is used in both hip screws (128) and helical blades (100). Placing cement into the hole drilled for SHSs before insertion has been effective. Inserting cement into the superior head and neck above the lag screw has reduced cut-outs in biomechanical studies (129). In an effort to prevent contralateral injury, cementing femoral necks through the lateral cortex to create a "V-shape" (the arms of the V extending up the inferior and superior neck) has the potential to limit hip fracture (130). In the distal femur, biochemical models of distal locking plates have shown increased anchorage to the bone with the constructs utilizing PMMA, decreasing implant failure. This has been trialed in conventional locking screws with cement injected into drill holes before screw insertion (131), and cement infiltration into cannulated, perforated locking screws (132). In the proximal tibia, perforated screws with cement augmentation are biomechanically superior, preventing varus deformation in an angular stability locking plate construct (133).

The role of systemic bisphosphonates preventing fragility fractures, but leading to atypical femoral fractures, has been well described (134). Despite being uncommon, the fracture is concerning in part due to long times to union (135), with most bisphosphonate treatment being ceased due to concern of subsequent bone healing. The application of intraosseous bisphosphonate preventing osteoclast activity has shown promise in animal models. Zoledronate absorbed on nanohydroxyapatite particles, when injected into a drill hole prescrew insertion, resulted in rapid mineralization (136). Such technology is promising for osteoporotic fracture fixation.

ARTHRODESIS

Arthrodesis is an uncommon but valid surgical option. In complex injuries with articular destruction and metaphyseal bone loss, it is preferable to avoid complex periarticular reconstruction that may take an extended period to unite (with high risk of nonunion), need a period of non-weight-bearing, and involve large soft-tissue dissection. These operative dilemmas usually exist in the lower limb where arthroplasty options are poor. Complex tibial plafond injuries have had predictable arthrodesis results of uniting without soft tissue complications through anterior plating (137). Primary management of ankle fractures with poor soft tissue envelopes and high risk for complication are suitable for tibiotalocalcaneal (hindfoot) fusion nails as primary management (138). Hindfoot fusion is also a reproducible salvage operation for failed osteosynthesis (139). In the setting of a complex calcaneal fracture, subtalar fusion has been described with good results (140).

ARTHROPLASTY

There are currently many fixation options for metaphyseal and periarticular fractures. The principle of mobilizing patients with osteoporotic fractures and giving the patient one definitive operation is vital. Arthroplasty, where suitable, can allow the patient immediate mobilization and avoid the risk of nonunion or failure of fixation.

Intracapsular fractures of the hip account for 50% of hip fractures (141). It is generally accepted that displaced intracapsular fractures receive arthroplasty due to high rates of avascular necrosis. Internal fixation of these patterns has higher revision rates than arthroplasty (142). Within what is thought to be "undisplaced," posterior tilt on lateral radiographs is a predictor of fixation failure (143), and replacement should be strongly considered. Randomized trials have demonstrated that fixation in an unstable pattern results in higher reoperation rates compared to total hip arthroplasty (144) or hemiarthroplasty (145). When internal fixation fails, total arthroplasty is a reliable salvage operation, with less displacement of the initial fracture being associated with less postarthroplasty complications (72).

Cemented techniques are generally thought to be superior in the osteoporotic fracture, leading to improved functional and quality of life scores, in addition to reduced risk of intraoperative fracture (146). Concerns regarding bone cement implantation syndrome in hip fracture have led to guidelines recommending minimal manual pressurization and vigilance in the operating room at the time of cementing (147). Modern cementing techniques show no difference in blood pressure changes between noncemented and cemented stems in canal preparation and stem insertion (148). Perioperative mortality rates are not increased with cementing (149); however, unsupported apprehension still exists, which explains the persistent use of press-fit stems.

The CHANCE RCT on uncemented total hip prostheses in a younger subset of fragility fractures (65–79 years) against cemented stems (150) was terminated early due to higher complications in the uncemented group (151).

In regard to implant choice, decision-making hinges on premorbid function and life expectancy rather than level of osteoporosis. Total hip arthroplasty (THA) is superior to hemiarthroplasty in a younger patient cohort that is less likely to be severely osteoporotic. RCTs have shown better mobility, quality of life, and pain scores (152), and reduced mortality and revision rates that favor THA in the medium term (153).

The majority of fragility fractures will however receive hemiarthroplasty. In osteoporotic bone, bipolar head components for hemiarthroplasty have theoretical advantages with reducing acetabular erosion, which subsequently should reduce pain and improve function. Less acetabular erosion is demonstrated with the use of bipolar heads in RCTs, but this does not reach statistical significance at the 4-year mark (154). Heterogeneous functional and pain outcomes do not allow for pooled data, despite individual RCTs showing improved quality of life (155). Overall, bipolar heads do not clearly show superior function to unipolar heads despite increased cost (154).

Fractures of the acetabulum are increasing in prevalence and challenging in the osteoporotic patient, commonly involving the anterior column more than young patients (156). Of those receiving internal fixation, over 50% are not anatomically reduced. THA is used in approximately 25% of patients as a salvage option. This however is an operation with greater complexity, and the revision rate of THA from acetabular ORIF salvage is 20% (157). A role exists for combining acetabular column fixation and primary arthroplasty in the osteoporotic patient. Either through one extensile posterior approach or combining with an anterior approach if the anterior column is involved, a stable acetabulum can be created for standard preparation of a primary total hip (158). At 4-year follow-up, the majority of patients have excellent results (159).

Comminuted distal femoral fractures involving the joint surface usually require rigid fixation achieved through plating constructs. The ability to weight-bear immediately is often delayed, despite emerging evidence suggesting otherwise (26). On the contrary, weight-bearing, load-sharing nail constructs are often inadequate at reducing complex intra-articular fractures. Total knee arthroplasty allows early weight-bearing and negates the need for anatomical articular reconstruction. Highly constrained modular prostheses allow for most distal fracture patterns to be suitable. The procedure is not without complications, with 1-year mortality up to 40%, reflecting the frailty of the cohort, and a reoperation rate of 18% over 3 years (160). More recent literature reports very few complications or deaths (161). There is a need for high-quality studies to define for which patient arthroplasty would be best suited.

Tibial plateau fractures are often complex intra-articular fracture patterns, in which full weight-bearing is unusual post osteosynthesis. These fractures are associated with an increased risk of needing subsequent total knee arthroplasty (hazard ratio: 5.29) (162). Complications tend to be increased after revision surgery (fixation converted to arthroplasty) compared to primary arthroplasty (163). Total knee replacement has been used as the primary procedure in tibial plateau fractures with low complications, attributed to early, full weight-bearing mobilization. Semiconstrained components can be used in simpler fracture patterns (B1–B3) with hinged prostheses used for more complex patterns (B3–C3) (164).

The comminuted proximal humerus has shown little advantage with fixation or hemiarthroplasty over nonoperative management in an elderly population (109). In the PROFHER study, only 10% received hemiarthroplasty, with the vast majority being plated. Reverse shoulder arthroplasty (RSA) is popular in current practice for proximal humerus fractures, possibly in an older patient subset (165). Traditionally there was no clear functional differences as shown in clinical scores between the two procedures (166), but now improved RCT evidence shows clinically superior function with RSA (167). Superior prosthesis migration of hemiarthroplasty, plus nonunion, malunion, and resorption of the tuberosities are cited as reasons for choosing RSA over hemiarthroplasty. Whether to operate at all is even questioned with RSA: nonrandomized cohort studies currently show equivalent functional results between RSA and nonoperative management (168). Further RCTs will define the role of arthroplasty compared with fixation (169), RSA versus hemiarthroplasty (NTR3028 [PROSHERE], ISRCTN21981284 [SHeRPA], NCT02075476), and RSA compared with no intervention (ReSHAPE) (170).

The distal humerus is a joint with complex anatomy and a propensity for postoperative stiffness. Total elbow arthroplasty (TEA) is not only a salvage option for failed fixation but a valid surgical option to address comminuted metaphyseal fracture patterns with joint incongruity in osteoporotic bone. Patients chosen for primary arthroplasty for fracture have shown good or excellent results (171), and utilization has steadily increased over the last decade, despite being more expensive than fixation (172) and with a similar complication profile (173). In the only RCT addressing these questions, TEA was superior to fixation in functional outcomes but not reoperation or range of motion. The study had an intraoperative conversion to arthroplasty in 25% of randomized fixation candidates, the authors concluding that 2% of osteoporotic distal humerus fractures are not amenable to fixation (174). Major and minor complications are similar to fixation, with approximately one in three patients having a complication in the medium term (175). Despite high rates of complications, survival in fracture patients is up to 90% at the 10-year mark (176).

Distal humeral hemiarthroplasty (DHH) is also an option in unreconstructable or failed osteosynthesis of distal humeral fractures, avoiding failure from ulna component loosening, periprosthetic fracture, or polyethylene wear. DHH is appropriate if the epicondyles, collateral ligaments, and proximal ulna and radius need to be intact or

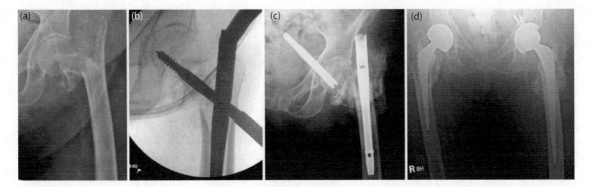

Figure 15.6 A comminuted proximal femur fracture (a) suitable for femoral nailing (b). The rotational moment exerted on the femoral neck with mobility has led the lag screw to wind through the osteoporotic acetabulum (c). The salvage option was a long stem cemented total hip replacement (d).

reconstructable. Furthermore, patient selection is important: even within the osteoporotic group, a low-level functioning patient is ideal (177). Cartilage wear from DHH is associated with worse functional and pain outcomes and is influenced by time after surgery but not age at surgery (178). Other medium-term results for DHH in small case series demonstrate instability and heterotopic ossification (179). Overall complication rates of DHH are similar to those of both TEA and fixation (180) and can be reduced via approaches that do not involve olecranon osteotomy in osteoporotic bone (181).

When initial osteosynthesis fails, arthroplasty is also advocated as a reliable and definitive solution in the periarticular area. With a "cut-out" or "cut-through" complication from femoral nailing of intertrochanteric fractures, several revision options exist: screw exchange, revision nailing, and joint replacement (Figure 15.6). Adhering to the principle of minimizing operative intervention in the osteoporotic patient, arthroplasty can have the most predictable outcome in a fragile population in certain fracture patterns. Despite the "predictability," functional outcomes after joint replacement still tend to be worse than those of patients who do not experience complications from primary fixation (182). This highlights the importance of making a concerted and calculated effort to plan and execute the most appropriate operation for this fragile patient cohort.

AFTERCARE

The postoperative course for surgical patients cannot be forgotten. Osteoporotic fractures occur in fragile patients, and it is well established that orthogeriatric units reduce morbidity and mortality and are generally cost-effective (183). Rehabilitation should be offered where cognition allows. Falls prevention and focusing on strength and functional performance give patients the best opportunity to remain at their previous level of care (184). During the time the consequences of trauma are dealt with, osteoporotic fractures are an opportunity to practice preventative medicine. A fracture liaison service can assess and commence

medical management in suitable patients, reducing major refracture rates by up to 40% (185).

After being discharged from surgical care, the frail patient is often difficult to follow up. Surgeons were the first group of physicians to audit their work, and it remains one of the quintessential surgical principles (186). Hip fracture patients are often not followed up in orthopedic clinics due to limited resources. It is only through the monitoring of patient outcomes that improved care can be provided. The UK National Hip Fracture Database has been operational for over a decade and shows improved patient outcomes from clinically based initiatives (187). When mortality will plateau in the United Kingdom is not known (188), but registries will allow evaluation of performance and inspire areas of clinical innovation.

CONCLUSION

The world's population is aging, and osteoporotic fractures will increase. The orthopedic surgeon needs to understand the patient, the injury, and what solution is best for the patient. When surgery is indicated, the fracture pattern and the benefits and limits of fixation need to be explored. The soft tissue envelope and timely medical optimization cannot be neglected. Augmentation of fixation where applicable can lead to a more robust and/or biologically active construct. The ability to fix a fracture is not always possible, and the principles of giving the patient one operation and early mobility with full weight-bearing should be maintained. Arthroplasty and primary arthrodesis are viable options. Most orthopedic departments and trauma centers are fortunate enough to have subspecialist orthopedic surgeons who can provide surgical expertise as necessitated.

Osteoporotic fractures are an opportunity to practice preventative medicine. A fracture liaison service can assess and commence medical management in suitable patients, reducing major refracture rates. Rehabilitation services need to be employed to return patients home where able, and a multidisciplinary team is necessary to help the surgical team make realistic discharge goals, which may include nursing home placement or even palliation.

The orthopedic evidence base is expanding, with the quality and number of trials increasing. The number of surgical devices and biologics is increasing, and technological innovations are often automatically viewed as better than existing practices. Orthopedic surgeons must keep abreast of this. When taking care of the osteoporotic patient with fracture, firm management principles will enable delivery of the highest standard of orthopedic service and provide leadership to the multidisciplinary hospital team.

REFERENCES

1. Cooper C, Cole ZA, Holroyd CR et al.; Epidemiology ICWGOF. Secular trends in the incidence of hip and other osteoporotic fractures. *Osteoporos Int.* 2011;22(5):1277–88.
2. Giannoudis P, Tzioupis C, Almalki T, Buckley R. Fracture healing in osteoporotic fractures: Is it really different? A basic science perspective. *Injury.* 2007;38(Suppl 1):S90–9.
3. Gibon E, Lu L, Goodman SB. Aging, inflammation, stem cells, and bone healing. *Stem Cell Res Ther.* 2016;7:44.
4. Loi F, Cordova LA, Pajarinen J, Lin TH, Yao Z, Goodman SB. Inflammation, fracture and bone repair. *Bone.* 2016;86:119–30.
5. Muller ME, Allgower M, Willenegger H. *Manual of Internal Fixation: Technique Recommended by the AO-Group.* 1970;1.
6. Lefaivre KA, Macadam SA, Davidson DJ, Gandhi R, Chan H, Broekhuyse HM. Length of stay, mortality, morbidity and delay to surgery in hip fractures. *J Bone Joint Surg Br.* 2009;91(7):922–7.
7. Moja L, Piatti A, Pecoraro V et al. Timing matters in hip fracture surgery: Patients operated within 48 hours have better outcomes. A meta-analysis and meta-regression of over 190,000 patients. *PLOS ONE.* 2012;7(10):e46175.
8. Arora R, Lutz M, Deml C, Krappinger D, Haug L, Gabl M. A prospective randomized trial comparing nonoperative treatment with volar locking plate fixation for displaced and unstable distal radial fractures in patients sixty-five years of age and older. *J Bone Joint Surg Am.* 2011;93(23):2146–53.
9. Sutherland AG, Cook A, Miller C et al. Older patients are immunocompromised by cytokine depletion and loss of innate immune function after HIP fracture surgery. *Geriatr Orthop Surg Rehabil.* 2015;6(4):295–302.
10. Fulop T, McElhaney J, Pawelec G et al. Frailty inflammation and immunosenescence. *Interdiscip Top Gerontol Geriatr.* 2015;41:26–40.
11. Girdlestone GR. Response of bone to stress: President's address. *Proc R Soc Med.* 1932;26(1):55–70.
12. Augat P, Goldhahn J. Osteoporotic fracture fixation—A biomechanical perspective. *Injury.* 2016; 47(Suppl 2):S1–2.
13. Egol KA, Kubiak EN, Fulkerson E, Kummer FJ, Koval KJ. Biomechanics of locked plates and screws. *J Orthop Trauma.* 2004;18(8):488–93.
14. Keene DJ, Lamb SE, Mistry D et al. Ankle injury management trial C. Three-year follow-up of a trial of close contact casting vs surgery for initial treatment of unstable ankle fractures in older adults. *JAMA.* 2018;319(12):1274–6.
15. Stromsoe K. Fracture fixation problems in osteoporosis. *Injury.* 2004;35(2):107–13.
16. Pesce V, Speciale D, Sammarco G, Patella S, Spinarelli A, Patella V. Surgical approach to bone healing in osteoporosis. *Clin Cases Miner Bone Metab.* 2009;6(2):131–5.
17. Marmor M, Alt V, Latta L et al. Osteoporotic fracture care: Are we closer to gold standards? *J Orthop Trauma.* 2015;29(Suppl 12):S53–6.
18. Perren SM. Evolution of the internal fixation of long bone fractures. The scientific basis of biological internal fixation: Choosing a new balance between stability and biology. *J Bone Joint Surg Br.* 2002;84(8):1093–110.
19. Larsson S, Procter P. Optimising implant anchorage (augmentation) during fixation of osteoporotic fractures: Is there a role for bone-graft substitutes? *Injury.* 2011;42(Suppl 2):S72–6.
20. Pidgeon TS, Johnson JP, Deren ME, Evans AR, Hayda RA. Analysis of mortality and fixation failure in geriatric fractures using quantitative computed tomography. *Injury.* 2018;49(2):249–55.
21. Tan SL, Balogh ZJ. Indications and limitations of locked plating. *Injury.* 2009;40(7):683–91.
22. Kolodziej P, Lee FS, Patel A et al. Biomechanical evaluation of the schuhli nut. *Clin Orthop Relat Res.* 1998;(347):79–85.
23. Fulkerson E, Egol KA, Kubiak EN, Liporace F, Kummer FJ, Koval KJ. Fixation of diaphyseal fractures with a segmental defect: A biomechanical comparison of locked and conventional plating techniques. *J Trauma.* 2006;60(4):830–5.
24. Freeman AL, Tornetta P 3rd, Schmidt A, Bechtold J, Ricci W, Fleming M. How much do locked screws add to the fixation of "hybrid" plate constructs in osteoporotic bone? *J Orthop Trauma.* 2010;24(3):163–9.
25. Ricci WM, Streubel PN, Morshed S, Collinge CA, Nork SE, Gardner MJ. Risk factors for failure of locked plate fixation of distal femur fractures: An analysis of 335 cases. *J Orthop Trauma.* 2014;28(2):83–9.
26. Poole WEC, Wilson DGG, Guthrie HC et al. "Modern" distal femoral locking plates allow safe, early weight-bearing with a high rate of union and low rate of failure: Five-year experience from a United Kingdom major trauma centre. *Bone Joint J.* 2017;99-B(7):951–7.
27. Helfet DL, Hotchkiss RN. Internal fixation of the distal humerus: A biomechanical comparison of methods. *J Orthop Trauma.* 1990;4(3):260–4.
28. Shin SJ, Sohn HS, Do NH. A clinical comparison of two different double plating methods for

intraarticular distal humerus fractures. *J Shoulder Elbow Surg.* 2010;19(1):2–9.

29. Kollias CM, Darcy SP, Reed JG, Rosvold JM, Shrive NG, Hildebrand KA. Distal humerus internal fixation: A biomechanical comparison of 90 degrees and parallel constructs. *Am J Orthop (Belle Mead NJ).* 2010;39(9):440–4.

30. Leigey DF, Farrell DJ, Siska PA, Tarkin IS. Bicolumnar 90-90 plating of low-energy distal humeral fractures in the elderly patient. *Geriatr Orthop Surg Rehabil.* 2014;5(3):122–6.

31. Steinberg EL, Elis J, Steinberg Y, Salai M, Ben-Tov T. A double-plating approach to distal femur fracture: A clinical study. *Injury.* 2017;48(10):2260–5.

32. Hoskins W, Sheehy R, Edwards ER et al. Nails or plates for fracture of the distal femur? data from the Victoria Orthopaedic Trauma Outcomes Registry. *Bone Joint J.* 2016;98-B(6):846–50.

33. Hoffmann MF, Jones CB, Sietsema DL, Tornetta P 3rd., Koenig SJ. Clinical outcomes of locked plating of distal femoral fractures in a retrospective cohort. *J Orthop Surg Res.* 2013;8:43.

34. Griffin XL, Parsons N, Zbaeda MM, McArthur J. Interventions for treating fractures of the distal femur in adults. *Cochrane Database Syst Rev.* 2015;(8):CD010606.

35. Rozell JC, Vemulapalli KC, Gary JL, Donegan DJ. Tibial plateau fractures in elderly patients. *Geriatr Orthop Surg Rehabil.* 2016;7(3):126–34.

36. Jiang R, Luo CF, Wang MC, Yang TY, Zeng BF. A comparative study of Less Invasive Stabilization System (LISS) fixation and two-incision double plating for the treatment of bicondylar tibial plateau fractures. *Knee.* 2008;15(2):139–43.

37. McNamara IR, Smith TO, Shepherd KL et al. Surgical fixation methods for tibial plateau fractures. *Cochrane Database Syst Rev.* 2015;(9):CD009679.

38. Jupiter JB, Ring D, Weitzel PP. Surgical treatment of redisplaced fractures of the distal radius in patients older than 60 years. *J Hand Surg Am.* 2002;27(4):714–23.

39. Wilcke MK, Hammarberg H, Adolphson PY. Epidemiology and changed surgical treatment methods for fractures of the distal radius: A registry analysis of 42,583 patients in Stockholm County Sweden: 2004–2010. *Acta Orthop.* 2013;84(3):292–6.

40. Chung KC, Shauver MJ, Birkmeyer JD. Trends in the United States in the treatment of distal radial fractures in the elderly. *J Bone Joint Surg Am.* 2009;91(8):1868–73.

41. Bartl C, Stengel D, Bruckner T, Gebhard F, Group OS. The treatment of displaced intra-articular distal radius fractures in elderly patients. *Dtsch Arztebl Int.* 2014;111(46):779–87.

42. Zhu Y, Lu Y, Shen J, Zhang J, Jiang C. Locking intramedullary nails and locking plates in the treatment of two-part proximal humeral surgical neck fractures:

A prospective randomized trial with a minimum of three years of follow-up. *J Bone Joint Surg Am.* 2011;93(2):159–68.

43. Olerud P, Ahrengart L, Ponzer S, Saving J, Tidermark J. Internal fixation versus nonoperative treatment of displaced 3-part proximal humeral fractures in elderly patients: A randomized controlled trial. *J Shoulder Elbow Surg.* 2011;20(5):747–55.

44. Jost B, Spross C, Grehn H, Gerber C. Locking plate fixation of fractures of the proximal humerus: Analysis of complications, revision strategies and outcome. *J Shoulder Elbow Surg.* 2013;22(4):542–9.

45. Schnetzke M, Bockmeyer J, Porschke F, Studier-Fischer S, Grutzner PA, Guehring T. Quality of reduction influences outcome after locked-plate fixation of proximal humeral type-C fractures. *J Bone Joint Surg Am.* 2016;98(21):1777–85.

46. Handoll HH, Brorson S. Interventions for treating proximal humeral fractures in adults. *Cochrane Database Syst Rev.* 2015;(11):CD000434.

47. Matar HE, Ali AA, Buckley S, Garlick NI, Atkinson HD. Surgical interventions for treating fractures of the olecranon in adults. *Cochrane Database Syst Rev.* 2014;(11):CD010144.

48. Ren YM, Qiao HY, Wei ZJ et al. Efficacy and safety of tension band wiring versus plate fixation in olecranon fractures: A systematic review and meta-analysis. *J Orthop Surg Res.* 2016;11(1):137.

49. Saeed ZM, Trickett RW, Yewlett AD, Matthews TJ. Factors influencing K-wire migration in tension-band wiring of olecranon fractures. *J Shoulder Elbow Surg.* 2014;23(8):1181–6.

50. Duckworth AD, Bugler KE, Clement ND, Court-Brown CM, McQueen MM. Nonoperative management of displaced olecranon fractures in low-demand elderly patients. *J Bone Joint Surg Am.* 2014;96(1):67–72.

51. Duckworth AD, Clement ND, McEachan JE, White TO, Court-Brown CM, McQueen MM. Prospective randomised trial of non-operative versus operative management of olecranon fractures in the elderly. *Bone Joint J.* 2017;99-B(7):964–72.

52. Symes M, Harris IA, Limbers J, Joshi M. SOFIE: Surgery for Olecranon Fractures in the Elderly: A randomised controlled trial of operative versus non-operative treatment. *BMC Musculoskelet Disord.* 2015;16:324.

53. Duckworth AD, Clement ND, White TO, Court-Brown CM, McQueen MM. Plate versus tension-band wire fixation for olecranon fractures: A prospective randomized trial. *J Bone Joint Surg Am.* 2017;99(15):1261–73.

54. Matta JM. Fractures of the acetabulum: Accuracy of reduction and clinical results in patients managed operatively within three weeks after the injury. *J Bone Joint Surg Am.* 1996;78(11):1632–45.

55. Spitler CA, Kiner D, Swafford R et al. Generating stability in elderly acetabular fractures-A biomechanical assessment. *Injury.* 2017;48(10):2054–9.

56. Crosby JM, Parker MJ. Femoral neck collapse after internal fixation of an intracapsular hip fracture: Does it indicate a poor outcome? *Injury.* 2016;47(12): 2760–3.

57. Knobe M, Gradl G, Ladenburger A, Tarkin IS, Pape HC. Unstable intertrochanteric femur fractures: Is there a consensus on definition and treatment in Germany? *Clin Orthop Relat Res.* 2013;471(9):2831–40.

58. Baumgaertner MR, Solberg BD. Awareness of tip-apex distance reduces failure of fixation of trochanteric fractures of the hip. *J Bone Joint Surg Br.* 1997;79(6):969–71.

59. O'Neill, F, Condon F, McGloughlin, T, Lenehan B, Coffey JC, Walsh M. Dynamic hip screw versus DHS blade: A biomechanical comparison of the fixation achieved by each implant in bone. *J Bone Joint Surg Br.* 2011;93(5):616–21.

60. Fang C, Lau TW, Wong TM, Lee HL, Leung F. Sliding hip screw versus sliding helical blade for intertrochanteric fractures: A propensity score-matched case control study. *Bone Joint J.* 2015;97-B(3):398–404.

61. Stern LC, Gorczyca JT, Kates S, Ketz J, Soles G, Humphrey CA. Radiographic review of helical blade versus lag screw fixation for cephalomedullary nailing of low-energy peritrochanteric femur fractures: There is a difference in cutout. *J Orthop Trauma.* 2017;31(6):305–10.

62. Chapman T, Zmistowski B, Krieg J, Stake S, Jones CM, Levicoff E. Helical blade versus screw fixation in the treatment of hip fractures with cephalomedullary devices: Incidence of failure and atypical "medial cutout." *J Orthop Trauma.* 2018;32(8):397–402.

63. Song HK, Choi HJ, Yang KH. Risk factors of avascular necrosis of the femoral head and fixation failure in patients with valgus angulated femoral neck fractures over the age of 50 years. *Injury.* 2016;47(12):2743–8.

64. Fixation using Alternative Implants for the Treatment of Hip fractures Investigators. Fracture fixation in the operative management of hip fractures (FAITH): An international, multicentre, randomised controlled trial. *Lancet.* 2017;389(10078):1519–27.

65. Yang JJ, Lin LC, Chao KH et al. Risk factors for nonunion in patients with intracapsular femoral neck fractures treated with three cannulated screws placed in either a triangle or an inverted triangle configuration. *J Bone Joint Surg Am.* 2013;95(1):61–9.

66. Jansen H, Frey SP, Meffert RH. Subtrochanteric fracture: A rare but severe complication after screw fixation of femoral neck fractures in the elderly. *Acta Orthop Belg.* 2010;76(6):778–84.

67. Schaefer TK, Spross C, Stoffel KK, Yates PJ. Biomechanical properties of a posterior fully threaded positioning screw for cannulated screw fixation of displaced neck of femur fractures. *Injury.* 2015;46(11):2130–3.

68. Weil YA, Qawasmi F, Liebergall M, Mosheiff R, Khoury A. Use of fully threaded cannulated screws decreases femoral neck shortening after fixation of femoral neck fractures. *Arch Orthop Trauma Surg.* 2018;138(5):661–7.

69. Zlowodzki M, Weening B, Petrisor B, Bhandari M. The value of washers in cannulated screw fixation of femoral neck fractures. *J Trauma.* 2005;59(4): 969–75.

70. Kain MS, Marcantonio AJ, Iorio R. Revision surgery occurs frequently after percutaneous fixation of stable femoral neck fractures in elderly patients. *Clin Orthop Relat Res.* 2014;472(12):4010–4.

71. Filipov O, Gueorguiev B. Unique stability of femoral neck fractures treated with the novel biplane double-supported screw fixation method: A biomechanical cadaver study. *Injury.* 2015;46(2):218–26.

72. Hernandez NM, Chalmers BP, Perry KI, Berry DJ, Yuan BJ, Abdel MP. Total hip arthroplasty after *in situ* fixation of minimally displaced femoral neck fractures in elderly patients. *J Arthroplasty.* 2018;33(1):144–8.

73. Anglen JO, Weinstein JN, American Board of Orthopaedic Surgery Research C. Nail or plate fixation of intertrochanteric hip fractures: Changing pattern of practice. A review of the American Board of Orthopaedic Surgery Database. *J Bone Joint Surg Am.* 2008;90(4):700–7.

74. Palm H, Jacobsen S, Sonne-Holm S, Gebuhr P, Hip Fracture Study G. Integrity of the lateral femoral wall in intertrochanteric hip fractures: An important predictor of a reoperation. *J Bone Joint Surg Am.* 2007;89(3):470–5.

75. Palm H, Lysen C, Krasheninnikoff M, Holck K, Jacobsen S, Gebuhr P. Intramedullary nailing appears to be superior in pertrochanteric hip fractures with a detached greater trochanter: 311 consecutive patients followed for 1 year. *Acta Orthop.* 2011;82(2):166–70.

76. Matre K, Havelin LI, Gjertsen JE, Vinje T, Espehaug B, Fevang JM. Sliding hip screw versus IM nail in reverse oblique trochanteric and subtrochanteric fractures. A study of 2716 patients in the Norwegian Hip Fracture Register. *Injury.* 2013;44(6):735–42.

77. Wirtz C, Abbassi F, Evangelopoulos DS, Kohl S, Siebenrock KA, Kruger A. High failure rate of trochanteric fracture osteosynthesis with proximal femoral locking compression plate. *Injury.* 2013;44(6):751–6.

78. Parker MJ, Handoll HH. Gamma and other cephalocondylic intramedullary nails versus extramedullary implants for extracapsular hip fractures in adults. *Cochrane Database Syst Rev.* 2010;(9):CD000093.

79. Queally JM, Harris E, Handoll HH, Parker MJ. Intramedullary nails for extracapsular hip fractures in adults. *Cochrane Database Syst Rev.* 2014;(9):CD004961.

80. Reindl R, Harvey EJ, Berry GK, Rahme E, Canadian orthopaedic trauma S. Intramedullary versus extramedullary fixation for unstable intertrochanteric fractures: A prospective randomized controlled trial. *J Bone Joint Surg Am.* 2015;97(23):1905–12.

81. Sanders D, Bryant D, Tieszer C et al. A multicenter randomized control trial comparing a novel intramedullary device (InterTAN) versus conventional treatment (Sliding Hip Screw) of geriatric hip fractures. *J Orthop Trauma*. 2017;31(1):1–8.

82. Hou Z, Bowen TR, Irgit KS et al. Treatment of pertrochanteric fractures (OTA 31-A1 and A2): Long versus short cephalomedullary nailing. *J Orthop Trauma*. 2013;27(6):318–24.

83. Vaughn J, Cohen E, Vopat BG, Kane P, Abbood E, Born C. Complications of short versus long cephalomedullary nail for intertrochanteric femur fractures, minimum 1 year follow-up. *Eur J Orthop Surg Traumatol*. 2015;25(4):665–70.

84. Zhang Y, Zhang S, Wang S et al. Long and short intramedullary nails for fixation of intertrochanteric femur fractures (OTA 31-A1, A2 and A3): A systematic review and meta-analysis. *Orthop Traumatol Surg Res*. 2017;103(5):685–90.

85. Abram SG, Pollard TC, Andrade AJ. Inadequate "three-point" proximal fixation predicts failure of the Gamma nail. *Bone Joint J*. 2013;95-B(6):825–30.

86. Gilat R, Lubovsky O, Atoun E, Debi R, Cohen O, Weil YA. Proximal femoral shortening after cephalomedullary nail insertion for intertrochanteric fractures. *J Orthop Trauma*. 2017;31(6):311–5.

87. Kuzyk PR, Zdero R, Shah S, Olsen M, Waddell JP, Schemitsch EH. Femoral head lag screw position for cephalomedullary nails: A biomechanical analysis. *J Orthop Trauma*. 2012;26(7):414–21.

88. De Bruijn K, den Hartog D, Tuinebreijer W, Roukema G. Reliability of predictors for screw cutout in intertrochanteric hip fractures. *J Bone Joint Surg Am*. 2012;94(14):1266–72.

89. Tosounidis TH, Castillo R, Kanakaris NK, Giannoudis PV. Common complications in hip fracture surgery: Tips/tricks and solutions to avoid them. *Injury*. 2015;46(Suppl 5):S3–11.

90. Haidukewych GJ, Berry DJ. Nonunion of fractures of the subtrochanteric region of the femur. *Clin Orthop Relat Res*. 2004;(419):185–8.

91. Muller T, Topp T, Kuhne CA, Gebhart G, Ruchholtz S, Zettl R. The benefit of wire cerclage stabilisation of the medial hinge in intramedullary nailing for the treatment of subtrochanteric femoral fractures: A biomechanical study. *Int Orthop*. 2011;35(8):1237–43.

92. Tomas J, Teixidor J, Batalla L, Pacha D, Cortina J. Subtrochanteric fractures: Treatment with cerclage wire and long intramedullary nail. *J Orthop Trauma*. 2013;27(7):e157–60.

93. Kim JW, Park KC, Oh JK, Oh CW, Yoon YC, Chang HW. Percutaneous cerclage wiring followed by intramedullary nailing for subtrochanteric femoral fractures: A technical note with clinical results. *Arch Orthop Trauma Surg*. 2014;134(9):1227–35.

94. Mingo-Robinet J, Torres-Torres M, Moreno-Barrero M, Alonso JA, Garcia-Gonzalez S. Minimally invasive clamp-assisted reduction and cephalomedullary nailing without cerclage cables for subtrochanteric femur fractures in the elderly: Surgical technique and results. *Injury*. 2015;46(6):1036–41.

95. Rothstock S, Plecko M, Kloub M, Schiuma D, Windolf M, Gueorguiev B. Biomechanical evaluation of two intramedullary nailing techniques with different locking options in a three-part fracture proximal humerus model. *Clin Biomech (Bristol Avon)*. 2012;27(7):686–91.

96. Tornetta P, 3rd. In Locked Plating vs. Retrograde Nailing for Distal Femur Fractures: A Multicenter Randomized Trial. *American Academy of Orthopaedic Surgeons Annual Meeting*. New Orleans Louisiana, 2014.

97. Li X, Heffernan MJ, Kane C, Leclair W. Medial pelvic migration of the lag screw in a short gamma nail after hip fracture fixation: A case report and review of the literature. *J Orthop Surg Res*. 2010;5:62.

98. Strauss E, Frank J, Lee J, Kummer FJ, Tejwani N. Helical blade versus sliding hip screw for treatment of unstable intertrochanteric hip fractures: A biomechanical evaluation. *Injury*. 2006;37(10):984–9.

99. Fensky F, Nuchtern JV, Kolb JP et al. Cement augmentation of the proximal femoral nail antirotation for the treatment of osteoporotic pertrochanteric fractures—A biomechanical cadaver study. *Injury*. 2013;44(6):802–7.

100. Kammerlander C, Gebhard F, Meier C et al. Standardised cement augmentation of the PFNA using a perforated blade: A new technique and preliminary clinical results. A prospective multicentre trial. *Injury*. 2011;42(12):1484–90.

101. Ito K, Hungerbuhler R, Wahl D, Grass R. Improved intramedullary nail interlocking in osteoporotic bone. *J Orthop Trauma*. 2001;15(3):192–6.

102. Niikura T, Lee SY, Sakai Y, Nishida K, Kuroda R, Kurosaka M. Retrograde intramedullary nailing for the treatment of femoral medial condyle fracture nonunion. *Strategies Trauma Limb Reconstr*. 2015;10(2):117–22.

103. Egol KA, Chang EY, Cvitkovic J, Kummer FJ, Koval KJ. Mismatch of current intramedullary nails with the anterior bow of the femur. *J Orthop Trauma*. 2004;18(7):410–5.

104. Karakas HM, Harma A. Femoral shaft bowing with age: A digital radiological study of Anatolian Caucasian adults. *Diagn Interv Radiol*. 2008;14(1):29–32.

105. Bazylewicz DB, Egol KA, Koval KJ. Cortical encroachment after cephalomedullary nailing of the proximal femur: Evaluation of a more anatomic radius of curvature. *J Orthop Trauma*. 2013;27(6):303–7.

106. Kanawati AJ, Jang B, McGee, R, Sungaran J. The influence of entry point and radius of curvature on femoral intramedullary nail position in the distal femur. *J Orthop*. 2014;11(2):68–71.

107. Collinge CA, Beltran CP. Does modern nail geometry affect positioning in the distal femur of elderly patients with hip fractures? A comparison of

otherwise identical intramedullary nails with a 200 versus 150 cm radius of curvature. *J Orthop Trauma*. 2013;27(6):299–302.

108. Schmutz B, Amarathunga J, Kmiec S Jr, Yarlagadda, P, Schuetz M. Quantification of cephalomedullary nail fit in the femur using 3D computer modelling: A comparison between 1.0 and 1.5 m bow designs. *J Orthop Surg Res* 2016;11(1):53.

109. Rangan A, Handoll H, Brealey S et al. Surgical vs nonsurgical treatment of adults with displaced fractures of the proximal humerus: The PROFHER randomized clinical trial. *JAMA*. 2015;313(10): 1037–47.

110. Giannoudis PV, Xypnitos FN, Dimitriou R, Manidakis N, Hackney R. Internal fixation of proximal humeral fractures using the Polarus intramedullary nail: Our institutional experience and review of the literature. *J Orthop Surg Res*. 2012;7:39.

111. Wong J, Newman JM, Gruson KI. Outcomes of intramedullary nailing for acute proximal humerus fractures: A systematic review. *J Orthop Traumatol*. 2016;17(2):113–22.

112. Davidovitch RI, Walsh M, Spitzer A, Egol KA. Functional outcome after operatively treated ankle fractures in the elderly. *Foot Ankle Int*. 2009;30(8):728–33.

113. Lamontagne J, Blachut PA, Broekhuyse HM, O'Brien PJ, Meek RN. Surgical treatment of a displaced lateral malleolus fracture: The antiglide technique versus lateral plate fixation. *J Orthop Trauma*. 2002;16(7):498–502.

114. Anderson SA, Li X, Franklin P, Wixted JJ. Ankle fractures in the elderly: Initial and long-term outcomes. *Foot Ankle Int*. 2008;29(12):1184–8.

115. Bugler KE, Watson CD, Hardie AR et al. The treatment of unstable fractures of the ankle using the Acumed fibular nail: Development of a technique. *J Bone Joint Surg Br*. 2012;94(8):1107–12.

116. White TO, Bugler KE, Appleton P, Will E, McQueen MM, Court-Brown CM. A prospective randomised controlled trial of the fibular nail versus standard open reduction and internal fixation for fixation of ankle fractures in elderly patients. *Bone Joint J*. 2016;98-B(9):1248–52.

117. Konstantinidis L, Helwig P, Hirschmuller A, Langenmair E, Sudkamp NP, Augat P. When is the stability of a fracture fixation limited by osteoporotic bone? *Injury*. 2016;47(Suppl 2):S27–32.

118. Russell TA, Leighton RK, Alpha BSM Tibeal Plateau Fracture Study Group. Comparison of autogenous bone graft and endothermic calcium phosphate cement for defect augmentation in tibial plateau fractures. A multicenter, prospective, randomized study. *J Bone Joint Surg Am*. 2008;90(10):2057–61.

119. Namdari S, Voleti PB, Mehta S. Evaluation of the osteoporotic proximal humeral fracture and strategies for structural augmentation during surgical treatment. *J Shoulder Elbow Surg*. 2012;21(12):1787–95.

120. Hildebrand GR, Wright DM, Marston SB, Switzer JA. Use of a fibular strut allograft in an osteoporotic distal humerus fracture: A case report. *Geriatr Orthop Surg Rehabil*. 2012;3(4):167–71.

121. Tsiridis E, Spence G, Gamie Z, El Masry MA, Giannoudis PV. Grafting for periprosthetic femoral fractures: Strut, impaction or femoral replacement. *Injury*. 2007;38(6):688–97.

122. Bajammal SS, Zlowodzki M, Lelwica A et al. The use of calcium phosphate bone cement in fracture treatment. A meta-analysis of randomized trials. *J Bone Joint Surg Am*. 2008;90(6):1186–96.

123. Stadelmann VA, Bretton E, Terrier A, Procter P, Pioletti DP. Calcium phosphate cement augmentation of cancellous bone screws can compensate for the absence of cortical fixation. *J Biomech*. 2010;43(15):2869–74.

124. Liu ZZ, Zhang GM, Ge T. Use of a proximal humeral internal locking system enhanced by injectable graft for minimally invasive treatment of osteoporotic proximal humeral fractures in elderly patients. *Orthop Surg*. 2011;3(4):253–8.

125. Goff T, Kanakaris NK, Giannoudis PV. Use of bone graft substitutes in the management of tibial plateau fractures. *Injury*. 2013;44(Suppl 1):S86–94.

126. Fliri L, Lenz M, Boger A, Windolf M. *Ex vivo* evaluation of the polymerization temperatures during cement augmentation of proximal femoral nail antirotation blades. *J Trauma Acute Care Surg*. 2012;72(4):1098–101.

127. Neuerburg C, Mehaffey S, Gosch M, Bocker W, Blauth M, Kammerlander C. Trochanteric fragility fractures: Treatment using the cement-augmented proximal femoral nail antirotation. *Oper Orthop Traumatol*. 2016;28(3):164–76.

128. Augat P, Rapp S, Claes L. A modified hip screw incorporating injected cement for the fixation of osteoporotic trochanteric fractures. *J Orthop Trauma*. 2002;16(5):311–6.

129. Stoffel KK, Leys T, Damen N, Nicholls RL, Kuster MS. A new technique for cement augmentation of the sliding hip screw in proximal femur fractures. *Clin Biomech (Bristol Avon)*. 2008;23(1):45–51.

130. Fliri L, Sermon A, Wahnert D, Schmoelz W, Blauth M, Windolf M. Limited V-shaped cement augmentation of the proximal femur to prevent secondary hip fractures. *J Biomater Appl*. 2013;28(1):136–43.

131. Wahnert D, Lange JH, Schulze M, Lenschow S, Stange R, Raschke MJ. The potential of implant augmentation in the treatment of osteoporotic distal femur fractures: A biomechanical study. *Injury*. 2013;44(6):808–12.

132. Wahnert D, Hofmann-Fliri L, Richards RG, Gueorguiev B, Raschke MJ, Windolf M. Implant augmentation: Adding bone cement to improve the treatment of osteoporotic distal femur fractures: A biomechanical study using human cadaver bones. *Medicine (Baltimore)*. 2014;93(23):e166.

133. Goetzen M, Nicolino T, Hofmann-Fliri L, Blauth M, Windolf M. Metaphyseal screw augmentation of the LISS-PLT plate with polymethylmethacrylate improves angular stability in osteoporotic proximal third tibial fractures: A biomechanical study in human cadaveric tibiae. *J Orthop Trauma*. 2014;28(5):294–9.

134. Kharwadkar N, Mayne B, Lawrence JE, Khanduja V. Bisphosphonates and atypical subtrochanteric fractures of the femur. *Bone Joint Res*. 2017;6(3):144–53.

135. Schilcher J, Michaelsson K, Aspenberg P. Bisphosphonate use and atypical fractures of the femoral shaft. *N Engl J Med*. 2011;364(18):1728–37.

136. Kettenberger U, Luginbuehl V, Procter P, Pioletti DP. *In vitro* and *in vivo* investigation of bisphosphonate-loaded hydroxyapatite particles for peri-implant bone augmentation. *J Tissue Eng Regen Med*. 2017;11(7), 1974–85.

137. Beaman DN, Gellman R. Fracture reduction and primary ankle arthrodesis: A reliable approach for severely comminuted tibial pilon fracture. *Clin Orthop Relat Res*. 2014;472(12):3823–34.

138. Taylor BC, Hansen DC, Harrison R, Lucas DE, Degenova D. Primary retrograde tibiotalocalcaneal nailing for fragility ankle fractures. *Iowa Orthop J*. 2016;36:75–8.

139. Houshian S, Bajaj SK, Mohammed AM. Salvage of osteoporotic ankle fractures after failed primary fixation with an ankle arthrodesis nail: A report on four cases. *Injury*. 2006;37(8):791–4.

140. Frangez I, Kasnik T, Cimerman M, Smrke DM. Guided tissue regeneration with heterologous materials in primary subtalar arthrodesis: A case report. *J Med Case Rep*. 2016;10(1):108.

141. Williams N, Hardy BM, Tarrant S et al. Changes in hip fracture incidence, mortality and length of stay over the last decade in an Australian major trauma centre. *Arch Osteoporos*. 2013;8(1–2):150.

142. Murphy DK, Randell T, Brennan KL, Probe RA, Brennan ML. Treatment and displacement affect the reoperation rate for femoral neck fracture. *Clin Orthop Relat Res*. 2013;471(8):2691–702.

143. Clement ND, Green K, Murray N, Duckworth AD, McQueen MM, Court-Brown CM. Undisplaced intracapsular hip fractures in the elderly: Predicting fixation failure and mortality. A prospective study of 162 patients. *J Orthop Sci*. 2013;18(4):578–85.

144. Chammout GK, Mukka SS, Carlsson T, Neander GF, Stark AW, Skoldenberg OG. Total hip replacement versus open reduction and internal fixation of displaced femoral neck fractures: A randomized long-term follow-up study. *J Bone Joint Surg Am*. 2012;94(21):1921–8.

145. Hedbeck CJ, Inngul C, Blomfeldt R, Ponzer S, Tornkvist H, Enocson A. Internal fixation versus cemented hemiarthroplasty for displaced femoral neck fractures in patients with severe cognitive dysfunction: A randomized controlled trial. *J Orthop Trauma*. 2013;27(12):690–5.

146. Inngul C, Blomfeldt R, Ponzer S, Enocson A. Cemented versus uncemented arthroplasty in patients with a displaced fracture of the femoral neck: A randomised controlled trial. *Bone Joint J*. 2015;97-B(11):1475–80.

147. Membership of Working Party, Griffiths R, White SM, Moppett IK et al., Association of Anaesthetists of Great Britain and Ireland; British Orthopaedic Association, British Geriatric Society. Safety guideline: Reducing the risk from cemented hemiarthroplasty for hip fracture 2015: Association of Anaesthetists of Great Britain and Ireland British Orthopaedic Association British Geriatric Society. *Anaesthesia*. 2015;70(5):623–6.

148. Miyamoto S, Nakamura J, Iida S et al. Intraoperative blood pressure changes during cemented versus uncemented bipolar hemiarthroplasty for displaced femoral neck fracture: A multi-center cohort study: The effect of bone cement for bipolar hemiarthroplasty in elderly patients. *Arch Orthop Trauma Surg*. 2017;137(4):523–9.

149. Costa ML, Griffin XL, Pendleton N, Pearson M, Parsons N. Does cementing the femoral component increase the risk of peri-operative mortality for patients having replacement surgery for a fracture of the neck of femur? Data from the National Hip Fracture Database. *J Bone Joint Surg Br*. 2011;93(10):1405–10.

150. Chammout G, Muren O, Boden H, Salemyr M, Skoldenberg O. Cemented compared to uncemented femoral stems in total hip replacement for displaced femoral neck fractures in the elderly: Study protocol for a single-blinded, randomized controlled trial (CHANCE-trial). *BMC Musculoskelet Disord*. 2016;17(1):398.

151. Chammout G, Muren O, Laurencikas E et al. More complications with uncemented than cemented femoral stems in total hip replacement for displaced femoral neck fractures in the elderly. *Acta Orthop*. 2017;88(2):145–51.

152. Wang F, Zhang H, Zhang Z, Ma C, Feng X. Comparison of bipolar hemiarthroplasty and total hip arthroplasty for displaced femoral neck fractures in the healthy elderly: A meta-analysis. *BMC Musculoskelet Disord*. 2015;16:229.

153. Avery PP, Baker RP, Walton MJ et al. Total hip replacement and hemiarthroplasty in mobile, independent patients with a displaced intracapsular fracture of the femoral neck: A seven- to ten-year follow-up report of a prospective randomised controlled trial. *J Bone Joint Surg Br*. 2011;93(8):1045–8.

154. Jia Z, Ding F, Wu Y et al. Unipolar versus bipolar hemiarthroplasty for displaced femoral neck fractures: A systematic review and meta-analysis of randomized controlled trials. *J Orthop Surg Res*. 2015;10:8.

155. Inngul C, Hedbeck CJ, Blomfeldt R, Lapidus G, Ponzer S, Enocson A. Unipolar hemiarthroplasty

versus bipolar hemiarthroplasty in patients with displaced femoral neck fractures: A four-year follow-up of a randomised controlled trial. *Int Orthop.* 2013;37(12):2457–64.

156. Ferguson TA, Patel R, Bhandari M, Matta JM. Fractures of the acetabulum in patients aged 60 years and older: An epidemiological and radiological study. *J Bone Joint Surg Br.* 2010;92(2):250–7.

157. Daurka JS, Pastides PS, Lewis A, Rickman M, Bircher MD. Acetabular fractures in patients aged >55 years: A systematic review of the literature. *Bone Joint J.* 2014;96-B(2):157–63.

158. Rickman M, Young J, Trompeter A, Pearce R, Hamilton M. Managing acetabular fractures in the elderly with fixation and primary arthroplasty: Aiming for early weightbearing. *Clin Orthop Relat Res.* 2014;472(11):3375–82.

159. Ortega-Briones A, Smith S, Rickman M. Acetabular fractures in the elderly: Midterm outcomes of column stabilisation and primary arthroplasty. *Biomed Res Int.* 2017;2017:4651518.

160. Appleton P, Moran M, Houshian S, Robinson CM. Distal femoral fractures treated by hinged total knee replacement in elderly patients. *J Bone Joint Surg Br.* 2006;88(8):1065–70.

161. Atrey A, Hussain N, Gosling O et al. A 3 year minimum follow up of endoprosthetic replacement for distal femoral fractures—An alternative treatment option. *J Orthop.* 2017;14(1):216–22.

162. Wasserstein D, Henry P, Paterson JM, Kreder HJ, Jenkinson R. Risk of total knee arthroplasty after operatively treated tibial plateau fracture: A matched-population-based cohort study. *J Bone Joint Surg Am.* 2014;96(2):144–50.

163. Saleh KJ, Sherman P, Katkin P et al. Total knee arthroplasty after open reduction and internal fixation of fractures of the tibial plateau: A minimum five-year follow-up study. *J Bone Joint Surg Am.* 2001;83-A(8):1144–8.

164. Haufe T, Forch S, Muller P, Plath J, Mayr E. The role of a primary arthroplasty in the treatment of proximal tibia fractures in orthogeriatric patients. *Biomed Res Int.* 2016;2016:6047876.

165. Dean BJ, Jones LD, Palmer AJ et al. A review of current surgical practice in the operative treatment of proximal humeral fractures: Does the PROFHER trial demonstrate a need for change? *Bone Joint Res.* 2016;5(5):178–84.

166. Ferrel JR, Trinh TQ, Fischer RA. Reverse total shoulder arthroplasty versus hemiarthroplasty for proximal humeral fractures: A systematic review. *J Orthop Trauma.* 2015;29(1):60–8.

167. Sebastia-Forcada E, Cebrian-Gomez R, Lizaur-Utrilla A, Gil-Guillen V. Reverse shoulder arthroplasty versus hemiarthroplasty for acute proximal humeral fractures. A blinded, randomized, controlled, prospective study. *J Shoulder Elbow Surg.* 2014;23(10):1419–26.

168. Roberson TA, Granade CM, Hunt Q et al. Nonoperative management versus reverse shoulder arthroplasty for treatment of 3- and 4-part proximal humeral fractures in older adults. *J Shoulder Elbow Surg.* 2017;26(6):1017–22.

169. Fjalestad T, Iversen P, Hole MO, Smedsrud M, Madsen JE. Clinical investigation for displaced proximal humeral fractures in the elderly: A randomized study of two surgical treatments: Reverse total prosthetic replacement versus angular stable plate Philos (The DELPHI-trial). *BMC Musculoskelet Disord.* 2014;15:323.

170. Smith GC, Bateman E, Cass B et al. Reverse Shoulder Arthroplasty for the treatment of Proximal humeral fractures in the Elderly (ReShAPE trial) : Study protocol for a multicentre combined randomised controlled and observational trial. *Trials.* 2017;18(1):91.

171. Frankle MA, Herscovici D Jr, DiPasquale TG, Vasey MB, Sanders RW. A comparison of open reduction and internal fixation and primary total elbow arthroplasty in the treatment of intraarticular distal humerus fractures in women older than age 65. *J Orthop Trauma.* 2003;17(7):473–80.

172. Rajaee SS, Lin CA, Moon CN. Primary total elbow arthroplasty for distal humeral fractures in elderly patients: A nationwide analysis. *J Shoulder Elbow Surg.* 2016;25(11):1854–60.

173. Lovy AJ, Keswani A, Koehler SM, Kim J, Hausman M. Short-term complications of distal humerus fractures in elderly patients: Open reduction internal fixation versus total elbow arthroplasty. *Geriatr Orthop Surg Rehabil.* 2016;7(1):39–44.

174. McKee MD, Veillette CJ, Hall JA et al. A multicenter, prospective, randomized, controlled trial of open reduction—Internal fixation versus total elbow arthroplasty for displaced intra-articular distal humeral fractures in elderly patients. *J Shoulder Elbow Surg.* 2009;18(1):3–12.

175. Githens M, Yao J, Sox AH, Bishop J. Open reduction and internal fixation versus total elbow arthroplasty for the treatment of geriatric distal humerus fractures: A systematic review and meta-analysis. *J Orthop Trauma.* 2014;28(8):481–8.

176. Barco R, Streubel PN, Morrey BF, Sanchez-Sotelo J. Total elbow arthroplasty for distal humeral fractures: A ten-year-minimum follow-up study. *J Bone Joint Surg Am.* 2017;99(18):1524–31.

177. Burkhart KJ, Nijs S, Mattyasovszky SG et al. Distal humerus hemiarthroplasty of the elbow for comminuted distal humeral fractures in the elderly patient. *J Trauma.* 2011;71(3):635–42.

178. Smith GC, Hughes JS. Unreconstructable acute distal humeral fractures and their sequelae treated with distal humeral hemiarthroplasty: A two-year to eleven-year follow-up. *J Shoulder Elbow Surg.* 2013;22(12):1710–23.

179. Heijink A, Wagener ML, de Vos MJ, Eygendaal D. Distal humerus prosthetic hemiarthroplasty:

Midterm results. *Strategies Trauma Limb Reconstr.* 2015;10(2):101–8.

180. Phadnis J, Banerjee S, Watts AC, Little N, Hearnden A, Patel VR. Elbow hemiarthroplasty using a "triceps-on" approach for the management of acute distal humeral fractures. *J Shoulder Elbow Surg.* 2015;24(8):1178–86.

181. Phadnis J, Watts AC, Bain GI. Elbow hemiarthroplasty for the management of distal humeral fractures: Current technique, indications and results. *Shoulder Elbow.* 2016;8(3):171–83.

182. Zielinski SM, Keijsers NL, Praet SF et al. Functional outcome after successful internal fixation versus salvage arthroplasty of patients with a femoral neck fracture. *J Orthop Trauma.* 2014;28(12):e273–80.

183. Sabharwal S, Wilson H. Orthogeriatrics in the management of frail older patients with a fragility fracture. *Osteoporos Int.* 2015;26(10):2387–99.

184. Pfeifer M, Sinaki M, Geusens P, Boonen S, Preisinger E, Minne HW, ASBMR Working Group on Musculoskeletal Rehabilitation. Musculoskeletal rehabilitation in osteoporosis: A review. *J Bone Miner Res.* 2004;19(8):1208–14.

185. Nakayama A, Major G, Holliday E, Attia J, Bogduk N. Evidence of effectiveness of a fracture liaison service to reduce the re-fracture rate. *Osteoporos Int.* 2016;27(3):873–9.

186. Trunkey DD. Invited commentary: Panel reviews of trauma mortality. *J Trauma.* 1999;47(Suppl 3): S44–5.

187. NHFD (NHFD). *National Report 2011-Summary;* 2011.

188. Giannoulis D, Calori GM, Giannoudis PV. Thirty-day mortality after hip fractures: Has anything changed? *Eur J Orthop Surg Traumatol.* 2016;26(4): 365–70.

16

Can we accelerate the osteoporotic bone fracture healing response?

MARTIJN VAN GRIENSVEN and ELIZABETH ROSADO BALMAYOR

INTRODUCTION

Osteoporosis is a systemic skeletal disease. It is characterized by a diminished bone mineral density and a change in the bone microarchitecture. These result in a reduction of the bone stiffness and thereby an increased risk for fractures (1). In women, decreased estrogen levels postmenopausal induce increased receptor activator of nuclear factor–κB ligand (RANKL) and lower osteoprotegerin secretion of osteoblasts. The higher presence of RANKL activates receptor activator of nuclear factor-κB (RANK) receptors in the surface of preosteoclasts. Subsequently, their differentiation and activation are induced. This in turn leads to a disbalance of the bone homeostasis related cells. The increased number of osteoclasts leads to an increased loss of bone mineral, and thereby the fracture risk is increased (2). When fractures are present, they show less intrinsic healing capacity. Moreover, as the structure of the bone per se is compromised, surgical treatment is also more difficult.

Current therapy concepts

Therapy concepts for osteoporosis are mainly systemic therapies with the goal of inhibiting bone resorption and thereby reducing the risk of fracture (3). Four groups of therapy can be distinguished (Table 16.1). The basic therapy consists of calcium carbonate to supplement the body with 40% of elementary calcium. This is mostly administered in combination with cholecalciferol as precursor for vitamin D. The cholecalciferol is metabolized by cytochrome P450 to calcitriol that induces an increased resorption of calcium in the intestines to the blood. From there the calcium is going to the bone, where osteoblasts exert their effects leading to an increased calcium deposition. This will lead to increased bone mineral density and stronger bones.

In the group of antiresorptive therapies, bisphosphonates, anti-RANKL, and specific estrogen receptor modulators can be found. Bisphosphonates bind to hydroxyapatite

in the bone tissue and are taken up by the osteoclasts during the process of bone resorption (4). This leads intracellularly to an inhibition of the osteoclast metabolism and thereby to apoptosis of the osteoclasts. This results in a suppression of bone resorption. As the anabolic bone activity is not impaired, the net effect is that bone mineral density and bone mass are increased.

Denosumab is an anti-RANKL antibody. Upon binding, osteoclast activity is diminished as is the production of new osteoclasts. Again, this leads to an inhibition of bone resorption, and with the concomitant normal anabolic bone activity, bone mineral density is increased (5).

Selective estrogen receptor modulators bind with high affinity to the estrogen receptor. This binding leads in bone tissue to an agonistic action, which leads to reduced RANKL and higher osteoprotegerin secretion from osteoblasts. This in turn leads to an inhibition of the differentiation and activation of osteoclasts. Thus, the net effect is again osteoanabolic. The effect of selective estrogen receptor modulators on bone relevant markers is, however, less measurable in comparison to the effects of bisphosphonates (6).

In the group of osteoanabolic drugs, mainly parathyroid hormone (PTH) is known. In particular, the first 34 amino acids of the parathyroid are used in the therapy as they are as effective as the complete molecule consisting of 84 amino acids (7). PTH stimulates osteoblasts and leads to a better interconnection of new trabeculae. The improved microarchitecture of the bone leads to better bone stiffness. A disadvantage of PTH therapy is that when administered for a long period of time, osteosarcomas can occur (8).

The last type of osteoporosis therapeutic drug has both osteoanabolic and antiresorptive characteristics. Strontium is well known to have these possibilities. It is used as ranelate and stimulates bone building and inhibits bone resorption. Each effect, per se, is less intense as seen for drugs that are purely antiresorptive or purely osteoanabolic.

Some small clinical studies show that combination therapies may have advantages over single drug therapies (9). Those studies mainly investigated bone mineral density

Table 16.1 Current therapy modalities for osteoporosis

Basic	Antiresorptive drugs	Osteoanabolic drugs	Osteoanabolic + antiresorptive drugs
Ca^{2+}	Bisphosphonates	PTH	Strontium ranelate
Vitamin D	• Alendronate	• 1–34 PTH analog	
	• Risedronate	• 1–84 PTH analog	
	• Ibandronate		
	• Zoledronate		
	RANKL-antibody		
	• Denosumab		
	SERMs		
	• Raloxifene		

Abbreviations: PTH, parathyroid hormone; RANKL, receptor activator of nuclear factor–κB ligand; SERM, selective estrogen receptor modulator.

by dual-energy x-ray absorptiometry (DEXA) analysis or by volumetric bone mineral density determination using quantitative computer tomography. None of those studies investigated the incidence of fractures.

LOCAL CELL THERAPY TO ACCELERATE FRACTURE HEALING

In order to accelerate fracture healing in osteoporotic patients, the basic treatment of fractures should be followed. However, besides the systemic therapies, local therapies to accelerate fracture healing can be taken into consideration. Locally stimulating fracture healing takes the same factors into consideration as for normal fracture healing or treatment of nonunions, e.g., the diamond concept (10,11). In the context of osteoporosis, adding mesenchymal stem cells may push the balance more toward an anabolic phenotype. Using biomaterials will provide a matrix that provides biomechanical stability. Growth factors will stimulate cells to differentiate and activate them to perform osteoanabolic actions. In this chapter, we focus on cells and growth factors.

Cell therapy for acceleration of fracture healing

In the field of regeneration, mesenchymal stem cells play an important role. They can be obtained autologously and are thereby in most countries a feasible means for therapy. It has been clinically proven that mesenchymal stem cells may have beneficial effects in pathologies such as graft-versus-host disease, myocardial infarction, amyotrophic lateral sclerosis, osteogenesis imperfecta, and Crohn fistula (12–16). The two main sources that are clinically used for obtaining mesenchymal stem cells are bone marrow and adipose tissue. Bone marrow mesenchymal stem cells have been claimed to be the gold standard for regeneration in the musculoskeletal field. Bone marrow mesenchymal stem cells can be isolated from bone marrow aspirates using gradient centrifugation. They have a relatively high frequency

in the bone marrow (17). Semiclosed centrifuges with gradients or ultraviolet light spectroscopy are available for use in the operating room. In the case of osteoporotic patients, attention needs to be given to the fact that the quality of mesenchymal stem cells that can be isolated diminishes with the age of the patient (18).

Besides the isolation of mesenchymal stem cells from bone marrow, adipose tissue can also be used that can be obtained from liposuction or liporesection procedures (19). The isolation of cells from adipose tissue is slightly more cumbersome than that from bone marrow. The fat tissue needs to be minced and digested by enzymes to allow the mesenchymal stem cells to be released from the tissue. The suspension of minced tissue and mesenchymal stem cells can then be passed through a cell strainer so that only the cell suspension remains. An automated procedure exists for clinical usage directly in the operating room.

For both procedures, it has to be taken into account that clinical good manufacturing practice procedures are necessary to ensure safety, reproducibility, and efficient use. Thus, all materials including the enzymes used must be well defined and validated.

Reamer-irrigator-aspirator

Mesenchymal stem cells obtained by the previously described methods can be implanted by either percutaneous injection or in combination with biomaterials. This ensures that the mesenchymal stem cells remain locally at the fracture site for a certain period. It is also known that the mesenchymal stem cells may migrate out of the defect area. However, it is important that they secrete locally osteoanabolic factors.

To avoid the use of biomaterials that have advantages and disadvantages themselves, one can also consider use of the reamer-irrigator-aspirator (RIA) method (20). In this method, complete bone marrow together with sawdust from the inner bone marrow channel is aspirated using a reaming procedure of a healthy long bone. The obtained material has a solid but smooth consistency and provides the optimal environment for the mesenchymal stem cells already embedded. The RIA material provides a natural extracellular matrix with growth factors and provides integration in the defects and natural bone.

LOCAL HUMORAL FACTORS TO ACCELERATE FRACTURE HEALING IN OSTEOPOROTIC PATIENTS

As stated in the diamond concept, growth factors are important for bone regeneration. Mesenchymal stem cells produce growth factors and the RIA material contains natural growth factors. Thus, recombinant growth factors may be used to accelerate fracture healing in osteoporotic patients. However, other factors may be used locally in the context of osteoporotic fracture healing.

Local release of parathyroid hormone

As stated previously (in the "Current therapy concepts" section), PTH is systemically used to treat osteoporosis. Its action results in a net gain in bone mineral density (21). As the mechanism is probably due to direct influence on osteoblasts and osteoclasts (22), a local treatment would probably also be beneficial. PTH is osteoinductive. Runx2 and osterix are expressed upon injection of PTH in mice with a fracture (21). In a diabetic rat model with a subcritical femur defect, similar effects with increased bone mineral density were observed (23). PTH may also stimulate mesenchymal stem cells to differentiate into osteoblasts (24).

In order to administer PTH locally, loading onto tricalcium phosphate scaffolds has been investigated in *in vivo* models. Implantation of tricalcium phosphate loaded with 30 μg/kg or 60 μg/kg PTH in a critically sized femur defect in rats, resulted in bone regeneration with a good bone quality (25,26). In order to optimize the release of parathyroid hormone, the tricalcium phosphate can be combined with collagen. Thereby, bone regeneration could be achieved with a lower dose of PTH (27).

Another possibility of achieving a slow release of PTH is coupling it via a transglutaminase substrate to fibrin. Implantation in drill-hole defects in femora and humeri of sheep resulted in increased bone percentage in a dose-dependent manner (28). This modified fibrin can be mixed with ceramic granules, thereby boosting even more bone regeneration (29).

MicroRNA for local treatment of osteoporotic fractures

Micro-Ribonucleicacids (MicroRNAs) are short, double-stranded, noncoding Ribonucleicacid (RNA) segments of 22 nucleotides. They are able to modulate important cellular biological functions such as proliferation, differentiation, and apoptosis (30,31). MicroRNAs are able to modulate these functions by inhibiting important protein translation. This occurs through either cleavage or direct repression of target messenger RNA (32). One microRNA can target several messenger RNAs. And one messenger RNA can be targeted by several microRNAs. This indicates the versatility and complexity of the microRNA modulating system. It has been calculated that microRNAs may regulate one-third of the human transcriptome, thereby regulating 50% of all human protein coding genes (33,34). MicroRNAs have been described to play a role in many different diseases. This also holds true for pathologies of the musculoskeletal system (35).

MICRORNA IN OSTEOPOROSIS

Osteoporosis has been associated with differentially regulated microRNAs in complete tissue, osteoblasts, osteoclasts, and the circulation as a free form (36–38). It was also shown that the expression levels of these microRNAs in serum from osteoporotic patients with fractures are gender independent. More interestingly, the level of microRNA expression in the serum correlates very well with bone mineral density values. For all investigated microRNAs, it was shown that the higher the microRNA level, the lower was the bone mineral density. This was highly significant for miR-21-5p, miR-24-3p, miR-93-5p, miR-100-5p, and miR-125b-5p (39). All of these microRNAs have targets that are crucial for bone formation or bone resorption (Figure 16.1).

Some of the microRNAs inhibit the transcription factors Runx2 and Osterix. These transcription factors are important for the activation of the osteogenic genes osteocalcin, osteopontin, bone sialoprotein, collagen Iα1, and matrix metalloproteinase (MMP)-13 (40). Other microRNAs are involved in the inhibition of growth factor effects by, for instance, inhibiting the translation of bone morphogenetic protein (BMP)-2 (41,42). This may also be conducted via inhibiting the expression of the receptor for BMPs (43–45).

Besides these osteoanabolic inhibiting microRNAs, microRNAs exist that inhibit inhibitors of osteoclast activity. Thereby, osteoclast activity and osteoclast production are increased, leading to bone resorption (36,46). For instance, miR-133a was highly upregulated in osteoporotic women, and this again showed an inverse correlation with bone mineral density (47).

USING ANTAGOMIRS AS LOCAL THERAPY IN OSTEOPOROTIC FRACTURES

Thus, in osteoporotic fractures, microRNAs can be upregulated that (1) inhibit the formation of bone-forming cells and/or bone-forming activity and (2) inhibit osteoclast-inhibiting proteins. Therefore, these microRNAs are detrimental for fracture healing in osteoporotic patients. Blocking these upregulated microRNAs would be a possible mechanism to ameliorate the negative effects and improve fracture healing. Inhibition of microRNAs can be achieved by using "antagomirs." Antagomirs are complementary RNA strands that bind to the active microRNA strand and then either degrade or block the binding to the target messenger RNA sequence. Subsequently, the microRNA cannot bind to its complementary messenger

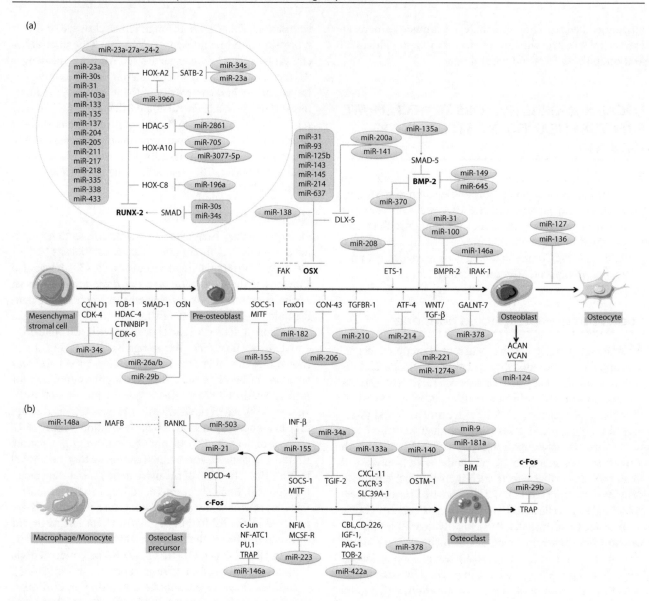

Figure 16.1 Presentation of microRNAs associated with osteoporosis. microRNAs related to either bone formation (a) or osteoclastic activity (b) are shown. The involved microRNAs regulate pathway components directly (solid lines) or indirectly (broken lines). (Reprinted with permission from Mary Ann Liebert, Inc., from Seeliger C et al. *Stem Cells Dev.* 2016;25[17]:1261–81.)

RNA, and there is no interference with the translation of the target messenger RNA into protein. The delivery of antagomirs is similar to the delivery in gene therapy. Antagomir delivery has been investigated in an array of different mammalian cells (48,49). It has also been used in *in vivo* models targeting different tissues such as brain and liver (50–52). The first clinical studies are being conducted using antagomir-122 for treating hepatitis C (53,54).

In a preliminary *in vitro* study for bone regeneration in an osteoporotic setting, we could show that transfecting osteoporotic osteoblasts using lipofectamine and antagomir for miR-100 was able to restore the transcription of BMP-R2. Thereby, osteoanabolic signals could be transferred again into the osteoblasts that started to produce collagen Iα1 as a typical protein of the bone extracellular matrix. Moreover, the osteoblasts increase the production of alkaline phosphatase and osteocalcin. Using

an antagomir against miR-148a increased MAFB (V-maf musculoaponeurotic fibrosarcoma oncogene homolog B) and thereby inhibited the maturation of osteoclasts. This resulted in less resorptive activity.

Therefore, it seems feasible to use antagomir therapy to accelerate fracture healing in osteoporotic patients. Nevertheless, it needs to be taken into account that several microRNAs are upregulated that have many different targets. The question is if blocking one microRNA is enough or if several microRNAs need to be antagonized. This drawback may be overcome by using microRNA "sponges" (55,56). They are also microRNA inhibitors; however, they contain multiple binding sites. Thereby, one microRNA sponge can target several microRNAs. They have been tested *in vivo* in neurological settings (57–59).

Another problematic aspect is delivering the antagomirs to the cells. The cells need to be transfected with the antagomir. Whether naked antagomirs can penetrate the cell membrane is not known at this moment. Clinically approved transfection agents are also not commonly on the market. Being 22 nucleotides large, the antagomirs are prone to fast degradation. This limits the feasibility of clinical use. However, modifications may improve this using 2′-O-methyl modifications, phosphorothioate bonds and adding a 3′ cholesterol tail (60).

Chemically modified ribonucleicacid for bone morphogenetic protein-2 to accelerate fracture healing

As mentioned earlier, growth factors like BMP-2 are important for inducing osteogenesis. Recombinant growth factors, however, need to be administered in supraphysiological concentrations in order to have a measurable effect in patients. This may also lead to unwanted side effects. The possibility to overcome these may lie in the possibility of presenting the BMP-2 gene to the cell.

As the typical plasmid gene delivery is not really feasible for a clinical setting, an innovative method was explored for clinical feasibility concerning gene therapy. In this case, the gene is introduced as messenger RNA to the cell, thereby preventing the need for the gene to enter the nucleus. The messenger RNA molecule is able to immediately be translated to protein once present in the cytoplasm. Messenger RNA molecules are, however, labile and immunogenic (61). Messenger RNA molecules may activate the immune system via toll-like receptors. In order to overcome this instability, a poly(A) tail of 120 nucleotides was added (62). Further stability and a decrease of immunogenicity were achieved by modifying uridine and cytidine nucleotides with thio- and methyl-groups, respectively (63).

It could be shown that this chemically modified messenger RNA encoding for BMP-2 was able to induce osteogenesis in adipose-derived mesenchymal stem cells (64). Furthermore, human tissue explants as a three-dimensional model could also be successfully transfected with proven translation of BMP-2 into protein that was secreted. As a proof of concept, this chemically modified messenger RNA encoding for BMP-2 was able to accelerate bone regeneration in a drill-hole model in rats (64).

The efficiency of the chemically modified messenger RNA was then further optimized concerning translation using different untranslated region elements (65). This optimized chemically modified messenger RNA for BMP-2 could be combined with tricalcium phosphate scaffolds and served as a transcript activated matrix. It was shown that this construction could effectively induce osteogenic pathways and differentiation in adipose-derived mesenchymal stem cells (66). Finally, such constructs were used in a critically sized femur defect model in rats. It was shown that bone regeneration with complete union could be induced in a dose-dependent manner (67).

Thus, chemically modified messenger RNA encoding for growth factors could be an innovative means to accelerate fracture healing in osteoporotic patients. In addition to using a messenger RNA encoding for BMP-2, other growth factors or combinations could be considered. For instance, chemically modified messenger RNA for BMP-9 was recently shown to accelerate bone regeneration in calvarial defects (68). This was a twofold higher result than treatment with chemically modified messenger RNA for BMP-2. This may be useful in the near future, as clinical studies with chemically modified messenger RNAs are being conducted in humans for other diseases (e.g., clinicaltrials.gov: NCT03323398, NCT00204516, NCT03480152, NCT03014089). It seems that these chemically modified messenger RNAs can adhere to the typical biomaterials used in bone regeneration. Therefore, the need for specific transfection agents would be omitted. However, whether this is true is the subject of ongoing investigations.

REFERENCES

1. Raisz LG. Pathogenesis of osteoporosis: Concepts, conflicts, and prospects. *J Clin Invest.* 2005;115(12):3318–25.
2. Maeda SS, Lazaretti-Castro M. An overview on the treatment of postmenopausal osteoporosis. *Arq Bras Endocrinol Metabol.* 2014;58(2):162–71.
3. Das S, Crockett JC. Osteoporosis—A current view of pharmacological prevention and treatment. *Drug Des Devel Ther.* 2013;7:435–48.
4. Reszka AA, Rodan GA. Mechanism of action of bisphosphonates. *Curr Osteoporos Rep.* 2003;1(2):45–52.
5. Silva-Fernandez L, Rosario MP, Martinez-Lopez JA, Carmona L, Loza E. Denosumab for the treatment of osteoporosis: A systematic literature review. *Reumatol Clin.* 2013;9(1):42–52.
6. Johnell O, Scheele WH, Lu Y, Reginster JY, Need AG, Seeman E. Additive effects of raloxifene and alendronate on bone density and biochemical markers of bone remodeling in postmenopausal women with osteoporosis. *J Clin Endocrinol Metab.* 2002;87(3):985–92.
7. Kimmel DB, Bozzato RP, Kronis KA et al. The effect of recombinant human (1–84) or synthetic human (1–34) parathyroid hormone on the skeleton of adult osteopenic ovariectomized rats. *Endocrinology.* 1993;132(4):1577–84.
8. Watanabe A, Yoneyama S, Nakajima M et al. Osteosarcoma in Sprague-Dawley rats after long-term treatment with teriparatide (human parathyroid hormone [1–34]). *J Toxicol Sci.* 2012;37(3):617–29.
9. Cosman F. Combination therapy for osteoporosis: A reappraisal. *Bonekey Rep.* 2014;3:518.
10. Giannoudis PV, Einhorn TA, Marsh D. Fracture healing: The diamond concept. *Injury.* 2007;38(Suppl 4):S3–6.
11. Giannoudis PV, Einhorn TA, Schmidmaier G, Marsh D. The diamond concept—Open questions. *Injury.* 2008;39(Suppl 2):S5–8.

12. Garcia-Olmo D, Garcia-Arranz M, Herreros D, Pascual I, Peiro C, Rodriguez-Montes JA. A phase I clinical trial of the treatment of Crohn's fistula by adipose mesenchymal stem cell transplantation. *Dis Colon Rectum.* 2005;48(7):1416–23.

13. Horwitz EM, Gordon PL, Koo WK et al. Isolated allogeneic bone marrow-derived mesenchymal cells engraft and stimulate growth in children with osteogenesis imperfecta: Implications for cell therapy of bone. *Proc Natl Acad Sci USA.* 2002;99(13):8932–7.

14. Erbs S, Linke A, Schachinger V et al. Restoration of microvascular function in the infarct-related artery by intracoronary transplantation of bone marrow progenitor cells in patients with acute myocardial infarction: The Doppler Substudy of the Reinfusion of Enriched Progenitor Cells and Infarct Remodeling in Acute Myocardial Infarction (REPAIR-AMI) trial. *Circulation.* 2007;116(4):366–74.

15. Mazzini L, Mareschi K, Ferrero I et al. Autologous mesenchymal stem cells: Clinical applications in amyotrophic lateral sclerosis. *Neurol Res.* 2006;28(5):523–6.

16. Ringden O, Uzunel M, Rasmusson I et al. Mesenchymal stem cells for treatment of therapy-resistant graft-versus-host disease. *Transplantation.* 2006;81(10):1390–7.

17. Mosna F, Sensebe L, Krampera M. Human bone marrow and adipose tissue mesenchymal stem cells: A user's guide. *Stem Cells Dev.* 2010;19(10):1449–70.

18. Barrilleaux B, Phinney DG, Prockop DJ, O'Connor KC. Review: *Ex vivo* engineering of living tissues with adult stem cells. *Tissue Eng.* 2006;12(11):3007–19.

19. Schneider S, Unger M, van Griensven M, Balmayor ER. Adipose-derived mesenchymal stem cells from liposuction and resected fat are feasible sources for regenerative medicine. *Eur J Med Res.* 2017;22(1):17.

20. Porter RM, Liu F, Pilapil C et al. Osteogenic potential of reamer irrigator aspirator (RIA) aspirate collected from patients undergoing hip arthroplasty. *J Orthop Res.* 2009;27(1):42–9.

21. Kaback LA, Soung do Y, Naik A et al. Teriparatide (1–34 human PTH) regulation of osterix during fracture repair. *J Cell Biochem.* 2008;105(1):219–26.

22. Gopalakrishnan R, Suttamanatwong S, Carlson AE, Franceschi RT. Role of matrix Gla protein in parathyroid hormone inhibition of osteoblast mineralization. *Cells Tissues Organs.* 2005;181(3–4):166–75.

23. Hamann C, Picke AK, Campbell GM et al. Effects of parathyroid hormone on bone mass, bone strength, and bone regeneration in male rats with type 2 diabetes mellitus. *Endocrinology.* 2014;155(4):1197–206.

24. Einhorn TA, Lee CA. Bone regeneration: New findings and potential clinical applications. *J Am Acad Orthop Surg.* 2001;9(3):157–65.

25. Tao ZS, Zhou WS, Tu KK et al. Treatment study of distal femur for parathyroid hormone (1–34) and β-tricalcium phosphate on bone formation in critical-sized defects in osteopenic rats. *J Craniomaxillofac Surg.* 2015;43(10):2136–43.

26. Tao ZS, Qiang Z, Tu KK et al. Treatment study of distal femur for parathyroid hormone (1–34) and β-tricalcium phosphate on bone formation in critical size defects in rats. *J Biomater Appl.* 2015;30(4):484–91.

27. Tao ZS, Zhou WS, Wu XJ et al. Single-dose local administration of parathyroid hormone (1–34, PTH) with β-tricalcium phosphate/collagen (β-TCP/COL) enhances bone defect healing in ovariectomized rats. *J Bone Miner Metab.* 2019;37:28–35.

28. Arrighi I, Mark S, Alvisi M, von Rechenberg B, Hubbell JA, Schense JC. Bone healing induced by local delivery of an engineered parathyroid hormone prodrug. *Biomaterials.* 2009;30(9):1763–71.

29. Goyenvalle E, Aguado E, Pilet P, Daculsi G. Biofunctionality of MBCP ceramic granules (TricOs) plus fibrin sealant (Tisseel) versus MBCP ceramic granules as a filler of large periprosthetic bone defects: An investigative ovine study. *J Mater Sci Mater Med.* 2010;21(6):1949–58.

30. Bartel DP. MicroRNAs: Genomics, biogenesis, mechanism, and function. *Cell.* 2004;116(2):281–97.

31. Wang WT, Zhao YN, Han BW, Hong SJ, Chen YQ. Circulating microRNAs identified in a genome-wide serum microRNA expression analysis as noninvasive biomarkers for endometriosis. *J Clin Endocrinol Metab.* 2013;98(1):281–9.

32. He L, Hannon GJ. MicroRNAs: Small RNAs with a big role in gene regulation. *Nat Rev Genet.* 2004;5(7):522–31.

33. Lewis BP, Burge CB, Bartel DP. Conserved seed pairing, often flanked by adenosines, indicates that thousands of human genes are microRNA targets. *Cell.* 2005;120(1):15–20.

34. Friedman RC, Farh KK, Burge CB, Bartel DP. Most mammalian mRNAs are conserved targets of microRNAs. *Genome Res.* 2009;19(1):92–105.

35. Seeliger C, Balmayor ER, van Griensven M. miRNAs related to skeletal diseases. *Stem Cells Dev.* 2016;25(17):1261–81.

36. Seeliger C, Karpinski K, Haug AT et al. Five freely circulating miRNAs and bone tissue miRNAs are associated with osteoporotic fractures. *J Bone Miner Res.* 2014;29(8):1718–28.

37. Panach L, Mifsut D, Tarin JJ, Cano A, Garcia-Perez MA. Serum circulating microRNAs as biomarkers of osteoporotic fracture. *Calcif Tissue Int.* 2015;97(5):495–505.

38. Li H, Wang Z, Fu Q, Zhang J. Plasma miRNA levels correlate with sensitivity to bone mineral density in postmenopausal osteoporosis patients. *Biomarkers.* 2014;19(7):553–6.

39. Kelch S, Balmayor ER, Seeliger C, Vester H, Kirschke JS, van Griensven M. miRNAs in bone tissue correlate to bone mineral density and circulating miRNAs are gender independent in osteoporotic patients. *Sci Rep.* 2017;7(1):15861.

40. Bruderer M, Richards RG, Alini M, Stoddart MJ. Role and regulation of RUNX2 in osteogenesis. *Eur Cell Mater.* 2014;28:269–86.

41. Li Z, Hassan MQ, Volinia S et al. A microRNA signature for a BMP2-induced osteoblast lineage commitment program. *Proc Natl Acad Sci USA.* 2008;105(37):13906–11.

42. Itoh T, Ando M, Tsukamasa Y, Akao Y. Expression of BMP-2 and Ets1 in BMP-2-stimulated mouse pre-osteoblast differentiation is regulated by microRNA-370. *FEBS Lett.* 2012;586(12):1693–701.

43. Cao Y, Lv Q, Lv C. MicroRNA-153 suppresses the osteogenic differentiation of human mesenchymal stem cells by targeting bone morphogenetic protein receptor type II. *Int J Mol Med.* 2015;36(3):760–6.

44. Zeng Y, Qu X, Li H et al. MicroRNA-100 regulates osteogenic differentiation of human adipose-derived mesenchymal stem cells by targeting BMPR2. *FEBS Lett.* 2012;586(16):2375–81.

45. Gao J, Yang T, Han J et al. MicroRNA expression during osteogenic differentiation of human multipotent mesenchymal stromal cells from bone marrow. *J Cell Biochem.* 2011;112(7):1844–56.

46. Sugatani T, Hruska KA. Down-regulation of miR-21 biogenesis by estrogen action contributes to osteoclastic apoptosis. *J Cell Biochem.* 2013;114(6):1217–22.

47. Wang Y, Li L, Moore BT et al. MiR-133a in human circulating monocytes: A potential biomarker associated with postmenopausal osteoporosis. *PLOS ONE.* 2012;7(4):e34641.

48. Grijalvo S, Alagia A, Puras G, Zarate J, Pedraz JL, Eritja R. Cationic vesicles based on non-ionic surfactant and synthetic aminolipids mediate delivery of antisense oligonucleotides into mammalian cells. *Colloids Surf B Biointerfaces.* 2014;119:30–7.

49. Lennox KA, Behlke MA. A direct comparison of anti-microRNA oligonucleotide potency. *Pharm Res.* 2010;27(9):1788–99.

50. Jan A, Karasinska JM, Kang MH et al. Direct intracerebral delivery of a miR-33 antisense oligonucleotide into mouse brain increases brain ABCA1 expression. *Neurosci Lett.* 2015;598:66–72.

51. Lanford RE, Hildebrandt-Eriksen ES, Petri A et al. Therapeutic silencing of microRNA-122 in primates with chronic hepatitis C virus infection. *Science.* 2010;327(5962):198–201.

52. Worm J, Stenvang J, Petri A et al. Silencing of microRNA-155 in mice during acute inflammatory response leads to derepression of c/ebp β and down-regulation of G-CSF. *Nucleic Acids Res.* 2009;37(17):5784–92.

53. van der Ree MH, van der Meer AJ, de Bruijne J et al. Long-term safety and efficacy of microRNA-targeted therapy in chronic hepatitis C patients. *Antiviral Res.* 2014;111:53–9.

54. van der Ree MH, van der Meer AJ, van Nuenen AC et al. Miravirsen dosing in chronic hepatitis C patients results in decreased microRNA-122 levels without affecting other microRNAs in plasma. *Aliment Pharmacol Ther.* 2016;43(1):102–13.

55. Ebert MS, Sharp PA. Emerging roles for natural microRNA sponges. *Curr Biol CB.* 2010;20(19):R858–61.

56. Ebert MS, Sharp PA. MicroRNA sponges: Progress and possibilities. *RNA.* 2010;16(11):2043–50.

57. Chen L, Zhang K, Shi Z et al. A lentivirus-mediated miR-23b sponge diminishes the malignant phenotype of glioma cells *in vitro* and *in vivo. Oncol Rep.* 2014;31(4):1573–80.

58. Bofill-De Ros X, Santos M, Vila-Casadesus M et al. Genome-wide miR-155 and miR-802 target gene identification in the hippocampus of Ts65Dn Down syndrome mouse model by miRNA sponges. *BMC Genomics.* 2015;16:907.

59. Otaegi G, Pollock A, Sun T. An optimized sponge for microRNA miR-9 affects spinal motor neuron development *in vivo. Front Neurosci.* 2011;5:146.

60. Lennox KA, Behlke MA. Chemical modification and design of anti-miRNA oligonucleotides. *Gene Ther.* 2011;18(12):1111–20.

61. Van Tendeloo VF, Ponsaerts P, Berneman ZN. mRNA-based gene transfer as a tool for gene and cell therapy. *Curr Opin Mol Ther.* 2007;9(5):423–31.

62. Holtkamp S, Kreiter S, Selmi A et al. Modification of antigen-encoding RNA increases stability, translational efficacy, and T-cell stimulatory capacity of dendritic cells. *Blood.* 2006;108(13):4009–17.

63. Kormann MS, Hasenpusch G, Aneja MK et al. Expression of therapeutic proteins after delivery of chemically modified mRNA in mice. *Nat Biotechnol.* 2011;29(2):154–7.

64. Balmayor ER, Geiger JP, Aneja MK et al. Chemically modified RNA induces osteogenesis of stem cells and human tissue explants as well as accelerates bone healing in rats. *Biomaterials.* 2016;87:131–46.

65. Ferizi M, Aneja MK, Balmayor ER et al. Human cellular CYBA UTR sequences increase mRNA translation without affecting the half-life of recombinant RNA transcripts. *Sci Rep.* 2016;6:39149.

66. Balmayor ER, Geiger JP, Koch C et al. Modified mRNA for BMP-2 in combination with biomaterials serves as a transcript-activated matrix for effectively inducing osteogenic pathways in stem cells. *Stem Cells Dev.* 2017;26(1):25–34.

67. Zhang W, De La Vega RE, Coenen MJ et al. An improved, chemically modified RNA encoding BMP-2 enhances osteogenesis *in vitro* and *in vivo. Tissue Eng Part A.* 2019;25(1-2):131–44.

68. Khorsand B, Elangovan S, Hong L, Dewerth A, Kormann MS, Salem AK. A comparative study of the bone regenerative effect of chemically modified RNA encoding BMP-2 or BMP-9. *AAPS J.* 2017;19(2):438–46.

17

Management of osteoporotic proximal humeral fractures

An overview

J.P.A.M. VERBRUGGEN

INTRODUCTION

Proximal humeral fractures are one of the most common fractures occurring in the older population that are related to osteoporosis. The frequency has been estimated between 63 and 105 per 100,000 per year. Proximal humeral fractures account for about 5% of all human fractures. With the aging of the world's population, the incidence increases by 13.7% per year of age in patients older than 60 years. It is expected that by the year 2030, the total amount of proximal humeral fractures will be tripled (1).

The highest incidence of proximal humeral fractures occurs with women older than 80 years of age. Osteoporotic women have a 5.3 times increase in risk of humeral fractures. Other risk factors are a history of falling and previous fractures, poor functional status, poor neuromuscular function, decreased physical activity, poor vision, insulin-dependent diabetes mellitus, and a history of hip fracture in the mother (2–4).

In general, persons sustaining a proximal humeral fracture tend to have poorer general health compared to other people of the same age. Patients sustaining a fracture of the proximal humerus appear to be more "fit" compared to patients sustaining a hip fracture but less healthy and active than patients sustaining a wrist fracture (3).

Not treating these patients optimally, meaning restoring their shoulder function properly, will lead to impairment of shoulder function and also of mobility. The elderly tend to use their hands and arms as "navigation tools," taking support on furniture and/or objects in their immediate surroundings while moving around. Losing a functional arm, they also might lose their ability to move around because they are less confident. A "fear of falling" develops. In 21% of patients, the ability to move freely diminished. This again leads to loss of independence. Up to 17% of all patients with a proximal humeral fracture had to give up their households and ended up in a nursing home (5,6). As with hip fractures, proximal humeral fractures are also associated with a higher mortality risk (2,7). A proximal humeral fracture is also an increased risk for other fractures. Sustaining a proximal humeral fracture increases the risk of experiencing a fracture of the proximal femur with a relative risk of 2.45 times more within 5 years and 3.1 times more within 10 years (2,5).

A proximal humeral fracture has significant impact on the patient, and proper treatment is necessary to give these patients a proper quality of life. This is even more important because not only is the incidence of fractures increasing, but also the population at risk is expanding. Due to the higher peri- and preoperative risk, it is mandatory to offer these patients the best treatment from the start, allowing them to mobilize and resume their former lives and activities as soon as possible.

DIAGNOSIS

In the elderly, a proximal humeral fracture occurs usually after a simple fall, mostly from standing height. The clinical image is clear with pain, swelling, and disturbed shoulder function. The fracture can be diagnosed easily by conventional radiology. A standard anteroposterior and trans-scapular view are sufficient. The (modified) axial view makes it possible to evaluate the position of the tuberosities. In case of more fragment fracture types, a computed tomography (CT) scan allows for better evaluation of the fracture and different fragments and their dislocation.

It is important to evaluate the neurovascular status of the arm. In case of proximal humeral fractures, the axillary nerve is at risk, and depending on the fracture mechanism, plexus lesions can occur. These are more common with fracture dislocations and also have a risk of combined vascular lesions. Due to collateral circulation, these might not always be obvious, but expanding hematoma, delayed anemia, or unexplained hypotension should be looked at with a high level of suspicion.

Osteoporosis cannot be defined in the acute situation. It is, however, important for the surgeon to have an idea about bone quality and hence of the stability of the osteosynthesis. A correlation exists between cortical thickness of the proximal humeral shaft and bone mineral density. A CT scan can be used to define bone density using the Hounsfield scale (8,9).

CLASSIFICATION

Fracture patterns are mostly classified according to the Neer classification. This classification is based on the descriptive classification described in 1934 by Codman who defined four main fragments: the head fragment, the greater and lesser tuberosities, and the shaft (10). The AO/ASIF classification is based on fracture patterns from simple to complex, defining A-, B-, and C-type fractures. Both classifications have a high inter- and intraobserver variability. Neither of these classification systems could demonstrate any correlation with healing or functional outcome or lead to a proper treatment proposition.

Hertel et al. proposed a more practical classification based on Codman's descriptive classification and the morphology of the fracture and not so much on dislocation itself. He described 12 different fracture types based on possible combinations of fracture lines between the different fragments of the proximal humerus. The length of the metaphyseal head extension (at least 8 mm), disruption of the medial hinge (more than 2 mm head dislocation), and basic fracture pattern with involvement of the anatomic neck were good predictors of head ischemia and therefore of the end result. Angulation of the head fragment and dislocation of more than 10 mm were poor predictors (11).

Description of the fracture pattern based on the four main fragments in combination with measuring dislocation of different fragments, and the criteria described by Hertel et al., help in deciding which treatment is best in a particular case, without necessarily providing a proper indication or prognosis.

MANAGEMENT

Nonoperative treatment

Lower demands and expectations in combination with osteoporosis and one or more comorbidities make nonoperative treatment an obvious choice. The standard technique is to provide the patient with a sling and adequate pain treatment. The first 2 weeks of relative rest is warranted, but as pain allows, early movement of the shoulder is stimulated, starting with pendulum exercises. This is followed by active and passive movement of the arm and shoulder under supervision of a physiotherapist.

In his publication in 1970, Neer reported that 85% of all proximal humeral fractures were minimally displaced according to his classification. Boolean et al. could confirm this number of about 80% in nonoperative treatment (12). However, more recently, percentages of only 14%–49% of minimally displaced fractures have been published (13,14). This suggests that fracture patterns have changed in the past 40 years but may also demonstrate the limitations of the Neer classification. Some authors mentioned displacement of more than 5 mm or even 3 mm and angulation of 20° or 30° as criteria for operative treatment and so increased operative indications (15,16).

RESULTS

Most series on nonoperative treatment report good healing and functional results. Gaebler et al. reviewed 507 patients with minimally or nondisplaced proximal humeral fractures; 88% had good to excellent results. Premorbid condition and age had a negative correlation with outcome (17). Yuksel et al. reviewed three- and four-part fractures. Patients with three-part fractures scored better than those with four-part fractures in the Constant score. Hanson et al. reported good functional results after nonoperative treatment, with a difference of 8 points in the Constant-Murley (CM) shoulder score and 10 points in the DASH (disabilities of the arm, shoulder, and hand) score comparing the affected shoulder with the healthy one. Court-Brown et al. specifically reported on treatment of 131 patients with varus impacted proximal humeral fractures. They found a correlation between decreasing function and older age but not with humeral head Mal-alignment. At 1 year, functional results were good with a mean Neer score of 84, regardless of amount of varus dislocation (18–20). However, Poeze et al. found a correlation between primary head shaft angle in the trans-scapular view and functional outcome as represented by CM and DASH scores (21).

In general, the earlier literature reports on nonoperative treatment of minimally displaced fractures and two-part fractures, whereas three- and four-part fractures are seen as an indication for operative treatment.

More recently a new interest in nonoperative treatment of these fracture has developed. This is also a consequence of the high complication rates described after operative treatment of these fractures (15,22). Good functional results have been mentioned. These results are generally not dependent on the fracture type or dislocation but correlate with age and comorbidities of the patients (17,20).

Several meta-analyses confirm that in the case of displaced proximal humeral fractures, nonoperative treatment is a valid option because at 2 years the functional results do not differ. A randomized controlled trial between operative and nonoperative treatments concluded that the functional result did not support operative treatment for proximal humeral fractures (23,24). In a subgroup analysis comparing different fracture types,

Sabharwal et al. concluded, however, that in the case of four-part fractures, surgery did lead to better quality of life and less osteoarthritis, osteonecrosis, and nonunion and malunion (25).

Nonoperative treatment of older patients with osteoporotic proximal humeral fractures is a valid option. However, there is still no concluding evidence that it is the only and best treatment. Therefore, decisions for treatment, whether operative or nonoperative, still must be made in view of the specific individual patient.

Operative treatment

The goal of operative treatment is to restore anatomy and allow for fast early active movement of the shoulder and arm through a stable osteosynthesis. Different techniques have been used for the operative treatment of proximal humeral fractures, from minimal invasive and percutaneous fixation to arthroplasty. However, no technique is currently being considered the standard of care.

The specific problem with operative treatment of osteoporotic proximal humeral fractures is the lack of cancellous bone in the head fragment. This fragment is often described as an "eggshell," with virtually no bone to allow sufficient purchase of screws or K-wires. To allow for a stable osteosynthesis, the implant needs enough "hold" in the humeral head. Different studies looked at the distribution of cancellous bone in the humeral head to make it possible to find the best position of screws and other implants. According to Frich et al., the highest density is located in the upper and medial parts of the humeral head; the posterior and lower parts are less dense (26).

The key is to reduce the different fracture fragments anatomically and then stabilize the fracture so forces are diverted over the bony structures. The tuberosities therefore have to be reduced anatomically first so the head fragment can rest on these fragments, allowing load sharing as much as possible (11). Important in this case is the medial support of the head. In case of medial comminution, the head fragment needs sufficient support provided by the implant to prevent varus dislocation (27). A postoperative head shaft angle of less than 130° may lead to a secondary varus dislocation of more than 10° (28). Depending on the technique used, K-wires or screws have to be introduced distally in the head fragment to support this fragment and prevent it from moving into varus. Alternatively, shortening with impaction of the head on the shaft may be necessary to create enough stability.

During follow-up, however, it is noticed that the fracture "settles" itself. In doing so, fragments can move or dislocate slightly. If fixation is too rigid, breaking out of the implant with secondary dislocation might occur. The ideal implant is a load-sharing device allowing guided impaction of the fragments (11). Stiff implants, be it plate or nail, are biomechanically not suited to stabilize osteoporotic fractures of the proximal humerus; elastic load-sharing devices should be used (29).

CLOSED REDUCTION AND PERCUTANEOUS FIXATION

By using a closed reduction and percutaneous fixation technique, the operative trauma to these already frail patients is minimized. Soft tissue damage is limited, reducing the risk of avascular head necrosis and infection. Operation time is shorter, so the impact of surgery on the patient is reduced. Retrograde flexible intramedullary nails like Ender or Prevot nails have been used to stabilize proximal humeral fractures. This technique is actually best suited for two-part fractures, but displaced tuberosities can be fixed by additional K-wires or screws. The main drawback of this technique is the high percentage of secondary displacement of these nails, with a high risk of secondary displacement of the fracture fragments, especially in osteoporotic bone (30).

Tension band wiring in combination with intramedullary Ender nails or K-wires has been considered the standard for a long time, and good results have been reported, but biomechanically these techniques are not stable (31–35).

Percutaneous K-wire fixation allows stabilization of more complex fracture types. The different fracture fragments are manipulated and reduced through small incisions with raspatory and hook. After closed reduction of the head fragment, this is fixed with two parallel K-wires introduced in a retrograde way, making sure the head fragment is supported at the medial calcar. After reduction, the greater tubercle is also fixed with one or more K-wires (36). In an anatomical study, Rowles et al. described the ideal positioning of K-wires to prevent damage to the axillary nerve. Good results have been obtained with this technique (37,38).

These techniques do not allow early functional treatment. Arms are immobilized for 2–3 weeks before active movements are allowed. In osteoporotic bone, these K-wires tend to slide or perforate the humeral head. Nho et al. considered osteoporosis as an absolute contraindication for K-wire fixation (39). Resch et al. combined K-wires with percutaneous screw fixation. To prevent the K-wires from sliding, he improved the technique and developed the "Humerus Block," a device fixed to the humeral shaft through which the K-wires are introduced and fixed by means of set screws preventing them from sliding (Figure 17.1). Good healing and functional results have been reported, also in the elderly, but results depend on the surgeon's experience (40–44).

PLATE OSTEOSYNTHESIS

The plate has been the standard for osteosynthesis of proximal humeral fractures until now. In a traditional plate osteosynthesis, stability depends on the friction between plate and bone provided by the compression exerted by screws fixing the plate to the bone. Conventional cancellous bone screws have less purchase in the osteoporotic bone of the humeral head fragment. This, in combination with higher stiffness of these implants, leads to plate loosening and secondary dislocations (45).

The locking plate has become the standard for plate osteosynthesis of osteoporotic proximal humeral fractures.

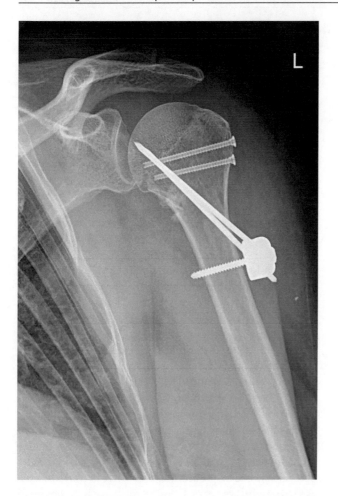

Figure 17.1 A proximal humeral fracture treated with Humerus Block technique.

These plates provide a stable fixation of two-, three-, and four-part fractures (Figure 17.2). Biomechanical studies have demonstrated its supremacy over conventional plates (46–48). The standard technique is through a deltopectoral approach. The alternative is a deltoid split incision, but here the axillary nerve is at risk, and expansion possibilities are restricted. The open technique allows for anatomical

reposition under direct sight followed by proper positioning and fixation of the plate. Due to stripping of the soft tissues, a higher risk of avascular head necrosis exists (49).

To prevent secondary dislocation, an anatomical reduction of all fragments is mandatory, creating a load sharing situation. For optimal fixation, screws should be placed in the subchondral bone taking care not to penetrate the articular surface (50–52). For medial support in case of comminution of the calcar, it is possible with most plates to introduce two or more "calcar screws," giving medial support to the head fragment (53,54). Alternatively, an intramedullary fibular strut graft can be used for medial support in combination with a plate (55). To enhance screw purchase, the head fragment can be filled with bone cement or a calcium phosphate cement (56–58).

Counteracting the forces of the rotator cuff is equally important to prevent varus dislocation. This is done by fixing the tuberosities with strong sutures to the plate (Figure 17.3). If not, varus dislocation with *en bloc* breakout of the head fragment can occur (59).

To prevent large incisions, minimal invasive plating techniques have been developed (60–62). A disadvantage of this technique is the indirect reposition of the fracture, which is technically more demanding. But more importantly, the axillary nerve prevents the use of the calcar screws because it lies directly over the plate holes provided for these screws (63). In case of medial comminution, this again increases the risk for varus dislocation.

Results

In general, functional results after plate osteosynthesis are acceptable. The published CM scores are between 70 and 80 points, indicating fair to good results. One has to take into account that in these series, younger patients are also included, thus influencing the functional results. In his publication on plate osteosynthesis of four-part proximal humeral fractures in patients older than 65 years, Kuhlmann et al. found a CM score of 61 points. Fjalestad et al. reported a CM score of only 52.3. Wanner et al. specifically made a distinction between patients younger and

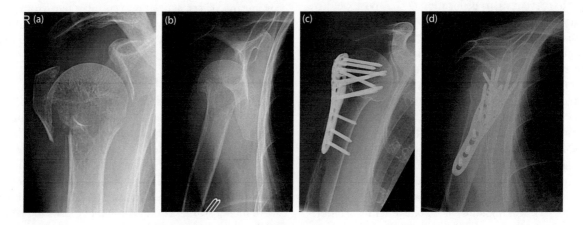

Figure 17.2 (a) A three-part fracture of the proximal humerus. (b) Trans-scapular view of this fracture. (c) Anteroposterior view after plate osteosynthesis with consolidation of the fracture. (d) Trans-scapular view after plate osteosynthesis.

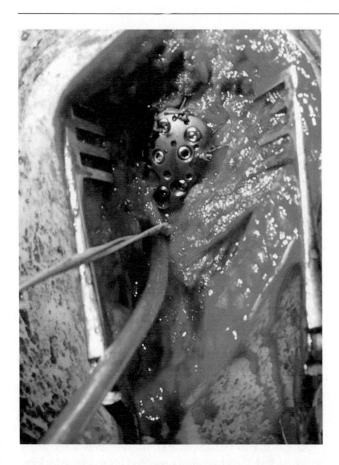

Figure 17.3 Plate osteosynthesis of the proximal humerus showing the wires fixing the tuberosities to the plate.

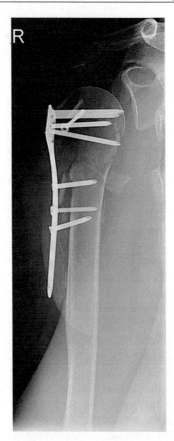

Figure 17.4 Plate loosening due to osteoporotic bone.

older than 60 years. The older patients had a CM score of 54 points. Clavert et al. found 54.7 points. Björkenheim et al. also saw a clear difference in function: patients between 60 and 70 years of age had a CM score of 72, between 70 and 80 years had a CM score of 66, and above 80 years had a CM score of only 59 points. Other studies confirm the negative correlation between functional score and old age (64–68).

The functional result seems to be more related to the fracture type than to the technique used. In a randomized controlled trial, Olerud et al. concluded that plate osteosynthesis leads to better functional results compared to nonoperative treatment, at an expense however of 30% reinterventions. Fjalestad et al. mentioned better functional results for nonoperative treatment, but anatomical results were better after surgery (68,69).

Complications

Complication rates for plate osteosynthesis in proximal humeral fractures are very high and occur in up to 36% of cases. The main complications are avascular head necrosis, screw perforation of the humeral head, plate loosening, and varus dislocation (Figure 17.4). Nonunion and infection occur in only 2% and 4%, respectively (70,71).

Avascular head necrosis (AVN) is thought to be related to devascularization of fragments due to the stripping of soft tissues. As AVN also occurs after nonoperative treatment, it may well be a general complication of the proximal humeral fracture caused by damage to the vessels of the humeral head.

Screw perforation may lead to damage of the joint and therefore is a major complication. Some authors describe primary screw perforation based on the fact that surgeons try to introduce the screws in the subchondral bone to have more purchase. Inadvertently, they might perforate the head surface, which is not noticed during surgery. Secondary perforation may be caused by AVN, but secondary displacement is a more important reason (45).

Varus dislocation is the most important complication. Lack of medial support due to comminution of the medial cortex or calcar may lead to moving of the head fragment in varus with secondary displacement of the fracture and loosening of the plate (27,53).

The risks of non-implant-related complications are correlated to age and fracture type.

INTRAMEDULLARY OSTEOSYNTHESIS

The use of an intramedullary nail has clear advantages in the treatment of the elderly with osteoporotic fractures. It is a minimally invasive technique that leads to less soft tissue damage and shorter operation times and may prevent peri- and postoperative complications (72). The nail is a load-sharing device. Stability does not depend on hold of screws in osteoporotic cancellous bone. It is the nail itself that provides the necessary reduction and stability of the head fragment; the locking bolts provide axial and rotational stability. Biomechanically, an intramedullary nail is superior to the locking plate (73–76).

As with the plate, an anatomical reduction is mandatory before introducing the nail, creating the correct head-shaft angle with reduction of the medial hinge to prevent varus dislocation (77,78).

Bended nails are designed to be introduced just lateral from the head fragment. Introduction, however, may cause dislocation of the head fragment or fracture of the greater tuberosity, and in case of metaphyseal comminution, there is a risk of varus dislocation (79). Postoperative pain and irritation of the rotator cuff that compromise function are possible complications (80). Therefore, it is advised to introduce both bended and straight nails through the head fragment. The nail has to be advanced into the subchondral bone so it does not protrude into the subacromial space, and at the same time, it is anchored in the subchondral bone plate of the head, fixing the head fragment and preventing varus dislocation. Locking screws provide for rotational and axial stability. As with the plate, locking bolts have to be advanced well into the subchondral bone plate for the best purchase (Figure 17.5). Extra bolts or sutures can be used to reduce and fix the tuberosities to counteract the varus forces of the rotator cuff (81,82). The nail also provides the necessary support for the head at the medial cortex in case of medial comminution. Depending on the nail design, locking bolts can be introduced as medial support screws for the head fragment (83).

Earlier nails like the Polaris led to good healing and functional results, but loosening of screws with secondary dislocation of the nail, and hence the fracture, were the main complications (84–86). After nails with angular stable locking bolts had been introduced, results became better (77).

Results

Healing and functional results are good and comparable for most series. Healing rates for most studies are well over 90% (77,78,82,85–90). Functional results are comparable with mean CM scores varying from 50 to 82 points (77,80,82,87,91). Most studies, however, are a mixture of younger and older patients. Results for the elderly are significantly lower. Popescu et al. specifically looked at the elderly patients in his total of 28 patients of which 64% were older than 70 years. The functional results in this group were significantly worse compared to the younger group with CM scores of 79.33 and 59 points, respectively (77). Giannoudis et al. reported a mean CM score of 74.5. Patients older than 60 years of age had a significantly lower CM score (87). Mathews et al. reported on the treatment of proximal humeral fractures in the geriatric patient. He treated 39 patients with a mean age of 81 years. The CM score was a mean of 57 points (90). Sosef reported a mean CM score of 62 (78).

Complications

Similar to plate osteosynthesis, for intramedullary osteosynthesis high rates of complications have been reported, like screw perforation of the head, AVN, and secondary displacement.

According to Giannoudis et al., the AVN after using this nail was 1.9% overall. Loosening of proximal locking screws varied from 3.7% to 15% (87).

Matthews reported implant-related complications in 15% of cases (91). Liu reported only four implant-related complications in 64 patients and two AVN complications (81). Hatzidakis et al. reported 11% reinterventions. Mittlemeier mentioned backing out of screws in 22.6% of cases with an AVN of 7.8%. Sosef had implant-related complications in 12%. Popescu mentioned implant-related complications in 17%.

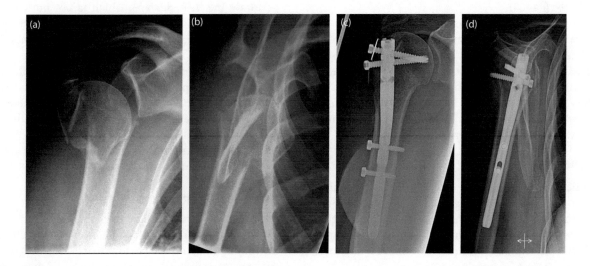

Figure 17.5   (a) A three-part fracture of the proximal humerus. (b) Trans-scapular view of the three-part fracture. (c) Anteroposterior view after intramedullary nailing. (d) Lateral view after nailing.

Evidence

No prospective randomized studies comparing nails and plates have been published. Most evidence is based on meta-analyses or retrospective comparative studies.

Lange et al. compared nonoperative treatment of proximal humeral fractures with intramedullary nailing. He could not find any difference in functional results, but nonoperative treatment led to less complications (92).

In comparative studies between nails and plates, no differences in function were found (93–97). Von Ruden et al. concluded that an intramedullary implant might be preferred because of biomechanical advantages and less soft tissue damage (94). Boudard et al. found more screw migration in the nail (95). According to Konrad et al., the patients in the nailing group had significantly less pain (97).

In a randomized trial, Lopiz et al. compared the straight Multiloc nail with the bended Polarus nail. The Polarus nail had significantly more symptoms related to rotator cuff disease. The reoperation rate was 42% for the Polarus and 11.5% for the Multiloc. Healing results were comparable (98).

In a meta-analysis including 615 patients comparing nails with plates, Wang et al. could not find evidence for either technique. Functional results and complications were comparable for both implants (99). In general, one can conclude that there is no evidence for superiority of either technique. Functional results appear to be determined by fracture complexity and age of the patient.

HEMIARTHROPLASTY

In case of three- and four-part proximal humeral fractures, there is a high risk of damage to the vascularization of the humeral head fragment. Neer advised primary hemiarthroplasty in all four-part fractures (100). Because of developments in osteosynthesis techniques and implants, the criteria for primary arthroplasty have changed throughout the years. With modern angular stable plates and locking nails, it is possible to fix three- and four-part fractures that would have been treated with an arthroplasty before.

According to the Hertel criteria, some fracture types carry a significantly higher risk of developing avascular head necrosis. In these cases, primary arthroplasty should be used (11). But despite the higher risk related to these criteria, AVN does not always develop (101). Depending on fracture type and patient demands and/or expectancies, the best treatment has to be chosen for each particular case. It is important to do it right the first time, because secondary hemiarthroplasties have worse results (102). In general, patients above 60 years of age do best with a prosthesis in case of a dislocated four-part fracture; other authors mention 70 years as the age limit (103,104).

To obtain good postoperative shoulder function, it is paramount to restore shoulder anatomy as much as possible. Proper retroversion and height of the prosthesis with fixation of the tuberosities at the proper height is necessary to restore rotator cuff function. Humeral height can be accurately restored by reconstructing the "gothic arc" formed by the lines of the medial cortex of the humeral shaft, the

calcar of the humerus, and the neck of the glenoid (Figure 17.6). Healing of the tuberosities and the position in which they heal are equally important, as secondary displacement and resorption of the tuberosities disturb function (105–109) (Figure 17.7). Healing of the tuberosities is significantly worse in older females with osteoporosis and in case of fractured tuberosities. Other factors influencing results are time to surgery and surgeon experience (106,110,111).

Results

Long-term survival rates of shoulder hemiarthroplasty are rather good, with a survival of almost 90% after 10 years (112). Infection rates are low with rates of superficial and deep infections of 1.6% and 0.6%, respectively (113).

Early reports on hemiarthroplasty reported very good functional results (100,114). Later functional results of hemiarthroplasties in general appeared to be disappointing (115,116). Recent studies reported that CM scores vary between 40 and 60 (107,113,117–120). Besides anatomical reconstruction and positioning of the prosthesis, age, time to definitive treatment (121), and fracture type have been reported as factors for functional results. Functional results for the elderly are worse than for the younger patients. Age appears to be the only determining factor for functional results (122). Elderly patients have lower functional demands, and more than 80% of patients appear to be satisfied due to sufficient pain relief (107,115,116).

Complications

Different complications have been reported at varying rates. Infection, loosening, heterotopic ossifications, and migration are the most important. They generally have minimal influence on the functional end result (104,107,117,123,124).

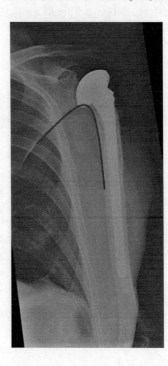

Figure 17.6 The "gothic arc" showing the correct positioning of the prosthesis.

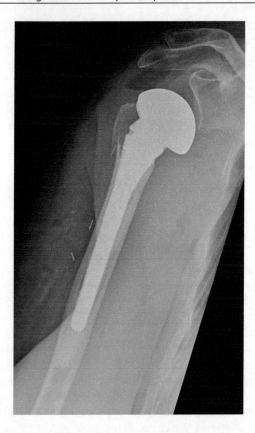

Figure 17.7 Hemiarthroplasty of the proximal humerus showing correct positioning of the tuberosities.

Evidence

In a large systemic review, Kontakis et al. found that the main complication was associated with failure of tuberosity healing, which occurred in 11.15% of cases. Heterotrophic ossification was found in 8.8% of cases, and proximal migration of the humerus head was found in 6.8% of cases (113).

In a randomized controlled trial comparing hemiarthroplasty with nonoperative treatment, Boons et al. (125) could not find a significant difference in function at 3 and 12 months. Abduction strength was better for the nonoperative group, but they experienced more pain at 3 months. Olerud et al. found a higher quality of life and less pain in the group with hemiarthroplasty after a 2-year follow-up but no difference in functional results (126).

Compared to plate osteosynthesis, functional results are better for the plate but at the expense of a high rate of reinterventions (127,128).

REVERSED SHOULDER ARTHROPLASTY

Results of hemiarthroplasty for proximal humeral fractures depend on the position and healing of the greater tuberosity. In case of osteoporosis, the bone quality of these fragments is often insufficient. Most tuberosity fragments are no more than a hollow shell, which is difficult to fix, let alone heal. Osteoporosis is correlated with bad results after hemiarthroplasty (105,122). Atrophy and fatty degeneration of rotator cuff muscles in the elderly also compromise eventual shoulder function (129). A reversed shoulder prosthesis is then a good alternative. Originally developed for irreparable rotator cuff pathology in the elderly, this prosthesis has found its place in the treatment of complex proximal humeral fractures in the elder patient group. By "bypassing" an afunctional rotator cuff, using the deltoid muscle instead, very good functional results can be achieved, especially in case of low-demand elderly patients. The procedure has been recommended for patients over 75 years (50). Replacing the glenoid with a head prevents further complaints from a possible degenerative joint. Though it is advised to fix the tuberosities to the prosthesis to improve functional results, function does not depend on the union or position of these tuberosities. Therefore, revalidation of these patients is much faster and leads to earlier satisfying results (130) (Figure 17.8).

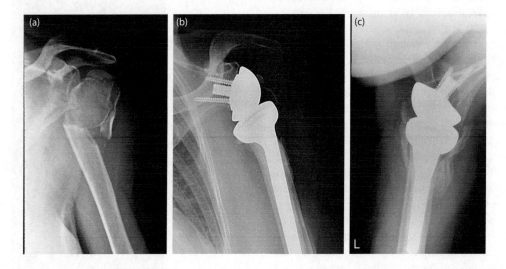

Figure 17.8 (a) A fracture dislocation of the proximal humerus. (b) Anteroposterior view of treatment with a reversed shoulder prosthesis. (c) Axial view of the reversed shoulder prosthesis. The healed tuberosities are clearly visible.

Results

Survival rate of the reversed shoulder arthroplasty is about 96% after 40 months (131). Infection rates are between 2% and 3% (130,132). Functional results with CM scores are comparable with hemiarthroplasty with a Constant score between 44 and 68 (50,130). Although refixation of tuberculi is not absolutely necessary, healing of the tuberculi does improve function (132). Also, age appears to be an important factor for functional results (133).

Complications

Complications after reversed shoulder prosthesis have been mentioned in high percentages. A variety of complications has been described: complex regional pain syndrome (CRPS), neurological complications, intraoperative fractures, dislocations, and infections. These complications do not appear to have a significant impact on the end results. Scapular notching is a specific complication of the reversed shoulder prosthesis. It can lead eventually to loosening of the base plate. Incidence can be up to 32% of cases (130,132). The clinical implications of it are not yet clearly understood. After 60 months, a correlation between pain and active range of motion exists (131). After a mean follow-up of 86 months, Cazeneuve et al. found only one patient with baseplate loosening due to scapular notching needing reintervention (134). Heterotopic ossifications up to 8.7% do not influence the results (132). Dislocations occur in up to 3.5% of cases (50,132).

Evidence

Comparative studies show a clear benefit for RSA for functional results. In a prospective, randomized controlled trial, Sebastia-Forcada et al. clearly demonstrated a significant difference in favor of RSA on functional results. There was no difference in healing or resorption of tuberosities. RSA resulted in less pain and revisions (131). For patients older than 70 years with a complex proximal humeral fracture, the RSA is the better treatment (129,135). This has been confirmed in other studies (130,136–140). Also, compared to osteosynthesis, RSA leads to faster revalidation with better function after 5 years, and this is at a significantly lower cost (136).

CONCLUSION

Recent literature does not show any evidence in favor of either treatment for fractures of the proximal humerus. Both operative and nonoperative treatments lead to good and comparable functional and healing results. There is also no evidence in favor of operative technique, be it plate, nail, or arthroplasty. Age appears to be the most decisive factor for the surgeon in deciding to operate or not. It appears also to be the most decisive factor for the functional results. Based on fracture type, expected demands of the patient, and comorbidities, it is up to the surgeon to decide which is the treatment of choice, taking into account his or her own experience and technical skills.

Based on the current literature, one could advise the following:

- In case of osteoporosis, proximal humeral fractures with little or no fracture dislocation should be treated nonoperatively.
- In case of dislocated three- and four-part fractures in patients younger than 70 years of age, an osteosynthesis is the first choice, taking into account the general condition of the patient. Results of plate and nail osteosyntheses do not differ, but a minimally invasive, biomechanically superior implant like the nail has preference. In case reconstruction is not possible (e.g., split head), a hemiarthroplasty is preferred depending on the quality of the tuberosities.
- Patients older than 70 years do best with an RSA because results do not depend on healing of the tuberosities, and recovery is faster.

REFERENCES

1. Kannus P, Palvanen M, Niemi S, Parkkari J, Jarvinen M, Vuori I. Osteoporotic fractures of the proximal humerus in elderly Finnish persons: Sharp increase in 1970–1998 and alarming projections for the new millennium. *Acta Orthop Scand.* 2000;71(5):465–70.
2. Guggenbuhl P, Meadeb J, Chales G. Osteoporotic fractures of the proximal humerus, pelvis, and ankle: Epidemiology and diagnosis. *Joint Bone Spine.* 2005;72(5):372–5.
3. Kelsey JL, Browner WS, Seeley DG, Nevitt MC, Cummings SR. Risk factors for fractures of the distal forearm and proximal humerus. The Study of Osteoporotic Fractures Research Group. *Am J Epidemiol.* 1992;135(5):477–89.
4. Nguyen TV, Center JR, Sambrook PN, Eisman JA. Risk factors for proximal humerus, forearm, and wrist fractures in elderly men and women: The Dubbo Osteoporosis Epidemiology Study. *Am J Epidemiol.* 2001;153(6):587–95.
5. Olsson C, Nordqvist A, Petersson CJ. Increased fragility in patients with fracture of the proximal humerus: A case control study. *Bone* 2004;34(6):1072–7.
6. Einsiedel T, Becker C, Stengel D et al. [Do injuries of the upper extremity in geriatric patients end up in helplessness? A prospective study for the outcome of distal radius and proximal humerus fractures in individuals over 65]. *Z Gerontol Geriatr.* 2006;39(6):451–61.
7. Shortt NL, Robinson CM. Mortality after low-energy fractures in patients aged at least 45 years old. *J Orthop Trauma.* 2005;19(6):396–400.
8. Tingart MJ, Apreleva M, von Stechow D, Zurakowski D, Warner JJ. The cortical thickness of the proximal humeral diaphysis predicts bone mineral density of the proximal humerus. *J Bone Joint Surg Br.* 2003;85(4):611–7.

9. Krappinger D, Roth T, Gschwentner M et al. Preoperative assessment of the cancellous bone mineral density of the proximal humerus using CT data. *Skeletal Radiol.* 2012;41(3):299–304.

10. Neer CS, 2nd. Displaced proximal humeral fractures. I. Classification and evaluation. *J Bone Joint Surg Am.* 1970;52(6):1077–89.

11. Hertel R. Fractures of the proximal humerus in osteoporotic bone. *Osteoporos Int.* 2005;16(Suppl 2):S65–72.

12. Boileau P, Chuinard C, Le Huec JC, Walch G, Trojani C. Proximal humerus fracture sequelae: Impact of a new radiographic classification on arthroplasty. *Clin Orthop Relat Res.* 2006;442:121–30.

13. Bahrs C, Bauer M, Blumenstock G et al. The complexity of proximal humeral fractures is age and gender specific. *J Orthop Sci.* 2013;18(3):465–70.

14. Court-Brown CM, Garg A, McQueen MM. The epidemiology of proximal humeral fractures. *Acta Orthop Scand.* 2001;72(4):365–71.

15. Lill H, Ellwein A, Katthagen C, Voigt C. [Osteoporotic fractures of the proximal humerus]. *Chirurg.* 2012;83(10):858–65.

16. Tepass A, Blumenstock G, Weise K, Rolauffs B, Bahrs C. Current strategies for the treatment of proximal humeral fractures: An analysis of a survey carried out at 348 hospitals in Germany, Austria, and Switzerland. *J Shoulder Elbow Surg.* 2013;22(1):e8–14.

17. Gaebler C, McQueen MM, Court-Brown CM. Minimally displaced proximal humeral fractures: Epidemiology and outcome in 507 cases. *Acta Orthop Scand.* 2003;74(5):580–5.

18. Yuksel HY, Yilmaz S, Aksahin E, Celebi L, Muratli HH, Bicimoglu A. The results of nonoperative treatment for three- and four-part fractures of the proximal humerus in low-demand patients. *J Orthop Trauma.* 2011;25(10):588–95.

19. Hanson B, Neidenbach P, de Boer P, Stengel D. Functional outcomes after nonoperative management of fractures of the proximal humerus. *J Shoulder Elbow Surg.* 2009;18(4):612–21.

20. Court-Brown CM, Cattermole H, McQueen MM. Impacted valgus fractures (B1.1) of the proximal humerus. The results of non-operative treatment. *J Bone Joint Surg Br.* 2002;84(4):504–8.

21. Poeze M, Lenssen AF, Van Empel JM, Verbruggen JP. Conservative management of proximal humeral fractures: Can poor functional outcome be related to standard transscapular radiographic evaluation? *J Shoulder Elbow Surg.* 2010;19(2):273–81.

22. Krettek C, Wiebking U. [Proximal humerus fracture: Is fixed-angle plate osteosynthesis superior to conservative treatment?]. *Unfallchirurg.* 2011;114(12):1059–67.

23. Handoll HH, Keding A, Corbacho B, Brealey SD, Hewitt C, Rangan A. Five-year follow-up results of the PROFHER trial comparing operative and non-operative treatment of adults with a displaced fracture of the proximal humerus. *Bone Joint J.* 2017;99-B(3):383–92.

24. Ghert M, McKee M. To operate or not to operate, that is the question: The proximal humerus fracture. *Bone Joint Res.* 2016;5(10):490–1.

25. Sabharwal S, Patel NK, Griffiths D, Athanasiou T, Gupte CM, Reilly P. Trials based on specific fracture configuration and surgical procedures likely to be more relevant for decision making in the management of fractures of the proximal humerus: Findings of a meta-analysis. *Bone Joint Res.* 2016;5(10):470–80.

26. Frich LH, Jensen NC. Bone properties of the humeral head and resistance to screw cutout. *Int J Shoulder Surg.* 2014;8(1):21–6.

27. Gardner MJ, Weil Y, Barker JU, Kelly BT, Helfet DL, Lorich DG. The importance of medial support in locked plating of proximal humerus fractures. *J Orthop Trauma.* 2007;21(3):185–91.

28. Ockert B, Siebenburger G, Kettler M, Braunstein V, Mutschler W. Long-term functional outcomes (median 10 years) after locked plating for displaced fractures of the proximal humerus. *J Shoulder Elbow Surg.* 2014;23(8):1223–31.

29. Lill H, Hepp P, Korner J et al. Proximal humeral fractures: How stiff should an implant be? A comparative mechanical study with new implants in human specimens. *Arch Orthop Trauma Surg.* 2003;123(2–3):74–81.

30. El-Alfy BS. Results of the percutaneous pinning of proximal humerus fractures with a modified palm tree technique. *Int Orthop.* 2011;35(9):1343–7.

31. Ruch DS, Glisson RR, Marr AW, Russell GB, Nunley JA. Fixation of three-part proximal humeral fractures: A biomechanical evaluation. *J Orthop Trauma.* 2000;14(1):36–40.

32. Ochsner PE, Ilchmann T. [Tension band osteosynthesis with absorbable cords in proximal comminuted fractures of the humerus]. *Unfallchirurg.* 1991;94(10):508–10.

33. Lu CC, Chang MW, Lin GT. Intramedullary pinning with tension-band wiring for surgical neck fractures of the proximal humerus in elderly patients. *Kaohsiung J Med Sci.* 2004;20(11):538–45.

34. Koval KJ, Blair B, Takei R, Kummer FJ, Zuckerman JD. Surgical neck fractures of the proximal humerus: A laboratory evaluation of ten fixation techniques. *J Trauma.* 1996;40(5):778–83.

35. Naranja RJ, Jr., Iannotti JP. Displaced three- and four-part proximal humerus fractures: Evaluation and management. *J Am Acad Orthop Surg.* 2000;8(6):373–82.

36. Fenichel I, Oran A, Burstein G, Perry Pritsch M. Percutaneous pinning using threaded pins as a treatment option for unstable two- and three-part fractures of the proximal humerus: A retrospective study. *Int Orthop.* 2006;30(3):153–7.

37. Jaberg H, Warner JJ, Jakob RP. Percutaneous stabilization of unstable fractures of the humerus. *J Bone Joint Surg Am.* 1992;74(4):508–15.

38. Rowles DJ, McGrory JE. Percutaneous pinning of the proximal part of the humerus. An anatomic study. *J Bone Joint Surg Am.* 2001;83-A(11):1695–9.

39. Nho SJ, Brophy RH, Barker JU, Cornell CN, MacGillivray JD. Management of proximal humeral fractures based on current literature. *J Bone Joint Surg Am.* 2007;89(Suppl 3):44–58.

40. Resch H, Povacz P, Frohlich R, Wambacher M. Percutaneous fixation of three- and four-part fractures of the proximal humerus. *J Bone Joint Surg Br.* 1997;79(2):295–300.

41. Brunner A, Weller K, Thormann S, Jockel JA, Babst R. Closed reduction and minimally invasive percutaneous fixation of proximal humerus fractures using the Humerusblock. *J Orthop Trauma.* 2010;24(7):407–13.

42. Tauber M, Hirzinger C, Hoffelner T, Moroder P, Resch H. Midterm outcome and complications after minimally invasive treatment of displaced proximal humeral fractures in patients younger than 70 years using the Humerusblock. *Injury.* 2015;46(10):1914–20.

43. Aschauer E, Resch H, Hubner C. Percutaneous osteosynthesis of humeral head fractures. *Oper Orthop Traumatol.* 2007;19(3):276–93.

44. Bogner R, Hubner C, Matis N, Auffarth A, Lederer S, Resch H. Minimally-invasive treatment of three- and four-part fractures of the proximal humerus in elderly patients. *J Bone Joint Surg Br.* 2008;90(12):1602–7.

45. Sudkamp N, Bayer J, Hepp P et al. Open reduction and internal fixation of proximal humeral fractures with use of the locking proximal humerus plate. Results of a prospective, multicenter, observational study. *J Bone Joint Surg Am.* 2009;91(6):1320–8.

46. Chudik SC, Weinhold P, Dahners LE. Fixed-angle plate fixation in simulated fractures of the proximal humerus: A biomechanical study of a new device. *J Shoulder Elbow Surg.* 2003;12(6):578–88.

47. Roderer G, AbouElsoud M, Gebhard F, Claes L, Aschoff AJ, Kinzl L. [Biomechanical investigation of fixed-angle plate osteosynthesis of the proximal humerus]. *Unfallchirurg.* 2010;113(2):133–8.

48. Walsh S, Reindl R, Harvey E, Berry G, Beckman L, Steffen T. Biomechanical comparison of a unique locking plate versus a standard plate for internal fixation of proximal humerus fractures in a cadaveric model. *Clin Biomech.* 2006;21(10):1027–31.

49. Kralinger F, Irenberger A, Lechner C, Wambacher M, Golser K, Sperner G. [Comparison of open versus percutaneous treatment for humeral head fracture]. *Unfallchirurg.* 2006;109(5):406–10.

50. Jordan RW, Modi CS. A review of management options for proximal humeral fractures. *Open Orthop J.* 2014;8:148–56.

51. Rothberg D, Higgins T. Fractures of the proximal humerus. *Orthop Clin North Am.* 2013;44(1):9–19.

52. Liew AS, Johnson JA, Patterson SD, King GJ, Chess DG. Effect of screw placement on fixation in the humeral head. *J Shoulder Elbow Surg.* 2000;9(5):423–6.

53. Lin SJ, Tsai YH, Yang TY, Shen SH, Huang KC, Lee MS. Medial calcar support and radiographic outcomes of plate fixation for proximal humeral fractures. *Biomed Res Int.* 2015;2015:170283.

54. Zhang L, Zheng J, Wang W et al. The clinical benefit of medial support screws in locking plating of proximal humerus fractures: A prospective randomized study. *Int Orthop.* 2011;35(11):1655–61.

55. Gardner MJ, Boraiah S, Helfet DL, Lorich DG. Indirect medial reduction and strut support of proximal humerus fractures using an endosteal implant. *J Orthop Trauma.* 2008;22(3):195–200.

56. Gradl G, Knobe M, Stoffel M, Prescher A, Dirrichs T, Pape HC. Biomechanical evaluation of locking plate fixation of proximal humeral fractures augmented with calcium phosphate cement. *J Orthop Trauma.* 2013;27(7):399–404.

57. Kwon BK, Goertzen DJ, O'Brien PJ, Broekhuyse HM, Oxland TR. Biomechanical evaluation of proximal humeral fracture fixation supplemented with calcium phosphate cement. *J Bone Joint Surg Am.* 2002;84-A(6):951–61.

58. Egol KA, Sugi MT, Ong CC, Montero N, Davidovitch R, Zuckerman JD. Fracture site augmentation with calcium phosphate cement reduces screw penetration after open reduction-internal fixation of proximal humeral fractures. *J Shoulder Elbow Surg.* 2012;21(6):741–8.

59. Micic ID, Kim KC, Shin DJ et al. Analysis of early failure of the locking compression plate in osteoporotic proximal humerus fractures. *J Orthop Sci.* 2009;14(5):596–601.

60. Roderer G, Erhardt J, Graf M, Kinzl L, Gebhard F. Clinical results for minimally invasive locked plating of proximal humerus fractures. *J Orthop Trauma.* 2010;24(7):400–6.

61. Smith J, Berry G, Laflamme Y, Blain-Pare E, Reindl R, Harvey E. Percutaneous insertion of a proximal humeral locking plate: An anatomic study. *Injury.* 2007;38(2):206–11.

62. Barco R, Barrientos I, Encinas C, Antuna SA. Minimally invasive poly-axial screw plating for three-part fractures of the proximal humerus. *Injury.* 2012;43(Suppl 2):S7–11.

63. Saran N, Bergeron SG, Benoit B, Reindl R, Harvey EJ, Berry GK. Risk of axillary nerve injury during percutaneous proximal humerus locking plate insertion using an external aiming guide. *Injury.* 2010;41(10):1037–40.

64. Kuhlmann T, Hofmann T, Seibert O, Gundlach G, Schmidt-Horlohe K, Hoffmann R. [Operative treatment of proximal humeral four-part fractures in elderly patients: Comparison of two angular-stable implant systems]. *Z Orthop Unfall.* 2012;150(2):149–55.

65. Wanner GA, Wanner-Schmid E, Romero J et al. Internal fixation of displaced proximal humeral fractures with two one-third tubular plates. *J Trauma.* 2003;54(3):536–44.

66. Clavert P, Adam P, Bevort A, Bonnomet F, Kempf JF. Pitfalls and complications with locking plate for proximal humerus fracture. *J Shoulder Elbow Surg.* 2010;19(4):489–94.

67. Bjorkenheim JM, Pajarinen J, Savolainen V. Internal fixation of proximal humeral fractures with a locking compression plate: A retrospective evaluation of 72 patients followed for a minimum of 1 year. *Acta Orthop Scand.* 2004;75(6):741–5.

68. Fjalestad T, Hole MO, Hovden IA, Blucher J, Stromsoe K. Surgical treatment with an angular stable plate for complex displaced proximal humeral fractures in elderly patients: A randomized controlled trial. *J Orthop Trauma.* 2012;26(2):98–106.

69. Olerud P, Ahrengart L, Ponzer S, Saving J, Tidermark J. Internal fixation versus nonoperative treatment of displaced 3-part proximal humeral fractures in elderly patients: A randomized controlled trial. *J Shoulder Elbow Surg.* 2011;20(5):747–55.

70. Thanasas C, Kontakis G, Angoules A, Limb D, Giannoudis P. Treatment of proximal humerus fractures with locking plates: A systematic review. *J Shoulder Elbow Surg.* 2009;18(6):837–44.

71. Sproul RC, Iyengar JJ, Devcic Z, Feeley BT. A systematic review of locking plate fixation of proximal humerus fractures. *Injury.* 2011;42(4):408–13.

72. Fazal MA, Baloch I, Ashwood N. Polarus nail fixation for proximal humeral fractures. *J Orthop Surg.* 2014;22(2):195–8.

73. Fuchtmeier B, May R, Hente R et al. Proximal humerus fractures: A comparative biomechanical analysis of -nd extramedullary implants. *Arch Orthop Trauma Surg.* 2007;127(6):441–7.

74. Yoon RS, Dziadosz D, Porter DA, Frank MA, Smith WR, Liporace FA. A comprehensive update on current fixation options for two-part proximal humerus fractures: A biomechanical investigation. *Injury.* 2014;45(3):510–4.

75. Hessmann MH, Hansen WS, Krummenauer F, Pol TF, Rommens P. Locked plate fixation and intramedullary nailing for proximal humerus fractures: A biomechanical evaluation. *J Trauma.* 2005;58(6):1194–201.

76. Kitson J, Booth G, Day R. A biomechanical comparison of locking plate and locking nail implants used for fractures of the proximal humerus. *J Shoulder Elbow Surg.* 2007;16(3):362–6.

77. Popescu D, Fernandez-Valencia JA, Rios M, Cune J, Domingo A, Prat S. Internal fixation of proximal humerus fractures using the T2-proximal humeral nail. *Arch Orthop Trauma Surg.* 2009;129(9):1239–44.

78. Sosef N, van Leerdam R, Ott P, Meylaerts S, Rhemrev S. Minimal invasive fixation of proximal humeral fractures with an intramedullary nail: Good results in elderly patients. *Arch Orthop Trauma Surg.* 2010;130(5):605–11.

79. Agel J, Jones CB, Sanzone AG, Camuso M, Henley MB. Treatment of proximal humeral fractures with Polarus nail fixation. *J Shoulder Elbow Surg.* 2004;13(2):191–5.

80. Liu QH, Sun W, Zhou JL et al. A new approach for the treatment of proximal humeral fractures using the TRIGEN proximal humeral nail. *Eur J Orthop Surg Traumatol.* 2014;24(4):467–74.

81. Stedtfeld HW, Mittlmeier T. Fixation of proximal humeral fractures with an intramedullary nail: Tips and tricks. *Eur J Trauma Emerg Surg.* 2007;33(4):367–74.

82. Mittlmeier TW, Stedtfeld HW, Ewert A, Beck M, Frosch B, Gradl G. Stabilization of proximal humeral fractures with an angular and sliding stable antegrade locking nail (Targon PH). *J Bone Joint Surg Am.* 2003;85-A(Suppl 4):136–46.

83. Hessmann MH, Nijs S, Mittlmeier T et al. Internal fixation of fractures of the proximal humerus with the MultiLoc nail. *Oper Orthop Traumatol.* 2012;24(4–5):418–31.

84. Adedapo AO, Ikpeme JO. The results of internal fixation of three- and four-part proximal humeral fractures with the Polarus nail. *Injury.* 2001; 32(2):115–21.

85. Sosef N, Stobbe I, Hogervorst M et al. The Polarus intramedullary nail for proximal humeral fractures: Outcome in 28 patients followed for 1 year. *Acta Orthop.* 2007;78(3):436–41.

86. Rajasekhar C, Ray PS, Bhamra MS. Fixation of proximal humeral fractures with the Polarus nail. *J Shoulder Elbow Surg.* 2001;10(1):7–10.

87. Giannoudis PV, Xypnitos FN, Dimitriou R, Manidakis N, Hackney R. Internal fixation of proximal humeral fractures using the Polarus intramedullary nail: Our institutional experience and review of the literature. *J Orthop Surg Res.* 2012;7:39.

88. Gradl G, Dietze A, Arndt D et al. Angular and sliding stable antegrade nailing (Targon PH) for the treatment of proximal humeral fractures. *Arch Orthop Trauma Surg.* 2007;127(10):937–44.

89. Koike Y, Komatsuda T, Sato K. Internal fixation of proximal humeral fractures with a Polarus humeral nail. *J Orthop Traumatol.* 2008;9(3):135–9.

90. Mathews J, Lobenhoffer P. The Targon PH nail as an internal fixator for unstable fractures of the proximal humerus. *Oper Orthop Traumatol.* 2007; 19(3):255–75.

91. Hatzidakis AM, Shevlin MJ, Fenton DL, Curran-Everett D, Nowinski RJ, Fehringer EV. Angular-stable locked intramedullary nailing of two-part surgical neck fractures of the proximal part of the humerus. A multicenter retrospective observational study. *J Bone Joint Surg Am.* 2011;93(23):2172–9.

92. Lange M, Brandt D, Mittlmeier T, Gradl G. Proximal humeral fractures: Non-operative treatment versus intramedullary nailing in 2-, 3- and 4-part fractures. *Injury.* 2016;47(Suppl 7):S14–9.

93. Gradl G, Dietze A, Kaab M, Hopfenmuller W, Mittlmeier T. Is locking nailing of humeral head fractures superior to locking plate fixation? *Clin Orthop Relat Res.* 2009;467(11):2986–93.

94. von Ruden C, Trapp O, Hierholzer C, Prohaska S, Wurm S, Buhren V. [Intramedullary nailing vs. locking plate osteosynthesis in proximal humeral fractures: Long-term outcome]. *Unfallchirurg.* 2015;118(8):686–92.

95. Boudard G, Pomares G, Milin L et al. Locking plate fixation versus antegrade nailing of 3- and 4-part proximal humerus fractures in patients without osteoporosis. Comparative retrospective study of 63 cases. *Orthop Traumatol Surg Res.* 2014;100(8):917–24.

96. Lekic N, Montero NM, Takemoto RC, Davidovitch RI, Egol KA. Treatment of two-part proximal humerus fractures: Intramedullary nail compared to locked plating. *HSS J.* 2012;8(2):86–91.

97. Konrad G, Audige L, Lambert S, Hertel R, Sudkamp NP. Similar outcomes for nail versus plate fixation of three-part proximal humeral fractures. *Clin Orthop Relat Res.* 2012;470(2):602–9.

98. Lopiz Y, Garcia-Coiradas J, Garcia-Fernandez C, Marco F. Proximal humerus nailing: A randomized clinical trial between curvilinear and straight nails. *J Shoulder Elbow Surg.* 2014;23(3):369–76.

99. Wang G, Mao Z, Zhang L et al. Meta-analysis of locking plate versus intramedullary nail for treatment of proximal humeral fractures. *J Orthop Surg Res.* 2015;10:122.

100. Neer CS 2nd. Displaced proximal humeral fractures. II. Treatment of three-part and four-part displacement. *J Bone Joint Surg Am.* 1970;52(6):1090–103.

101. Bastian JD, Hertel R. Initial post-fracture humeral head ischemia does not predict development of necrosis. *J Shoulder Elbow Surg.* 2008;17(1):2–8.

102. Norris TR, Green A, McGuigan FX. Late prosthetic shoulder arthroplasty for displaced proximal humerus fractures. *J Shoulder Elbow Surg.* 1995;4(4):271–80.

103. Valenti P, Aliani D, Maroun C, Werthel JD. A new stem guide and a tuberosity anchoring "Lasso" system for shoulder hemiarthroplasty in the treatment of complex proximal humerus fractures. *Tech Hand Up Extrem Surg.* 2017;21(4):131–6.

104. Park YK, Kim SH, Oh JH. Intermediate-term outcome of hemiarthroplasty for comminuted proximal humerus fractures. *J Shoulder Elbow Surg.* 2017;26(1):85–91.

105. Boileau P, Krishnan SG, Tinsi L, Walch G, Coste JS, Mole D. Tuberosity malposition and migration: Reasons for poor outcomes after hemiarthroplasty for displaced fractures of the proximal humerus. *J Shoulder Elbow Surg.* 2002;11(5):401–12.

106. Liu J, Li SH, Cai ZD et al. Outcomes, and factors affecting outcomes, following shoulder hemiarthroplasty for proximal humeral fracture repair. *J Orthop Sci.* 2011;16(5):565–72.

107. Gronhagen CM, Abbaszadegan H, Revay SA, Adolphson PY. Medium-term results after primary hemiarthroplasty for comminute proximal humerus fractures: A study of 46 patients followed up for an average of 4.4 years. *J Shoulder Elbow Surg.* 2007;16(6):766–73.

108. Hoel S, Jensen TG, Falster O, Ulstrup A. Hemiarthroplasty for proximal humerus fracture and consequences of a comminuted greater tubercle fragment. *Musculoskelet Surg.* 2016;100(1):9–14.

109. Reuther F, Muhlhausler B, Wahl D, Nijs S. Functional outcome of shoulder hemiarthroplasty for fractures: A multicentre analysis. *Injury.* 2010;41(6):606–12.

110. Demirhan M, Kilicoglu O, Altinel L, Eralp L, Akalin Y. Prognostic factors in prosthetic replacement for acute proximal humerus fractures. *J Orthop Trauma.* 2003;17(3):181–8; discussion 8–9.

111. Becker R, Pap G, Machner A, Neumann WH. Strength and motion after hemiarthroplasty in displaced four-fragment fracture of the proximal humerus: 27 patients followed for 1–6 years. *Acta Orthop Scand.* 2002;73(1):44–9.

112. Robinson CM, Page RS, Hill RM, Sanders DL, Court-Brown CM, Wakefield AE. Primary hemiarthroplasty for treatment of proximal humeral fractures. *J Bone Joint Surg Am.* 2003;85-A(7):1215–23.

113. Kontakis G, Koutras C, Tosounidis T, Giannoudis P. Early management of proximal humeral fractures with hemiarthroplasty: A systematic review. *J Bone Joint Surg Br.* 2008;90(11):1407–13.

114. Tanner MW, Cofield RH. Prosthetic arthroplasty for fractures and fracture-dislocations of the proximal humerus. *Clin Orthop Relat Res.* 1983 (179):116–28.

115. Zyto K, Wallace WA, Frostick SP, Preston BJ. Outcome after hemiarthroplasty for three- and four-part fractures of the proximal humerus. *J Shoulder Elbow Surg.* 1998;7(2):85–9.

116. Wretenberg P, Ekelund A. Acute hemiarthroplasty after proximal humerus fracture in old patients. A retrospective evaluation of 18 patients followed for 2–7 years. *Acta Orthop Scand.* 1997;68(2):121–3.

117. Castricini R, De Benedetto M, Pirani P, Panfoli N, Pace N. Shoulder hemiarthroplasty for fractures of the proximal humerus. *Musculoskelet Surg.* 2011;95(Suppl 1):S49–54.

118. Mighell MA, Kolm GP, Collinge CA, Frankle MA. Outcomes of hemiarthroplasty for fractures of the proximal humerus. *J Shoulder Elbow Surg.* 2003;12(6):569–77.

119. Prakash U, McGurty DW, Dent JA. Hemiarthroplasty for severe fractures of the proximal humerus. *J Shoulder Elbow Surg.* 2002;11(5):428–30.

120. Shah N, Iqbal HJ, Brookes-Fazakerley S, Sinopidis C. Shoulder hemiarthroplasty for the treatment of three and four part fractures of the proximal humerus using Comprehensive Fracture stem. *Int Orthop.* 2011;35(6):861–7.

121. Bosch U, Skutek M, Fremerey RW, Tscherne H. Outcome after primary and secondary hemiarthroplasty in elderly patients with fractures of the proximal humerus. *J Shoulder Elbow Surg.* 1998;7(5):479–84.

122. Nijs S, Broos P. Outcome of shoulder hemiarthroplasty in acute proximal humeral fractures: A frustrating meta-analysis experience. *Acta Orthop Belg.* 2009;75(4):445–51.

123. Fialka C, Stampfl P, Arbes S, Reuter P, Oberleitner G, Vecsei V. Primary hemiarthroplasty in four-part fractures of the proximal humerus: Randomized trial of two different implant systems. *J Shoulder Elbow Surg.* 2008;17(2):210–5.

124. Antuna SA, Sperling JW, Cofield RH. Shoulder hemiarthroplasty for acute fractures of the proximal humerus: A minimum five-year follow-up. *J Shoulder Elbow Surg.* 2008;17(2):202–9.

125. Boons HW, Goosen JH, van Grinsven S, van Susante JL, van Loon CJ. Hemiarthroplasty for humeral four-part fractures for patients 65 years and older: A randomized controlled trial. *Clin Orthop Relat Res.* 2012;470(12):3483–91.

126. Olerud P, Ahrengart L, Ponzer S, Saving J, Tidermark J. Hemiarthroplasty versus nonoperative treatment of displaced 4-part proximal humeral fractures in elderly patients: A randomized controlled trial. *J Shoulder Elbow Surg.* 2011;20(7):1025–33.

127. Dietrich M, Meier C, Lattmann T, Zingg U, Gruninger P, Platz A. [Complex fracture of the proximal humerus in the elderly. Locking plate osteosynthesis vs hemiarthroplasty]. *Chirurg.* 2008;79(3):231–40.

128. Dai J, Chai Y, Wang C, Wen G. Meta-analysis comparing locking plate fixation with hemiarthroplasty for complex proximal humeral fractures. *Eur J Orthop Surg Traumatol.* 2014;24(3):305–13.

129. Jones KJ, Dines DM, Gulotta L, Dines JS. Management of proximal humerus fractures utilizing reverse total shoulder arthroplasty. *Curr Rev Musculoskelet Med.* 2013;6(1):63–70.

130. Mata-Fink A, Meinke M, Jones C, Kim B, Bell JE. Reverse shoulder arthroplasty for treatment of proximal humeral fractures in older adults: A systematic review. *J Shoulder Elbow Surg.* 2013;22(12):1737–48.

131. Sebastia-Forcada E, Cebrian-Gomez R, Lizaur-Utrilla A, Gil-Guillen V. Reverse shoulder arthroplasty versus hemiarthroplasty for acute proximal humeral fractures. A blinded, randomized, controlled, prospective study. *J Shoulder Elbow Surg.* 2014;23(10):1419–26.

132. Anakwenze OA, Zoller S, Ahmad CS, Levine WN. Reverse shoulder arthroplasty for acute proximal humerus fractures: A systematic review. *J Shoulder Elbow Surg.* 2014;23(4):e73–80.

133. Lopiz Y, Garcia-Coiradas J, Serrano-Mateo L, Garcia-Fernandez C, Marco F. Reverse shoulder arthroplasty for acute proximal humeral fractures in the geriatric patient: Results, health-related quality of life and complication rates. *Int Orthop.* 2016;40(4):771–81.

134. Cazeneuve JF, Cristofari DJ. Grammont reversed prosthesis for acute complex fracture of the proximal humerus in an elderly population with 5 to 12 years follow-up. *Orthop Traumatol Surg Res.* 2014;100(1):93–7.

135. Jobin CM, Galdi B, Anakwenze OA, Ahmad CS, Levine WN. Reverse shoulder arthroplasty for the management of proximal humerus fractures. *J Am Acad Orthop Surg.* 2015;23(3):190–201.

136. Chalmers PN, Slikker W, 3rd, Mall NA et al. Reverse total shoulder arthroplasty for acute proximal humeral fracture: Comparison to open reduction-internal fixation and hemiarthroplasty. *J Shoulder Elbow Surg.* 2014;23(2):197–204.

137. Baudi P, Campochiaro G, Serafini F et al. Hemiarthroplasty versus reverse shoulder arthroplasty: Comparative study of functional and radiological outcomes in the treatment of acute proximal humerus fracture. *Musculoskelet Surg.* 2014;98(Suppl 1):19–25.

138. Wang J, Zhu Y, Zhang F, Chen W, Tian Y, Zhang Y. Meta-analysis suggests that reverse shoulder arthroplasty in proximal humerus fractures is a better option than hemiarthroplasty in the elderly. *Int Orthop.* 2016;40(3):531–9.

139. Shukla DR, McAnany S, Kim J, Overley S, Parsons BO. Hemiarthroplasty versus reverse shoulder arthroplasty for treatment of proximal humeral fractures: A meta-analysis. *J Shoulder Elbow Surg.* 2016;25(2):330–40.

140. Longo UG, Petrillo S, Berton A, Denaro V. Reverse total shoulder arthroplasty for the management of fractures of the proximal humerus: A systematic review. *Musculoskelet Surg.* 2016;100(2):83–91.

18

Distal humerus fractures in the elderly

To fix or to replace?

JON B. CARLSON, CRAIG S. ROBERTS, and DAVID SELIGSON

INTRODUCTION

The goal for treatment of fractures in the geriatric population is early definitive treatment and restoration of function. Restoration of function is achieved with anatomical reduction, stable internal fixation, and early motion. However, bone mineral density has a linear correlation with the holding power of screws, and osteoporotic bone may lack the strength to hold screws in the setting of early functional motion.

Distal humerus fractures account for 5% of osteoporotic fractures in patients older than 60 years (1). Most of these fractures occur in women and are complete articular injuries. Surgical fixation is challenging because standard techniques of internal fixation fail in osteoporotic bone. In addition, the older patient often has multiple medical comorbidities and very thin skin necessitating meticulous handling of the soft tissues throughout any proposed surgical procedure.

The treatment options for fractures extending into the elbow joint in the elderly include nonoperative treatment, open osteosynthesis, and elbow replacement.

Nonoperative treatment using the "bag of bones" technique is reserved for patients thought to be too high risk to undergo anesthesia or who have very low functional demands. This treatment typically involves immobilization of the elbow in about 60°–70° of flexion for 2–3 weeks followed by gentle range of motion (2), or either immobilization at 100°–125° of flexion with progressive extension over 3 weeks versus active motion 2 weeks following immobilization of the elbow at 90° of flexion (3). Application of a hinged external fixator may also provide acceptable outcomes in terms of function, rate, and type of complications and reoperation rate versus conservative treatment, open reduction and internal fixation (ORIF), and total elbow arthroplasty (4).

Distal humerus fractures in the elderly can be challenging injuries to treat. For example, an active 74-year-old female who sustained a supracondylar humerus fracture with intra-articular extension and minimal comminution may be best managed with ORIF. However, an 82-year-old male sustaining a "smashed" distal humerus fracture is best managed with total elbow replacement. Treatment should be guided both by the characteristics of the particular patient and the personality of the injury.

The incidence of all fragility fractures continues to increase markedly as the population ages. An important component of managing these injuries is reducing the risk of future fragility fractures. Low-energy falls are a common mechanism, and every effort should be undertaken to reduce this risk. Strategies for reducing the fall risk include modification of the home environment to one suited for the patient and physical therapy for gait and balance training. The use of an assistive device such as a walker should also be considered. Patients should also be evaluated for possible pharmacologic treatment for osteoporosis as well as regular weight-bearing exercise and nutritional education (5).

Palvanen et al. (6) reported a marked increase in distal humerus fractures in elderly females older than age 65 years from 1970 to 1988. The incidence increased from 12 per 100,000 to 34 per 100,000 during that time period, and the absolute number of such fractures increased from 42 to 224. However, during the time period from 1988 to 2007, the incidence and the absolute number decreased slightly to 25 per 100,000 and 192, respectively. In patients 65 years of age and older, most fractures are AO/OTA C-type fractures and occur in women more than 80% of the time. Most patients sustaining these injuries have high levels of autonomy and live at home. Greater than 90% of these injuries were reported to have been treated surgically (7).

Figure 18.1a,b shows the radiographs of an active, right-hand dominant 74-year-old male who sustained a fall from 3 feet off a ladder sustaining a fracture of the medial and lateral columns of the right elbow, making this an AO/OTA 13.C1 injury. His bone quality was fairly good; he

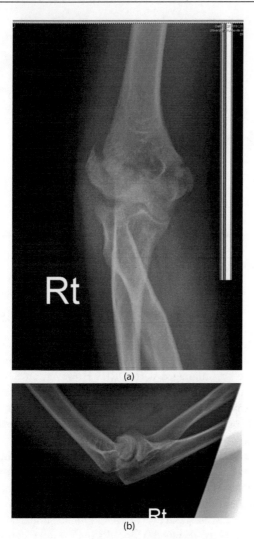

(a)

(b)

Figure 18.1 (a and b) Anteroposterior and lateral injury radiographs of a 74-year-old male who fell from a standing height sustaining a low T-type fracture.

was relatively healthy and did not smoke. This injury was treated with ORIF as shown in Figure 18.2a,b. Figure 18.3 demonstrates the radiographs of a right-hand dominant 82-year-old female who lives independently and fell in her apartment after tripping. The patient does not smoke. Her left distal humerus fracture shows a marked degree of comminution involving both the medial and lateral columns of the elbow with poor bone quality. This injury is an AO/OTA 13.C3 fracture and was treated with a total elbow replacement as shown in Figure 18.4a,b.

The primary failure mode of internal fixation in osteoporotic bone typically results from failure of the bone to hold the implants rather than failure of the construct itself (8). Bone mineral density has a linear correlation with the holding power of screws, and osteoporotic bone may lack the strength to hold screws in the setting of early functional motion. Osteoporosis is associated with reduced cortical thickness with overall increasing diameter of the medullary canal in diaphyseal bone. The metaphyseal bone, composed primarily of cancellous bone, has reduction of the

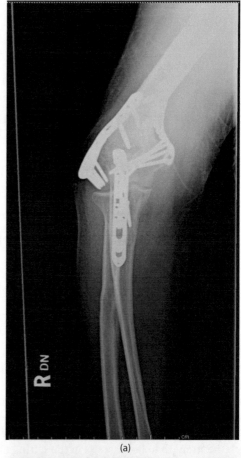

(a)

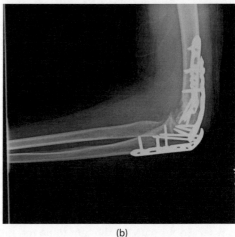

(b)

Figure 18.2 (a and b) Postoperative anteroposterior and lateral radiographs demonstrating reduction and fixation of the low T-type fracture.

trabeculae and overall loss of bone mineral density (9). In severely osteoporotic bone, screw fixation is obtained only in the thin cortical margins with minimal fixation in the weakened cancellous bone. Some of these concerns may be alleviated with the use of more modern implants. However, even with newer implants, fixation is limited, especially in the lateral column where fixation of the capitellar fragment is held with unicortical screws.

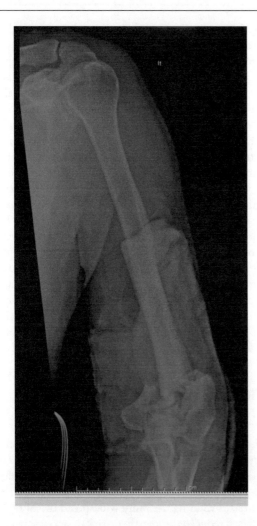

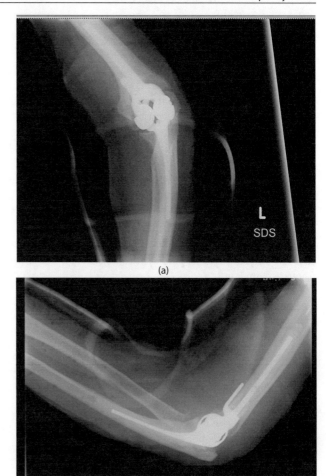

Figure 18.3 Anteroposterior injury radiograph of an 82-year-old female who sustained a comminuted intra-articular distal humerus fracture after a mechanical fall from a standing height.

Figure 18.4 (a and b) Anteroposterior and lateral injury radiographs demonstrating placement of a total elbow arthroplasty.

CLASSIFICATIONS

Several classification systems have been described for fractures of the distal humerus. The OA/OTA system is composed of three main groups with a total of nine subtypes (10). A-type fractures are extra-articular, B-type fractures are partial articular, and C-type fractures are complete articular injuries. Further subclassification is based on the amount of intra- or extra-articular comminution. In our experience, this classification system is most useful for discussion of fractures only when used in a very broad sense such as A-type, B-type, and C-type fractures. Mehne and Jupiter (11) described seven types of bicolumnar distal humerus fractures: high T, low T, Y fractures, H fracture, medial and lateral lambda fractures, and multiplane fractures. Coronal sheer fractures are not well described by the previous classification systems. Bryan and Morrey described coronal sheer fractures in 1985 (12), and this classification was modified by McKee in 1996 (13). The first type of fracture, also known as a Hahn-Steinthal fracture,

is a coronal fracture of the capitellum. An osteochondral lesion of the capitellum, also known as a Kocher-Lorenz fracture, is the second type. The third type is a comminuted fracture of the capitellum, and the fourth type has extension of the capitellar fracture into the trochlea.

The AO descriptions of A-type, B-type, and C-type fractures are useful as a way to describe these fractures, but no single classification system provides much guidance when it comes to development of the surgical tactic. Each fracture is best understood individually. Delineating the relationship of multiple fracture lines to the articular margins and their orientations in the axial, coronal, and sagittal planes is critical.

RATIONALE FOR TOTAL ELBOW ARTHROPLASTY

Total elbow arthroplasty (TEA) should be considered as an alternative in patients with fracture comminution and osteoporosis who do not have other contraindications for surgery (1,14). A summary of the historical progression of TEA used in the primary treatment of distal humerus fractures in the elderly is provided by Mansat et al. (1).

The use for TEA for elderly patients with fractures of the distal humerus was initially published by Cobb and Morrey in 1997 (15). Their study was a retrospective review of 20 consecutive patients (21 elbows) collected over a 10-year period. The mean follow-up was 3.3 years with a minimum 2-year follow up, except for three patients who had died prior to the 2-year mark. Twenty implants were intact at latest follow-up, and one patient underwent a revision due to fracture secondary to a fall. Their results showed 15 excellent results and 5 good results according to the Mayo Elbow Performance Score (MEPS). No fair or poor results were found. Mean flexion arc was reported as 25°–130°. The authors noted that the presence of rheumatoid arthritis was a factor in decision-making in about half of their patients. Complications included three ulnar nerve injuries, one case of complex regional pain syndrome (CRPS), and one fracture from a fall.

In 2004, Kamineni and Morrey (16) published a retrospective review of 49 acute distal humerus fractures in 48 patients. The average age of the patients in this study was 67 years, and all were treated with primary TEA. Forty-three fractures had a minimum follow-up of 2 years, with an average follow-up of 7 years and average MEPS of 93/100. Fracture patterns according to the AO system included most C-type fractures with five A-type and five B-type fractures. The results for all 49 patients at the time of the latest follow-up showed an average flexion arc of 24°–131°. MEPS averaged 93/100. Sixty-five percent of patients had no complications and no further surgeries. Fourteen elbows (29%) had a single complication, most of which did not require surgery. Complications included five revision arthroplasties and five soft tissue procedures. Fourteen patients died during the review period. The authors concluded that TEA may be considered when osteosynthesis is not considered feasible, especially in patients who are physiologically older and place low demands on the joint.

Multiple subsequent studies confirmed that TEA was a reasonable option for older, low-demand patients with intra-articular distal humerus fractures (17–21). Range of motion was reported to be 25°–125° of flexion. Most fractures were AO/OTA C-type fractures. The average age was approximately 70 years. MEPS were consistently above 90/100. There were five complications reported that included superficial infection, triceps insufficiency, heterotopic ossification, CRPS, and one case of aseptic loosening. Of note, the prosthesis used in all of these studies was the semiconstrained Coonrad-Morrey implant that does not depend on healing of the humeral condyles. Additionally, excision of the humeral condyles along with the use of this prosthesis has been shown to have an effect on forearm strength and wrist or hand function, and no effect on the MEPS (22).

In 2013, Mansat et al. (23) published the largest series of patients evaluating TEA as primary treatment for elderly patients with distal humerus fractures. This study was a retrospective, multicenter study of 87 patients (80 women) over the age of 65 years (average age 79 years; range, 65–93 years) demonstrating satisfactory results with stable and painless elbow function and relatively low (9%) revision rate. Most fractures (70/87) were AO/OTA C-type injuries. After mean follow-up of 37.5 months, most patients had either a pain-free (63%) or slightly painful (24%) elbow. Function was reported as normal in 69/87 patients.

In 2016, Prasad et al. (24) published a series involving 37 patients with no indication of rheumatoid arthritis who were treated with TEA and followed for 10 years. Of the 19 patients available for follow-up, two had undergone revision, with another patient requiring two-stage revision for infection. Six other patients had evidence of loosening or wear, but only two were clinically symptomatic. Using revision and definite loosening as endpoints, survivorship of the prosthesis was 89.5% in patients with minimum 10-year follow-up and 86% in the entire group of 36 patients (excluding one patient lost to follow-up). Another important finding is that 17 (53%) had died before the 10th anniversary of their surgery (24). The authors concluded that TEA provides acceptable function and implant survival for those patients who survive to 10-year follow-up.

RATIONALE FOR OPEN REDUCTION WITH INTERNAL FIXATION

Until the 1960s, most methods of open reduction and internal fixation were applied infrequently. In the 1960s, and 1970s, with better implants and newer techniques, management shifted toward open techniques. Advances in anesthesia, including the more widespread use of regional anesthesia, reduced the anesthetic risk in sicker patients (5).

In 2005, Srinivasan et al. (25) examined 29 fractures in 28 elderly patients (age 75–100 years; mean, 85 years) who underwent surgery versus 8 who were treated nonsurgically due to either medical comorbidities or patient preference for nonoperative management. They found reported better range of motion in the operatively treated group (23.5°–99° versus 33.5°–71°). In addition, operatively treated patients had better pain relief with 52% reporting mild or no pain. Only 25% of the nonoperatively treated group reported mild or no pain. Radiographic results were also superior in the operatively treated group, while complication rates were found to be equivalent to those seen in younger patients. Additionally, poor results were seen in 3 of 8 elbows in the nonoperative group (37.5%) versus only 2 of the 21 elbows treated surgically (10%). Pain, loss of reduction, and nonunion were also more commonly seen in the group treated nonoperatively.

In 2005, Korner et al. (26) performed a retrospective review of 45 patients with a mean age of 73 years (range, 61–92 years) who underwent ORIF for distal humerus fractures. Clinical and radiographic follow-up was a minimum of 2 years with an average follow-up of 87 months. Functional results were evaluated according to the MEPS. Using the AO/OTA classification, they found that fractures with complete joint involvement according to the AO/

OTA classification were the most common, and functional results deteriorated with degree of joint involvement. Plates were applied either dorsally or in perpendicular fashion depending on the fracture pattern (A2, A3, and all type C fractures had 90–90 plating). A posterior approach was used for all A, B3, and C fractures, with olecranon osteotomy performed for C-type fractures only. A lateral approach was used for B2-type fractures. The ulnar nerve was anteriorly transposed in 29 (64%) cases. The authors described a high rate of complications including screw loosening and/or implant failure at the lateral column in the 4 months following surgery. However, clinical results were good or excellent in 26 (58%) patients. Most patients lost some amount of flexion, extension, or both. Only seven patients had no loss of extension, and nine had full flexion. Loss of extension ranged from 10° to 50°, and loss of flexion ranged from 5° to 45°. Twenty-five patients had no loss of pronation or supination, with the remaining 20 patients having a median loss of 30° (range, 15°–80°). Development of postsurgical arthrosis was common (32 patients) but was not found to correlate to either pain or range of motion. The authors noted that poorer results found in patients with C-type fractures could have been due to longer periods of immobilization and concluded that immobilization should be no longer than 10 days in duration. The authors also recommend against the use of 1/3 tubular plates, as they were found to have a relatively high rate of failure in this population. Overall, the authors recommended ORIF over TEA with the goal of preservation of the elbow, since good functional results can be obtained.

If the decision to fix the fracture has been made, Park et al. (27) examined the bone mineral density in 14 cadaveric specimens at three levels with quantitative computed tomography (CT) scan to determine regional differences in bone density. They found the highest cancellous volume in the anterior aspect of the lateral condyle and the least in the posterior aspect of the lateral condyle. Cortical thickness was greatest posteromedially and thinnest anteriorly followed by laterally. The authors caution that plate fixation is potentially weak if screws are placed into these areas of weak bone.

In another biomechanical study, Stoffel et al. (28) compared parallel versus perpendicular plating in AO/OTA-type C2 fractures of the distal humerus in paired, osteoporotic distal humerus samples. The parallel locking plate system was shown to provide significantly higher stability in compression and external rotation, as well as a greater ability to resist axial plastic deformation. Stability was found to be dependent on bone quality in both constructs, but the perpendicular system was more sensitive to bone mineral density. The authors suggested that a parallel construct may be indicated in osteoporotic bone.

Another construct that may be considered is the use of a small medial T-plate combined with a transcondylar screw passed from the lateral to the medial wall of the trochlea. Imatani et al. (29) described a series of 17 elderly (older than 70 years of age) patients treated with this construct

with a minimum 2-year follow-up, and reported radiographic union in all but one patient. They had three excellent results, 11 good results, and 3 fair results according to Kundel's modification (30) of Cassebaum's range of motion criteria (31). This outcome measure combines pain; return to work; range of motion in flexion, extension, pronation, and supination; and complications, with an emphasis on return of flexion and extension.

Principles of reduction and fixation in the setting of a "smashed" distal humerus have been described in the literature by O'Driscoll et al. (32), but poor bone stock in osteoporotic fractures makes the management of these injuries with ORIF particularly challenging. In general, the authors recommend four basic goals of treatment: soft tissue healing without infection, restoration of diaphyseal bone stock, union between the distal fragments and the shaft, and a stable and mobile articulation.

When sufficient bone loss leads to the inability to restore a stable anatomical reduction, they recommend the restoration of nonanatomical, stable reduction that achieves the four goals as a reasonable, and even preferable, plan (32). The authors offer several pearls to aid in achieving the four goals mentioned earlier, such as extensive debridement to minimize risk of infection in open fractures, shortening the limb if needed to relax the soft tissues, extending one plate proximal to the fracture to obtain eight cortices of fixation with each screw engaging a fragment on the opposite side that is also fixed to a plate, placing as many screws as possible in the distal fragments, applying plates such that compression is achieved at the supracondylar level for both columns, and using plates that are strong enough to resist breaking or bending before union at the supracondylar level.

Supporting the case for attempted ORIF, in 2008 a study by Prasad and Dent (21) examined the differences between patients treated acutely with TEA versus those with delayed conversion to TEA from either nonoperative treatment or attempted ORIF. Twenty-seven patients were retrospectively reviewed after excluding those with inflammatory arthropathy or posttraumatic osteoarthrosis. The sample size and mean ages in both groups were similar: 15 patients aged 78 years and 17 patients aged 73 years, respectively. The patients in the late conversion group were referred for painful nonunion following ORIF (13) or after closed treatment in plaster (4). The mean time between injury and TEA was approximately 1 year after injury (range, 16–96 months). Fracture classification had a relatively even distribution with six AO/OTA-type A3, six B3, and five C3 fractures. A Coonrad-Morrey prosthesis was used. Mean follow-up was 56 months (range, 18–88 months). All elbows were stable at time of final follow-up. No differences were found between the groups for mean flexion arc, MEPS scores, subjective pain scores, or subjective satisfaction rates. Survivorship was noted to be 93% at 88 months for the acute group compared to 76% at 84 months for the late group, but these differences were not statistically significant. Good or excellent results were found in 84.6% of the patients in the acute group versus 78.5% of the patients in the delayed group. These results were not statistically significant. Overall, the series showed that 93% of patients were satisfied with their results, and 87.5% reported no pain or only mild pain. Good and excellent results were found in 82% of the patients. The authors concluded that TEA provides a predictable and reproducible result with respect to pain relief and function in elderly osteoporotic patients with difficult fractures of the distal humerus. Problems with this study included small sample size and lack of power analysis. It is entirely possible that with a larger sample size, differences in function and other outcomes would become statistically significant.

RATIONALE FOR SURGEON PREFERENCE: OPEN REDUCTION AND INTERNAL FIXATION VERSUS TOTAL ELBOW ARTHROPLASTY

Egol et al. (33) published a retrospective cohort study looking at functional outcomes in women over the age of 60 years following TEA versus ORIF. Of the 20 patients in the study, 9 underwent cemented semiconstrained TEA and 11 underwent ORIF. Mean follow-up was 14.8 months. There were no differences in total flexion arc or disabilities of the arm, shoulder, and hand (DASH) scores between the groups. Two patients in each group died. Four of the TEAs showed radiographic loosening with one going on to revision with a good outcome. Ten of the 11 patients with ORIF went on to radiographic union with the one remaining nonunion being asymptomatic. Of note, two patients in the ORIF group went on to have contracture releases for limited range of motion. The authors concluded that good outcomes may be obtained following either TEA or ORIF, and they recommended that implant choice be based on bone quality, expected outcome, and surgeon experience.

AUTHORS' PREFERRED TREATMENT

The authors of this chapter favor open reduction with internal fixation for the majority of fractures of the distal humerus. Our surgeons have extensive experience with open osteosynthesis, and modern locked implants provide adequate fixation in most cases. In the instance of the truly "smashed" C3 injury in an elderly low-demand patient, TEA is a good option and should be considered.

The authors have five additional components of surgical strategy:

1. The patient is positioned laterally with a bean bag and axillary roll. The arm is draped over a radiolucent plastic cylinder attached to the side of the bed ("paint roller"). The down-side arm is positioned on a well-padded, radiolucent cardiac board with the shoulder flexed at 90° and the elbow flexed 90°. A C-arm is brought in from the head of the table, and anteroposterior (AP) and lateral views are confirmed prior to the prep and drape. With correct setup, the lateral view is possible with minimal manipulation of the extremity. Only after verification of adequate intraoperative fluoroscopic views is the prep and drape undertaken. The skin is first washed with a dilute chlorhexidine solution. Alcohol is then applied, and a towel is used to ensure that it has dried. Finally, a commercial product containing isopropyl alcohol and chlorhexidine gluconate is applied. Drapes and use of a tourniquet are at the preference of the surgeon.

2. If there is a chance that intraoperative conversion to arthroplasty is a possibility, we avoid an olecranon osteotomy. A modified posterior approach to the humerus as described by Gerwin et al. (34) allows access to 94% of the posterior and distal aspect of the humerus if needed.

3. The ulnar nerve is routinely exposed, mobilized, and protected. A vessel loop is passed around the nerve, but no knots or surgical instruments are used to "close the loop." We do not routinely transpose the ulnar nerve, as the literature has not demonstrated a clear benefit (35,36), and it may increase the incidence of postoperative ulnar nerve symptoms (37). Transposition would be considered in the setting of preoperative symptoms or possible irritation from the plate if left *in situ*. Newer, lower-profile implants make the latter finding rare in our experience, and transposition in this setting remains only a theoretical advantage (38).

4. We do not routinely offer postoperative prophylaxis against heterotopic ossification (HO). HO is a known complication of distal humerus fractures occurring in 3%–49% of cases with an average incidence of 9% (39–43). Heterotopic ossification is not common in the elbow in the absence of risk factors such as a head injury. Fixation within 48 hours has been shown to decrease the risk (44). Other risks in AO/OTA C-type fracture-dislocations include severe trauma and delay in fixation (45). Low-dose radiation has been shown to be effective in some studies (46). One prospective trial was stopped when the group receiving prophylaxis was found to have a higher nonunion rate with no decrease in the formation of heterotopic bone (47). HO excision can be performed as soon as 6–9 months following injury and should be performed along with the appropriate capsular and/or ligamentous releases, taking care to maintain a stable elbow. A small series of nine patients showed good clinical results with postoperative radiation prophylaxis following HO excision (48).

5. Most patients are placed in a soft dressing and allowed early active range of motion. Passive range of motion with physical therapy is avoided postoperatively for the first 2 weeks as this places excessive stress on the implants and may lead to the formation of HO (38). If a splint is used, it is placed on the anterior aspect of the arm, removed on postoperative day 2, and not replaced. Follow-up is at the 2-week, 6-week, and 3-month time intervals unless more frequent visits are needed for wound checks.

REFERENCES

1. Mansat P, Bonnevialle N, Rongières M, Bonnevialle P. Bone, Joint Trauma Study Group (GETRAUM). The role of total elbow arthroplasty in traumatology. *Orthop Traumatol Surg Res*. 2014;100(Suppl 6):S293–8.

2. Brown RF, Morgan RG. Intercondylar T-shaped fractures of the humerus. Results in ten cases treated by early mobilisation. *J Bone Joint Surg Br*. 1971;53(3):425–8.

3. Ring D, Jupiter JB. Complex fractures of the distal humerus and their complications. *J Shoulder Elbow Surg*. 1999;8(1):85–97.

4. Maniscalco P, Pizzoli AL, Renzi Brivio L, Caforio M. Hinged external fixation for complex fracture-dislocation of the elbow in elderly people. *Injury*. 2014;45(Suppl 6):S53–7.

5. Popovic D, King GJW. Fragility fractures of the distal humerus: What is the optimal treatment? *J Bone Joint Surg Br*. 2012;94(1):16–22.

6. Palvanen M, Kannus P, Niemi S, Parkkari J. Secular trends in distal humeral fractures of elderly women: Nationwide statistics in Finland between 1970 and 2007. *Bone*. 2010;46(5):1355–8.

7. Charissoux J-L, Vergnenegre G, Pelissier M, Fabre T, Mansat P, SOFCOT. Epidemiology of distal humerus fractures in the elderly. *Orthop Traumatol Surg Res*. 2013;99(7):765–9.

8. Helfet DL, Hotchkiss RN. Internal fixation of the distal humerus: A biomechanical comparison of methods. *J Orthop Trauma*. 1990;4(3):260–4.

9. King GJ, Faber KJ. Posttraumatic elbow stiffness. *Orthop Clin North Am*. 2000;31(1):129–43.

10. Müller M, Schneider R, Willenegger H. In Allgöwer M, ed. *Manual of Internal Fixation: Techniques Recommended by the AO-ASIF Group*. 3rd ed. Berlin, New York: Springer-Verlag, 1991.

11. Mehne DK, Jupiter JB. Fractures of the distal humerus. In Browner BD, Jupiter JB, Trafton PG, eds. *Skeletal Trauma: Fractures, Dislocations, Ligamentous Injuries*. 3rd ed. Philadelphia, PA: WB Saunders, 1992.

12. Bryan RS, Morrey BF. Fractures of the distal humerus. In Morrey BF, ed. *The Elbow and Its Disorders*. Philadelphia, PA: WB Saunders, 1985, pp. 302–39.

13. McKee MD, Jupiter JB, Bamberger HB. Coronal shear fractures of the distal end of the humerus. *J Bone Joint Surg Am*. 1996;78(1):49–54.

14. Bégué T. Articular fractures of the distal humerus. *Orthop Traumatol Surg Res*. 2014;100(Suppl 1):S55–63.

15. Cobb TK, Morrey BF. Total elbow arthroplasty as primary treatment for distal humeral fractures in elderly patients. *J Bone Joint Surg Am*. 1997;79(6):826–32.

16. Kamineni S, Morrey BF. Distal humeral fractures treated with noncustom total elbow replacement. *J Bone Joint Surg Am*. 2004;86-A(5):940–7.

17. Ray PS, Kakarlapudi K, Rajsekhar C, Bhamra MS. Total elbow arthroplasty as primary treatment for distal humeral fractures in elderly patients. *Injury*. 2000;31(9):687–92.

18. Gambirasio R, Riand N, Stern R, Hoffmeyer P. Total elbow replacement for complex fractures of the distal humerus. An option for the elderly patient. *J Bone Joint Surg Br*. 2001;83(7):974–8.

19. Garcia JA, Mykula R, Stanley D. Complex fractures of the distal humerus in the elderly. The role of total elbow replacement as primary treatment. *J Bone Joint Surg Br*. 2002;84(6):812–6.

20. Lee KT, Lai CH, Singh S. Results of total elbow arthroplasty in the treatment of distal humerus fractures in elderly Asian patients. *J Trauma*. 2006;61(4):889–92.

21. Prasad N, Dent C. Outcome of total elbow replacement for distal humeral fractures in the elderly: A comparison of primary surgery and surgery after failed internal fixation or conservative treatment. *J Bone Joint Surg Br*. 2008;90(3):343–8.

22. McKee MD, Pugh DMW, Richards RR, Pedersen E, Jones C, Schemitsch EH. Effect of humeral condylar resection on strength and functional outcome after semiconstrained total elbow arthroplasty. *J Bone Joint Surg Am*. 2003;85-A(5):802–7.

23. Mansat P, Nouaille Degorce H, Bonnevialle N, Demezon H, Fabre T, SOFCOT. Total elbow arthroplasty for acute distal humeral fractures in patients over 65 years old—Results of a multicenter study in 87 patients. *Orthop Traumatol Surg Res*. 2013;99(7):779–84.

24. Prasad N, Ali A, Stanley D. Total elbow arthroplasty for non-rheumatoid patients with a fracture of the distal humerus: A minimum ten-year follow-up. *Bone Joint J*. 2016;98-B(3):381–6.

25. Srinivasan K, Agarwal M, Matthews SJE, Giannoudis PV. Fractures of the distal humerus in the elderly: Is internal fixation the treatment of choice? *Clin Orthop Relat Res*. 2005;(434):222–30.

26. Korner J, Lill H, Müller LP et al. Distal humerus fractures in elderly patients: Results after open reduction and internal fixation. *Osteoporos Int*. 2005;16(Suppl 2):S73–79.

27. Park SH, Kim SJ, Park BC et al. Three-dimensional osseous micro-architecture of the distal humerus: Implications for internal fixation of osteoporotic fracture. *J Shoulder Elbow Surg*. 2010;19(2):244–50.

28. Stoffel K, Cunneen S, Morgan R, Nicholls R, Stachowiak G. Comparative stability of perpendicular versus parallel double-locking plating systems in osteoporotic comminuted distal humerus fractures. *J Orthop Res Off Publ Orthop Res Soc*. 2008;26(6):778–84.

29. Imatani J, Ogura T, Morito Y, Hashizume H, Inoue H. Custom AO small T plate for transcondylar fractures of the distal humerus in the elderly. *J Shoulder Elbow Surg*. 2005;14(6):611–5.

30. Kundel K, Braun W, Wieberneit J, Rüter A. Intraarticular distal humerus fractures. Factors affecting functional outcome. *Clin Orthop Relat Res.* 1996;(332):200–8.

31. Cassebaum WH. Open reduction of T & Y fractures of the lower end of the humerus. *J Trauma.* 1969;9(11):915–25.

32. O'Driscoll SW, Sanchez-Sotelo J, Torchia ME. Management of the smashed distal humerus. *Orthop Clin North Am.* 2002;33(1):19–33, vii.

33. Egol KA, Tsai P, Vazques O, Tejwani NC. Comparison of functional outcomes of total elbow arthroplasty vs plate fixation for distal humerus fractures in osteoporotic elbows. *Am J Orthop Belle Mead NJ.* 2011;40(2):67–71.

34. Gerwin M, Hotchkiss RN, Weiland AJ. Alternative operative exposures of the posterior aspect of the humeral diaphysis with reference to the radial nerve. *J Bone Joint Surg.* 1996;78(11):1690–5.

35. Wang KC, Shih HN, Hsu KY, Shih CH. Intercondylar fractures of the distal humerus: Routine anterior subcutaneous transposition of the ulnar nerve in a posterior operative approach. *J Trauma.* 1994;36(6):770–3.

36. Gupta R. Intercondylar fractures of the distal humerus in adults. *Injury.* 1996;27(8):569–72.

37. Chen RC, Harris DJ, Leduc S, Borrelli JJ, Tornetta P, Ricci WM. Is ulnar nerve transposition beneficial during open reduction internal fixation of distal humerus fractures? *J Orthop Trauma.* 2010;24(7):391–4.

38. Stannard JP, Schmidt AH. *Surgical Treatment of Orthopaedic Trauma.* 2nd ed. New York: Thieme, 2016.

39. Nauth A, McKee MD, Ristevski B, Hall J, Schemitsch EH. Distal humeral fractures in adults. *J Bone Joint Surg Am.* 2011;93(7):686–700.

40. Helfet DL, Schmeling GJ. Bicondylar intraarticular fractures of the distal humerus in adults. *Clin Orthop.* 1993;(292):26–36.

41. Sanchez-Sotelo J, Torchia ME, O'Driscoll SW. Principle-based internal fixation of distal humerus fractures. *Tech Hand Up Extrem Surg.* 2001;5(4):179–87.

42. Athwal GS, Hoxie SC, Rispoli DM, Steinmann SP. Precontoured parallel plate fixation of AO/OTA type C distal humerus fractures. *J Orthop Trauma.* 2009;23(8):575–80.

43. Mighell MA, Harkins D, Klein D, Schneider S, Frankle M. Technique for internal fixation of capitellum and lateral trochlea fractures. *J Orthop Trauma.* 2006;20(10):699–704.

44. Ilahi OA, Strausser DW, Gabel GT. Post-traumatic heterotopic ossification about the elbow. *Orthopedics* 1998;21(3):265–8.

45. Douglas K, Cannada LK, Archer KR, Dean DB, Lee S, Obremskey W. Incidence and risk factors of heterotopic ossification following major elbow trauma. *Orthopedics* 2012;35(6):e815–22.

46. Stein DA, Patel R, Egol KA, Kaplan FT, Tejwani NC, Koval KJ. Prevention of heterotopic ossification at the elbow following trauma using radiation therapy. *Bull Hosp Jt Dis.* 2003;61(3–4):151–4.

47. Hamid N, Ashraf N, Bosse MJ et al. Radiation therapy for heterotopic ossification prophylaxis acutely after elbow trauma: A prospective randomized study. *J Bone Joint Surg Am.* 2010;92(11):2032–8.

48. Heyd R, Strassmann G, Schopohl B, Zamboglou N. Radiation therapy for the prevention of heterotopic ossification at the elbow. *J Bone Joint Surg Br.* 2001;83(3):332–4.

19

Distal radius osteoporotic features

My preferred method of treatment

DONATO PERRETTA and JESSE B. JUPITER

INTRODUCTION

Distal radius fractures in elderly patients are very common with an estimated 80,000 occurring every year in the United States (1). The majority of these fractures are related to postmenopausal or senile osteoporosis and are the result of low-energy injuries, such as a fall from standing height. Low bone density has been shown to increase the risk of distal radius fracture (2). Osteoporosis also affects the treatment of distal radius fractures in several ways. It decreases fracture stability after closed reduction. In addition, fixation methods are dependent on bone quality. The approach to the management of distal radius fracture has undergone an evolution over the past two decades with an increasing percentage of osteoporotic fractures undergoing internal fixation due to the development of angular stable plate and screw fixation.

Outcome measures

Radiographic measures of alignment and healing do not tell the full story since their relationship to function is not clear, especially in the elderly. Patient-reported outcome measures based on elements such as pain, disability, and ability to perform tasks independently are perhaps more useful. These tools include the SF-36 (3), DASH (disabilities of the arm, shoulder, and hand) score (4), and the patient-rated wrist evaluation (PRWE) (5).

The SF-36 contains 36 questions and is a general measure of health and well-being. It lacks specificity for upper extremity disability and is not geared toward a specific age group; therefore, it is not a useful measure of function after distal radius fracture.

The DASH is a 30-point questionnaire specific for the upper extremity and is likely the most commonly used patient-reported outcome measure for the upper extremity in the literature. However, its use has not been validated in patients older than 65 years. Some of its questions may not be geared toward the actual required activities of this age group. Lower scores indicate lower disability.

The PRWE score contains five questions about pain and functional ability and is specific to the wrist, which makes it ideal for patients with distal radius fracture. Equal weight is given to pain and disability. Lower scores indicate lower degree of impairment. Additionally, it has been validated for use in multiple age groups.

The Physical Activity Scale for the Elderly (PASE) (6) can be used to assess the preinjury activity level of the patient, as well as follow the patient's progression after injury. It reports on the patient's activity level in the prior 7 days. Additionally, it has been demonstrated to be an effective outcome measure in the surgical treatment of osteoporotic fractures (7). The preinjury score may also be useful in surgical decision-making.

DECISION-MAKING

Imaging

High-quality radiographs, both pre- and postreduction, are necessary for making informed decisions about distal radius fracture. CT scans are recommended after reduction of intra-articular fractures as they can provide a clearer delineation of the fracture fragments and level of comminution.

Closed reduction

Injury radiographs provide a good deal of information about the stability of the fracture pattern. Lafontaine (8) retrospectively reviewed 112 consecutive distal radius fractures treated with closed reduction and immobilization. The prereduction radiographs were analyzed for the presence of dorsal angulation greater than 20°, dorsal comminution, intra-articular radiocarpal fracture, and associated ulnar fracture. These characteristics, along with age greater than 60 years, were each independently found to be associated with radiographic displacement at the time of healing. The average radiographic position improved significantly after closed reduction; however, the average healed position of the fracture returned to the prereduction position. It was concluded that the presence of three factors should lead to consideration of surgical management.

Despite the tendency of osteoporotic distal radius fractures to return to their prereduction position, we believe that closed reduction of displaced fractures is beneficial. This is based on the belief that improved alignment of the wrist may improve soft tissue swelling and lessen the likelihood of nerve compression.

OPTIONS FOR TREATMENT

Closed treatment

With the enthusiasm of treating osteoporotic fractures growing due to the technological advance of angular stable internal fixation, a number of evidence-based studies have compared the outcomes of closed reduction to operative treatment. There is a significant body of literature that suggests that nonoperative treatment of displaced distal radius fracture yields acceptable results in the elderly, low-demand population. Functional outcome is not correlated to radiographic outcome in this population group as opposed to a younger, more active one (9). Egol et al. performed a case-controlled study with 90 patients comparing operative to nonoperative treatment of distal radius fractures in patients older than 65 years. The operative interventions included external and internal fixation techniques. The operative group had better radiographic measures and better grip strength; however, there was no difference in DASH score between the groups at 1 year. These findings were confirmed by Arora et al. (10) in a randomized study comparing closed reduction and immobilization to volar plating of unstable distal radius fractures. Grip strength and radiographic alignment were better in the operative group. DASH and PRWE scores were improved in the early postoperative period in the operative group; however, at 6 months and 1 year, there were no significant differences.

The decision to proceed with closed treatment should be accompanied by close attention to the soft tissue. The use of a constrictive cast or one that does not allow for digital range of motion can lead to a poor functional outcome. Figure 19.1 is an example of a patient placed in a tight cast who developed intrinsic tightness and reduced digital range of motion.

The fact that objective measures of outcomes such as radiographic appearance and grip strength are better after operative treatment of unstable fractures, while subjective measures such as DASH and PRWE are similar, would suggest that the functional demands may reduce the need for anatomical alignment.

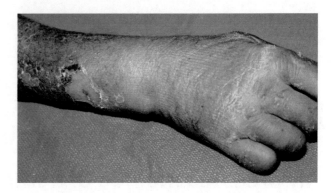

Figure 19.1 Swelling and digital stiffness secondary to cast placement.

Additionally, it is broadly reported that operative treatment leads to a higher complication rate than closed treatment (10,11). Pin site infection is common with external fixation and Kirshner wires. Tendon irritation is common with volar and dorsal plating techniques (11,12). Carpal tunnel syndrome and reflex sympathetic dystrophy can occur after closed or operative treatment.

Indications for operative treatment

There are no absolute indications for the operative treatment of osteoporotic distal radius fractures. In the authors' opinion, the most important factor in decision-making is the preinjury activity level of the elderly patient with osteoporosis. Chronological age alone should not dictate treatment. With advances in medical care, there is significant variability in functional ability and demands among patients older than 65 years. Accordingly, in 2002 Jupiter et al. (7) retrospectively reviewed 20 patients who underwent open reduction and internal fixation of a distal radius fracture after initial reduction was lost. All patients had significant preinjury functional demands due to work, hobbies, or independent living. The radiographic parameters that signified unacceptable alignment were volar radiocarpal subluxation, articular incongruity greater than 2 mm, or greater than 20° of dorsal tilt. If one of these radiographic parameters is present in an active patient, we recommend surgery regardless of the chronological age. In addition, operative treatment is indicated in cases of acute carpal tunnel syndrome and multiply injured patient.

TECHNOLOGY

Internal fixation

Internal fixation of distal radius fractures is based on the presumption that restoration of the anatomy of the distal radius will improve the ultimate outcome. Early mobilization of the digits and wrist is another positive aspect of internal fixation. With an increasing amount of displacement, the biomechanics of the wrist joint become significantly altered. Dorsal tilt and radial shortening increase the amount of load borne by the ulna (13). Excessive dorsal angulation of the distal radius can lead to compensatory changes in the carpus and adaptive carpal instability.

Angular stable plate and screw fixation

Angular stable plate and screw fixation has significantly improved the orthopedic surgeon's ability to operatively manage metaphyseal fractures in osteoporotic bone, such as in the distal radius, proximal humerus, distal femur, and proximal tibia. Screw thread purchase in osteoporotic metaphyseal bone is decreased, which limits the ability to obtain adequate fixation with conventional non-locked plate and screw constructs. Angular stable fixation is obtained when screws or pegs lock into the plate. This transforms shear stress to compressive stress. Since bone is able to resist compressive stress more effectively, fixation is improved. Additionally, strain at the fracture site is reduced since there is no motion at the plate-screw interface. The plates and screws essentially act as one device, spreading the stress over a larger area.

Pi plate

The first implant to provide angular stable fixation specifically for fractures of the distal radius was the "Pi" plate system, which was available for volar and dorsal application.

Dorsal plating of dorsally displaced distal radius fractures using the low-profile "Pi" plate was a significant advance in a surgeon's ability to accurately restore anatomy (14). It was first released in the United States in 1995 and was contoured to fit the dorsal aspect of the distal radius and could be further customized with bending irons and trimming (Figure 19.2). Most osteoporotic distal radius fractures are the result of a bending force and are displaced dorsally, so the dorsal location of the plate could effectively resist displacement. The angle stable buttress pin inserted through the distal aspect of the plate was especially important in treating osteoporotic distal radius fractures with poor metaphyseal bone quality. Ring et al. (14) reported on its use in 22 patients with complex fracture of the distal radius. Radiographic parameters at healing were excellent with an average palmar tilt of 5°, radial inclination of 18.5°, no radial shortening, and maximum articular incongruity of 0.5 mm. There was no loss of reduction between the initial postoperative radiographs and healing. No infections, nonunions, wound problems, or plate failures occurred. Five patients developed extensor tendon irritation, and four had their plates removed. Later studies reported extensor tendon ruptures (15). Due to these complications, alternative internal fixation methods were developed.

Current indications for dorsal plating

Design modifications and low-profile construction have substantially limited problems with the overlying extensor tendons. The approach allows for direct visualization of

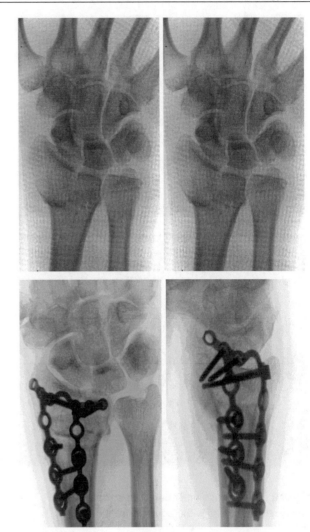

Figure 19.2 Pi plate dorsal application in an active 81-year-old oral surgeon.

the articular surface, which is particularly important when addressing the dorsal ulnar fragment (16). It may be used in conjunction with other plates in a fragment-specific manner as in Figure 19.3. In addition, dorsal shear fractures are most appropriately addressed with dorsal fixation.

Volar plating

The initial design of the volar Pi plate was further adapted for fixation of dorsally displaced radius fractures. In 2002, Orbay and Ferndandez (17) reported the successful treatment of 31 distal radius fractures fixed with this method. The technique relies on indirect reduction of the dorsal fragments and provides locking screw fixation of the distal fragments. Interposition of the pronator quadratus between the flexor tendons and the plate decreases the chance of tendon irritation. Further investigation revealed that this technique was extremely useful in the elderly population as volar plates could successfully fixate osteopenic bone. This allowed early motion and good final results, with a

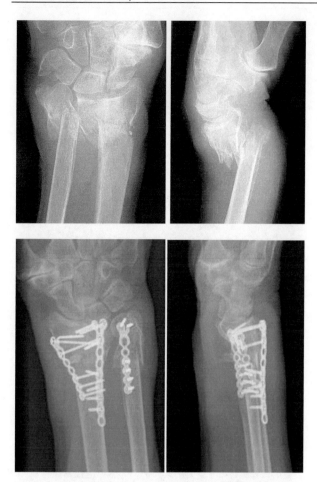

Figure 19.3 Grade one open intra-articular fracture in an elderly female treated with fragment specific fixation.

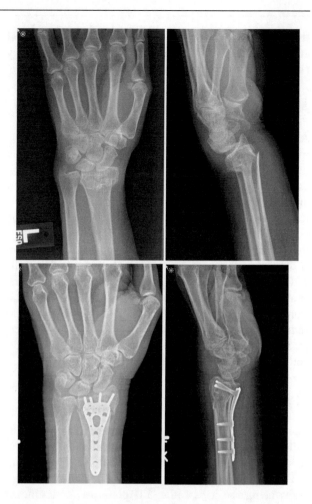

Figure 19.4 Dorsally displaced osteoporotic distal radius fracture treated with volar plate.

low complication profile (18). The clinical success of the volar plate has led to its increased use over the past 15 years (1). The likelihood of tendon irritation is lower with volar plating as compared to dorsal plating, making it preferable.

The volar locking plate can be used for the majority of displaced osteoporotic distal radius fractures for which open reduction and internal fixation are recommended. Volar plating is necessary in volar shear fractures. Small volar lunate facet fragments may not be captured by standard volar plating techniques and may require more distal plate placement (19) or hook plate fixation. Figure 19.4 shows an example of volar plating of a dorsally displaced distal radius fracture in an osteoporotic 68-year-old female.

Bone cement

Synthetic calcium phosphate bone cement (20) was developed in the mid-1990s as a method to support the structural characteristics of weak and comminuted bone, especially to compressive loads. Norian (Synthes) is a commercially available, fiber-reinforced calcium phosphate void filler. Once injected into bone, it is converted into carbonated apatite, which closely mimics the mineral phase of bone. Ultimately, it is remodeled into bone. Cassidy et al. investigated its use in a randomized

study of 323 distal radius fractures in 2003 (21). Figure 19.5 demonstrates closed reduction and pinning with calcium phosphate injection into the fracture site. Patients received standard treatment, which included closed reduction, pinning, and/or external fixation with or without injection of calcium phosphate into the fracture site. Improved grip strength and range of motion were noted at 6–8 weeks in the calcium phosphate group. There were no clinical or radiographic differences noted at 1 year. The use of injectable cements proved technically challenging when used along with closed reduction as the viscosity of the cement made it difficult to fill the void created by the fracture. However, if delivery systems are improved, the structural stability added by calcium phosphate cement might make it a useful adjunct to closed or percutaneous management of osteoporotic fractures.

Calcium phosphate has also been shown to be safe and effective when used during distal radius osteotomies after malunion (22).

Dorsal bridge plating

In the setting of highly comminuted intra-articular fractures, temporary bridge plating may be used to align the distal radius and carpus. In this technique, a plate is affixed

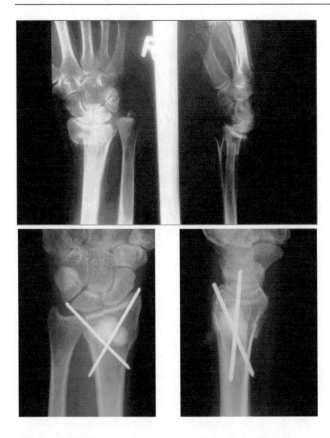

Figure 19.5 Fracture treated with pinning and calcium phosphate bone cement.

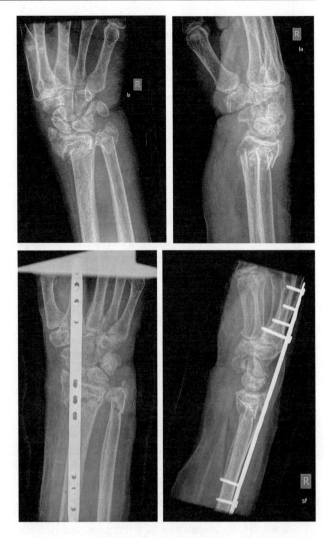

Figure 19.6 Dorsal spanning plate in grade one elderly osteoporotic open fracture.

to the second or third metacarpal and the radial shaft underneath the extensor tendons. It also allows for early weight-bearing on the affected extremity, which is useful in a multiply injured patient. Similar to external fixation, the fracture is held out to length with ligamentotaxis as seen in Figure 19.6. However, plate fixation is more stable, and there is no chance of pin site infection. It does require a second operation for plate removal.

Lauder et al. (23) reported on 18 patients who received dorsal bridge plating for comminuted and intra-articular distal radius fractures. The average age was 61 years, and plates were removed at an average of 2.4 months. At final follow-up more than 1 year after plate removal, the average flexion-extension arc was 89°, and grip strength was 88% of the noninjured wrist.

Bridging external fixation

Prior to the advent of internal fixation techniques, external fixation with or without supplemental K-wires was the standard of care for the operative management of osteoporotic distal radius fractures. The reduction relied on ligamentotaxis to maintain the alignment of the carpus to the radial shaft. The results of this technique have been shown to be ultimately equivalent to open reduction and internal fixation (24). However, there is a high incidence of minor pin tract problems. Currently, there is a limited

role for bridging external fixation in low-energy osteoporosis distal radius fractures. Its use is reserved for higher-energy injuries in which there is significant damage to the soft tissue envelope. It also may be used as a supplement to internal fixation in the rare circumstances when the carpus remains unstable after appropriate plate and screw fixation.

CONCLUSION

Our approach to treatment of osteoporotic distal radius fracture takes into account patient factors and fracture characteristics. In low-demand patients and those with significant medical comorbidities, closed treatment with care to avoid hand swelling or nerve compression remains a fundamental approach supported by evidence-based studies.

In active patients, however, restoration of anatomy is the critical factor in later function. The criteria described by Lafontaine (8) predict that many osteoporotic distal radius fractures will be unstable after reduction. Understanding the high likelihood of displacement after fracture reduction, our indications to perform surgical intervention will generally be based on the patient's activity level and medical status. Angular stable plate fixation has become popular, but we would also consider injectable bone cement as this technology improves. Some osteoporotic fractures are so highly comminuted and displaced that they preclude treatment with periarticular plate and screws. These can be treated effectively with dorsal bridge plate fixation with a limited surgical exposure.

REFERENCES

1. Chung KC, Shauver MJ, Birkmeyer JD. Trends in the United States in the treatment of distal radial fractures in the elderly. *J Bone Joint Surg Am.* 2009;91(8):1868–73.
2. Bouxsein ML, Palermo L, Yeung C, Black DM. Digital x-ray radiogrammetry predicts hip, wrist and vertebral fracture risk in elderly women: A prospective analysis from the study of osteoporotic fractures. *Osteoporos Int.* 2002;13(5):358–65.
3. Ware JE, Jr., Sherbourne CD. The MOS 36-item short-form health survey (SF-36). I. Conceptual framework and item selection. *Med Care.* 1992;30(6):473–83.
4. Hudak PL, Amadio PC, Bombardier C. Development of an upper extremity outcome measure: The DASH (disabilities of the arm, shoulder and hand). The Upper Extremity Collaborative Group (UECG). *Am J Ind Med.* 1996;29(6):602–8.
5. MacDermid JC, Turgeon T, Richards RS, Beadle M, Roth JH. Patient rating of wrist pain and disability: A reliable and valid measurement tool. *J Orthop Trauma.* 1998;12(8):577–86.
6. Washburn RA, Smith KW, Jette AM, Janney CA. The Physical Activity Scale for the Elderly (PASE): Development and evaluation. *J Clin Epidemiol.* 1993;46(2):153–62.
7. Jupiter JB, Ring D, Weitzel PP. Surgical treatment of redisplaced fractures of the distal radius in patients older than 60 years. *J Hand Surg Am.* 2002;27(4):714–23.
8. Lafontaine M, Hardy D, Delince P. Stability assessment of distal radius fractures. *Injury.* 1989;20(4):208–10.
9. Young BT, Rayan GM. Outcome following nonoperative treatment of displaced distal radius fractures in low-demand patients older than 60 years. *J Hand Surg Am.* 2000;25(1):19–28.
10. Arora R, Lutz M, Deml C, Krappinger D, Haug L, Gabl M. A prospective randomized trial comparing nonoperative treatment with volar locking plate fixation for displaced and unstable distal radial fractures in patients sixty-five years of age and older. *J Bone Joint Surg Am.* 2011;93(23):2146–53.
11. Lutz K, Yeoh KM, MacDermid JC, Symonette C, Grewal R. Complications associated with operative versus nonsurgical treatment of distal radius fractures in patients aged 65 years and older. *J Hand Surg Am.* 2014;39(7):1280–6.
12. Arora R, Lutz M, Hennerbichler A, Krappinger D, Espen D, Gabl M. Complications following internal fixation of unstable distal radius fracture with a palmar locking-plate. *J Orthop Trauma.* 2007;21(5):316–22.
13. Pogue DJ, Viegas SF, Patterson RM et al. Effects of distal radius fracture malunion on wrist joint mechanics. *J Hand Surg Am.* 1990;15(5):721–7.
14. Ring D, Jupiter JB, Brennwald J, Buchler U, Hastings H 2nd. Prospective multicenter trial of a plate for dorsal fixation of distal radius fractures. *J Hand Surg Am.* 1997;22(5):777–84.
15. Kambouroglou GK, Axelrod TS. Complications of the AO/ASIF titanium distal radius plate system (pi plate) in internal fixation of the distal radius: A brief report. *J Hand Surg Am.* 1998;23(4):737–41.
16. Benson LS, Minihane KP, Stern LD, Eller E, Seshadri R. The outcome of intra-articular distal radius fractures treated with fragment-specific fixation. *J Hand Surg Am.* 2006;31(8):1333–9.
17. Orbay JL, Fernandez DL. Volar fixation for dorsally displaced fractures of the distal radius: A preliminary report. *J Hand Surg Am.* 2002;27(2):205–15.
18. Orbay JL, Fernandez DL. Volar fixed-angle plate fixation for unstable distal radius fractures in the elderly patient. *J Hand Surg Am.* 2004;29(1):96–102.
19. Kachooei AR, Tarabochia M, Jupiter JB. Distal radius volar rim fracture fixation using DePuy-Synthes volar rim plate. *J Wrist Surg.* 2016;5(1):2–8.
20. Constantz BR, Ison IC, Fulmer MT et al. Skeletal repair by *in situ* formation of the mineral phase of bone. *Science* 1995;267(5205):1796–9.
21. Cassidy C, Jupiter JB, Cohen M et al. Norian SRS cement compared with conventional fixation in distal radial fractures. A randomized study. *J Bone Joint Surg Am.* 2003;85-A(11):2127–37.
22. Lozano-Calderon S, Moore M, Liebman M, Jupiter JB. Distal radius osteotomy in the elderly patient using angular stable implants and Norian bone cement. *J Hand Surg Am.* 2007;32(7):976–83.
23. Lauder A, Agnew S, Bakri K, Allan CH, Hanel DP, Huang JI. Functional outcomes following bridge plate fixation for distal radius fractures. *J Hand Surg Am.* 2015;40(8):1554–62.
24. Leung F, Tu YK, Chew WY, Chow SP. Comparison of external and percutaneous pin fixation with plate fixation for intra-articular distal radial fractures. A randomized study. *J Bone Joint Surg Am.* 2008;90(1):16–22.

20

Management of osteoporotic pelvic fractures

POL M. ROMMENS, DANIEL WAGNER, and ALEXANDER HOFMANN

INTRODUCTION

Thanks to longer life expectancy, the incidence of elderly persons is steadily increasing in industrialized countries. The number of age-related diseases and injuries is increasing accordingly. Particularly in elderly women, osteoporosis is a very common medical condition and a significant health-care problem (1–3). Osteoporotic fractures are most frequently situated in the hip and spine, yet a constantly rising number of fragility fractures of the pelvic ring (FFP) has also been reported (4). A nationwide inpatient sample from the United States that recorded more than 600 million Medicare-paid hospital discharges from 1993 to 2010 showed a 24% increase in pelvic fractures, while the incidence of hip fractures declined in this 18-year period (5). A recent Finnish study reported similar data: the age-adjusted incidence of pelvic fractures increased from 73 to 364 per 100,000 persons 80 years and older in the period between 1970 and 2013 (6). Clinical picture, radiological morphology, and loss of stability of FFP represent a spectrum of pathologies, which has not been described in detail so far. There also is still no consensus on the treatment strategy of these lesions. Recently, a new classification system has been developed that provides a framework for analysis of instability of FFP. General recommendations for treatment and indications for specific, less-invasive surgical techniques for stabilization are given for the different types and subtypes of instability (7).

ANAMNESIS AND CLINICAL PICTURE AT ADMISSION

The leading symptom and primary reason for presentation in the emergency department is *pain in the pelvic region*. Pain came up after a domestic fall or another low-energy trauma. Sometimes, a traumatic event is not memorable. Repetitive harmless incidents, such as short transfers, sneezing, and crouching, which may not be regarded as traumatic, have also been described as causing "pelvic pain" (8). The pain is immobilizing; most patients are not able to walk. Some patients complain of chronic pain that started after a previous event—that was the cause of FFP—which has been underestimated, underdiagnosed, or undertreated.

Pain is localized at the pubic symphysis, in the groin, and/or at the posterior pelvis or low back. When pain in the low back is dominant, physicians may focus diagnostic examinations on the lumbar spine and overlook a sacral pathology (9). Direct palpation of the symphysis pubis, the groin, and the sacrum will provoke pain. Manual compression on both iliac wings enhances pain intensity substantially. Gross pelvic instability is not detectable. With the exception of a hematoma, which may be visible at the fracture site, the skin and soft tissue envelope around the pelvis are not altered. Nevertheless, local skin infections or decubitus, which may influence treatment protocol, must be excluded. The neurological status and vascular status of the lower extremities are not changed by the injury but should be documented in all patients.

The hemodynamic condition of the patient is not altered by the fracture, as there is no significant bleeding. Yet, there must be a high index of suspicion for bleeding in patients who take anticoagulants. The hemodynamic condition of these patients should be monitored for at least 24 hours. In case of active and continuing bleeding, arteriography with selective embolization is chosen as the first-line, damage control procedure. Delay will enhance mortality (10).

Comorbidities increase the risk of suffering an FFP. Many patients have a history of osteoporosis, which causes rarefication of bone mass (11). Other findings are vitamin D depletion (12), long-term immobilization, rheumatoid arthritis (13), long-term cortisone intake, pelvic irradiation for treatment of a malignancy (14), or bone harvesting at the posterior ilium for lumbar spine surgery (15).

RADIOLOGICAL EXAMINATIONS

Conventional pelvic overviews

Conventional pelvic overviews are taken in all patients with a clinical suspicion of FFP. On the *anteroposterior view* (AP view), fractures of the pubic bone or of the superior and inferior pubic rami are easily recognized. The fracture line runs horizontally at the superior pubic ramus in case there was a lateral compression. We then see a slight overriding of the fracture fragments, the lateral fracture fragment being displaced medially. Fractures of the posterior pelvic ring are less easily detected, unless there is marked displacement.

Pelvic inlet and outlet views are obtained when a pelvic fracture is confirmed on the AP pelvic overview. The *inlet view* best depicts any internal rotation of the innominate bone. The integrity of the anterior sacral cortex and of the inner curve of the innominate bone can also be analyzed. The *outlet view* provides information on the shape and symmetry of the sacrum, neuroforamina, and sacroiliac joints. These views will serve as reference for later controls.

Conventional pelvic overviews have a low sensitivity for fractures of the posterior pelvic ring, especially in older patients. The large, often very obese soft tissue envelope, bowel content, and bowel gas are overlying the bony structures and joints of the posterior pelvis. Moreover, due to rarefaction of cortical and cancellous bone, fissures and nondisplaced fractures may not be recognized. This leads to underestimation of the severity of the fragility fracture pattern and results in inadequate treatment and aftertreatment (16).

Computed tomography scan and multiplanar reconstructions

We recommend always performing a pelvic computed tomography (CT) scan when a fracture of the anterior pelvic ring has been confirmed on pelvic overviews. In a cohort of 245 patients with FFP, more than 80% had a posterior pelvic ring fracture. When only a pelvic overview would have been taken at admission, there would have been a very high risk of overlooking posterior pelvic ring fractures (7). Axial transections and coronal and sagittal reconstructions should be made and analyzed to get a complete understanding of the fractures of the posterior pelvic ring. In coronal reconstructions, a fracture of the lateral mass of the sacrum is sometimes better visible than in axial transections. The horizontal component of an H-type sacral fracture is difficult to identify in axial CT transections but is much more easily visible on sagittal CT reconstructions.

In case of chronic instability, radiological signs include callus formation at the edges of the fracture margins and bone defects as the result of persistent movement between fracture fragments. Joint instability leads to an irregular joint space, zones of sclerosis, and intra-articular nitrogen bubbles.

Magnetic resonance imaging

Magnetic resonance imaging (MRI) of the pelvic ring is the most sensitive examination for detecting occult fractures. Bone bruise in the sacrum is already visible when fissures or fractures are not yet detectable on pelvic overviews or CT. MRI is not part of our diagnostic workup of FFP. We recommend using MRI if conventional radiographs and CT cannot explain the clinical picture of the patient, especially low back and posterior pelvic pain. A positive MRI finding does not mean that an FFP is already present. Differentiation between bone marrow edema and malignancy is possible with MRI (17).

CLASSIFICATION

The Tile (18), AO/OTA (19), and Young-Burgess (20) classifications of pelvic ring injuries have been developed for high-energy trauma. The classifications distinguish different types of instability, being the result of different directions of traumatizing force. The different types of high-energy pelvic trauma are combined with specific concomitant injuries (neurological, vascular, hollow organs, skin) that influence outcome. Low-energy FFPs have completely different trauma mechanisms. Concomitant injuries of the soft tissues are seldom seen. Not the direction of the traumatic force but rather the areas of very low bone density are responsible for the fracture morphology (21). This leads to fracture morphologies that do not exist in high-energy trauma. In some patients with FFP, the instability of their lesion increases over time. This happens when new fractures add to the already existing fractures in case of inadequate treatment. This phenomenon is unique for FFP. The previously mentioned characteristics of FFP formed the reason and basis for the development of a new comprehensive classification system.

The classification system is based on an analysis of both conventional x-rays and CT data of 245 patients, 65 years or older, with FFP (7). The leading criterion is the *degree of instability*. *Instability* is defined as the inability of a structure to withstand physiologic loads without displacement. As in younger adults, this criterion is crucial for setting an indication for surgical stabilization. Fracture displacement is the clearest proof of instability. Nondisplaced lesions are characterized by a crush zone or a fracture without deformation. Displaced lesions are characterized by a crush or a fracture with deformation of the anatomical landmarks. The second criterion of the classification system is the *localization of the fracture in the posterior pelvis*. The localization of the instability will be decisive for the type and invasiveness of operative treatment.

Four categories with increasing instability are distinguished: lesions with slight, moderate, high, and highest instability. These categories are named FFP type I, FFP type II, FFP type III, and FFP type IV. The subtypes are characterized by the alphabetic characters a, b, or c (Figure 20.1).

FFP type III - displaced unilateral posterior pelvic ring fracture

FFP type I - anterior pelvic ring fracture only

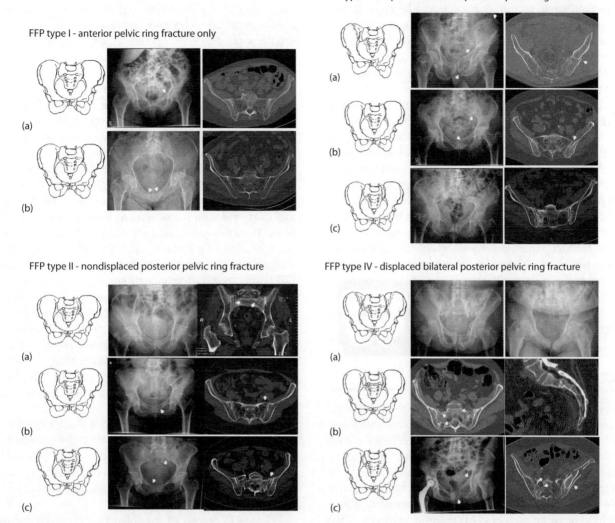

Figure 20.1 Classification of fragility fracture of the pelvis (FFP) type I: anterior pelvic ring fracture only. FFP type II: posterior nondisplaced pelvic ring fracture. FFP type III: posterior unilaterally displaced pelvic ring fracture. FFP type IV: posterior bilaterally displaced pelvic ring fracture. (Reprinted with permission from Rommens PM and Hofmann A. *Injury*. 2013;44[12]:1733–44.)

FFP type I lesions have the lowest degree of instability; patients have anterior pelvic ring fractures only. There is no lesion of the posterior pelvic ring. FFP type Ia is a unilateral anterior lesion. FFP type Ib is a bilateral anterior lesion. In the series of 245 patients, which forms the basis of this classification, FFP type I comprised 17.5% (7). More than 80% of patients had a fracture in the posterior pelvic ring. These data support recommending a CT evaluation of all patients with low-energy pelvic ring trauma, where an anterior pelvic ring fracture has been diagnosed on conventional pelvic overviews. Bilateral fractures of the anterior pelvic ring without fracture of the posterior pelvic ring (FFP type Ib) are very rare. They nearly always are combined with a posterior pelvic ring fracture.

FFP type II is a nondisplaced posterior pelvic ring fracture. There is more instability than in isolated anterior lesions but less than in displaced posterior lesions. FFP type IIa is a nondisplaced and isolated posterior pelvic ring fracture. FFP type IIb is a sacral crush with anterior disruption. FFP type IIc is a nondisplaced sacral, sacroiliac, or iliac

fracture with anterior disruption. FFP type II accounted for more than half of FFP in the observed series of 245 patients (7). Sacral fractures or crush zones of the sacral ala without displacement are the most typical fracture patterns; they are much more frequent than nondisplaced sacroiliac dislocations or fractures of the posterior ilium. The fractures through the sacrum have unique and consistent fracture patterns. The fractures typically run vertically through the sacral ala, whereas transforaminal fractures, or fractures through the sacral body are exceptional (22). The reason for this is the consistent decrease of bone mass in the sacral ala, which is detected in all elderly patients. This was calculated in a statistical model of the sacrum by Wagner et al. from CT data of 92 older Europeans (21,23). FFP type II must be regarded as posterior pelvic ring fractures before completion and displacement. The traumatizing vector of FFP type IIb and FFP type IIc comes from a lateral lesion, reflecting a lateral compression injury.

FFP type III is a displaced unilateral posterior combined with an anterior pelvic ring lesion. FFP type IIIa involves a displaced unilateral ilium fracture. FFP type IIIb is a displaced unilateral sacroiliac disruption. FFP type IIIc is a displaced unilateral sacral fracture. Displaced unilateral posterior lesions formed the smallest group of 245 FFPs, comprising 11% of FFPs (7).

FFP type IV has displaced bilateral posterior injuries. FFP type IVa has bilateral iliac fractures or bilateral sacroiliac disruptions. FFP type IVb is a U- or H-type sacral fracture containing a bilateral vertical fracture through the sacral ala with a horizontal component connecting them. FFP type IVc is a combination of different posterior instabilities. The incidence of U- or H-type sacral fractures (FFP type IVb), being 15%, was striking in our series of 245 patients (7). This fracture morphology is the progress of bilateral nondisplaced vertical sacral ala fractures, seen in FFP type II lesions. The horizontal component of the U- or H-type sacral fracture is hardly visible on conventional pelvic overviews. It therefore is strongly recommended to look at the sagittal reconstructions of CT to detect or exclude this fracture. Typically, a small kink in the anterior sacral cortex with slight flexion of the proximal sacral fragment is visible.

DECISION-MAKING

The leading symptom of FFP is pain in the pelvic ring region. This pain is due to the fracture, which brings instability. Pain leads to immobilization. Immobilization leads to deterioration of the physical condition of any elderly patient, with higher morbidity and mortality due to secondary complications (24). Consequently, the main goal of treatment is the restoration of prefracture mobility. This is achieved by restoration of stability in the pelvic ring. The decisions of whether an operation is needed and which type of osteosynthesis should be performed are based on the severity of complaints and the degree of instability. It therefore is of utmost importance to thoroughly analyze the characteristics of the fractures and classify them correctly. The new classification system forms the basis for recommendations on treatment.

The management of FFP includes a team approach, with the input of several specialists such as orthopedic surgeons, geriatricians, and specialists in bone metabolism. The general condition of the patient should be optimized in the short term and any metabolic disorder addressed. The underlying bone disease must be addressed in accordance with established guidelines, including bisphosphonates and parathyroid hormone (25–27). The patient is monitored during his or her hospital stay, and management is adapted to the physical condition and progress of recovery.

FFP type I lesions are treated nonoperatively. We recommend hospitalizing the patient and performing a hemodynamic monitoring for the first 24 hours (10). Treatment is based on pain therapy, physiotherapy, and monitoring. Mobilization out of bed should be obtained within days after admission. When mobilization is not possible or delayed due to uncontrollable pain, the amount of pelvic

instability should be reevaluated radiologically. A further displacement of pubic rami fractures may be a sign of a concomitant posterior ring fracture. In case additional fractures are detected or primary nondisplaced fractures show displacement, management may change from nonoperative to operative.

Also in FFP type II lesions, nonoperative treatment is recommended at first. As the pelvic ring is broken posteriorly and anteriorly, we may expect more severe pain and a longer rehabilitation time compared to FFP type I. Monitoring is needed to control recovery in an acceptable time period. If mobilization is impossible because of nonrelenting or increasing pain intensity, operative instead of nonoperative therapy must be taken into consideration and discussed with the patient. As the fracture fragments of the posterior pelvic ring are not displaced, percutaneous procedures for screw fixation are most useful. Before surgery, pelvic instability should be controlled with a new CT. Displacement of previously nondisplaced fractures of the posterior pelvic ring may be discovered. Displacement of fractures in the posterior pelvic ring leads to a higher degree of instability and to a shift in the classification toward a higher FFP type (28). Nonoperative management becomes obsolete in this case. Operative therapy must be adapted to the degree of displacement and can differ from a percutaneous procedure to open reduction and internal fixation.

In FFP type III lesions, only operative fixation can guarantee restoration of stability and quick mobilization. The operation should be performed as an elective procedure but without delay. The type of internal fixation depends on the localization of the displacement: ilium, iliosacral joint, or sacral ala.

FFP type IV lesions ask for a bilateral fixation procedure. The lumbar spine and sacral segments, which are broken out, have to be reconnected with the posterior pelvic ring. The construct prevents further intrusion of the lumbosacral spine into the small pelvis. In case of left and right instabilities of different morphologies, the best fixation technique for each type of instability must be chosen.

NONOPERATIVE MANAGEMENT

Nonoperative management of pelvic ring fractures in older patients does not mean that nothing has to be done. As stated earlier, a multidisciplinary approach is needed to improve the physiologic and psychologic status of the patient, to monitor progress of treatment, and to prevent further fragility fractures.

The cornerstones of nonoperative treatment are pain therapy and physiotherapy. Pain management must be individualized and adapted to the needs and subjective findings of the patient. Choice of drugs will follow the guidelines of the World Health Organization (WHO) and intensive monitoring brings the team to the optimal effect with minimal side effects (29). The search for the optimal pain therapy is one of several reasons to keep the

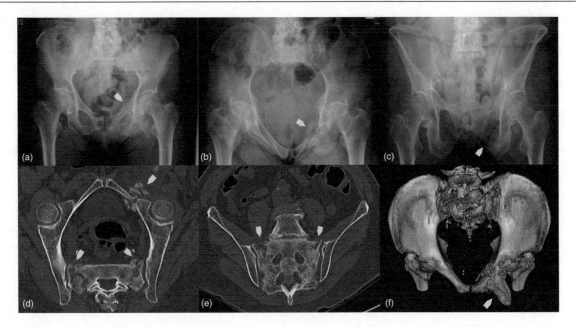

Figure 20.2 A 75-year-old female with history of pelvic pain after a fall at home. Conservative treatment consisting of pain reduction, bed rest, and careful out-of-bed mobilization was carried out. (a) Anteroposterior pelvic overview. (b) Pelvic inlet view. (c) Pelvic outlet view taken after 6 weeks shows abundant callus formation at the left superior and inferior pubic ramus. (d) Computed tomography (CT) reconstruction showing the pelvic inlet plane confirms the existence of a bilateral sacral ala fracture and a left pubic ramus fracture (FFP type IIc). There is a large callus mass around the left pubic ramus fracture. There also is callus formation at the anterior cortex of the sacral ala fractures (arrows). (e) Callus formation is also visible on the CT reconstruction along the longitudinal axis of the sacrum (arrows). (f) The three-dimensional reconstruction of the pelvic ring shows a massive callus mass in front of the left superior pubic ramus fracture.

patient in the hospital during the first days after trauma. Physiotherapy starts with the patient still in bed. Breathing therapy and mobilization of the extremities are performed. The patient is set up, when he or she allows. Standing and consecutively walking follow. Walking aids such as a high roller are very useful (30). The physiotherapist monitors progress and communicates this in the team discussions. Out-of-bed mobilization should be possible within 1 week after trauma. Radiographs before discharge ensure that there is no secondary displacement in the fracture site. After discharge, close monitoring of the progress of recovery remains necessary. Conventional pelvic overviews at 3, 6, and 12 weeks are recommended to ensure uneventful healing. In doubt, CT control is recommended (Figure 20.2a–f).

OPERATIVE TREATMENT

The techniques for reduction and fixation of posterior and anterior pelvic ring instabilities, which have been developed for the treatment of high-energy pelvic trauma, are only partially valid for the surgical treatment of FFPs (7). The main goals of treatment of FFPs are restoring stability to minimize pain and enable quick mobilization, while being as minimally aggressive as possible. Restoring perfect anatomy is of less importance than in younger adult patients. Consequently, minimally invasive, percutaneous procedures are especially attractive because they take less

operative time, involve less blood loss, and allow for quick recovery. Long-lasting surgery, as in open reduction and internal fixation, combined with associated blood loss and higher risk of infection and thromboembolism should be avoided (31).

The type of stabilization depends on the localization of instability, the amount of displacement of the fractures, and the individual anatomy of the posterior pelvis. Timing depends on the general condition of the patient and the planning of the surgical team. There is no need for emergent or urgent surgery. Preoperative planning must include positioning of the patient, the instruments needed, the sequence of surgical procedures, and the type of implants.

Preoperatively, the bowels should be cleared to assure good intraoperative visualization of bony landmarks with the image intensifier. This is of special interest for all cases in which a percutaneous procedure is planned.

Posterior pelvic ring

In the following paragraphs, the most accepted techniques for fixation of posterior pelvic ring fractures in FFPs are presented and discussed.

ILIOSACRAL SCREW FIXATION

This technique is widely accepted for fixation of sacral fractures and iliosacral dislocations in high-energy pelvic trauma. It can also be used in fragility fractures of the pelvis (32). As shown earlier, the majority of patients with FFPs have a fracture of the sacral ala, which is not or only slightly displaced. Iliosacral screw insertion allows stable fixation, if a good anchorage of the screw(s) is guaranteed. Biomechanical studies have proven that stability of an iliosacral screw fixation is significantly higher with two screws (33). Surgical anatomy of the broken pelvis must be analyzed thoroughly preoperatively. Corridors for optimal screw placement are sometimes very narrow (34). In dysmorphic sacra, it is advantageous to use computer navigation for exact screw placement (35).

The patient is placed with the injured side on the edge of a radiolucent table enabling free orientation of the drill. Before starting the surgical procedure, high-quality image intensifier views of the injured pelvic side must be obtained. The anatomical landmarks of the sacrum and the iliosacral joints must clearly be visible on the three pelvic overviews and on the lateral view of the lumbosacral junction. The ideal insertion point for iliosacral screw placement in S1

is identified on the lateral view. Through a small skin incision, the tip of the drill is placed at this point. Short drilling perforates the outer cortex of the posterior ilium. The image intensifier is now turned back for AP inlet and outlet views for further drilling and screw insertion. The tip of the drill is inserted as far as the opposite sacral ala. A large fragment cannulated screw of 7.3 or 8 mm diameter with a long or continuous thread is inserted over the drill. The tip of the screw should cross the midline and reach the opposite ala. This ensures that the thread of the screw is situated in the sacral body, which has the highest trabecular density (21,23) (Figure 20.3a–h).

The screw direction is perpendicular to the plane of the sacral ala fracture. Tightening a screw with long thread will put some compression on the fracture site by direct pressure of the screw head against the lateral cortex of the posterior ilium. The surgeon feels increasing resistance when continuing torque of the screw and stops there (36). Washers help to avoid screw perforation through the lateral

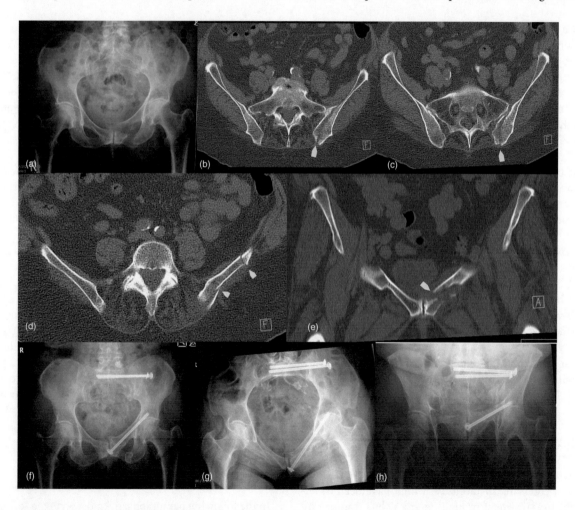

Figure 20.3 An 82-year-old female suffered a left proximal humerus fracture and a FFP type IIIb. (a) The anteroposterior (AP) pelvic overview demonstrates a displaced left superior pubic ramus fracture. (b–d) Axial computed tomography (CT) cuts through the posterior pelvis show a fracture-dislocation starting at the left iliosacral joint and extending superiorly and laterally through the posterior ilium. (e) Coronal CT reconstruction through the anterior pelvic ring showing the left superior pubic ramus fracture, which is displaced and has a horizontal fracture plane. (f) AP pelvic overview. (g) Pelvic inlet view. (h) Pelvic outlet view taken 1 year after operative treatment. Two long iliosacral screws have been inserted in S1 and one retrograde transpubic screw for the left transpubic instability. There is complete healing with excellent functional recovery.

cortex of the posterior ilium. When too much force is used, the screw may perforate the near cortex despite the washer. In case a screw with continuous thread is used, it is sufficient to insert it until its head with the washer gets in contact with the lateral cortex of the posterior ilium. The screw has the function of a positioning screw. When two screws are inserted in S1, they should be parallel or slightly converging. A second screw can also be placed in the body of S2, but the S2 corridor is smaller than the S1. This gives a higher risk of damaging neurological structures.

Iliosacral screw fixation can be done with the patient in supine or prone position. A disadvantage of the prone position is that the fragile patient has to be turned on the table. The most important advantage of the prone position concerns accessibility of the posterior pelvic ring. Due to gravity, the soft tissue mass of the buttocks falls down, which makes it easier to access the posterior ilium and enhances the precision of screw placement. In obese persons, this is of significant importance.

ILIOSACRAL SCREW FIXATION WITH CEMENT AUGMENTATION

Iliosacral screw insertion in osteoporotic bone increases local stiffness and diminishes pain. But there is a higher risk of secondary screw loosening due to low anchorage in trabecular bone. Changes in the screw design, which enable cement augmentation for better anchorage, have therefore been developed. Several perforations were made in the screw near the tip. After screw insertion, a few cubic centimeters of low-viscosity cement are injected through the cannulated screw. The cement leaves the screw through its perforations and is distributed in the cancellous bone around the tip of the screw. Once the cement is hardened, the pull-out force of the screw is much higher than without cement (37). When nonperforated cannulated screws are used, an alternative technique for cement augmentation is possible. The screw is turned back for about 1 cm after complete insertion. Then, the canal of the screw beyond the tip is filled with liquid cement and the screw reinserted as before (37). Cement injection has to be done very carefully and under continuous image intensifier control in order to avoid leakage into the sacral canal or the canal of the nerve roots. Data from first clinical results are promising, yet further critical analysis is still needed to recommend it as a standard procedure (38,39).

SACROPLASTY

This technique is a minimally invasive procedure in which a few cubic centimeters of cement are directly injected into the sacral fracture or alar void (40). There is no fixation with titanium or steel implants. After the procedure, pain intensity goes down, and mobilization can be started quickly. Cement leakage outside the fracture gap is the most important complication. Out of 243 procedures, Kortman et al. describe only one cement leakage that needed surgical revision (0.4%) (41). Bastian observed cement leakage into veins and neuroforamina in 27% of 33 patients, with the need for surgical revision in one patient (3.3%) (42).

Short-term outcome data for sacroplasty are gratifying (43,44). Nevertheless, some critical remarks must be made. Although adequate stability seems to be restored, it remains unclear what happens with the sacral fracture itself. The cement, which is a foreign body located between the fracture fragments, may hinder bone healing. Moreover, vertical load while standing and walking leads to shearing forces in the vertical sacral fracture, which may hinder bone healing as well. Sacroplasty restores some stability in the posterior pelvic ring but not in the anterior. The vast majority of fragility fractures of the pelvis have a combination of a fracture of the posterior pelvic ring with a fracture of the anterior pelvic ring. The anterior pelvic ring remains interrupted and unstable. Stabilization of the anterior pelvic ring should at least be taken into consideration when the posterior pelvis is treated surgically. When another intervention is needed in case of a recurrent ipsilateral or new contralateral sacral fracture, the cement may hinder iliosacral screw insertion.

ANTERIOR PLATE FIXATION OF ILIUM

Fractures of the ilium comprise a minority of fractures of the posterior pelvic ring in FFP. The fracture typically starts at the inner curve of the innominate bone and runs laterally and proximally through the ilium wing toward the iliac crest (45). As instability is high, ilium fractures need open reduction and internal fixation. The fracture is approached via the first window of the ilioinguinal approach. The fracture area is debrided and reduction and compression of the fracture gap is performed with the help of reduction forceps and a Faraboeuf clamp placed on top of the iliac crest. Fixation is obtained with a preshaped and twisted large fragment angular stable plate, which is placed along the pelvic brim. At least two angular stable screws should be used at each side of the fracture. The screws must take the longest possible trajectory through the bone: parallel to the iliosacral joint for the proximal screws and through the ilium body above the acetabulum for the distal screws. At the iliac crest, the fracture is additionally stabilized with a long lag screw, which runs between the inner and outer cortexes (Figure 20.4a–g). Alternatively, a small fragment plate that bridges the fracture is placed on top of the iliac crest.

TRANS-SACRAL BAR OSTEOSYNTHESIS

Trans-sacral bar osteosynthesis is a modification of transiliac bar osteosynthesis. The latest osteosynthesis has been described as one of the alternative stabilization techniques for high-energy pelvic disruptions (46).

In trans-sacral bar osteosynthesis, a threaded bar is inserted through the sacral corridor of S1. With the image intensifier, a lateral view of the lumbosacral junction is obtained, and the sacral corridor in S1 and the ideal entry portal for the sacral bar are identified. Two skin incisions of 4–5 cm are made in line with the central axis of the transsacral corridor of S1. Drilling is done through the corridor in a strict coronal plane and strictly parallel to the L5-S1 junction. Depending on the design of the implant, the bar is

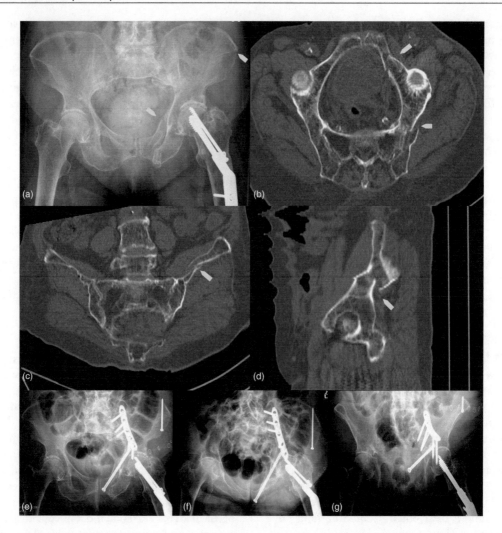

Figure 20.4 An 85-year-old female with a FFP type IIIa after a fall in a nursing home. (a) Anteroposterior (AP) pelvic overview showing a left ilium fracture and left superior and inferior pubic ramus fracture with medial displacement (arrows). (b) Computed tomography (CT) reconstruction in the pelvic inlet plane. (c) Coronal CT reconstruction. (d) Sagittal CT reconstruction. CT reconstructions show severe osteoporosis, the displaced ilium fracture, and the anterior pelvic ring instability. (e) AP pelvic overview. (f) Pelvic inlet view. (g) Pelvic outlet view. The ilium fracture was fixed with an angular stable plate, which was inserted along the pelvic brim through the first window of the ilioinguinal approach. Length and direction of the angular stable screws are nicely visible. An additional small fragment screw was inserted along the pelvic crest and a retrograde transpubic screw was inserted for stabilization of the left anterior pelvic ring instability. Good functional recovery.

inserted over the drill or separately. On both sides, washers and nuts are placed over the threaded bar ends. Tightening the nuts creates compression on the vertical sacral fracture (47,48). Preoperative analysis of conventional radiographs and CT data is of utmost importance for assessment of the dimension of the sacral corridor of S1. The incidence of dysmorphic sacra, in which the trans-sacral corridor is very small or inexistent, was low in a Caucasian but higher in an Asian population (23).

This osteosynthesis creates adequate stability in non- or minimally displaced fractures of the sacral ala or sacroiliac joint. The technique can also be used for bilateral sacral fractures and as a preventive stabilization of the nonfractured contralateral side. The stability of the construct does not depend on the strength of the anchorage in the cancellous bone in the body of S1, as is the case in iliosacral

screw osteosynthesis. The stability depends on the strength of the external cortex of the posterior ilium, against which the nuts and washers are tightened. Literature data are rare. Reported outcomes in two small series of patients treated with this technique were promising (Figure 20.5a–i) (48,49).

POSTERIOR BRIDGING PLATE OSTEOSYNTHESIS

This technique has been used for stabilization of posterior pelvic ring instabilities in high-energy trauma. It can be done as a less-invasive procedure in FFP (50). The patient needs to be placed in prone position. Two small vertical incisions are made parallel to the posterior iliac crests. A subcutaneous tunnel is developed between the two incisions behind the sacrum. A bowed plate of adapted length, which is curved at its ends, is inserted through the tunnel. The curved ends of the plate lay just behind the outer cortex of

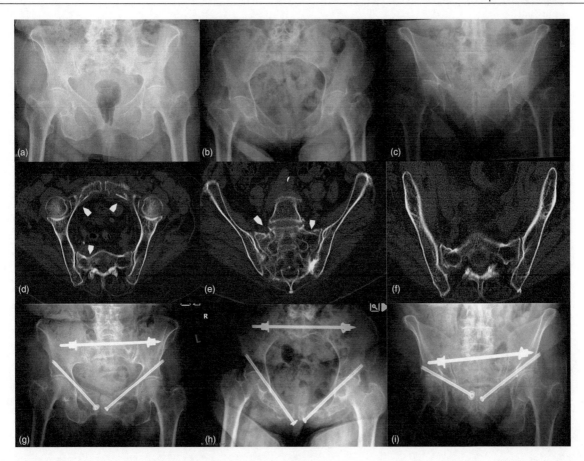

Figure 20.5 An 82-year-old female with FFP type IIc after a domestic fall. (a) Anteroposterior (AP) pelvic overview. (b) Pelvic inlet view. (c) Pelvic outlet view. The conventional pelvic overviews show bilateral pubic ramus fractures. There is no clear lesion of the posterior pelvic ring visible. (d) Computed tomography (CT) reconstruction in the pelvic inlet plane. (e) Coronal CT reconstruction. (f) Axial CT reconstruction. A bilateral anterior pelvic ring instability and bilateral sacral ala fractures can be detected (green arrows). There is no displacement. (g) AP pelvic overview. (h) Pelvic inlet view. (i) Pelvic outlet view 2 months after operative treatment. The posterior instabilities were fixed with a trans-sacral bar, the anterior instabilities with retrograde transpubic screws. Good functional outcome.

the left and right posterior inferior iliac spines. Long screws are inserted through the two marginal plate holes on each side. One screw goes in the anterior direction parallel to the sacroiliac joint, the other screw in the superior direction parallel to the iliac crest. The posterior bridging plate does not create compression on the fracture site but takes the function of a tension band. Bilateral sacral ala fractures can be stabilized in one procedure with this technique. In case of unilateral fractures, the bridging plate prevents development of a contralateral fracture. An angular stable plate with a specific design has been developed for this procedure (51).

POSTERIOR TRANSILIAC INTERNAL FIXATION

Another minimally invasive technique for bridging the posterior pelvic ring in FFP is posterior transiliac internal fixation (52). The patient is placed in prone position. Two small vertical incisions are made just medial to the posterior superior iliac spines. The medial and posterior aspects of the spines are exposed. One long pedicle screw is placed in the left and one in the right posterior ilium. Their trajectory starts from the posterior superior iliac spine and goes laterally and anteriorly in the direction of the anterior

superior iliac spine, passing just above the greater sciatic notch. The screws are located between the inner and outer cortexes of the ilium and have a diameter of up to 7 mm and a length of up to 100 mm. The screw heads are connected with a slightly bowed rod with a diameter of 5 or 6 mm, which has been placed in a subcutaneous tunnel connecting both crests. To avoid protruding hardware, which may lead to wound disturbances, a bone block with the width of a pedicle screw head is removed from the posterior iliac crest before screw insertion. This enables countersinking of the screw head below or at the level of the iliac crest (Figure 20.6a–i). Stiffness of the posterior transiliac internal fixator was higher as in double iliosacral screw osteosynthesis in a transforaminal fracture model (53). Recently, promising clinical data with a cement augmented transiliac internal fixator were published (54). Other outcome data with the posterior transiliac internal fixator in FFP have not yet been published.

LUMBOPELVIC FIXATION

The lumbopelvic fixator creates a tight connection between the lumbar spine and the posterior ilium. The patient is

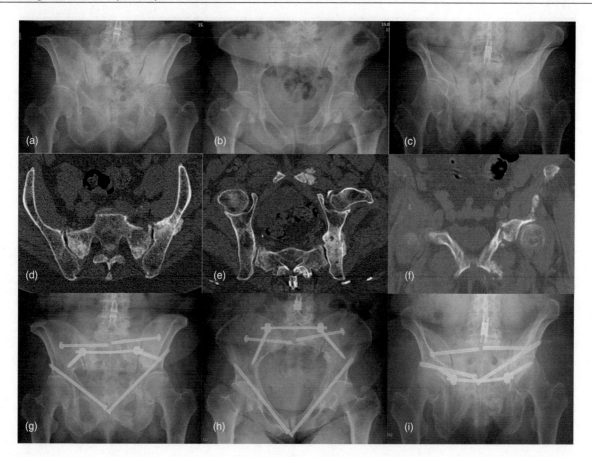

Figure 20.6 A 73-year-old female with history of continuous pain after a fall 6 months ago. Treatment with pain therapy and mobilization has been unsuccessful. (a) Anteroposterior (AP) pelvic overview. (b) Pelvic inlet view. (c) Pelvic outlet view. On conventional pelvic overviews, callus formation without healing of the left superior and inferior pubic ramus fractures is visible. There also is an irregularity at the inner cortex of the innominate bone near to the left iliosacral joint. (d) Axial computed tomography (CT) reconstruction. (e) Oblique CT reconstruction. (f) Coronal CT reconstruction. On the CT images, a healed left ilium fracture is visible. Left and right sacral ala are fractured. There also is a bilateral instability of the anterior pelvic ring. The sacral corridor is too small for a safe trans-sacral bar placement. (g) Postoperative AP pelvic overview. (h) Pelvic inlet view. (i) Pelvic outlet view. The anterior instabilities were transfixed with two retrograde transpubic screws. The posterior instabilities were fixed with a transiliac internal fixator and two iliosacral screws.

placed prone. A vertical incision starts medial to the posterior superior iliac spine and goes up to the level of L4 or L5. At the side of the posterior pelvic fracture, one pedicle screw is placed in the pedicle of L5; alternatively, the pedicle of L4 is used. The second pedicle screw is inserted in the posterior ilium in the same technique, which has been described for posterior transiliac internal fixation. A curved rod connects the heads of the two screws. When a distractor is used, the distance between the screws can be increased and a vertically displaced hemipelvis pushed down. Experience shows that this is hardly necessary in FFP, as the amount of displacement usually is low. Unilateral lumbopelvic fixation can be combined with a transverse fixation like iliosacral screw fixation or a trans-sacral bar. The construct then looks like a triangular osteosynthesis (55). A bilateral lumbopelvic fixation with transverse connection between both rods is performed for stabilization of a U- or H-type sacral fracture (55). The construct prevents intrusion of the broken out S1 body into the small pelvis. When bilateral distraction between the pedicles is used, a displacement

in flexion of the broken out sacral fracture is corrected. Lumbopelvic fixation does not create compression in the sacral fracture sites. It therefore is often combined with an iliosacral or trans-sacral osteosynthesis (Figure 20.7a–f). Stability of such a triangular osteosynthesis is very high and full weight-bearing can be allowed immediately (56). Specific data about complications and results in FFP are not yet published.

Anterior pelvic ring

Fractures of the anterior pelvic ring are the most frequent fractures in FFP. They were isolated fractures in only 20% and combined with posterior pelvic ring fractures in 80% of the patients in the series of Rommens and Hofmann (7). In the series of Lau and Leung, anterior pelvic ring fractures were combined with posterior pelvic ring lesions in 60% of the patients (16). Biomechanical studies by Tile et al. showed that stability of a pelvic ring is diminished

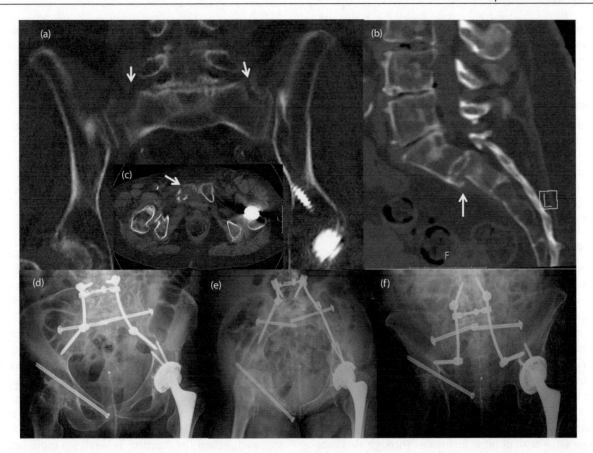

Figure 20.7 A 77-year-old female with FFP type IVb after a domestic fall. Patient is admitted in our trauma unit 1 month later. (a) Coronal computed tomography (CT) reconstruction through the posterior pelvic ring. (b) Axial CT reconstruction through the anterior pelvic ring. (c) Sagittal CT reconstruction through the midline of the sacrum. CT reconstructions reveal a bilateral sacral ala fracture, a horizontal fracture component between the sacral body S1 and S2, and a translation of the body of S1 toward anterior and inferior (arrows). There is no neurological deficit. (d) Postoperative anteroposterior overview. (e) Pelvic inlet view. (f) Pelvic outlet view. Iliolumbar fixation prevents further intrusion of the lumbosacral segment into the small pelvis. The pedicle screws have been put in the L4 pedicles and in the posterior ilium. A transverse rod connects the left and right fixation. Two iliosacral screws enhance the stability and put some compression on the sacral ala fractures. A right retrograde transpubic screw stabilizes the anterior pelvic ring instability.

by 30% when the anterior pelvic ring is ruptured (57). Consequently, sole stabilization of the posterior pelvic ring in FFP may not restore adequate stability. When loading an incompletely reconstructed pelvic ring during mobilization, there is a higher risk of implant loosening or secondary fracture displacement. We therefore recommend additionally stabilizing the anterior pelvic ring for restoring a stable and pain-free pelvic ring.

Different techniques, devices, and implants are available. The choice of which osteosynthesis is the most appropriate depends on the localization of the instability fracture and the extent of displacement. Whenever possible, a minimally invasive procedure is preferred.

EXTERNAL FIXATION

External fixation is well known as a provisional treatment of high-energy pelvic disruptions. It can be used for pain control in FFP (58). At each side, one or two pins are inserted from the anterior inferior iliac spine toward the posterior superior iliac spine. The skin incisions run

vertically just laterally to the anterior superior iliac spine downward. Care has to be taken not to injure the lateral cutaneous femoral nerve, that is localized just medially of the anterior superior iliac spine. The screws may have a length of up to 100 mm. They are connected to each other and to the other side with rods that are arranged in the form of a tent (59). Biomechanical studies have proven that external fixation is stable enough to control fractures of the anterior pelvic ring but not of the posterior pelvic ring (60). External fixation therefore should always be used as an adjunct to posterior fixation.

Personally, we do not recommend external fixation of FFP as a treatment of first choice. Several disadvantages make its use uncomfortable and cumbersome. Pin track infections are seen frequently, especially in obese persons (61). Because the trajectory between the skin and the bone is long and the soft tissue envelope mobile, wound margins around the pins very quickly show areas of inflammation due to continuous pressure. Soft tissue irritation leads to swelling, pain, drainage, and infection. In many patients, there is a conflict between the soft tissues and external fixator rods while sitting. Finally, there is a high risk of pin loosening due to the lower holding power of the pins in the weaker bone and due to pin track infections.

INTERNAL FIXATION

The stability of internal fixation is more predictable and higher than with external fixation. The choice of procedure mainly depends on the localization of the instability.

Whereas superior pubic ramus fractures can be splinted with a retrograde transpubic screw, plate osteosynthesis is the treatment of choice in pubic bone fractures and symphysis pubis diastasis.

Retrograde transpubic screw fixation

Optimal indications are superior pubic ramus fractures, situated above the obturator foramen or at the anterior lip of the acetabulum. The retrograde transpubic screw is also called an anterior column screw as it can be inserted antegrade as part of the osteosynthesis of acetabular fractures. Retrograde insertion is done in a percutaneous technique if the fracture is minimally displaced.

The corridor for the screw is analyzed on pelvic overviews and CT pictures preoperatively. A small skin incision is made near the pubic symphysis. Through the subcutaneous tissue, the trajectory to the pubic tubercle is prepared. The drill bit is forwarded through this tunnel until it reaches bone. It is held in 45° inclination to the sagittal plane pointing toward lateral, and in 45° inclination to the transverse plane pointing toward superior. These values of the orientation of the anterior column screw corridor have been identified as averages in a CT study on 58 normal pelvises (62). In a similar study, inclinations of about 35° and 60° to the sagittal and transverse planes were observed in eight pelvic specimens lying in the supine position (63). Under image intensification using obturator-outlet and the inlet views, the location of the drill tip is adjusted until it lies precisely in line with the optimal trajectory of the screw (64). While carefully oscillating drilling, the drill bit enters the canal and progresses cranially and laterally through the anterior column screw corridor. Special attention is paid to avoid penetration of the drill bit through the cortex or into the acetabulum. The drilling procedure is continued until the tip of the drill bit reaches and perforates the posterolateral cortex of the ilium body. The length of the trajectory in the bone may reach up to 130 mm (65) (Figure 20.6a-i). The anterior part of the trajectory is overdrilled. A large fragment cannulated screw of appropriate length is inserted over the drill bit. The use of a washer is not necessary. The screw head lies in the thick tendinous attachments of the adductor muscles at the pubic bone. The screw primarily splints the superior pubic ramus fracture; stability is lower than in plate osteosynthesis (66). Only when the tip of the screw passes the posterolateral cortex of the ilium is compression brought about when tightened. When the drill bit cannot pass the acetabulum without perforating the joint, a shorter screw must be chosen. This will lead to

lower stability and a higher risk of loosening. In a series of 158 retrograde transpubic screw fixations, the incidence of complications was very low and bony union of the anterior pelvic ring more than 90% (67).

When the superior pubic ramus fracture is displaced but appropriate for retrograde transpubic screw fixation, open reduction can be done. The skin incision is the same but can be smaller than in the case of plate fixation. The displaced ramus superior pubic fracture is reduced by direct means, and the trajectory for the screw drilled under control of finger touch on the retropubic bone surface and image intensification.

Plate and screw osteosynthesis

This well-known technique can be used for stabilization of superior pubic rami fractures, fractures in the pubic bone near the pubic symphysis, pubic symphysis instabilities, and nonunions or bone defects due to chronic instabilities of the anterior pelvic ring (Figure 20.8a–i). A Pfannenstiel or an infraumbilical midline incision is chosen for the approach to the anterior pelvic ring. The linea alba is exposed and split over a length of less than 10 cm. The retropubic space is opened; the peritoneum and bladder are carefully retracted with a broad malleable valve. The anterior curve of the pelvic ring can be exposed further lateral following the modified Stoppa approach, when the fracture is localized more laterally (68). A curved plate is placed above the fracture plane and should allow for minimally two, and better three, screws on each side of the instability. When two screws cannot be placed lateral of the fracture and medial of the acetabulum, a longer plate is inserted along the pelvic brim with two screws above the acetabulum. Small fragment curved plates are used, which allow variable screw directions (69). The screws should all have the longest possible length. Long trajectories in the bone ensure good purchase and high pull-out force. Near to the pubic symphysis, screw lengths of 60 mm should be obtained. The infra-acetabular corridor with the screw passing lateral to the obturator foramen and medial to the acetabulum going into the posterior column should be used, when possible. The infra-acetabular screw can have a length of more than 100 millimeters and doubles the fixation strength (70,71). The modified Stoppa approach is well tolerated as it uses anatomical layers without the need for muscle or tendon detachments (72).

Anterior subcutaneous pelvic internal fixation

External fixation in FFP is connected with major disadvantages such as pin loosening, pin track infection, and discomfort. To avoid these complications, a minimally invasive alternative, called the anterior subcutaneous pelvic internal fixator or pelvic bridge, with the same biomechanical working mechanism, has been developed (73). The concept of the internal fixator is similar to that of the transiliac internal fixator on the posterior pelvis. One large and long pedicle screw is inserted from the anterior inferior iliac spine toward the posterior superior iliac spine on

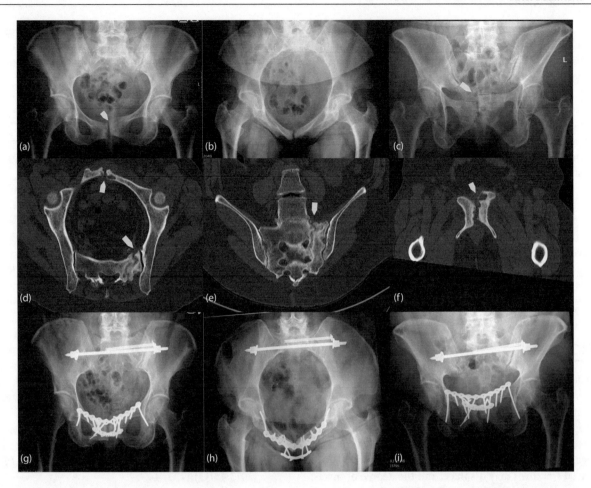

Figure 20.8 A 78-year-old female with an FFP type IIIc after a fall from a chair 5 months ago. (a) Anteroposterior (AP) pelvic overview. The pubic symphysis has an irregular shape with the left pubic bone slightly higher than the right. The bone structure of the left sacral ala also seems irregular (green arrow). (b) Pelvic inlet view. (c) Pelvic outlet view. The pubic symphysis is unstable with the position of the left pubic bone being clearly higher than the right pubic bone (arrow). Irregularities of the left sacral bone mass are also visible. (d) Computed tomography (CT) reconstruction through the pelvic inlet plane. A complete fracture of the left sacral ala and bone resorption at the pubic symphysis are visible (arrows). (e) Coronal reconstruction through the posterior pelvic ring. The vertical left sacral ala fracture is clearly visible. (f) Coronal reconstruction through the pubic symphysis area. Irregularities of the pubic bone margins and instability can be seen. (g) Postoperative AP pelvic overview. (h) Pelvic inlet view. The direct contact of the washers and nuts on the sacral bar with the outer cortex of the left and right posterior ilium is nicely visible. (i) Pelvic outlet view. The posterior pelvic ring has been stabilized with a trans-sacral bar and an iliosacral screw in S1. The anterior pelvic ring has been stabilized with a double-plate osteosynthesis. A debridement of the pubic symphysis and bone grafting were performed. The double-plate osteosynthesis was meant to counteract the stress forces on the pubic symphysis during the long healing process. On both sides, the long infra-acetabular corridor was used for optimal purchase in the dense bone of the ischium (posterior column). Excellent functional outcome.

each side. The skin incisions and pathways for insertion of the pedicle screws are the same as those for the pins of the external fixator. The length of the screws goes up to 100 mm. A transverse subcutaneous tunnel anterior to the abdominal wall is prepared between the two screw heads. A bended rod is inserted in this tunnel and connected with the screws (73). The stability of the construct is similar to that of external fixation. The femoral and lateral cutaneous femoral nerves are the structures most at risk in this procedure (74). A case series of 6 patients with 8 femoral nerve palsies has been presented in the literature (75). Implant removal must be considered in patients with complaints of prominent hardware.

AFTERTREATMENT

The main goals of treatment in FFP are diminishing pain, early out-of-bed mobilization, and return to activities of daily life similar to the period before the fracture (76). Prerequisites for a successful outcome are sufficient pain therapy, a stable bone-implant construct, and active but adapted muscle training. Also, treatment of comorbidities such as cognitive impairment or depressive symptoms must be given high priority (77). The frequency and intensity of physiotherapy are adapted to the general condition of the patient, to the level of activity before admission, and to the amount of pelvic ring stability obtained after surgical fixation. Being non-weight-bearing is not realistic in this patient population.

In patients with FFP type I and type II who are treated nonoperatively, standing up and walking is allowed as tolerated. A high index of suspicion is needed to sort out those patients who are not doing well and express continuing or increasing pain (31). A possible increase of instability must be ruled out with new radiological examinations.

In patients who have been treated operatively, immediate short transfers, from the bed to a chair or from the bed to the lavatory, are allowed, but further mobilization is restricted for the first 6 weeks. If the general condition of the patient allows, walking with walking aids is started from the seventh week on. This recommendation is meant to prevent early implant loosening with secondary fracture displacement due to early full weight-bearing. Radiological studies after 3, 6, and 12 weeks confirm stability and ongoing fracture healing.

CONCLUSION

FFPs comprise a clinical picture with increasing frequency. Their trauma mechanism, fracture morphology, and natural course are not comparable with those of pelvic ring lesions in adolescents and younger adults. When not treated adequately, fracture configuration of an FFP changes over time, additional fractures may occur, nondisplaced fractures may displace, and the degree of instability may increase from a lower to a higher level. A novel comprehensive classification of FFPs has been developed to take these specific properties into account. Four degrees of instability form the major categories: anterior pelvic ring lesions only, nondisplaced posterior lesions, displaced unilateral posterior lesions, and displaced bilateral posterior lesions. The localization of the fracture forms the criterion for the subcategories. Recommendations for treatment are given for every type of FFP. FFP type I and type II lesions are treated nonoperatively. In case nonoperative treatment is not successful; a percutaneous stabilization is recommended. FFP type III and type IV lesions need surgical stabilization. When treated operatively, the less invasive procedure should be preferred. Stability has a higher priority than anatomy. The most appropriate technique depends on the localization of the instability, the quality of the bone, the degree of fracture displacement, and the condition of the soft tissues. Aftertreatment is adapted to the general condition of the patient, the level of activity before the fracture occurred, and the amount of pelvic ring stability obtained. Multidisciplinary geriatric comanagement, including pain therapy, adapted physiotherapy, and treatment of cognitive impairment and other comorbidities, as well as osteoporotic and anabolic drug therapy, is imperative and will improve long-term outcomes.

Although increasing, literature data on treatment and long-term follow-up of nonoperatively and operatively treated FFP are still rare. More clinical and biomechanical research work on minimally invasive techniques and implants is urgently needed to find optimal solutions for the management of these lesions.

REFERENCES

1. Dhanwal DK, Dennison EM, Harvey NC, Cooper C. Epidemiology of hip fracture: Worldwide geographic variation. *Indian J Orthop.* 2011;45(1):15–22.
2. Watts NB. The Fracture Risk Assessment Tool (FRAX®): Applications in clinical practice. *J Womens Health (Larchmt).* 2011;20(4):525–31.
3. Johnell O, Kanis JA. An estimate of the worldwide prevalence and disability associated with osteoporotic fractures. *Osteoporos Int.* 2006;17(12):1726–33.
4. Dodge G, Brison R. Low-impact pelvic fractures in the emergency department. *CJEM.* 2010;12(6):509–13.
5. Sullivan MP, Baldwin KD, Donegan DJ, Metha S, Ahn J. Geriatric fractures about the hip: Divergent patterns in the proximal femur, acetabulum, and pelvis. *Orthopedics.* 2014;37:151–7.
6. Kannus P, Parkkari J, Niemi S, Sievänen H. Low-trauma pelvic fractures in elderly Finns in 1970–2013. *Calc Tissue Int.* 2015;97:577–80.
7. Rommens PM, Hofmann A. Comprehensive classification of fragility fractures of the pelvic ring. Recommendations for surgical treatment. *Injury.* 2013;44(12):1733–44.
8. Finiels H, Finiels PJ, Jacquot JM, Strubel D. Fractures of the sacrum caused by bone insufficiency. Meta-analysis of 508 cases. *Presse Med.* 1997;26:1568–73.
9. Weber M, Hasler P, Gerber H. Sacral insufficiency fractures as an unsuspected cause of low back pain. *Rheumatology.* 1999;38:90–1.
10. Dietz SO, Hofmann A, Rommens PM. Haemorrhage in fragility fractures of the pelvis. *Eur J Trauma Emerg Surg.* 2015;41:363–7.
11. Krappinger D, Kammerlander C, Hak DJ, Blauth M. Low-energy osteoporotic pelvic fractures. *Arch Orthop Trauma Surg.* 2010;130(9):1167–75.
12. McCabe MP, Smyth MP, Richardson DR. Current concept review: Vitamin D and stress fractures. *Foot Ankle Int.* 2012;33:526–33.
13. Dreher R, Buttgereit F, Demary W et al. Insufficiency fractures in rheumatology. Case report and overview. *Z Rheumatol.* 2006;65:417–23.
14. Tokumaru S, Toita T, Oguchi M et al. Insufficiency fractures after pelvic radiation therapy for uterine cervical cancer: An analysis of subjects in a prospective multi-institutional trial, and cooperative study of the Japan Radiation Oncology Group (JAROG) and Japanese Radiation Oncology Study Group (JROSG). *Int J Radiat Oncol Biol Phys.* 2012;84(2):e195–200.
15. Chan K, Resnick D, Pathria M, Jacobson J. Pelvic instability after bone graft harvesting from posterior iliac crest: Report of nine patients. *Skeletal Radiol.* 2001;30:278–81.

16. Lau TW, Leung F. Occult posterior pelvic ring fractures in elderly patients with osteoporotic pubic rami fractures. *J Orthop Surg*. 2010;18(2):153–7.

17. Lyders EM, Whitlow CT, Baker MD, Morris PP. Imaging and treatment of sacral insufficiency fractures. *Am J Neuroradiol*. 2010;31(2):201–10. Review.

18. Tile M. Pelvic ring fractures. Should they be fixed? *J Bone Joint Surg*. 1988;70B:1–12.

19. Fracture and dislocation compendium. Orthopaedic Trauma Association Committee for Coding and Classification. *J Orthop Trauma*. 1996;10(Suppl 1):v–ix, 1–154.

20. Dalal SA, Burgess AR, Siegel JH et al. Pelvic fracture in multiple trauma: Classification by mechanism is key to pattern of organ injury, resuscitative requirements, and outcome. *J Trauma*. 1989;29(7):981–1000; discussion 1000–2.

21. Wagner D, Kamer L, Sawaguchi T, Richards GR, Noser H, Rommens PM. Bone mass distribution of the sacrum assessed by 3D CT statistical models—Implications for pathogenesis and treatment of fragility fractures of the sacrum. *J Bone Joint Surg*. 2016;98(7):584–90.

22. Linstrom NJ, Heiserman JE, Kortman KE et al. Anatomical and biomechanical analyses of the unique and consistent locations of sacral insufficiency fractures. *Spine*. 2009;34(4):309–15.

23. Wagner D, Kamer L, Rommens PM, Sawaguchi T, Richards RG, Noser H. 3D statistical modeling techniques to investigate the anatomy of the sacrum, its bone mass distribution, and the trans-sacral corridors. *J Orthop Res*. 2014;32(11):1543–8.

24. Van Dijk WA, Poeze M, Van Helden SH, Brink PRG, Verbruggen JPAM. Ten-year mortality among hospitalized patients with fractures of the pubic rami. *Injury*. 2010;41(4):411–4.

25. Black DM, Rosen CJ. Postmenopausal osteoporosis. *N Engl J Med*. 2016;374:254–62.

26. Peichl P, Holzer LA, Maier R, Holzer G. Parathyroid hormone 1–84 accelerates fracture-healing in pubic bones of elderly osteoporotic women. *J Bone Joint Surg Am*. 2011;93:1583–7.

27. Babu S, Sandiford NA, Vrahas M. Use of teriparatide to improve fracture healing: What is the evidence? *World J Orthop*. 2015;6(6):457–61.

28. Rommens PM, Arand C, Hopf JC, Mehling I, Dietz SO, Wagner D. Progress of instability in fragility fractures of the pelvis: An observational study. *Injury*. 2019;50(11):1966–73.

29. World Health Organization. *Cancer Pain Relief*. Geneva, Switzerland: World Health Organization, 1986.

30. Babayev M, Lachmann E, Nagler W. The controversy surrounding sacral insufficiency fractures: To ambulate or not to ambulate? *Am J Med Rehabil*. 2000;79:404–9.

31. Rommens PM, Wagner D, Hofmann A. Fragility fractures of the pelvis. *JBJS Rev*. 2017;5(3).

32. Hopf JC, Krieglstein CF, Müller LP, Koslowsky TC. Percutaneous iliosacral screw fixation after osteoporotic posterior ring fractures of the pelvis reduces pain significantly in elderly patients. *Injury*. 2015;46(8):1631–6.

33. van Zwienen CM, van den Bosch EW, Snijders CJ, Kleinrensink GJ, van Vugt AB. Biomechanical comparison of sacroiliac screw techniques for unstable pelvic ring fractures. *J Orthop Trauma*. 2004;18:589–95.

34. Goetzen M, Ortner K, Lindtner RA, Schmid R, Blauth M, Krappinger D. A simple approach for the preoperative assessment of sacral morphology for percutaneous SI screw fixation. *Arch Orthop Trauma Surg*. 2016;136(9):1251–7.

35. Zwingmann J, Konrad G, Kotter E, Südkamp NP, Oberst M. Computer-navigated iliosacral screw insertion reduces malposition rate and radiation exposure. *Clin Orthop Relat Res*. 2009;467(7):1833–8.

36. Bastian JD, Bergmann M, Schwyn R, Keel MJ, Benneker LM. Assessment of the breakaway torque at the posterior pelvic ring in human cadavers. *J Invest Surg*. 2015;28(6):328–33.

37. Oberkircher L, Masaeli A, Bliemel C, Debus F, Ruchholtz S, Krüger A. Primary stability of three different iliosacral screw fixation techniques in osteoporotic cadaver specimens—A biomechanical investigation. *Spine J*. 2016;16(2):226–32.

38. Wähnert D, Raschke MJ, Fuchs T. Cement augmentation of the navigated iliosacral screw in the treatment of insufficiency fractures of the sacrum: A new method using modified implants. *Int Orthop*. 2013;37(6):1147–50.

39. König MA, Hediger S, Schmitt JW, Jentzsch T, Sprengel K, Werner CM. In-screw cement augmentation for iliosacral screw fixation in posterior ring pathologies with insufficient bone stock. *Eur J Trauma Emerg Surg*. 2018;44(2):203–10.

40. Garant M. Sacroplasty: A new treatment for sacral insufficiency fracture. *J Vasc Interv Radiol*. 2002;13(12):1265–7.

41. Kortman K, Ortiz O, Miller T et al. Multicenter study to assess the efficacy and safety of sacroplasty in patients with osteoporotic sacral insufficiency fractures or pathologic sacral lesions. *J Neurointerv Surg*. 2013;5(5):461–6.

42. Bastian JD, Keel MJ, Heini PF, Seidel U, Benneker LM. Complications related to cement leakage in sacroplasty. *Acta Orthop Belg*. 2012;78(1):100–5.

43. Frey ME, DePalma MJ, Cifu DX, Bhagia SM, Carne W, Daitch JS. Percutaneous sacroplasty for osteoporotic sacral insufficiency fractures: A prospective, multicenter, observational pilot study. *Spine J*. 2008;8(2):367–73.

44. Bayley E, Srinivas S, Boszczyk BM. Clinical outcomes of sacroplasty in sacral insufficiency fractures: A review of the literature. *Eur Spine J*. 2009;18(9):1266–71.

45. Lee SW, Kim WY, Koh SJ, Kim YY. Posterior locked lateral compression injury of the pelvis in geriatric patients: An infrequent and specific variant of the fragility fracture of pelvis. *Arch Orthop Trauma Surg.* 2017;137(9):1207–1218.

46. Gorczyca JT, Varga E, Woodside T, Hearn T, Powell J, Tile M. The strength of iliosacral lag screws and transiliac bars in the fixation of vertically unstable pelvic injuries with sacral fractures. *Injury.* 1996;27:561–4.

47. Vanderschot P, Kuppers M, Sermon A, Lateur L. Transiliac-sacral-iliac-bar procedure to treat insufficiency fractures of the sacrum. *Indian J Orthop.* 2009;43:245–52.

48. Mehling I, Hessmann MH, Rommens PM. Stabilisation of fatigue fractures of the dorsal pelvis with a trans-sacral bar. Operative technique and outcome. *Injury.* 2012;43:446–51.

49. Vanderschot P. Treatment options of pelvic and acetabular fractures in patients with osteoporotic bone. *Injury.* 2007;38:497–508.

50. Krappinger D, Larndorfer R, Struve P, Rosenberger R, Arora R, Blauth M. Minimally invasive transiliac plate osteosynthesis for type C injuries of the pelvic ring: A clinical and radiological follow-up. *J Orthop Trauma.* 2007;21:595–602.

51. Kobbe P, Hockertz I, Sellei RM, Reilmann H, Hockertz T. Minimally invasive stabilization of posterior pelvic-ring instabilities with a transiliac locked compression plate. *Int Orthop (SICOT).* 2012;36:159–64.

52. Dienstknecht T, Berner A, Lenich A, Nerlich M, Fuechtmeier B. A minimally invasive stabilizing system for dorsal pelvic ring injuries. *Clin Orthop Rel Res.* 2011;469:3209–17.

53. Salášek M, Jansová M, Křen J, Pavelka T, Weisová D. Biomechanical comparison of a transiliac internal fixator and two iliosacral screws in transforaminal sacral fractures: A finite element analysis. *Acta Bioeng Biomech.* 2015;17(1):39–49.

54. Schmitz P, Baumann F, Grechenig S, Gaensslen A, Nerlich M, Müller MB. The cement-augmented transiliacal internal fixator (caTIFI): An innovative surgical technique for stabilization of fragility fractures of the pelvis. *Injury.* 2015;46(Suppl 4):S114–20.

55. Schildhauer TA, Bellabarba C, Nork SE, Barei DP, Rout ML, Chapman J. Decompression and lumbopelvic fixation for sacral fracture-dislocations with spinopelvic dissociation. *J Orthop Trauma.* 2006;20:447–57.

56. Schildhauer T, Josten C, Muhr G. Triangular osteosynthesis of vertically unstable sacrum fractures: A new concept allowing early weight-bearing. *J Orthop Trauma.* 1998;12:307–14.

57. Tile M, Hearn T, Vrahas M. Biomechanics of the pelvic ring. Chapter 4. In: Tile M, Helfet D, Kellam J, eds. *Fractures of the Pelvis and Acetabulum.* 3rd ed. Philadelphia, PA: Lippincott Williams and Wilkins, 2003, pp. 32–45.

58. Gänsslen A, Hildebrand F, Krettek C. Supraacetabular external fixation for pain control in geriatric type B pelvic injuries. *Acta Chir Orthop Traumatol Cech.* 2013;80(2):101–5.

59. Lidder S, Heidari N, Gänsslen A, Grechenig W. Radiological landmarks for the safe extra-capsular placement of supra-acetabular half pins for external fixation. *Surg Radiol Anat.* 2013;35(2):131–5.

60. Bircher MD. Indications and techniques of external fixation of the injured pelvis. *Injury.* 1996;27 (Suppl 2):B3–19. Review.

61. Mason WT, Khan SN, James CL, Chesser TJ, Ward AJ. Complications of temporary and definitive external fixation of pelvic ring injuries. *Injury.* 2005;36(5):599–605.

62. Feng X, Fang J, Lin C, Zhang S, Lei W, Li Y, Tang S, Chen B. Axial perspective to find the largest intraosseous space available for percutaneous screw fixation of fractures of the acetabular anterior column. *Int J Comput Assist Radiol Surg.* 2015;10(8):1347–53.

63. Zheng Z, Wu W, Yu X, Pan J, Latif M, Hou Z, Zhang Y. Axial view of acetabular anterior column: A new X-ray projection of percutaneous screw placement. *Arch Orthop Trauma Surg.* 2015;135(2):187–92.

64. Rommens PM. Is there a role for percutaneous pelvic and acetabular reconstruction? *Injury.* 2007;38(4):463–77.

65. Gänsslen A, Krettek C. Retrograde transpubic screw fixation of transpubic instabilities. *Oper Orthop Traumatol.* 2006;18(4):330–40.

66. Acklin YP, Zderic I, Buschbaum J et al. Biomechanical comparison of plate and screw fixation in anterior pelvic ring fractures with low bone mineral density. *Injury.* 2016;47(7):1456–60.

67. Rommens PM, Graafen M, Arand C, Mehling I, Hofmann A, Wagner D. Minimal-invasive stabilization of anterior pelvic ring fractures with retrograde transpubic screws. *Injury* 2020 (51). DOI: https://doi.org/10.1016/j.injury.2019.12.018

68. Bible JE, Choxi AA, Kadakia RJ, Evans JM, Mir HR. Quantification of bony pelvic exposure through the modified Stoppa approach. *J Orthop Trauma.* 2014;28(6):320–3.

69. Grimshaw CS, Bledsoe JG, Moed BR. Locked versus standard unlocked plating of the pubic symphysis: A cadaver biomechanical study. *J Orthop Trauma.* 2012;26(7):402–6.

70. Culemann U, Marintschev I, Gras F, Pohlemann T. Infra-acetabular corridor—Technical tip for an additional screw placement to increase the fixation strength of acetabular fractures. *J Trauma.* 2011;70(1):244–6.

71. Gras F, Marintschev I, Schwarz CE, Hofmann GO, Pohlemann T, Culemann U. Screw-versus plate-fixation strength of acetabular anterior column fractures: A biomechanical study. *J Trauma Acute Care Surg.* 2012;72(6):1664–70.

72. Bastian JD, Ansorge A, Tomagra S et al. Anterior fixation of unstable pelvic ring fractures using the modified Stoppa approach: Mid-term results are independent on patients' age. *Eur J Trauma Emerg Surg.* 2016;42(5):645–50.

73. Hiesterman TG, Hill BW, Cole PA. Surgical technique: A percutaneous method of subcutaneous fixation for the anterior pelvic ring: The pelvic bridge. *Clin Orthop Relat Res.* 2012;470(8):2116–23.

74. Apivatthakakul T, Rujiwattanapong N. Anterior subcutaneous pelvic internal fixator (INFIX), Is it safe? A cadaveric study. *Injury.* 2016;47(10):2077–80.

75. Hesse D, Kandmir U, Solberg B et al. Femoral nerve palsy after pelvic fracture treated with INFIX: A case series. *J Orthop Trauma.* 2015;29(3):138–43.

76. Bukata SV, Digiovanni BF, Friedman SM et al. A guide to improving the care of patients with fragility fractures. *Geriatr Orthop Surg Rehabil.* 2011; 2:5–37.

77. Buecking B, Bohl K, Eschbach D et al. Factors influencing the progress of mobilization in hip fracture patients during the early postsurgical period? A prospective observational study. *Arch Gerontol Geriatr.* 2015;60(3):457–63.

78. Rommens PM, Hofmann A. Comprehensive classification of fragility fractures of the pelvic ring: Recommendations for surgical treatment. *Injury.* 2013;44(12):1733–44.

Management of osteoporotic acetabular fractures
Fix or replace?

PETER V. GIANNOUDIS and PANAGIOTIS DOURAS

INTRODUCTION

Acetabular fractures presenting either in isolation or in the context of polytrauma remain challenging injuries. High-energy trauma following road traffic accidents is the most common etiological factor in patients under 50 years of age. In contrast, a low-energy fall, usually from standing height, is the dominant mechanism in the elderly. Usually a fall on the greater trochanter causes a certain type of fracture (comminution of anterior column, anterior wall, and quadrilateral plate fracture). Another mechanism of injury in the elderly is the vehicle against pedestrian, where the fracture pattern is more complex.

The prevalence of acetabular fractures in the elderly is ever increasing. Ferguson et al. reported that the number of these fractures will increase at least twofold during the next two decades (1).

Initial assessment is performed according to the advanced trauma life support (ATLS) guidelines. Lifesaving procedures take priority in the polytrauma setting with the focus being to restore hemodynamic stability and preservation of function of vital organs. Emergency interventions in acetabulum injuries are rare and usually involve fracture dislocations with or without neurological compromise, requiring prompt reduction and management of hypovolemic shock that may be secondary to an arterial lesion in close proximity to the hip joint, requiring interventional radiology (embolization) or surgical homeostasis. Usually, acetabular fractures are managed with planned reconstruction procedures following the acquisition of standard radiographs (anteroposterior pelvis and Judet views) and computed tomography (CT) scan. A CT scan of the pelvis with 2 mm cuts is of paramount importance in order to evaluate accurately the fracture pattern and to identify the presence of concomitant injuries.

Distinct radiological features of acetabulum fractures in the elderly include the "Gull-Sign" (Figure 21.1), roof impaction (14%–56%), femoral head injury (20%), posterior wall comminution (60%–71%), posterior hip dislocation (47%–79%), and anteriocentral hip dislocation (20%) (1).

The most common classification system used to describe the type of fracture sustained and to guide treatment remains the Letournel classification (2).

The management of acetabulum fractures in the elderly requires careful assessment and consideration of several parameters in order to make the right decision for the patient.

Elderly patients usually suffer from a variety of comorbidities, poor bone stock, and functional impairment. The presence of "frailty," the so-called "independent geriatric syndrome," requires careful screening as it can have a negative impact on outcome. Clinical characteristics include anorexia, sarcopenia, osteoporosis, fatigue, risk of falls, and poor physical health in general (3).

The decision concerning the therapeutic strategy is therefore far more perplexing. In the authors' opinion, a standardized approach should be followed in order to reach the optimum decision for the patient waiting for a plan by the treating physician. Analysis of three important facets that could influence the outcome is essential prior to decision-making. These three facets include the following:

1. Patient factors (age, number, and severity of comorbidities; preexisting arthritic changes in the acetabulum; mobility status prior to injury; degree of osteoporosis and mental capacity)
2. Injury factors (fracture type, open or closed fracture, degree of comminution, presence of impaction, concomitant injury to femoral head, other associated injuries)
3. Therapeutic factors (timing of presentation since injury sustained [i.e., delayed presentation], approach required for reconstruction and length of surgery, risk of complications)

Overall, the aim of treatment is to reduce anatomically the affected hip joint and to achieve a stable fixation

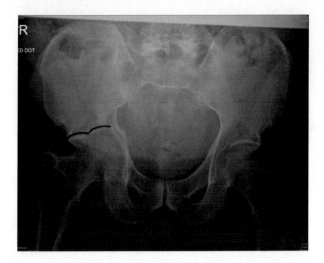

Figure 21.1 Anteroposterior radiograph in a 79-year-old female patient obtained following a fall showing a fracture of right acetabulum with the radiological feature of the "Gull-Sign" (black line).

allowing early mobilization with a timely recovery of function and level of preinjury mobility. Surgical reconstruction, however, may not be possible due to the degree of comminution, articular impaction, and bone quality, thus pointing to the option of a total hip arthroplasty (THA). Selection of which one of these two surgical options may be more appropriate for the patient can be difficult. However, careful assessment of all of the facets discussed and detailed discussion with the patient would help in reaching the most sensible, "safe," long-lasting option for the patient.

Treatment options can be divided into nonoperative and surgical treatment.

NONOPERATIVE TREATMENT

Candidates for this therapeutic approach are usually patients with nondisplaced or minimally displaced fractures (less than 2 mm), with no subluxation of the hip joint, and having "secondary congruity." Also, patients unfit for surgical intervention due to severe medical comorbidities and patients with reduced functional capacity (i.e., wheelchair bound) and reduced mental capacity (dementia) could be considered for this treatment option (Figure 21.2).

Nonoperative treatment includes adequate pain relief management and immobilization of the affected joint, particularly if the fracture pattern is prone to displacement. In these circumstances and assuming that the patient is cooperative, simple bed rest is usually adequate without the need of either distal femoral skeletal traction or skin traction. Functional physical therapy can be initiated with bed-to-chair transfers through a special board (banana board) and pivoting on the nonfractured lower extremity. Usually a period of immobilization of 6–8 weeks is adequate to facilitate sufficient healing to allow progression of mobilization to partial weight-bearing and eventually to full weight-bearing. Thromboprophylaxis is mandatory. Radiographs taken initially weekly (first 2–3 weeks) will allow monitoring of potential fracture displacement.

Application of skeletal traction or skin traction is not recommended in the elderly due to skin-related complications, bed sores, and infection of the pin sites. Pin disengagement and pull-out in osteoporotic bones have also been reported.

A few studies report on the results of nonoperative treatment. Spencer treated 25 acetabular fractures in elderly patients (age range 65–95 years) (4): 17 patients did not have significant displacement; 9 were treated with traction

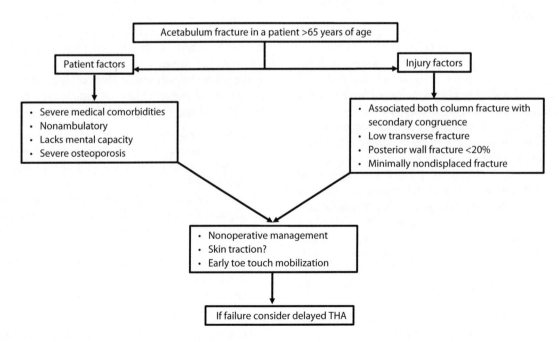

Figure 21.2 Indications for nonoperative treatment in patients above the age of 65 years.

for 6 weeks; and 2 succumbed because of the concomitant injuries. Seven patients (30%) out of the 23 survivors demonstrated unacceptable functional results. Poor results were associated with displaced posterior column fractures, femoral head injuries, too-brief traction, and early weight-bearing.

Sen and Veerappa evaluated 32 patients with displaced acetabular fractures (greater than 3 mm displacement) involving the weight-bearing dome and not associated with unstable pelvic ring injuries with a minimum of 2 years of follow-up evaluation (5). The reducibility by conservative management stood at 18 of 32 (56.3%), synchronizing with 18 of 32 (56.3%) good to excellent clinical scores. In patients with good fracture reduction, good to excellent results were seen in 83.3% cases. The radiological grade was good to excellent in 50% of cases with good clinicoradiological correlation ($P = 0.0001$). The authors concluded that acetabular fractures involving the weight-bearing dome if reduced by closed means can be maintained by heavy lateral and longitudinal traction, resulting in good outcome comparable with operative management (5).

In another study, Magu et al. reported the results of treatment in 69 patients out of which 15 developed complications (6 cases avascular necrosis of the femoral head [AVN], 5 pin site infections, 2 cases of knee stiffness, 1 bed sore, and 1 permanent popliteal nerve injury) (6). Fracture patterns associated with poor results included four displaced transverse fractures (two both column, two T-shaped) and two transverse with posterior wall (6).

SURGICAL TREATMENT

Operative treatment can be categorized as follows:

1. Open reduction and internal fixation (ORIF)
2. Open reduction and internal fixation with acute THA
3. Delayed THA

Open reduction and internal fixation

ORIF remains the most common treatment modality of acetabular fracture management in the young and middle-aged patient. However, in the elderly population, two important issues must be considered prior to contemplating ORIF:

1. Is the patient fit enough to tolerate the surgical stress induced by the procedure and mentally able to follow the postoperative instructions?
2. Can the surgeon reduce the fracture pattern and retain the fixation and the congruity of the hip joint and completion of fracture union?

In general terms, conditions must be favorable on all the previously discussed parameters (patient factors, injury factors, and treatment factors) for surgery to be the selected option of treatment. Indications for ORIF are based on a fracture with a pattern amenable to fixation through a single nonextensile exposure, adequate bone quality for fixation, no femoral head injury or substantial articular impaction, and whether the reconstruction may be performed in a reasonable surgical time (Figure 21.3). Any delay of surgery is important as well. It has been reported that if the operation is performed after a period of 11 days, the success rate is decreased due to callus formation, granulated tissue, and hematoma formation preventing easy reduction. The usual approaches for ORIF are the ilioinguinal, the modified Stoppa, and the Kocher-Langenbeck. New approaches have also been introduced, such as the pararectus approach by Bastian et al. (7) and the two-incision minimally invasive technique by Ruchholtz et al. (8). Percutaneous techniques for fixation may be of use in certain cases, but they lack strength and rigidity in comparison to the plating technique.

Factors that influence the result of the operation include a successful anatomical reduction, maintenance of reduction with the presence of good bone quality, and obeying the protocol prescribed for rehabilitation (Figure 21.4a, b).

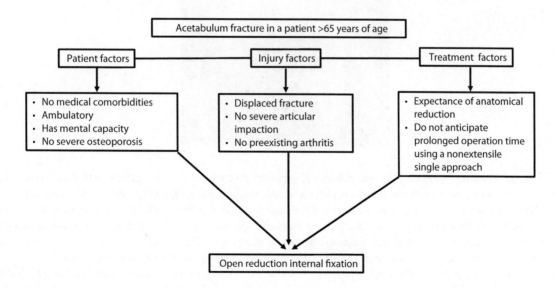

Figure 21.3 Indications for open reduction and internal fixation for acetabulum fractures in patients over 65 years of age.

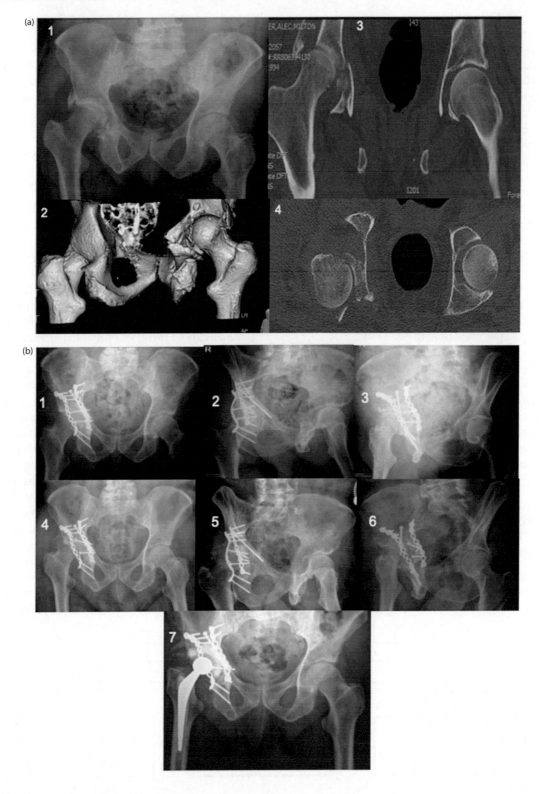

Figure 21.4 (a) 1. Anteroposterior (AP) radiograph in a 72-year-old male who sustained a right acetabulum fracture. 2. Three-dimensional reconstruction showing the degree of posterior wall comminution. 3. Computed tomography (CT) cuts showing degree of comminution. 4. Axial CT cuts showing the presence of articular impaction (arrow). (b) 1. AP pelvic postoperative radiograph showing anatomical reduction using a Kocher-Langenbeck approach (impaction was addressed with a cement bone substitute). 2. Obturator oblique postoperative radiograph showing anatomical reduction. 3. Iliac oblique postoperative radiograph showing anatomical. 4. AP pelvic postoperative radiograph 8 weeks after fixation showing loss of reduction and femoral head subluxation due to early weight-bearing (patient did not follow post-op instructions). 5. Obturator oblique post-operative radiograph at 8 weeks showing loss of reduction. 6. Iliac oblique postoperative radiograph at 8 weeks showing loss of reduction. 7. AP pelvic radiograph showing total hip arthroplasty 5 months after original fixation.

A recent systematic review of the literature analyzed the results of 354 patients with a mean age of 71.6 years (55–96 years) and a mean follow-up of 43 months (20–188 months) (9). Complex fractures were reported in 70.1% of patients. Seven studies presented the results of ORIF. The mean operation time was 236 minutes, mean blood loss was 707 mL, and mean mortality rate at 1 year was 22.6%. In the patients who underwent ORIF, conversion to THA was performed at a mean of 25.5 months with anatomical reduction in 11.6% and imperfect and poor reduction in 22.3%.

ORIF of acetabular fractures is connected to several complications, even when the fixation result is considered successful. These include loss of reduction, failure of metalwork, development of posttraumatic arthritis, heterotopic ossification, infection, and AVN of the femoral head. Overall, Capone et al. reported a nonfatal complication rate in the elderly of 30.3% (9).

With the introduction of new implants to address the issue of poor bone quality, it is expected that the results of treatment are going to improve. Implants with angular stability and quadrilateral extension can provide better fixation. Future studies will provide the evidence as to whether this indeed would be the case.

ACUTE TOTAL HIP ARTHROPLASTY

There is a great debate regarding the role of acute THA in elderly patients with acetabulum fractures. Advocates of this approach argue that this option is favorable because it is "one shot" surgery, is associated with a less extensile approach, and offers easier ambulation and faster recovery time. Disadvantages that must be discussed with the patient are risk of dislocation, especially in patients with cognitive or neurological impairment, inability to achieve stable fixation, risk of aseptic loosening, and risk of heterotopic ossification. Overall, acute THA is challenging taking into consideration that the important aim is to provide primary stability of the acetabular component, an objective that is threatened by unstable bony fragments/columns.

Indications for acute THR are preexisting osteoarthritis in the affected hip joint, fracture of the femoral head, severe comminution of the acetabulum, severe impaction, wide abrasion of the femoral head, multipartite acetabular fracture, and bone with a great degree of osteoporosis (Figures 21.5 and 21.6). Relative indications include delayed presentation and no medical comorbidities. Two strategic pathways can be selected. First, to perform THR after an ORIF of the acetabular fracture, and second to perform THR without attempting to reduce the fracture.

In the first case, depending on the elements of the acetabulum that are fractured, one surgical approach might be sufficient, both for the fixation step and the arthroplasty (i.e., a Kocher-Langenbeck for fracture of the posterior column). If one approach is not adequate, a dual approach could be used. The patient is positioned supine and the anterior column is addressed through a modified Stoppa approach. Then, the patient is re-draped, and the arthroplasty is performed through a Kocher-Langenbeck approach. In any case, the main issue is the ability to provide a stable bed and sufficient bone stock for the acetabular component. Otherwise the stability is compromised, and as such the prosthesis may subside or migrate. For this reason, it is essential to define the boundaries of the socket and to plan how to manage the bone loss, the volume of graft needed, and how containment can be optimized. The femoral head can be used as an osseous graft, impacted at the bottom of the acetabular socket. A standard arthroplasty acetabular component can be implanted or a special reinforcement ring can be used (Müller, Burch-Schneider antiprotrusion cage, or new type cage with an iliac extension).

DELAYED TOTAL HIP ARTHROPLASTY

Delayed THA following acetabular fracture is used either as a staged procedure following initial treatment or as a

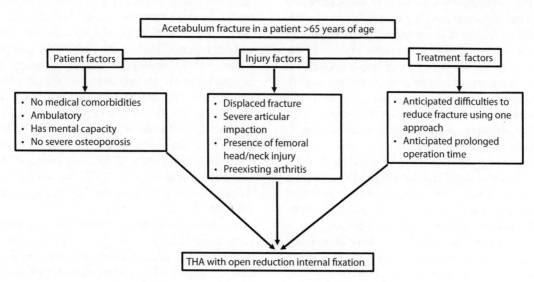

Figure 21.5 Indications for total hip arthroplasty for acetabulum fractures in patients over 65 years of age.

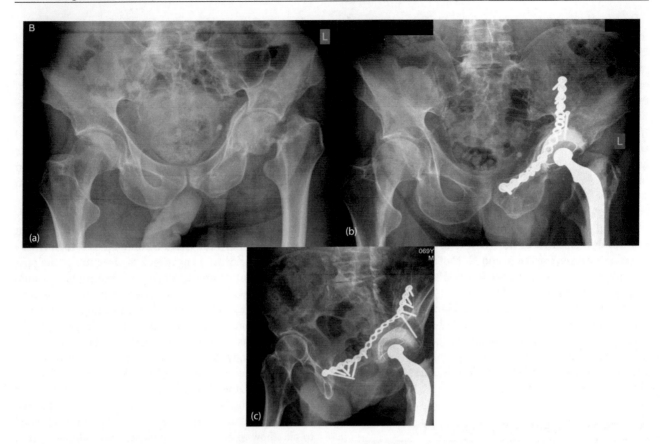

Figure 21.6 (a) Anteroposterior (AP) radiograph in a male patient 74 years of age who sustained a combined left acetabulum (anterior column) and femoral neck fracture. (b) Postoperative AP radiograph showing acute treatment with a cemented total hip arthroplasty (THA). (c) Postoperative obturator oblique radiograph showing the left THA.

1salvage procedure to failed ORIF or posttraumatic degenerative arthritis. Delayed THA after conservative treatment may involve difficulties due to a malunion or nonunion at the fracture site. Salvage THA following ORIF can be complicated by extended scar tissue formation, underlying low-grade infection, hardware penetrating the joint from the previous ORIF, or heterotopic ossification. Bone stock loss and disruption of normal anatomy are predictors of a difficult procedure. In case of low-grade infection, which can be diagnosed with bone biopsies, bone scan, and biochemical investigations, the dilemma for the surgeon is removal or not of the extra-articular metalwork previously used to fix the fracture. If there is clear evidence of involvement, then the metalwork must be removed. Otherwise, careful consideration of the pros and cons must be discussed with the patient prior to decision-making.

Delayed THA surgery is an elective procedure. Careful planning is critical to avoid any surprises in the operating room. Selection of the appropriate approach, type of implant to be implanted, and need for bone grafting, among others, must be well analyzed and executed. Usually more than a plan must have been formulated in order to be able to deal with any eventuality. Advantages of a delayed THA option include a defined bone stock and consolidated fracture and availability of the desired type and volume of bone graft needed, as well as of cemented and uncemented standard and custom-made implants, including acetabular reinforcement rings. Disadvantages are the difficulty of the surgical approach due to scar tissue, heterotopic ossification, avascularity or infection, malunion, higher risk of bleeding, and difficulty removing any *in situ* metalwork.

In terms of the results of treatment, Makridis et al. analyzed 654 patients with a systematic review approach (10). An uncemented acetabular and femoral component was used in 80.1% and 59.8% of the cases, respectively. The authors reported that in the early THA group, Kaplan-Meier survivorship analysis with any loosening, osteolysis, or revision as the endpoint revealed that the 10-year cup survival was 81%, whereas in the late THA group it was 76% ($P = 0.287$). The 10-year survival was 95% for the early stems and 85% for the late ones ($P = 0.001$). The median Harris hip score was 88 points. The authors concluded that due to their complexity of the cases analyzed, these fractures should be managed in highly specializing units where the expertise of arthroplasty and trauma reconstruction is available.

In conclusion, treatment of osteoporotic acetabular fractures in the elderly remains a challenging issue. Factors affecting the decision-making are divided into severity of injury, patient profile, and treatment options. Treatment has to be individualized for every patient, taking into consideration comorbidities and the ability of the patient to undergo a prolonged procedure. Nonoperative treatment is selected when there is no gross pelvic deformity and subluxation of the hip joint is not an issue. Minimally invasive stabilization techniques may be considered as a compromise but do not offer stable fixation. Even though ORIF remains the workhorse of reconstruction, high failure rates have been reported in patients with advanced osteoporosis. An acute THA would yield satisfactory results, if the fracture pattern is thoroughly evaluated, the patient risk and prognostic factors are properly assessed, and the right implant is selected.

Delayed THA has the advantage of a consolidated fracture and a defined bone stock. Proper initial management is of paramount importance, as an early failure may result in a protracted postoperative course, subsequent salvage surgery, and significant morbidity.

REFERENCES

1. Ferguson TA, Patel R, Bhandari M, Matta JM. Fractures of the acetabulum in patients aged 60 years and older: An epidemiological and radiological study. *J Bone Joint Surg.* 2010;92-B:250–57.
2. Letournel E. Acetabulum fractures: Classification and management. *Clin Orthop Relat Res.* 1980;(151):81–106.
3. Strandberg TE, Pitkälä KH. Frailty in elderly people. *Lancet.* 2007;369(9570):1328–9.
4. Spencer RF. Acetabular fractures in older patients. *J Bone Joint Surg Br.* 1989;71(5):774–6.
5. Sen RK, Veerappa LA. Long-term outcome of conservatively managed displaced acetabular fractures. *J Trauma.* 2009;67(1):155–9.
6. Magu NK, Rohilla R, Arora S. Conservatively treated acetabular fractures: A retrospective analysis. *Indian J Orthop.* 2012;46(1):36–45.
7. Bastian JD, Savic M, Cullmann JL, Zech WD, Djonov V, Keel MJ. Surgical exposures and options for instrumentation in acetabular fracture fixation: Pararectus approach versus the modified Stoppa. *Injury.* 2016;47(3):695–701
8. Ruchholtz S, Buecking B, Delschen A et al. The two-incision, minimally invasive approach in the treatment of acetabular fractures. *J Orthop Trauma.* 2013;27(5):248–55.
9. Capone A, Peri M, Mastio M. Surgical treatment of acetabular fractures in the elderly: A systematic review of the results. *EFORT Open Rev.* 2017;2(4):97–103.
10. Makridis KG, Obakponovwe O, Bobak P, Giannoudis PV. Total hip arthroplasty after acetabular fracture: Incidence of complications, reoperation rates and functional outcomes: Evidence today. *J Arthroplasty.* 2014;29(10):1983–90.

Management of osteoporotic proximal intertrochanteric/subtrochanteric femoral fractures

AVADHOOT KANTAK and GEORGE TSELENTAKIS

INTRODUCTION

As the elderly population grows, the number of hip fractures continues to increase. The elderly have weaker bone and are more likely to fall due to poorer balance, medication side effects, and difficulty maneuvering around environmental hazards.

Worldwide, the total number of hip fractures is expected to surpass 6 million by the year 2050 (1).

Hip fractures substantially increase the risk of death and major morbidity in the elderly (2,3). These risks are especially high among nursing home residents, particularly men, patients over age 90 years, those with cognitive impairment and other comorbidities, individuals treated nonoperatively, and those who cannot ambulate independently (4,5). In-hospital mortality rates range from approximately 1%–10% depending on the location and patient characteristics, but rates are typically higher in men, although this discrepancy appears to be declining in some areas (6,10). One-year mortality rates have ranged from 12% to 37% (2,11–13) but may be declining (14). Approximately one-half of patients are unable to regain their ability to live independently (15). A meta-analysis of prospective studies found the relative hazard for mortality during the first 3 months following a hip fracture to be 5.75 (95% confidence interval [CI] 4.94–6.67) in older women and 7.95 (95% CI 6.13–10.30) in older men (16). Although it decreases over time, the increased risk of death likely persists, according to this review and other studies (12).

Approximately 60% of fractures of the hip in the elderly are intracapsular (17). Intracapsular fractures occur about three times more often in women. The highest rates were found among white women. Extracapsular fractures also occur in a 3:1 female-to-male ratio. Subtrochanteric fractures show a bimodal distribution (20–40 years and over 60 years) (18).

Fractures of the hip have a high morbidity and mortality in the elderly with up to 10% of patients dying within 30 days of surgery and 30% dying within 1 year (19).

OSTEOPOROSIS AND THE PROXIMAL FEMUR

The World Health Organization (WHO) defines osteoporosis as a bone mineral density (BMD) of 2.5 standard deviations (SDs) or more below the young normal mean (20). However, this definition applies only to postmenopausal women assessed by dual-energy x-ray absorptiometry (DEXA) scan, and no such definition exists for men. Previous attempts to estimate the degree of osteoporosis include the Singh index, which involves fitting the pattern of proximal femoral trabecular lines into six separate categories; however, this has been shown to have poor inter- and intraobserver reliability (21), and moreover, it does not correlate with BMD as measured by DEXA scanning. Perhaps the most useful description of fragility fractures is that recently proposed by Kanis et al. (22) in defining osteoporotic fractures as those that occur at a site associated with low BMD and that increase in incidence over the age of 50 years. About 30% of fractures in men, 66% of fractures in women, and 70% of inpatient fractures are potentially osteoporotic.

Orthopedic concerns of osteoporotic proximal fractures

When dealing with osteoporotic fractures, the bone behaves as the weaker link. If we consider the fracture fixation to be a composite of metal (fixation device) and bone, it becomes apparent that any weakness in the bone will cause the entire composite to be deficient. In osteoporosis there is general reduction of bone mass and hence chances of inadequate fixation are higher. We discuss some of the pitfalls routinely encountered due to failure of fixation of osteoporotic fractures.

FIXATION FAILURE

With regard to peritrochanteric fractures of the femur, the results of randomized controlled trials (RCTs) demonstrate a failure rate of 5% and a reoperation rate of 4.9% (23). Failure rates will vary, however, depending on the stability of the fracture type. While most studies included both stable and unstable fracture patterns, Varela-Egocheaga (24) solely focused on stable fracture types, noting a failure rate of 3.8%; this can be contrasted with the findings of Sadowski et al. (25) who investigated only the most unstable fracture patterns (reverse oblique and transverse intertrochanteric) and noted a significant increase in failure rate to 22.9% (Figure 22.1).

PROLONGED HOSPITAL STAY

On average, the failures of fixation result in a twofold increase in the length of hospital stay (23). Thakar et al. (26) divided total hospital stay into acute—and community— stay periods and found that the majority of the 37-day difference in mean total time spent in UK National Health Service (NHS) care for failed fixations was due to an increase in acute hospital bed days rather than community hospital days.

INABILITY TO ACHIEVE PREOPERATIVE STATUS OF ACTIVITY

Several studies have noted a downgrade in patients' discharge destination following the failure of internal fixation compared to that of uncomplicated cases. Eastwood (27) noted that patients requiring revision surgery were 35 times more likely to be referred to continuing care, with a consequent increase in social dependency. Other studies support these findings with patients less likely to return to their own homes and more likely to be referred for

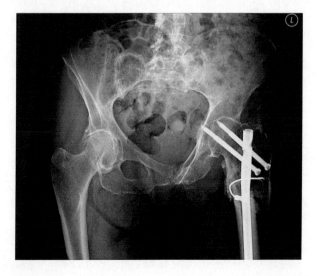

Figure 22.1   Failure of fixation in a proximal femoral fracture.

continuing rehabilitation (26,28). It appears, however, that this downgrade of residential status is limited to the short term, and several authors have noted no difference at long-term follow-up (29,30).

QUALITY OF LIFE

While all patients suffer a decrease in their quality of life (QoL) after hip fracture, this is particularly evident in patients who have a failed fixation. Tidermark et al. (31) noted that mean quality of life (EQ-5D index score) was higher at each follow-up assessment for those with healing fractures than for those who suffered a failure of fixation: at 4 months, 0.66 versus 0.49 ($P < 0.05$) and at 17 months, 0.62 versus 0.31 ($P < 0.005$). At inclusion, there had been no difference between the groups. They also noted a more profound decrease in body weight and lean body mass at 6 months in the fixation failure group. Other studies support this additional impact on quality of life in the short term, noting lower QoL scores and increased use of walking aids at 4–6-month follow-up (30,32,33).

MORTALITY

As hip fractures—and their surgical treatment—carry a well-documented increased mortality (7–9) risk, it is of particular interest to examine the effect of additional surgery in the same patient group. While Thakar et al. (26) did note a significant increase in the probability of mortality following reoperation, other studies have observed only transient increases in mortality during either the initial period of hospitalization (34) or during the first 6 months (35). Revision procedures after this did not increase mortality risk, and at long-term follow-up, several authors noted no overall difference in mortality between the groups (27–30,36,37). It is likely, however, that patients fit enough to undergo a secondary operation are a subgroup within this population with a bias toward better survival.

BIOLOGY OF OSTEOPOROSIS

The two most important determinants in the development of osteoporosis are peak bone mass and the rate of bone loss thereafter. Peak bone mass generally is achieved in the early part of the fourth decade of life. Thereafter, bone is lost at a rate that depends on several factors. These factors include (a) the normal aging process; (b) the accelerated bone loss associated with menopause; and (c) genetic, environmental, and nutritional conditions and chronic disease states. The mechanism of bone loss resulting from normal aging is poorly understood. Based solely on normal aging, the rate of bone loss in women is nearly equivalent to that of men. This bone loss is independent of menopausal bone mass loss. Factors that contribute to bone loss include decreased activity, a calcium-deficient diet, inherited characteristics, and factors related to childbirth, premature menopause, and alcoholism. Estrogen deficiency is directly implicated in the etiology of osteoporosis. Although postmenopausal women produce estrogen, the levels are below those of premenopausal women and age-matched men. Twenty percent of postmenopausal women have a marked paucity of estrogen. In addition, smoking enhances estrogen degradation, and low body fat results in insufficient estrogen production. The primary consequences of postmenopausal bone loss are fractures of the hip, distal radius, and vertebrae. Calcium intake and absorption have been identified as key factors in fracture incidence. Individuals ingesting physiologic levels of calcium have one-fourth to one-third the rate of hip fractures experienced by individuals with low calcium intake. Excess calcium intake may be harmful and is less effective than estrogen in preventing osteoporosis (38). Recent attention has also demonstrated that eating disorders such as anorexia and excessive exercise leading to amenorrhea may also result in profound osteoporosis. This particular type of osteoporosis is especially worrisome because it affects women at a relatively early age, when their bone mass should be reaching its peak. Excessive loading or overuse can also lead to stress fractures, a special problem in military recruits as well as athletes. Whether the cause of these fractures is purely structural such as decreased moment of inertia of the bone or also the result of poor calcium intake and decreased bone mass is not known (38).

Basic pathology

Skeletal fragility can result from

- Failure to produce a skeleton of optimal mass and strength during growth.
- Excessive bone desorption resulting in decreased bone mass and microarchitectural deterioration of the skeleton.
- An inadequate formation response to increased resorption during bone remodelling. In addition, the incidence of fragility fractures, particularly of the hip and wrist, is further determined by the frequency and direction of falls.

To understand how excessive bone resorption and inadequate formation result in skeletal fragility, it is necessary to understand the process of bone remodeling, which is the major activity of bone cells in the adult skeleton. The bone remodeling or bone multicellular units (BMUs) described many years ago by Frost (39) can occur either on the surface of trabecular bone as irregular Howship lacunae or in cortical bone as relatively uniform cylindrical haversian systems. The process begins with the activation of hematopoietic precursors to become osteoclasts, which normally requires an interaction with cells of the osteoblastic lineage. Because the resorption and reversal phases of bone remodeling are short and the period required for osteoblastic replacement of the bone is long, any increase in the rate of bone remodeling will result in a loss of bone mass. Moreover, the larger number of unfilled Howship lacunae and haversian canals will further weaken the bone. Excessive resorption can also result in complete loss of trabecular structures, so that there is no template for

bone formation. Thus, there are multiple ways in which an increase in osteoclastic resorption can result in skeletal fragility. However, high rates of resorption are not always associated with bone loss, for example, during the pubertal growth spurt. Hence, an inadequate formation response during remodeling is an essential component of the pathogenesis of osteoporosis (38).

Central role of estrogen

The concept that estrogen deficiency is critical to the pathogenesis of osteoporosis was based initially on the fact that postmenopausal women, whose estrogen levels naturally decline, are at the highest risk for developing the disease. Morphologic studies and measurements of certain biochemical markers have indicated that bone remodeling is accelerated at the time of menopause, as both markers of resorption and formation are increased (39,40). Hence, contrary to Albright's original hypothesis, an increase in bone resorption, and not impaired bone formation, appears to be the driving force for bone loss in the setting of estrogen deficiency. But the rapid and continuous bone loss that occurs for several years after menopause must indicate an impaired bone formation response, since in younger individuals going through a pubertal growth spurt, even faster rates of bone resorption can be associated with an increase in bone mass. However, the increased bone formation that normally occurs in response to mechanical loading is diminished in estrogen deficiency, suggesting that estrogen is both anticatabolic and anabolic (41). Estrogen deficiency continues to play a role in bone loss in women in their 70s and 80s, as evidenced by the fact that estrogen treatment rapidly reduces bone breakdown in these older women (42). Moreover, recent studies in humans have shown that the level of estrogen required to maintain relatively normal bone remodeling in older postmenopausal women is lower than that required to stimulate classic target tissues such as the breast and uterus (43). Fracture risk is inversely related to estrogen levels in postmenopausal women, and as little as one-quarter of the dose of estrogen that stimulates the breast and uterus is sufficient to decrease bone resorption and increase bone mass in older women (44). This greater sensitivity of the skeleton may be age related. In 3-month-old mice, the uterus appeared to be more responsive to estrogen than bone, whereas in 6-month-old mice, the reverse was found (45). Estrogen is critical for epiphyseal closure in puberty in both sexes and regulates bone turnover in men as well as in women. In fact, estrogen has a greater effect than androgen in inhibiting bone resorption in men, although androgen may still play a role (46). Estrogen may also be important in the acquisition of peak bone mass in men (47). Moreover, osteoporosis in older men is more closely associated with low estrogen than with low androgen levels (48). Estrogen deficiency increases and estrogen treatment decreases the rate of bone remodeling, as well as the amount of bone lost with each remodeling cycle. Studies in animal models and in cell cultures have suggested that this involves multiple sites of estrogen action, not only on the cells of the BMU but also on other marrow cells. Estrogen acts through two receptors: estrogen receptor α (ERα) and ERβ. ERα appears to be the primary mediator of estrogen's actions on the skeleton (41). Osteoblasts do express ERβ, but the actions of ERβ agonists on bone are less clear. Some studies suggest that the effects of estrogen signaling through ERα and ERβ are in opposition, while other studies suggest that activation of these two receptors has similar effects on bone (49,50). Single nucleotide polymorphisms (SNPs) of ERα may affect bone fragility. The SNPs for this receptor were associated with a significant reduction in fracture risk, independent of BMD. Other studies have suggested that SNPs of ERα can affect BMD and rates of bone loss as well as fracture risk in both men and women (51,52). An orphan nuclear receptor, estrogen receptor–related receptor α (ERRα), with sequence homology to ERα and ERβ, is also present in bone cells (53). Despite its inability to bind estrogens, this receptor may interact with ERα and ERβ or act directly to alter bone cell function. A regulatory variant of the gene encoding ERRα was recently found to be associated with a significant difference between lumbar spine and femoral neck BMD in premenopausal women (54). Sex hormone-binding globulin (SHBG), the major binding protein for sex steroids in plasma, may not only alter the bioavailability of estrogen to hormone-responsive tissues but may also affect its entry into cells. Epidemiologic studies suggest that SHBG may have an effect on bone loss and fracture risk independent of the effect as a binding protein (55). Local formation of estradiol from aromatase could play an additional role (56). While estrogen can act on cells of the osteoblastic lineage, its effects on bone may also be dependent on actions on cells of the hematopoietic lineage, including osteoclast precursors, mature osteoclasts, and lymphocytes. Local cytokines and growth factors may mediate these effects. Bone loss after oophorectomy in rodent models can be prevented by inhibiting interleukin (IL)-1 or tumor necrosis factor (TNF)-α and does not occur in mice deficient in the IL-1 receptor or TNF-α (57,58). The effects of estrogen on cytokine production may be mediated by T cells (59). A direct effect of estrogen in accelerating osteoclast apoptosis has been attributed to increased transforming growth factor (TGF)-β production (60). Another possibility is that estrogen exerts its beneficial effects by suppressing reactive oxygen species (ROS) (61). In estrogen deficiency, thiol antioxidant defenses may be diminished, and the resultant increase in ROS may induce TNF-α (62). The relevance of these findings for human osteoporosis has yet to be determined.

Calcium, vitamin D, and parathyroid hormone

The concept that osteoporosis is due primarily to calcium deficiency, particularly in the elderly, was initially put forward as a counterproposal to Albright's estrogen deficiency theory. Decreased calcium intake, impaired intestinal absorption of calcium due to aging or disease, as well as vitamin D deficiency can result in secondary hyperparathyroidism. The active hormonal form, 1,25-dihydroxy vitamin D (calcitriol), is not only necessary for optimal intestinal absorption of calcium and phosphorus but also exerts a tonic inhibitory effect on parathyroid hormone (PTH) synthesis, so that there are dual pathways that can lead to secondary hyperparathyroidism (63). Vitamin D deficiency and secondary hyperparathyroidism can contribute not only to accelerated bone loss and increasing fragility but also to neuromuscular impairment that can increase the risk of falls (64,65). Clinical trials involving older individuals at high risk for calcium and vitamin D deficiency indicate that supplementation of both can reverse secondary hyperparathyroidism, decrease bone resorption, increase bone mass, decrease fracture rates, and even decrease the frequency of falling (63). However, in a large recent study, calcium and vitamin D supplementation did not reduce fracture incidence significantly, perhaps because this population was less deficient in vitamin D (66). Polymorphisms of the vitamin D receptor (VDR) have been studied extensively, but the results have been variable. This may be in part because the effect of a given polymorphism in this receptor is dependent on an interaction with the environment, particularly with calcium (67). VDR polymorphisms are also associated with differences in the response to therapy with calcitriol (68). There is also evidence for an effect on fracture risk independent of bone density and bone turnover, which might be due to an alteration in the frequency of falls (69). Secondary hyperparathyroidism presents when there is relative insufficiency of vitamin D—that is, where the levels of the circulating form, 25-hydroxy vitamin D fall below 30 ng/mL, suggesting that the target for vitamin D supplementation should be at this level or higher (70). The seasonal decrease in vitamin D level and increase in PTH level during the winter months is associated with an increase in fractures, independent of the increase in rate of falls (71). In addition, increased PTH levels are associated with increased mortality in the frail elderly, independent of bone mass and vitamin D status. The precise mechanisms underlying this relationship have not yet been determined, but the risk of cardiovascular death was increased (72). Polymorphisms of the calcium sensing receptor, which regulates calcium secretion by suppression of *PTH* translation and PTH secretion, have not yet been associated with any alteration in bone phenotype (73,74).

BIOMECHANICS OF PROXIMAL FEMORAL FRACTURES

Because of its shape, the femur is subjected to eccentric loading. The proximal end of the femur has been likened to a cantilevered arch that transfers the force of weight-bearing to the hip and pelvis (75). *In vivo* this bending force loads the medial cortex in compression and lateral cortex in tension; the forces are not in equilibrium. There are high stresses acting in the subtrochanteric area, up to 0.351168 kg/m². There is high compressive stress on the medial side and high tensile stress on the lateral side (76). Although lateral muscles partly compensate for the high compressive medial forces, the proximal femur is still eccentrically loaded as the compressive medial forces are considerably greater than the lateral tensile forces (77). Major compressive stresses in the femur are greatest in the medial cortex 2.5–7.6 cm below the lesser trochanter. If the medial buttress is not intact or cannot be reestablished, the internal fixation devices are subjected mainly to bending stresses, and the loads are concentrated in this high stress area resulting in implant failure or loss of fixation. This is the most highly stressed region in the body (78). This dissimilar loading pattern is of great importance in selecting internal fixation devices and in understanding the causes and prevention of failure of internal fixation devices.

The loading pattern further emphasizes the importance of integrity of the medial half of the column as well as the importance of prestressing of the implant in tension. This in turn increases axial compression, which increases the stability of the fixation and restores the fractured fragment as a functional unit. If the medial cortex can be reconstituted at the time of surgery, a plate placed laterally acts as a tension band, allowing impaction with protected weight-bearing. If the medial cortical contact is not restored, bending stresses are concentrated in one small area of the plate, which often results in mechanical failure of the internal fixation device with delayed union, nonunion, or malunion of the fracture. Until recently, restoration of the continuity of the medial cortex of the proximal femur has been the key to success (78).

The proximal femur is surrounded by large and powerful muscles. These together with the interplay of gravity result in characteristic deformities in the case of subtrochanteric fractures. The iliopsoas flexes, abducts, and externally rotates the proximal fragment. The adductors lead to adduction of the shaft. This deformity complicates attempts at closed reduction. Shortening, of course, occurs as a result of the contraction of all the long muscles that span the length of the shaft. Thus, the characteristic deformity is an anterior and lateral bowing of the femoral shaft combined with considerable shortening (Figure 22.2). The angle formed by the axis of femoral neck and femoral shaft is 130 ± 7. If the angle is reduced as would occur with varus reduction of fracture, the distance between the head and shaft is increased, with the increased moment arm and the bending forces across the fracture, and may produce varus collapse (77).

CLASSIFICATION

A classification is useful only if it considers the severity of the bone lesion and serves as a basis for treatment and for evaluation of the results.

Maurice Müller

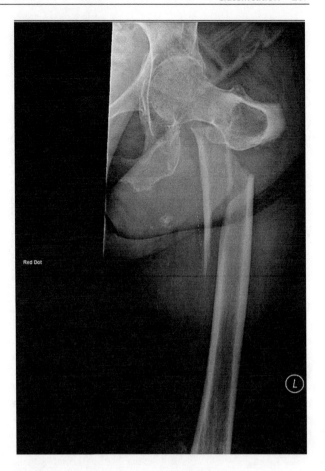

Figure 22.2 Deformity in subtrochanteric fractures.

Intertrochanteric

Commonly, fractures are described by the number of "parts" (fragments) and instability. The presence of certain fracture characteristics, such as displaced posteromedial fragment shattered lateral wall, indicates instability.

There are several classifications (79–82). Evans (79) has based his classification on stability of the fracture. Jansen has modified Evans classification into three groups: stable, unstable, and very unstable (Figure 22.3). Gotfried and Kyle et al. each have added a new variety of intertrochanteric fracture (80,81).

Gotfried has described the important lateral trochanteric wall as a key element of instability (80). The lateral trochanteric wall acts as a buttress to the proximal fragment. A shattered lateral wall allows excessive collapse of the proximal fragment over the sliding screw. Excessive collapse results in pain, reduced mobility of the hip, inability to walk sometimes, and nonunion and failure. It is important to prevent lateral wall fracture during surgery. If fractured, it should be reconstructed by tension band wiring or lateral buttress plate or lag screws.

Basi-cervical neck fracture may be included in intertrochanteric fracture. This fracture is prone to avascular necrosis of the head of the femur. There is also rotational instability. Therefore, an additional derotation screw should be used.

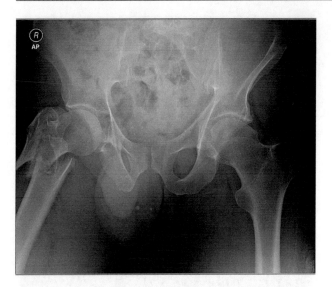

Figure 22.3 Unstable reverse trochanteric fracture.

The AO Foundation/Orthopaedic Trauma Association (AO/OTA) classification has attempted to standardize the way fractures are classified and is a system that is now most commonly utilized in all literature. The classification describes fractures in ascending severity with regard to stability and ease of reconstruction (Table 22.1) (82).

Subtrochanteric

The earliest classification system identified was the trochanteric classification of Murray and Frew, whose patients were treated conservatively with traction (83). They simply classified subtrochanteric fractures into oblique subtrochanteric (type 4) and transverse subtrochanteric (type 5) fractures.

Watson et al. did not classify the fracture into a limited number of categories; instead, three numbers were used to describe the fracture (84). The first (reference line) referred to the distance from the notch at the base of the superior neck to the beginning of the fracture, the second (fracture length line) was the distance from the most proximal to the most distal point of the fracture, and the third (comminution Digit) was the number of fragments. The reference line in their series was 9 cm in all but two fractures. There was a tendency toward long comminuted fractures to be associated with delayed union.

Fielding and Magliato used three groups, those with a fracture at the level of the lesser trochanter (type 1), those within 2.5 cm below the lesser trochanter (type 2), and those from 2.5 to 5 cm below the lesser trochanter (type 3) (85). In their series, most patients were treated with plated Jewett nails, and they found that nonunion was more prevalent in the more distally located fractures.

Cech and Sosna had four main types and included fractures with extension into the trochanteric region, true subtrochanteric (simple and comminuted), pathologic fractures, and subtrochanteric fractures in children (86).

Zickel used an intramedullary device to treat his patients and included six groups based on the morphology of the fracture, short oblique (with or without comminution), long oblique (with or without comminution), and high or low transverse fractures (87). He found that the long oblique comminuted fractures required more surgical exposure and mobilization of fragments to achieve reduction, and no association was found between the level of the fracture and implant failure.

Table 22.1 AO/Orthopaedic Trauma Association (OTA) classification of extracapsular proximal femur fractures

Simple pertrochanteric (stable) A1 1. Two part 2. Greater trochanter involvement 3. Lesser trochanter involvement **Multifragmented pertrochanteric A2 (partially stable)** 1. One intermediate fragment 2. Two intermediate fragments 3. More than two intermediate fragments **Intertrochanteric (unstable) A3** 1. Oblique fracture 2. Transverse fracture 3. With medial fragment/s	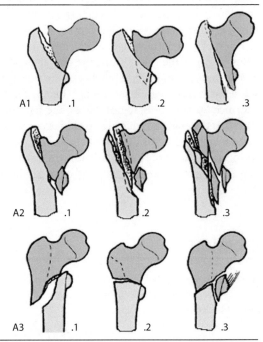

Waddell used three types, transverse or short oblique with minimal or no comminution (type I), long oblique or spiral fractures with minimal or no comminution (type II), and fractures with a significant degree of comminution including those with an intertrochanteric component (type III) (88). Following fixation of these fractures mostly with a plate, he found that metal fatigue and nonunions were minimal in the type I and II fractures.

Pankovich and Tarabishy treated their subtrochanteric fractures with Ender nails and divided these fractures into simple/short oblique (type I), long oblique/spiral (type II), fractures with unicortical comminution (type III), and fractures with comminution at the entire cortical circumference (type IV) (89). They defined subtrochanteric fractures as those distal to the lesser trochanter but no more than 5 cm distal to it at their most proximal point. Harris divided fractures into stable subtrochanteric (horizontal or short oblique) at a level between the lower margin of the lesser trochanter and 5 cm distally and unstable subtrochanteric (horizontal or short oblique with posteromedial comminution or long oblique fractures) (90).

Malkawi divided subtrochanteric fractures into noncomminuted (IA, transverse type; IB, oblique type) and comminuted (IIA, with medial cortex comminution; IIB, with medial cortical and greater trochanteric comminution; IIC, with lateral cortical comminution) (91). He suggested that type I (A and B) and type IIC fractures be treated with compression internal fixation alone, with type IIA and IIB fractures supplemented with bone grafting.

Zain Elabdien et al. divided subtrochanteric fractures into simple transverse (type I), oblique with long or short fracture lines (type II), and comminuted with involvement of lesser trochanter or greater trochanter or both (type III) (92). The proximal border of the subtrochanteric area was defined as a line crossing from the base of the greater trochanter to the base of the lesser trochanter and the subtrochanteric zone 7.5 cm distal to it. In type II and III fractures, the Ender nails were supplemented with nylon or cerclage-wire fixation, and there was a tendency toward increased delayed union in the type III group as compared with the other groups.

Winquist et al., who reported on the results of intramedullary nailing of femur fractures, divided proximal one-third femur fractures into transverse, oblique, and comminuted with further classification of comminuted fractures from I to IV types (93).

Ungar et al. used five groups, type I (two fragments, transverse or short oblique), type II (two fragments, long oblique or spiral), type III (three fragments), type IV (comminuted), and type V (combined per- and subtrochanteric) (94). They defined the subtrochanteric zone as the area between the lower margin of the lesser trochanter and 5 cm distally.

Russell and Taylor devised a classification based on lesser trochanteric continuity and involvement of the piriformis fossa (95). Type I fractures do not extend into the piriformis fossa, whereas type II fractures do involve the piriformis fossa. In types IA and IIA, the lesser trochanter is intact; in fracture types IB and IIB, the lesser trochanter is fractured. They defined the subtrochanteric zone as the area of bone below the lesser trochanter to the femoral isthmus.

The two most commonly used systems are those from Seinsheimer (96) and the AO (82). Seinsheimer in his series of patients found a 44% failure of fixation in the type IIIA fractures. The AO system aims to standardize the description of these fractures. The system also gives a good indication of prognosis due to recognition of mechanical stability in the fracture classification (Table 22.2).

Table 22.2 AO/ASIF classification of subtrochanteric fractures

A. *Simple fracture (two part)*
1. Spiral
2. Oblique
3. Transverse

A1.1   A2.1   A3.1

B. *Wedge fracture (with a butterfly fragment)*
1. Spiral wedge
2. Bending wedge
3. Comminuted wedge

B1.1   B2.1   B3.1

C. *Multifragmented*
1. Complex spiral
2. Complex segmental
3. Complex irregular

C1. ≤ 1 2 3   C2. ≤ 1 2 3   C3. ≤ 1 2 3

SURGICAL TREATMENT

The best outcome with proximal femur fractures is with surgical stabilization. Due to the comorbidities in the patient cohort, a stable fixation device that will allow immediate weight-bearing is desirable. It can be challenging at times to achieve this kind of fixation in osteoporotic bone.

In stable intertrochanteric fractures, a standard sliding hip screw fixation is satisfactory. Subtrochanteric fractures require intramedullary nailing with a Recon option available for proximal locking. It is of paramount importance to obtain anatomical reduction or at least a stable reduction prior to nailing. In case of the unstable intertrochanteric fractures and the reverse oblique fractures, an intramedullary nail is a better biomechanical device with less chance of failure.

Trochanteric fracture associated with fracture of the shaft of the femur may be treated by Recon, long Gamma, or proximal femoral nail. Pathological fracture forms a separate variety (97–100). In reverse oblique fractures, use of a dynamic hip screw may cause excessive collapse leading to failure. Excessive collapse occurs due to shearing forces and to powerful muscles acting on fragments. In fracture with shattered lateral wall, treated by dynamic hip screw (DHS), excessive collapse occurs due to the loss of a buttressing effect of the lateral wall. Excessive collapse can result in functional deficit due to reduced mobility of the hip, pain resulting in inability to walk, and nonunion or implant failure. This may be prevented by trochanteric plate, reconstruction of lateral wall, and intramedullary nail. Some modifications of the dynamic hip screw that can be utilized in reverse oblique fracture patterns are as follows:

1. *Medoff plate* (101): Medoff designed a device that allows axial compression. Medoff recommends the axial compression for unstable fractures.
2. *Trochanteric stabilizing plate*: The trochanteric stabilizing plate construct buttresses the greater trochanter and prevents lateral displacement and excessive fracture collapse, which results in limb shortening. When the lateral wall is shattered, it is reconstructed using a lag screw or tension band wire passing through tendon of abductor muscles. A trochanteric stabilizing plate is useful when the lateral wall is fractured.
3. *Augmentation*: Tricalcium phosphate cement or polymethyl methacrylate cement can be injected into the void in the posteromedial area in unstable fractures. This increases stability (102).
4. *Hydroxyapatite-coated screw*: This achieves better fixation in osteoporotic bone.

Technical tips

Though a major part of the outcome in these fractures is due to host factors (i.e., fracture pattern, osteoporosis, etc.), a surgeon can prevent further damage and improve the outcome by following certain basic principles during osteosynthesis. We identified some essential principles that could help in the surgical treatment of these complex injuries.

REDUCTION

In a stable intertrochanteric fracture, reduction is achieved with gentle traction to the limb. A slight flexion and internal rotation of the limb align the distal fragment to the proximal fragment with a near anatomical reduction in most cases.

In unstable fractures, due to a complete detachment of the trochanters, the sag-down effect is noticed at the fracture. Traction alone is not effective in reducing these fractures. In such circumstances, a vertically applied force in the posterior to anterior direction to the fracture site allows adequate alignment of the fracture site. A guidewire is then passed with the reduction held. A further lateral wall reconstruction may be necessary in these fractures.

In some unstable fractures, a closed reduction is not possible, and open reduction becomes imperative. An indirect open reduction suffices in most cases with the use of bone-holding forceps. It is noticed that in most cases the proximal fragment is flexed and internally rotated due to the effect of iliopsoas pull. Attention also needs to be given to soft tissue (anterior capsule, iliopsoas, rectus muscle, etc.) interposition, which impedes reduction. If anatomical reduction is unstable (due to comminution), we aim to stabilize the reduction by shortening and/or fragment impaction. In rare circumstances, a Dimon-Hughston type of osteotomy can be utilized (103).

In subtrochanteric fractures, closed reduction is more difficult, and open reduction is required more often to achieve stability. We aim to reduce by maneuvering the distal fragment to align with the proximal fragment and hold the reduction with bone-holding forceps. Reaming is done with the reduction forceps holding the reduction to avoid losing the alignment. We also have a low threshold to pass a cerclage wire around the fracture site to ease reduction and reaming (Figure 22.4). There is some concern raised regarding loss of periosteal blood circulation following cerclage wiring, but there is evidence suggesting no significant difference in healing time when cerclage wires are used (104).

TIP-TO-APEX DISTANCE

The tip-to-apex distance has been described by Baumgaertner et al. (105,106) as a useful intraoperative indicator of deep and central placement of the lag screw in the femoral head, regardless of whether a nail or a plate is chosen to fix the fracture. This is perhaps the most important measurement of accurate hardware placement and has been shown in multiple studies to be predictive of success after the treatment of standard oblique intertrochanteric fractures. Older theories about screw placement favored a low and occasionally a posterior position of the lag screw, thereby leaving more bone superior and anterior to the screw. This effectively lengthens the tip-to-apex distance

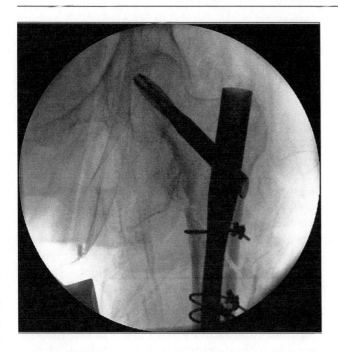

Figure 22.4 Use of cerclage wires to reduce subtrochanteric fractures.

and should be avoided. The ideal position for a lag screw in both planes is deep and central in the femoral head within 10 mm of the subchondral bone (107,108). A tip-to-apex distance of less than 25 mm has been shown to be generally predictive of a successful result; however, most traumatologists aim for a tip-to-apex distance of less than 20 mm.

LATERAL WALL

Fractures that involve the lateral wall of the proximal part of the femur are, by definition, either reverse oblique fractures or transtrochanteric fractures (Figure 22.5). These

fractures do not have any lateral osseous buttress; therefore, if a sliding hip screw is used, medial translation of the femoral shaft and lateralization of the proximal femoral fragment can occur. This results in deformity, nonunion, and screw cut-out. In some series there was a 56% failure rate when a sliding hip screw had been used for reverse oblique fractures of the proximal part of the femur (109). Although devices with a trochanteric stabilizing plate, those with a proximal trochanteric flare, and those that allow axial compression and locking of the sliding hip screw (such as the Medoff device) are reported to have reasonably good results, on balance, if there is no lateral wall, a hip screw should not be used (107–113). Locking plates and 95 condylar blade-plates may function as prosthetic lateral cortices, but the results of using these devices for more problematic fractures of the proximal part of the femur are not available. Intramedullary nails seem to be superior to dynamic condylar screws for reverse oblique fractures (113–115).

NAIL THE UNSTABLE FRACTURE

The unstable patterns include reverse oblique fractures, transtrochanteric fractures, fractures with a large posteromedial fragment implying loss of the calcar buttress, and fractures with subtrochanteric extension (107–109,113, 116–120). These fractures, in general, should be treated with an intramedullary nail because of the more favorable biomechanical properties of an intramedullary nail compared with a sliding hip screw (Figures 22.6 and 22.7).

MIND THE BOW

As a person ages, the femoral diaphysis enlarges and the femoral bow increases (121). Most commercial intramedullary nails have gradually evolved into a more bowed design,

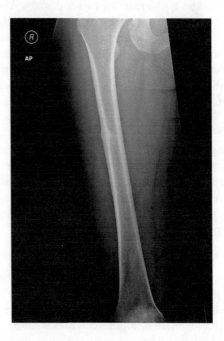

Figure 22.6 Anterior-posterior x-ray of right femur demonstrating atypical fracture related to bisphosphonate medication intake.

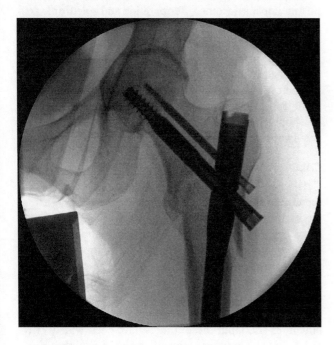

Figure 22.5 Fractured lateral wall.

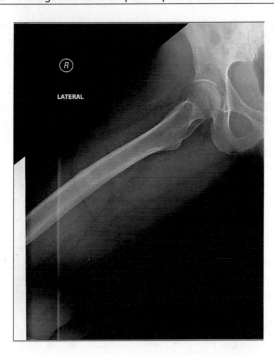

Figure 22.7 Lateral x-ray of right femur demonstrating atypical fracture related to bisphosphonate medication intake.

and many of them now have a radius of curvature of around 2 m. The concern with using a straight intramedullary nail in a bowed osteopenic femur is that the nail can impinge on, and in some cases even perforate, the anterior femoral metaphyseal cortex distally.

CHOOSE APPROPRIATE ENTRY POINT

Avoid being too posterior with the entry, as it can cause the nail to be close to the anterior cortex distally. Also keeping the entry slightly medial on the trochanter rather than lateral helps prevent a lateral wall blowout. An improper entry point can also be an important reason for malreduction of fractures. In most cases, an entry point at the junction of the anterior one-third and posterior two-thirds of the trochanter in the lateral view is recommended by us.

AVOID VARUS ANGULATION

Varus angulation at the fracture site substantially increases the tensile forces across the fracture site, increasing the chances of fixation failure. Aim for anatomical fixation, if this is unstable; achieve stability in the reduction by giving more valgus than varus at the fracture site and by maintaining good fragment contact.

USE DISTAL LOCKING SCREWS

Osteoporotic bones have a wide femoral canal with ill-defined isthmus. Hence, intramedullary devices have little hold in the isthmus. Distal locking screws are needed for control of rotation, alignment, and stability of fixation. As the nail may have very little isthmic contact, interlocking screws become necessary. Also aim to choose an implant that can cater to the large diameters found in osteoporotic femurs.

ACHIEVE COMPRESSION AND STABILITY ACROSS FRACTURE SITE

Compression across the fracture site improves stability and aids healing.

MEDICAL TREATMENT

Antiresorptive medications

Major pharmacologic interventions are the bisphosphonates, denosumab, PTH peptides, and raloxifene and strontium ranelate. All of these interventions have been shown to reduce the risk of vertebral fracture, and some have been shown to also reduce the risk of nonvertebral fractures, in some cases specifically at the hip.

These drugs work by altering the osteoclastic activity and hence reducing net bone desorption.

The low cost of generic alendronate, which has a broad spectrum of antifracture efficacy, makes this the first-line treatment in the majority of cases. In individuals who are intolerant of alendronate or in whom it is contraindicated, ibandronate, risedronate, zoledronic acid, denosumab, raloxifene, or strontium ranelate may provide appropriate treatment options. The high cost of PTH peptides restricts their use to those at very high risk, particularly for vertebral fractures. Other approved pharmacologic interventions for postmenopausal women include calcitriol, etidronate, and hormone replacement therapy. Alendronate, risedronate, zoledronic acid, strontium ranelate, and teriparatide are approved for the treatment of men at increased risk of fracture.

Individuals taking oral glucocorticoids alendronate, etidronate, and risedronate are approved for the prevention and treatment of glucocorticoid-induced osteoporosis in postmenopausal women. Teriparatide and zoledronic acid are approved for the treatment of glucocorticoid-induced osteoporosis in men and women at increased risk of fracture. Bone-protective treatment should be started at the onset of glucocorticoid therapy in patients at increased risk of fracture. Alendronate remains the first choice of treatment. In individuals who are intolerant of these agents or in whom it is contraindicated, etidronate, risedronate, and zoledronic acid are appropriate options.

CALCIUM AND VITAMIN D SUPPLEMENTATION

Calcium and vitamin D supplementation is widely recommended in older people who are housebound or living in residential or nursing homes, where vitamin D deficiency and low dietary calcium intake are common. Supplementation is also often advocated as an adjunct to other treatments for osteoporosis, as the clinical trials of these agents were performed in patients who were calcium and vitamin D replete. It has been suggested that calcium supplementation may potentially be associated with adverse cardiovascular outcomes (122), but these studies have been widely criticized, and the putative association requires further clarification (123). Although a longitudinal cohort study also suggested an increased risk of cardiovascular events with calcium supplementation, this was not seen with a high dietary intake of calcium (124). It may therefore be prudent to increase dietary calcium intake and use vitamin D alone, where the use of calcium and vitamin D supplementation might otherwise be considered (125).

Duration and monitoring of therapy

In most patients at increased risk of fracture, treatment needs to be continued long term. The beneficial effects of treatment with drugs other than bisphosphonates wear off soon after therapy is discontinued but may be maintained for longer periods of time after cessation of bisphosphonate therapy. This, together with concerns over possible adverse effects of long-term bisphosphonate therapy, particularly osteonecrosis of the jaw and atypical femoral fractures (AFFs) (126), has raised questions over the optimal duration of bisphosphonate treatment and whether, in some individuals, treatment should be discontinued for a period of time (the "drug holiday").

Based on the data available, it is recommended that treatment review should be performed after 5 years for alendronate, risedronate, or ibandronate and after 3 years for zoledronic acid. Withdrawal of treatment with these bisphosphonates is associated with decreases in BMD and bone turnover after 2–3 years for alendronate and 1–2 years for ibandronate and risedronate (127–129). Continuation of treatment without the need for further assessment can generally be recommended in the following groups:

- Those aged 75 years or older.
- Those who have previously sustained a hip or vertebral fracture.
- Those who are taking continuous oral glucocorticoids in a dose of 7.5 mg/d or greater of prednisolone or equivalent.
- Individuals who sustain one or more low trauma fractures during treatment, after exclusion of poor adherence to treatment (e.g., less than 80% of treatment has been taken) and after causes of secondary osteoporosis have been excluded. In such cases, the treatment option should be reevaluated.
- If the total hip or femoral neck BMD T-score is –2.5 SD or less, continuation of treatment should generally be advised.

In these individuals in whom treatment is continued, treatment review should be performed every 5 years, including assessment of renal function.

If treatment is discontinued, fracture risk should be reassessed

- After a new fracture regardless of when this occurs
- If no new fracture occurs, after 2 years

As a part of risk assessment, a statistical tool can be utilized to determine fracture risk. There is a well-validated tool developed for this purpose. FRAX is a computer-based algorithm that provides models for the assessment of fracture probability in men and women (126). The approach uses easily obtained clinical risk factors (CRFs) to estimate 10-year fracture probability.

ATYPICAL FEMUR FRACTURES SECONDARY TO OSTEOPOROSIS TREATMENT

Bisphosphonate treatment increases the bone mass and reduces the risk of fractures in patients with osteoporosis by suppressing bone desorption. In spite of its clinical benefits, the long-term use of bisphosphonates has been linked to the occurrence of AFFs. Although the evidence has been controversial regarding the association between the occurrence of these fractures and bisphosphonate use, more recent studies with radiographic adjudication have indicated the significant associations between them (130).

These fractures were first described by Odvina and colleagues in 2005 (131). They suggested that long-term bisphosphonate therapy may lead to oversuppression of bone remodeling, resulting in an impaired ability to repair skeletal microcracks and increased skeletal fragility. The incidence of these fractures is quite variable with a significant difference in the results. Lenart and colleagues reported that radiographic features of AFFs were present in 31.7% of ST/FS cases (132). In Australia, Girgis and colleagues reviewed the radiographs of 152 patients with ST/FS fractures and confirmed that 20 patients (13%) had AFFs (133). In the Netherlands, Giusti and colleagues reported that the patients with AFFs comprised 16% (10/63) of subtrochanteric (ST)/femoral shaft (FS) fracture patients (134). In Sweden, Schilcher and colleagues reviewed the radiographs of 1234 of the 1271 female patients who had a ST/FS fracture in 2008 and identified 59 (4.8%) patients with AFFs (135). In the United Kingdom, Thompson and colleagues investigated 3515 patients with femoral fractures and identified 27 individuals with 29 AFFs, representing 0.8% of all hip fractures and 7% of FS fractures (136). According to the radiographic adjudication studies and large database studies, the incidence of AFFs can be estimated at between 0.3 and 11 per 100,000 person-years (137). Similarly, in the United States, Feldstein and others investigated the incidence of new femur fractures between 1996 and 2009 in female patients over 50 years old and male patients over 65 years old, and revealed that the incidence of AFFs was 5.9 per 100,000 person-years (95% CI 4.6–7.4), with 1,271,575 person-years observed (138). In Switzerland, Meier and colleagues reported that the incidence rate of AFFs was 3.2 cases per 100,000 person-years (139).

The American Society for Bone and Mineral Research (ASBMR) task force published its report regarding AFFs (140). They identified major and minor features of these fractures to standardize diagnosis. The fracture must be located along the femoral diaphysis from just distal to the lesser trochanter to just proximal to the supracondylar flare.

In addition, at least four of five major features must be present. None of the minor features is required, but they have sometimes been associated with these fractures.

Major features include the following:

- The fracture is associated with minimal or no trauma, as in a fall from a standing height or less.
- The fracture line originates at the lateral cortex and is substantially transverse in its orientation, although it may become oblique as it progresses medially across the femur.
- Complete fractures extend through both cortices and may be associated with a medial spike; incomplete fractures involve only the lateral cortex.
- The fracture is noncomminuted or minimally comminuted.
- Localized periosteal or endosteal thickening of the lateral cortex is present at the fracture site ("beaking" or "flaring").

Minor features include the following:

- Generalized increase in cortical thickness of the femoral diaphysis
- Unilateral or bilateral prodromal symptoms such as dull or aching pain in the groin or thigh
- Bilateral incomplete or complete femoral diaphysis fractures
- Delayed fracture healing

The mechanisms underlying the development of AFFs have not been fully understood. The characteristics of radiological features of AFFs, such as focal hypertrophy of the lateral cortex, periosteal and endosteal callus formation, and the transverse fracture line at the lateral cortex, suggest that fatigue damage accumulates within the bone cortex for a long period and that AFFs are stress or insufficiency fractures. A concentration of mechanical stress on the bone leads to the formation of microcracks, which heal by bone remodeling *via* the initiation of osteoclastic bone desorption, followed by osteoblastic bone formation to replace new bone. The pathogenesis of bisphosphonate-associated fractures seems to be related to the alterations of this tissue repair process as a result of the continuous suppression of the bone turnover rate (141). Ettinger and others proposed the mechanisms underlying the pathogenesis of AFFs by reviewing the evidence that supports suppression of bone turnover contributing to reduce bone material quality (142). They hypothesized that long-term decreased bone turnover causes tissue brittleness that initiates cracks, increases homogeneity of osteonal and interstitial structures, and impairs targeted repair by bone metabolic units. These pathogenic changes result in unimpeded crack progression and lead to the development of AFFs.

The surgical treatment of these fractures is not dissimilar to any other femur fractures, but physician input is important to evaluate the osteoporosis therapy. It is also useful to have some tissue histopathology of the bone tissue at the time of surgery.

CONCLUSION

Osteoporotic fractures are an extremely important public health concern now and will be in the decades to come. With a considerable increase in the aging population, the incidence of such fractures will continually rise. These fractures pose challenges both medically and surgically.

The exact scientific basis for osteoporosis is still being studied, and knowledge is constantly updated. Advances are also made in the surgical management of these fractures. As new evidence pours in, it is important to appraise the situation frequently.

A multidisciplinary approach is of paramount importance in treating these injuries. Ideally the team treating these fractures should have contributions from an ortho-geriatric physician, a rheumatologist, a specialist physiotherapist, and nurses and orthopedic surgeons interested in treating trauma. The medical comorbidities in these patients need regular input by physicians and affect the outcome more than the surgical intervention.

Having a protocol to treat these injuries helps to streamline their management. It minimizes the failure of fixation. Surgery should be well planned, and due diligence must be given to stable reduction, appropriate implant choice, and sound biomechanical fixation. Correct treatment not only restores the patient's quality of life but also reduces mortality and morbidity.

REFERENCES

1. Kannus P, Parkkari J, Sievänen H et al. Epidemiology of hip fractures. *Bone.* 1996;18:57S.
2. Wolinsky FD, Fitzgerald JF, Stump TE. The effect of hip fracture on mortality, hospitalization, and functional status: A prospective study. *Am J Public Health.* 1997;87:398.
3. Bentler SE, Liu L, Obrizan M et al. The aftermath of hip fracture: Discharge placement functional status change, and mortality. *Am J Epidemiol.* 2009;170:1290.
4. Neuman MD, Silber JH, Magaziner JS et al. Survival and functional outcomes after hip fracture among nursing home residents. *JAMA Intern Med.* 2014;174:1273.
5. Mariconda M, Costa GG, Cerbasi S et al. The determinants of mortality and morbidity during the year following fracture of the hip: A prospective study. *Bone Joint J.* 2015;97-B:383.
6. Frost SA, Nguyen ND, Black DA et al. Risk factors for in-hospital post-hip fracture mortality. *Bone.* 2011;49:553.
7. Orces CH. In-hospital hip fracture mortality trends in older adults: The National Hospital Discharge Survey, 1988–2007. *J Am Geriatr Soc.* 2013;61:2248.
8. Wu TY, Jen MH, Bottle A et al. Admission rates and in-hospital mortality for hip fractures in England 1998 to 2009: Time trends study. *J Public Health.* 2011;33:284.

9. Alzahrani K, Gandhi R, Davis A, Mahomed N. In-hospital mortality following hip fracture care in southern Ontario. *Can J Surg.* 2010;53:294.

10. Alvarez-Nebreda ML, Jiménez AB, Rodríguez P, Serra JA. Epidemiology of hip fracture in the elderly in Spain. *Bone.* 2008;42:278.

11. LaVelle DG. Fractures of hip. In: Canale ST, ed. *Campbell's Operative Orthopaedics.* 10th ed. Philadelphia, PA: Mosby, 2003, p. 2873.

12. Panula J, Pihlajamäki H, Mattila VM et al. Mortality and cause of death in hip fracture patients aged 65 or older: A population-based study. *BMC Musculoskelet Disord.* 2011;12:105.

13. LeBlanc ES, Hillier TA, Pedula KL et al. Hip fracture and increased short-term but not long-term mortality in healthy older women. *Arch Intern Med.* 2011;171:1831.

14. Brauer CA, Coca-Perraillon M, Cutler DM, Rosen AB. Incidence and mortality of hip fractures in the United States. *JAMA.* 2009;302:1573.

15. Morrison RS, Chassin MR, Siu AL. The medical consultant's role in caring for patients with hip fracture. *Ann Intern Med.* 1998;128:1010.

16. Haentjens P, Magaziner J, Colón-Emeric CS et al. Meta-analysis: Excess mortality after hip fracture among older women and men. *Ann Intern Med.* 2010;152:380.

17. Court-Brown CM, Caesar B. Epidemiology of adult fractures: A review. *Injury.* 2006;37:691–7.

18. Brunner LC, Eshilian-Oates L, Kuo TY. Hip fractures in adults. *Am Fam Physician.* 2003;67:537.

19. Gardner MJ, Lorich DG, Lane JM. Osteoporotic femoral neck fractures: Management and current controversies. *Instr Course Lect.* 2004;53:427–39.

20. World Health Organization Study Group. *Assessment of fracture risk and its application to screening for postmenopausal osteoporosis.* Report of a WHO study group. World Health Organization Technical Report Series; 1994, vol. 843, pp. 1–129.

21. Koot VCM, Kesselaer SMMJ, Clevers GJ, de Hooge P, Weits T, van der Werken C. Evaluation of the Singh index for measuring osteoporosis. *J Bone Joint Surg Series B.* 1996;78(5):831–4.

22. Kanis JA, Oden A, Johnell O, Jonsson B, de Laet C, Dawson A. The burden of osteoporotic fractures: A method for setting intervention thresholds. *Osteoporosis Int.* 2001;12(5):417–27.

23. Broderick JM, Bruce-Brand R, Stanley E, Mulhall KJ. Osteoporotic hip fractures: The burden of fixation failure. *Sci World J.* 2013;2013:515197.

24. Varela-Egocheaga JR, Iglesias-Colao R, Suárez-Suárez MA, Fernández-Villán M, González-Sastre V, Murcia-Mazon A. Minimally invasive osteosynthesis in stable trochanteric fractures: A comparative study between Gotfried percutaneous compression plate and Gamma 3 intramedullary nail. *Arch Orthop Trauma Surg.* 2009;129(10):1401–7.

25. Sadowski C, Lubbeke A, Saudan M, Riand N, Stern R, Höffmeyer P. Treatment of reverse oblique and transverse intertrochanteric fractures with use of an intramedullary nail or a 95° screw-plate: A prospective, randomized study. *J Bone Joint Surg Series A.* 2002;84(3):372–81.

26. Thakar C, Alsousou J, Hamilton TW, Willett K. The cost and consequences of proximal femoral fractures which require further surgery following initial fixation. *J Bone Joint Surg Series B.* 2010;92(12):1669–77.

27. Eastwood HDH. The social consequences of surgical complications for patients with proximal femoral fractures. *Age Ageing.* 1993;22(5):360–4.

28. Palmer SJ, Parker MJ, Hollingworth W. The cost and implications of reoperation after surgery for fracture of the hip. *J Bone Joint Surg Series B.* 2000;82(6):864–6.

29. Bjørgul Kand Reikeras O. Outcome after treatment of complications of Gamma nailing: A prospective study of 554 trochanteric fractures. *Acta Orthop.* 2007;78(2):231–5.

30. Sipila J, Hyvönen P, Partanen J, Ristiniemi J, Jalovaara P. Early revision after hemiarthroplasty and osteosynthesis of cervical hip fracture: Short-term function decreased, mortality unchanged in 102 patients. *Acta Orthop Scand.* 2004;75(4):402–7.

31. Tidermark J. Quality of life and femoral neck fractures. *Acta Orthop Scand Suppl.* 2003;74(309):1–42.

32. Frihagen F, Nordsletten L, Madsen JE. Hemiarthroplasty or internal fixation for intracapsular displaced femoral neck fractures: Randomised controlled trial. *Br Med J.* 2007;335(7632):1251–4.

33. Blomfeldt R, Tornkvist H, Ponzer S, Söderqvist A, Tidermark J. Displaced femoral neck fracture: Comparison of primary total hip replacement with secondary replacement after failed internal fixation: A 2-year follow-up of 84 patients. *Acta Orthop.* 2006;77(4):638–43.

34. Kopp L, Edelmann K, Obruba P, Prochazka B, Blstakova K, Dzupa V. Mortality risk factors in the elderly with proximal femoral fracture treated surgically. *Acta Chir Orthop Traumatol Cech.* 2009;76(1):41–6.

35. Soreide O, Lillestol J. Mortality patterns following internal fixation for acute femoral neck fractures in the elderly with special emphasis on potential excess mortality following reoperations. *Age Ageing.* 1980;9(1):59–63.

36. Foss NB, Palm H, Krasheninnikoff M, Kehlet H, Gebuhr P. Impact of surgical complications on length of stay after hip fracture surgery. *Injury.* 2007;38(7):780–4.

37. Hoelsbrekken SE, Opsahl JH, Stiris M, Paulsrud O, Stromsoe K. Failed internal fixation of femoral neck fractures. *Tidsskr Nor Laegeforen.* 2012;132(11):1343–7.

38. Raisz LG. Pathogenesis of osteoporosis: Concepts, conflicts, and prospects. *J Clin Investig.* 2005;115(12):3318–25.

39. Frost HM. Bone "mass" and the "mechanostat": A proposal. *Anat Rec.* 1987 Sep;219(1):1–9.

40. Ebeling PR, Atley LM, Guthrie JR, Burger HG, Dennerstein L, Hopper JL, Wark JD. Bone turnover

markers and bone density across the menopausal transition. *J Clin Endocrinol Metab.* 1996;81:3366–71.

41. Lee K, Jessop H, Suswillo R, Zaman G, Lanyon L. Endocrinology: Bone adaptation requires oestrogen receptor-alpha. *Nature.* 2003;424:389.

42. Prestwood KM. et al. The short-term effects of conjugated oestrogen on bone turnover in older women. *J Clin Endocrinol Metab.* 1994;79:366–71.

43. Prestwood KM, Kenny AM, Unson C, Kulldorff M. The effect of low dose micronized 17ss-estradiol on bone turnover, sex hormone levels, and side effects in older women: A randomized, double blind, placebo-controlled study. *J Clin Endocrinol Metab.* 2000;85:4462–9.

44. Prestwood KM, Kenny AM, Kleppinger A, Kulldorff M. Ultralow-dose micronized 17β-estradiol and bone density and bone metabolism in older women: A randomized controlled trial. *JAMA.* 2003;290:1042–8.

45. Modder UI. et al. Dose-response of oestrogen on bone versus the uterus in ovariectomized mice. *Eur J Endocrinol.* 2004;151:503–10.

46. Falahati-Nini A, Riggs BL, Atkinson EJ, O'Fallon WM, Eastell R, Khosla S. Relative contributions of testosterone and oestrogen in regulating bone desorption and formation in normal elderly men. *J Clin Invest.* 2000;106:1553–60.

47. Khosla S, Melton LJ, 3rd, Atkinson EJ, O'Fallon WM. Relationship of serum sex steroid levels to longitudinal changes in bone density in young versus elderly men. *J Clin Endocrinol Metab.* 2001;86:3555–61.

48. Van Pottelbergh I, Goemaere S, Zmierczak H, Kaufman JM. Perturbed sex steroid status in men with idiopathic osteoporosis and their sons. *J Clin Endocrinol Metab.* 2004;89:4949–53.

49. Windahl SH. et al. Female oestrogen receptor β⁻ mice are partially protected against age-related trabecular bone loss. *J Bone Miner Res.* 2001;16:1388–98.

50. Sims NA, Dupont S, Krust A et al. Deletion of oestrogen receptors reveals a regulatory role for oestrogen receptors-β in bone remodelling in females but not in males. *Bone.* 2002;30:18–25.

51. Albagha OM. et al. Association of oestrogen receptor α gene polymorphisms with postmenopausal bone loss, bone mass, and quantitative ultrasound properties of bone. *J Med Genet.* 2005;42:240–6.

52. Khosla S. et al. Relationship of oestrogen receptor genotypes to bone mineral density and to rates of bone loss in men. *J Clin Endocrinol Metab.* 2004;89:1808–16.

53. Bonnelye E, Aubin JE. Oestrogen receptor-related receptor α: A mediator of oestrogen response in bone. *J Clin Endocrinol Metab.* 2005;90:3115–21.

54. Laflamme N. et al. A frequent regulatory variant of the oestrogen-related receptor α gene associated with BMD in French-Canadian premenopausal women. *J Bone Miner Res.* 2005;20:938–44.

55. Goderie-Plomp HW. et al. Endogenous sex hormones, sex hormone-binding globulin, and the risk of incident vertebral fractures in elderly men and women: The Rotterdam Study. *J Clin Endocrinol Metab.* 2004;89:3261–9.

56. Van Pottelbergh I, Goemaere S, Kaufman JM. Bioavailable estradiol and an aromatase gene polymorphism are determinants of bone mineral density changes in men over 70 years of age. *J Clin Endocrinol Metab.* 2003;88:3075–81.

57. Kimble RB. et al. Simultaneous block of interleukin-1 and tumor necrosis factor is required to completely prevent bone loss in the early postovariectomy period. *Endocrinology.* 1995;136:3054–61.

58. Lorenzo JA. et al. Mice lacking the type I interleukin-1 receptor do not lose bone mass after ovariectomy. *Endocrinology.* 1998;139:3022–25.

59. Gao Y et al. Oestrogen prevents bone loss through transforming growth factor beta signaling in T cells. *Proc Natl Acad Sci USA.* 2004;101:16618–23.

60. Hughes DE. et al. Oestrogen promotes apoptosis of murine osteoclasts mediated by TGF-beta. *Nat Med.* 1996;2:1132–6.

61. Lean JM. et al. A crucial role for thiol antioxidants in oestrogen-deficiency bone loss. *J Clin Invest.* 2003;112:915–23.

62. Lean JM, Jagger CJ, Kirstein B, Fuller K, Chambers TJ. Hydrogen peroxide is essential for oestrogen-deficiency bone loss and osteoclast formation. *Endocrinology.* 2005;146:728–35.

63. Lips P. Vitamin D deficiency and secondary hyperparathyroidism in the elderly: Consequences for bone loss and fractures and therapeutic implications. *Endocrinol Rev.* 2001;22:477–501.

64. Bischoff-Ferrari HA. et al. Effect of vitamin D on falls: A meta-analysis. *JAMA.* 2004;291:1999–2006.

65. Sambrook PN et al. Serum parathyroid hormone predicts time to fall independent of vitamin D status in a frail elderly population. *J Clin Endocrinol Metab.* 2004;89:1572–6.

66. Grant AM. et al. Oral vitamin D3 and calcium for secondary prevention of low-trauma fractures in elderly people (Randomised Evaluation of Calcium Or vitamin D, RECORD): A randomised placebo-controlled trial. *Lancet.* 2005;365:1621–8.

67. Ferrari SL, Rizzoli R, Slosman DO, Bonjour JP. Do dietary calcium and age explain the controversy surrounding the relationship between bone mineral density and vitamin D receptor gene polymorphisms? *J Bone Miner Res.* 1998;13:363–70.

68. Morrison NA. et al. 2005. Vitamin D receptor genotypes influence the success of calcitriol therapy for recurrent vertebral fracture in osteoporosis. *Pharmacogenet Genomics.* 15:127–35.

69. Garnero P, Munoz F, Borel O, Sornay-Rendu E, Delmas PD. Vitamin D receptor gene polymorphisms are associated with the risk of fractures in postmenopausal women, independently of bone mineral density. The OFELY study. *J Clin Endocrinol Metab.* 2005;90:4829–35.

70. Lips P. Which circulating level of 25-hydroxyvitamin D is appropriate? *J. Steroid Biochem Mol Biol.* 2004;89–90:611–4.

71. Pasco JA. et al. Seasonal periodicity of serum vitamin D and parathyroid hormone, bone desorption, and fractures: The Geelong Osteoporosis Study. *J Bone Miner Res.* 2004;19:752–8.

72. Sambrook PN. et al. Serum parathyroid hormone is associated with increased mortality independent of 25-hydroxy vitamin D status, bone mass, and renal function in the frail and very old: A cohort study. *J Clin Endocrinol Metab.* 2004;89:5477–81.

73. Bollerslev J. et al. Calcium-sensing receptor gene polymorphism A986S does not predict serum calcium level, bone mineral density, calcaneal ultrasound indices, or fracture rate in a large cohort of elderly women. *Calcif Tissue Int.* 2004;74:12–17.

74. Suda T. et al. Modulation of osteoclast differentiation and function by the new members of the tumor necrosis factor receptor and ligand families. *Endocr Rev.* 1999;20:345–57.

75. Koch J. The laws of bone architecture. *Am J Anat.* 1917;21:177–298.

76. Rybicki EF, Simonen FA, Weis EB Jr. On the mathematical analysis of stress in the human femur. *J Biomech.* 1972;5(2):203–15.

77. Wani M, Wani M, Sultan A, Dar T. Subtrochanteric fractures—Current management options. *Internet J Orthop Surg.* 2009;17(2):1–8.

78. Joglekar SB, Lindvall EM, Martirosian A. Contemporary management of subtrochanteric fracture. *Orthop Clin North Am.* 2015;46(1):21–35.

79. Evans EM. The treatment of trochanteric fracture of femur. *J Bone Joint Surg.* 1949;31:190–203.

80. Gotfried Y. The lateral trochanteric wall. *Clin Orthop.* 2004;425:82–6.

81. Kyle RF, Gustilo RB, Premer RF. Analysis of 622 intertrochanteric hip fractures-a retrospective and prospective study. *J Bone Joint Surg.* 1979;61:216–21.

82. Muller ME, Nazarian S, Koch P, Schatzker J. *The AO Classification of Fractures of Long Bones.* Berlin, Heidelberg: Springer-Verlag, 1990.

83. Murray RC, Frew JFM. Trochanteric fractures of the femur: A plea for conservative treatment. *J Bone Joint Surg Br.* 1949;31:204–19.

84. Watson HK, Campbell RD, Wade PA. Classification, treatment, and complications of the adult subtrochanteric fracture. *J Trauma.* 1964;4:457–80.

85. Fielding JW, Magliato HJ. Subtrochanteric fractures. *Surg Gynecol Obstet.* 1966;122:555–60.

86. Cech O, Sosna A. Principles of the surgical treatment of subtrochanteric fractures. *Orthop Clin North Am.* 1974;5:651–62.

87. Zickel RE. An intramedullary fixation device for the proximal part of the femur. Nine years' experience. *J Bone Joint Surg Am.* 1976;58:866–72.

88. Waddell JP. Subtrochanteric fractures of the femur: A review of 130 patients. *J Trauma.* 1979;19:582–91.

89. Pankovich AM, Tarabishy IE. Ender nailing of intertrochanteric and subtrochanteric fractures of the femur: Complications, failures and errors. *J Bone Joint Surg Am.* 1980;62:635–45.

90. Harris LJ. Closed retrograde intramedullary nailing of peritrochanteric fractures of the femur with a new nail. *J Bone Joint Surg Am.* 1980;62:1185–93.

91. Malkawi H. Bone grafting in subtrochanteric fractures. *Clin Orthop.* 1982;168:69–72.

92. Zain Elabdien BS, Olerud S, Karlstrom G. Subtrochanteric fractures: Classification and results of Ender nailing. *Arch Orthop Trauma Surg.* 1984;103:241–50.

93. Winquist RA, Hansen ST, Clawson DK. Closed intramedullary nailing of femoral fractures. A report of five hundred and twenty cases. *J Bone Joint Surg Am.* 1984;66:529–53.

94. Ungar F, Cossi CG, Papliazzi A et al. Osteosynthesis of subtrochanteric fractures; a review of different methods. *Ital J Orthop Traumatol.* 1985;11:419–26.

95. Russell TA, Taylor JC. Subtrochanteric fractures of the femur. In: Browner BD, Jupiter JB, Levine AM, Trafton PG, eds. *Skeletal Trauma. Fractures, Dislocations, Ligamentous Injuries.* Philadelphia, PA: WB Saunders, 1992, pp. 1485–524.

96. Seinsheimer F. Subtrochanteric fractures of the femur. *J Bone Joint Surg Am.* 1978;60:300–6.

97. Goldhaggen PR, O'Connor DR, Schumarze D et al. Prospective comparative study of compression hip screw in the Gamma nail. *J Orthop Trauma.* 1994;8:367–72.

98. Leung K, So WS, Shung WY et al. Gamma nails and dynamic hip screws for peritrochanteric fractures—A randomized prospective in the elder patients. *J Bone Joint Surg.* 1992;74:345–51.

99. Radford PJ, Needoff M, Webb JK. A prospective prolonged comparison of the dynamic hip screw and the Gamma locking nail. *J Bone Joint Surg.* 1993;75B:789–93.

100. Williams WW, Parker BC. Complications associated with use of the Gamma nail. *Injury.* 1992;23:291.

101. Medoff RJ, Maes K, Mitsunaga M, Chappuis JL. Axial compression screw: A new implant for the fixation of the high subtrochanteric and unstable intertrochanteric fractures of the hip. *Poster exhibit at the 53rd Annual Meeting of the American Academy of Orthopaedic Surgeons*, New Orleans, LA, 1990.

102. Cheug CL, Chow SP, Leons TCV. Long term results and complications of cement augmentation in the treatment of unstable trochanteric fractures. *Injury.* 1989;20(3):134–8.

103. Dimon JH, Hughston JC. Unstable intertrochanteric fractures of the hip. *J Bone Joint Surg.* 1967;49-A:440–50.

104. Ban I, Birkelund L, Palm H, Brix M, Troelsen A. Circumferential wires as a supplement intramedullary nailing in unstable trochanteric hip fractures: 4 reoperations in 60 patients followed for 1 year. *Acta Orthop.* 2012;83(2):240–3.

105. Baumgaertner MR, Curtin SL, Lindskog DM, Keggi JM. The value of the tip-apex distance in predicting failure of fixation of peritrochanteric fractures of the hip. *J Bone Joint Surg Am.* 1995;77:1058–64.

106. Baumgaertner MR, Solberg BD. Awareness of tip-apex distance reduces failure of fixation of trochanteric fractures of the hip. *J Bone Joint Surg Br.* 1997;79:969–71.

107. Kyle RF, Cabanela ME, Russell TA et al. Fractures of the proximal part of the femur. *Instr Course Lect.* 1995;44:227–53.

108. Kyle RF, Gustilo RB, Premer RF. Analysis of six hundred and twenty-two intertrochanteric hip fractures. *J Bone Joint Surg Am.* 1979;61:216–21.

109. Haidukewych GJ, Israel TA, Berry DJ. Reverse obliquity fractures of the intertrochanteric region of the femur. *J Bone Joint Surg Am.* 2001;83:643–50.

110. Janzing HM, Houben BJ, Brandt SE et al. The Gotfried percutaneous compression plate versus the dynamic hip screw in the treatment of pertrochanteric hip fractures: Minimal invasive treatment reduces operative time and postoperative pain. *J Trauma.* 2002;52:293–8.

111. Knight WM, DeLee JC. Nonunion of intertrochanteric fractures of the hip: A case study and review [abstract]. *Orthop Trans.* 1982;6:438.

112. Kosygan KP, Mohan R, Newman RJ. The Gotfried percutaneous compression plate compared with the conventional classic hip screw for the fixation of intertrochanteric fractures of the hip. *J Bone Joint Surg Br.* 2002;84:19–22.

113. Sadowski C, Lübbeke A, Saudan M, Riand N, Stern R, Hoffmeyer P. Treatment of reverse oblique and transverse intertrochanteric fractures with use of an intramedullary nail or a 95° screw-plate: A prospective, randomized study. *J Bone Joint Surg Am.* 2002;84:372–81.

114. Kinast C, Bolhofner BR, Mast JW, Ganz R. Subtrochanteric fractures of the femur. Results of treatment with the 95° condylar blade-plate. *Clin Orthop Relat Res.* 1989;238:122–30.

115. Sanders R, Regazzoni P. Treatment of subtrochanteric femur fractures using the dynamic condylar screw. *J Orthop Trauma.* 1989;3:206–13.

116. Haidukewych GJ, Berry DJ. Hip arthroplasty for salvage of failed treatment of intertrochanteric hip fractures. *J Bone Joint Surg Am.* 2003;85:899–904.

117. Haidukewych GJ, Berry DJ. Salvage of failed internal fixation of intertrochanteric hip fractures. *Clin Orthop Relat Res.* 2003;412:184–8.

118. Koval KJ, Sala DA, Kummer FJ, Zuckerman JD. Postoperative weight-bearing after a fracture of the femoral neck or an intertrochanteric fracture. *J Bone Joint Surg Am.* 1998;80:352–6.

119. van Doorn R, Stapert JW. The long Gamma nail in the treatment of 329 subtrochanteric fractures with major extension into the femoral shaft. *Eur J Surg.* 2000;166:240–6.

120. Wu CC, Shih CH, Chen WJ, Tai CL. Treatment of cutout of a lag screw of a dynamic hip screw in an intertrochanteric fracture. *Arch Orthop Trauma Surg.* 1998;117:193–6.

121. Ostrum RF, Levy MS. Penetration of the distal femoral anterior cortex during intramedullary nailing for subtrochanteric fractures: A report of three cases. *J Orthop Trauma.* 2005;19:656–60.

122. Bolland MJ, Grey A, Avenell A, Gamble GD, Reid IR. Calcium supplements with or without vitamin D and risk of cardiovascular events: Reanalysis of the Women's Health Initiative limited access dataset and meta-analysis. *BMJ.* 2011;342:d2040.

123. Abrahamsen B, Sahota O. Do calcium plus vitamin D supplements increase cardiovascular risk? *BMJ.* 2011;342:d2080.

124. Li K, Kaaks R, Linseisen J, Rohrmann S. Associations of dietary calcium intake and calcium supplementation with myocardial infarction and stroke risk and overall cardiovascular mortality in the Heidelberg cohort of the European Prospective Investigation into Cancer and Nutrition study (EPIC Heidelberg). *Heart.* 2012;98:920–5.

125. National Osteoporosis Society. Vitamin D and bone health: A practical clinical guideline for patient management; 2013. Available from https://theros.org.uk

126. National Osteoporosis Guideline Group. Osteoporosis, Clinical guideline for prevention and treatment, Available from: http://www.shef.ac.uk/NOGG, Updated May 2013.

127. Black DM, Schwartz AV, Ensrud KE et al. Effects of continuing or stopping alendronate after 5 years of treatment: The Fracture Intervention Trial Long-Term Extension (FLEX): A randomized trial. *JAMA.* 2006;296:2927–38.

128. Ravn P, Christensen JO, Baumann M, Clemmesen B. Changes in biochemical markers and bone mass after withdrawal of ibandronate treatment: Prediction of bone mass changes during treatment. *Bone.* 1998;22:559–64.

129. Watts NB, Chines A, Olszynski WP et al. Fracture risk remains reduced one year after discontinuation of risedronate. *Osteoporos Int.* 2008;19:365–72.

130. Saita Y, Ishijima M, Kaneko K. Atypical femoral fractures and bisphosphonate use: Current evidence and clinical implications. *Ther Adv Chronic Dis.* 2015;6(4):185–93.

131. Odvina C, Zerwekh J, Rao D, Maalouf N, Gottschalk F, Pak C. Severely suppressed bone turnover: A potential complication of alendronate therapy. *J Clin Endocrinol Metab.* 2005;90:1294–301.

132. Lenart B, Neviaser A, Lyman S et al. Association of low-energy femoral fractures with prolonged bisphosphonate use: A case control study. *Osteoporos Int.* 2009;20:1353–62.

133. Girgis C, Sher D, Seibel M. Atypical femoral fractures and bisphosphonate use. *N Engl J Med.* 2010;362:1848–9.

134. Giusti A, Hamdy N, Dekkers O, Ramautar S, Dijkstra S, Papapoulos S. Atypical fractures and

bisphosphonate therapy: A cohort study of patients with femoral fracture with radiographic adjudication of fracture site and features. *Bone.* 2011;48:966–71.

135. Schilcher J, Michaelsson K, Aspenberg P. Bisphosphonate use and atypical fractures of the femoral shaft. *N Engl J Med.* 2011;364:1728–37.

136. Thompson R, Phillips J, McCauley, S, Elliott J, Moran C. Atypical femoral fractures and bisphosphonate treatment: Experience in two large United Kingdom teaching hospitals. *J Bone Joint Surg Br.* 2012;94:385–90.

137. Saita Y, Ishijima M, Mogami A et al. The incidence of and risk factors for developing atypical femoral fractures in Japan. *J Bone Miner Metab.* 2015 May;33(3):311–8

138. Feldstein A, Black D, Perrin N et al. Incidence and demography of femur fractures with and without atypical features. *J Bone Miner Res.* 2012;27:977–86.

139. Meier R, Perneger T, Stern R, Rizzoli, R, Peter R. Increasing occurrence of atypical femoral fractures associated with bisphosphonate use. *Arch Intern Med.* 2012;172:930–6.

140. Shane E, Burr D, Abrahamsen B et al. Atypical subtrochanteric and diaphyseal femoral fractures: Second report of a task force of the American Society for Bone and Mineral Research. *J Bone Miner Res.* 2014;29:1–23.

141. Mashiba T, Hirano T, Turner C, Forwood M, Johnston C, Burr D. Suppressed bone turnover by bisphosphonates increases microdamage accumulation and reduces some biomechanical properties in dog rib. *J Bone Miner Res.* 2000;15:613–20.

142. Ettinger B, Burr D, Ritchie R. Proposed pathogenesis for atypical femoral fractures: Lessons from materials research. *Bone.* 2013;55:495–500.

23

Osteoporotic distal femoral fractures

When to fix and how

CYRIL MAUFFREY and NICHOLAS A. ALFONSO

INTRODUCTION

Osteoporotic distal femur fractures are often challenging injuries to manage and treat. They commonly are intra-articular and comminuted, which makes reduction and maintenance of alignment/fixation arduous. The problem in most cases is poor bone quality and subsequent insufficient implant anchorage. This ultimately can lead to implant cutout, malunion, nonunion, and failure of fixation (1). In addition, several options exist in terms of fixation strategies and implant designs with limited prospective guidance from the literature.

Distal femur fractures account for less than 1% of all fractures and about 3%–6% of all femoral fractures (2,3). A simple mechanical fall is the most common etiology of distal femur fractures in osteoporotic bone, with studies showing peak incidence in elderly women (3,4). Periprosthetic distal femoral fractures are estimated to be 5.5% after primary total knee arthroplasty (TKA) and 30% after revision TKA (5). These incidences will likely increase with the aging population and subsequent knee arthroplasty surgeries (6). Simply put, orthopedic surgeons will be managing more distal femoral fractures with or without a periprosthetic component in the next decade.

The AO/Orthopaedic Trauma Association (OTA) fracture classification system is the most universally used for distal femur fractures (7). Fracture patterns are classified as type A (extra-articular), type B (partial articular/unicondylar), and type C (complete articular/bicondylar). Subclassification within fracture types A through C reflects the degree of comminution and instability. Of note, coronal plane partial articular fractures (Hoffa fractures) are designated as type B3. Type C fractures can also have coronal plane fracture lines.

WHEN TO FIX

Conservative management can be considered for stable and minimally displaced extra-articular fractures. These are treated with restricted weight-bearing in a hinged knee brace. Ambulation and early range of motion are encouraged. Weight-bearing can be advanced once radiographic evidence of healing is obtained, typically between 4 and 6 weeks.

In the younger patient, relative contraindications to surgery include nonambulatory status, medical unsuitability, and severe comminuted fractures that cannot be reconstructed (6). Treatment in these situations involves splinting or bracing with protected weight-bearing or skin/skeletal traction. Routine interval radiographs need to be obtained to monitor healing progress. However, these contraindications are exceedingly rare and even the most comminuted distal femur fractures can be reconstructed or even staged, with arthroplasty as the end goal.

In the elderly patient, conservative management of distal femoral fractures should seldom be selected. Weight-bearing restrictions in the elderly are associated with higher morbidity and mortality from various causes that include loss of knee function, deconditioning, pressure sores, pneumonia, and pulmonary embolus (6,8). Some literature supports surgical intervention even in nonambulatory patients to reduce the risk of such complications (8). In addition, similarly to hip fractures, a delay in surgery of more than 4 days may be associated with an increased risk of mortality (9). With this in mind, we recommend managing distal femoral fractures in elderly patients with a similar treatment philosophy as hip fractures—early surgical fixation allowing for early mobilization and return to function with lower morbidity and mortality.

In our opinion, an absolute contraindication for surgery in the osteoporotic patient is when the medical risk of undergoing anesthesia and surgery greatly outweighs the surgical benefits of early ambulation. Severely comminuted fractures that are un-reconstructable due to osteoporosis and/or degree of comminution may benefit from early mobilization with a distal femoral replacement.

Table 23.1 Factors surgeons need to consider between healthy and osteoporotic bone when deciding surgical indications and planning

Factors	Young healthy bone	Elderly osteoporotic bone
Restricted weight-bearing	Better tolerated	Higher morbidity/mortality rates
Reserve to undergo surgery	Better Less medical comorbidities	Limited and higher risks More medical comorbidities
Boney quality	Normal	Poor, soft
Reduction and stabilization	Less difficult Better fixation	More difficult (more comminution) Harder fixation Higher rates of implant cutout
Healing potential	Better biology Healthy skin	Higher malunion/nonunion rates Fragile skin

The decision to surgically fix osteoporotic distal femur fractures carries multiple important ramifications that need to be discussed with the patient and family. Osteoporotic distal femoral fractures will have less healing potential, are typically more comminuted, and will be more difficult to fix and stabilize than their nonosteoporotic counterparts. Additionally, the osteoporotic patient typically has less physiological reserve and may not be able to withstand lengthy surgeries without medical compromise. However, it is our opinion that the majority of elderly patients with a

distal femoral fracture benefit from surgical management and early mobilization. See Table 23.1 for differences in patients with healthy versus osteoporotic bone.

Surgical options can be broken down into five basic strategies depending on fracture pattern: minimally invasive plate osteosynthesis (MIPO), open reduction and internal fixation (ORIF) with locked plating systems, retrograde intramedullary nailing, a combination of plate/screw fixation with intramedullary nailing, or arthroplasty. Regardless of the strategy, the basic principles of length, alignment, and rotation must be followed. For intra-articular fractures, the aim is to obtain anatomical reduction, a task that is arduous in osteoporotic bone. TKA or distal femoral replacement are last-resort options. They may be considered in the setting of preexisting knee arthritis or fractures that are not amenable to fixation due to severe comminution and/or bone loss (10). See Figure 23.1 for our suggested treatment algorithm for osteoporotic distal femoral fractures.

HOW TO FIX

Initial management

Before proceeding to the operating room, a complete medical and surgical workup should be performed. Typically, patients with osteoporotic bone have other medical comorbidities that need to be addressed by a consulting medical service. Both knee and full-length femur radiographs should be obtained for fracture visualization. It is important to get full-length femoral films to rule out any proximal hardware that may be present. Advanced imaging is

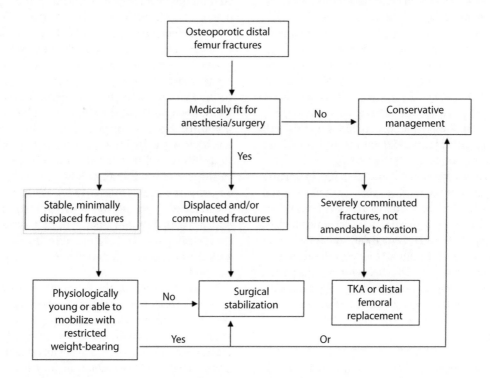

Figure 23.1 Suggested treatment algorithm for osteoporotic distal femoral fractures.

commonly ordered for these fractures since comminution is common. A computed tomography (CT) scan is often recommended in high-mechanism injuries or patients with osteoporosis to help identify intercondylar splits or coronal plane fractures that may not be obvious on plain radiographs. One study found the prevalence of associated coronal plane fractures to be 38% in a retrospective review of high-energy supracondylar-intercondylar distal femoral fractures (11). CT can further assist the surgeon with pre-operative planning, such as lag screw placement.

If the patient is medically unstable on arrival, a damage control orthopedic strategy should likely be utilized. Spanning external fixation can be quickly placed to restore length with minimal soft tissue damage and provide stability for the extremity until definitive fixation is more appropriate. In cases with severe comminution or if the patient remains physiologically unstable, external fixation can remain as a definitive treatment, but these circumstances are rare. External fixation does not allow for fixation of articular components and increases the risk for knee stiffness since bridging the knee is required.

Anatomy

Understanding the unique geometry of the distal femur in all three planes is important for preoperative planning. The normal anatomical axis of the femoral shaft is oriented between 6° and 11° of valgus in relation to the joint. This is an important factor to keep in mind to help restore the normal mechanical axis of the limb, prevent varus collapse, and maintain joint function. Additionally, the medial and lateral cortices of the distal femur taper anteriorly toward the midline. This trapezoidal shape needs to be taken into consideration when placing screws and determining screw length. Internal rotation views can be used to help confirm lengths and prevent hardware irritation from prominent screws medially. Intra-articular placement of screws anteriorly in the trochlea or within the notch posteriorly also needs to be avoided. An intercondylar notch view can also help assess appropriate placement of hardware. Anatomically precontoured locking plates are usually designed to fit along a specific aspect of the femur to help avoid screw penetration in these areas. This is often on the anterior half of the distal femur and approximating the border of the articular surface. Regardless, a detailed understanding of the distal femur anatomy and proper placement of your chosen implant are crucial for success.

Positioning

In almost all cases the patient is positioned supine on a radiolucent table. Care should be taken to pad all bony prominences, since patients with osteoporotic bone are likely to have fragile soft tissues and are prone to skin breakdown. A bump underneath the hip on the ipsilateral side of the fracture helps keep the injured extremity from falling into external rotation. Fluoroscopy is often placed perpendicular to the long axis of the table and on the contralateral side of the injured extremity in order to get anteroposterior (AP) and lateral views. A sterile bump underneath the knee or radiolucent triangle can be a very helpful tool not only for extremity positioning but also for assistance with fracture reduction. Keep in mind that retrograde intramedullary nailing requires at least 70° of knee flexion in order to obtain a correct nail entry point. Lateral positioning can also be considered, especially for extra-articular fractures. A lateral position can also help with exposure in cases with patients that have large body habitus, as soft tissue will fall away from the wound.

Approaches

There are several approaches to the distal femur and knee that can be utilized. The approach or combination of approaches is dependent on fracture pattern and implant choice. A direct lateral approach can often be used in simple, extra-articular fractures. With this approach, the iliotibial band is split in line with the incision, and the vastus lateralis is subsequently reflected anteriorly to gain access to the femur. Since a majority of fracture patterns in osteoporotic bone will be intra-articular, a lateral parapatellar arthrotomy is commonly the workhorse approach for osteoporotic patients. Swashbuckler and Mini-swashbuckler approaches have also been described for distal femoral fractures (12,13). These approaches also expose the articular surface via a lateral parapatellar arthrotomy but with arguably less invasive skin and soft tissue dissection.

The medial approach to the distal femur can be considered with isolated medial condyle or severely comminuted bicondylar fractures. An incision is made straight medially and centered over the fracture site, with distal extension made anterior to the adductor tubercle. Fascia is then divided in line with the skin incision with the interval between the sartorius and vastus medialis to expose the femur. The superficial femoral artery should be identified and retracted posteriorly in this approach. Although a medial parapatellar arthrotomy is the workhorse approach in knee arthroplasty, it is less useful in distal femur fixation given difficulty with proximal extension. Regardless, accessory medial incisions can be made if necessary in combination with lateral-sided approaches to help visualize and reduce fracture fragments.

For retrograde intramedullary nailing, a longitudinal anterior incision is used, with either a tendon split or parapatellar arthrotomy. Since the patella and tibial tuberosity are more lateral structures, a medial arthrotomy usually allows for easier access to the nail start point. In the coronal plane, the starting point is in the center of the femoral notch, just anterior to the posterior cruciate ligament. The tip of the guidewire in the sagittal plane is on the superior margin of Blumensaat's line on a true lateral fluoroscopic view. Before advancing the guide pin, guidewire trajectory toward the center of the intramedullary canal and starting point is finally confirmed on both AP and lateral views using fluoroscopy. A soft tissue protector is then used while reaming to protect the patella tendon and other intra-articular structures.

Plating surgical strategy

In healthy bone, simple fracture patterns can be addressed with absolute stability using AO techniques of compressive plating or lag screw fixation with neutralization plating. Unfortunately, this is usually not feasible in osteoporotic bone that has poor fixation quality and comminution. In this environment, even simple osteoporotic fractures will require indirect reduction and bridge plating to preserve fracture biology.

MIPO can be a powerful strategy in the setting of simple and extra-articular metaphyseal fracture patterns. An indirect reduction can be obtained and confirmed using fluoroscopy. The skin incision is just a shorter version of an open lateral approach to the distal femur. In general, blade plates have fallen out of favor, especially when treating osteoporotic bone given the lack of fixation properties with bad quality bone. Additionally, new-generation locking plates have shown to be biomechanically superior to blade plates (14). New-generation Condylar LCP hardware is anatomically designed and precontoured to match the distal femur. These plates have both nonlocking and locking screw-hole options. Straight plates are available for shorter constructs where curve plates are precontoured to mimic the anterior convexity of the femoral shaft and can be used for longer constructs.

The plate is then inserted underneath the belly of the vastus lateralis through a submuscular tunnel along the lateral femur. Assembling the guides to the distal aspect of the plate can help control and maneuver the plate as you advance it proximally. It is pertinent on lateral views to confirm that the plate is appropriately placed and not off the bone either anteriorly or posteriorly along the femur. K-wires can be placed both proximally and distally to help hold the plate in place once in appropriate position. Many plates have a central guidewire at the distal end that can also help with plate positioning and should be placed parallel to the joint line. Stab incisions can then be made proximally in line with the screw holes on the plate with the help of fluoroscopy. Be sure to sharply cut through skin down to bone so that soft tissue and fascia do not become problematic with screw insertion. A common pitfall is making the stab incisions too small.

New-generation locking plates are typically required once fracture patterns become more comminuted, more distal, and intra-articular. Most plates are designed to fit on the lateral side of the femur with an open lateral approach to the distal femur. These new-generation plates offer the versatility of multiple distal screw-hole options with the ability to either compress or use locking screws. This versatility creates the opportunity to capture multiple fracture fragments while maintaining rigid reductions of comminuted fracture patterns. Proximal

screw insertion can be either open or using the MIPO technique.

Many manufacturers are now offering polyaxial plates, which offer even greater versatility with screw positioning. These plates are ideal in the setting of comminuted intra-articular fractures. With the polyaxial component, screws can be angled away from the articular surface, a prosthesis already implanted, or lag screws that have already been placed in the articular block.

Medial plating can be used as well, but typically only in the setting of an isolated medial condyle fracture or an adjunct to lateral plating. Fractures with severe metaphyseal comminution and bone loss are at a higher rate of failure and fall into varus collapse. In these cases, supplemental medial plate fixation in addition to a lateral plate can be used to gain greater stability and strengthen the construct (15).

Finally, carbon-fiber-reinforced implants are gaining popularity due to material advantages. This implant trend can also be used in the setting of osteoporotic distal femur fractures. These implants have the advantage of being able to assess the quality of reduction in the sagittal plane, something difficult to assess using traditional metal implants. They also do not create metal artifact typically seen on CT and magnetic resonance imaging (MRI). Additionally, these carbon-fiber-reinforced implants can be manufactured to have properties more compliant than metal, better matching the modulus of elasticity of bone. Keep in mind that too much flexibility can potentially lead to pseudarthrosis, and the radiolucent nature of the material precludes direct visualization of the implants radiographically (although radiopaque markers are often added to help with visualization) (16). Pitfalls with the locking mechanisms of these implant have been highlighted in our personal experience. In addition, prospective studies will be required to support their use.

Intramedullary nailing surgical strategy

Extra-articular fracture patterns are a great indication for intramedullary nailing (IMN) fixation. There are several theoretical advantages to IMN in the osteoporotic patient given that it is a load-sharing device. It often allows for minimal disruption of soft tissue and periosteum around the fracture site, an important quality if the patient already has diminished healing potential and poor skin quality.

With the advent of newer implants, the indications for the use of IMN for intra-articular distal femur fractures have greatly expanded. These new devices now offer multiple distal screw position options that allow for fixation of articular reconstruction in multiple planes. Additionally, some or all of the distal screws can be locked to the nail, creating fixed-angle constructs. The 33C AO/OTA type fractures are no longer a contraindication with these newer-generation nails. If this strategy is used, nailing should follow ORIF with lag screw fixation of the articular surface. A medial or lateral parapatellar approach can be used to reconstruct the articular block (consider the need for future total knee arthroplasty). The IMN can typically also use this same incision for retrograde nail insertion. With this in mind, it becomes important to preoperatively plan and critically think about lag screw placement in order to prepare for IMN passage.

Both standard and short length nail options exist depending on fracture type. Shorter options should allow for placement of at least two interlock screws proximally. Standard length nails should extend to the level of the lesser trochanter. Longer nails increase the working length of the construct and can use isthmal fit to aid in nail stability. They also have the theoretical advantage of preventing future periprosthetic fractures. Regardless of nail length, multiple distal screws are necessary to control alignment and stability of the construct. Using clinical evaluation and fluoroscopy is essential in confirming final nail positioning before placing interlocking screws. Overseating the nail can limit interlocking options in the articular block, while underseating the nail can leave prominent hardware in the knee joint leading to articular erosion.

Plating versus nailing

Currently, there is no "gold standard" that has been identified in the orthopedic literature as to which implant should be used in osteoporotic distal femoral fractures. There is no study thus far demonstrating that one implant choice is clearly superior compared to the other. Published reports over the past decade looking at titanium alloy retrograde nails and modern-day plates for distal femur fractures all report mostly good results (17). The largest randomized study, thus far, by Tornetta et al. described marginally improved results with nails over plates in a prospective, randomized, multicenter study on 126 patients with distal femur fractures (18). Since no clear guidelines exist in the literature, the decision of plating versus nailing often comes down to surgeon preference and comfort.

Although no absolute indications exist, there are some general considerations and relative indications when choosing between plating versus nailing. Plating is often needed if a condylar segment is too short to allow nailing or the fracture pattern is too distal for interlocking screw fixation. In periprosthetic fractures around a TKA femoral component with a closed box design (posterior cruciate ligament substituting), a locking plate is likely the only option. Finally, retrograde nailing may not be an option when preexisting total hips or anterograde femoral nails have already been implanted. If a retrograde nail is chosen in this setting, a plate needs to be placed to bridge the two intramedullary implants with the intent of avoiding a stress riser.

One of the main drawbacks to using plating as the surgical implant is that it may allow early knee range of motion, but not necessarily early weight-bearing. This is a crucial component when managing patients with osteoporotic distal femur fractures. Since a retrograde intramedullary nail is a load-sharing construct, it may allow for immediate weight-bearing. As previously discussed, early mobilization is what can decrease morbidity and mortality in these patients and why we argue that surgical management is indicated in almost every case. One disadvantage of nailing is that it does violate the knee joint, with a theoretical increased risk of septic arthritis and damage to intra-articular structures during nail placement when compared to plating.

Combination of plating and nailing surgical strategy

Taking advantage of the strengths of both implant designs by creating a combination plate-nail construct has been described and can be useful in some circumstances (19). Even the new-generation nails designed for distal femur fixation may not offer enough fixation in very distal fracture patterns. In this case, a distal femoral locking plate can be used to create a fixed-angle construct capturing distal fragments, while adding the nail component offers the potential for early weight-bearing. Replacing a medial plate with an IMN for additional fixation to a lateral plate construct already in place can be considered in the setting of severe comminution or bone loss. The IMN once again adds the potential advantages of early weight-bearing and decreased soft tissue disruption compared to dual-plate fixation.

Periprosthetic distal femur fracture considerations

As mentioned earlier, the incidence of osteoporotic, periprosthetic distal femur fractures will likely increase as the elderly population continues to grow with subsequent increases in knee arthroplasty. Similar to fractures without previously placed implants, surgical intervention is indicated in almost all periprosthetic fractures. We would once again argue that the only contraindication is a patient who is medically unsuitable for surgery. Operative management offers the ability to correct alignment, restore implant stability, begin early knee range of motion, and possibly begin early weight-bearing. If the implant is found to be stable, then the implant type and fracture pattern will determine what options are possible for fixation.

If the fracture occurs around a TKA, the exact type of femoral component should be retrieved if possible. This is important in order to determine if a retrograde nail is able to pass through the intercondylar notch (typically seen in posterior cruciate ligament substituting implants with an open box design). An opening equal to or greater than 1 mm larger than the size of the intended nail is recommended, and the component must allow appropriate passage and seating of the nail within the medullary canal (6). A previously published study can be accessed that lists components that allow retrograde nail passage (20).

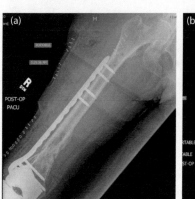
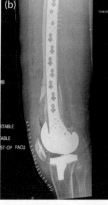

Figure 23.2 (a) AP radiograph. (b) lateral radiograph of a periprosthetic distal femoral fracture stabilised with a locking plate.

Retrograde nailing through a femoral component is not without risks. The starting point of a retrograde femoral nail in relation to the femoral component design (especially cruciate retaining) can inherently deviate the guide pin posterior to Blumensaat's line, predisposing to recurvatum deformity (21). Finally, it has also been shown that increasing the number of distal interlocking screws reduces the risk of nonunion and reoperation (22,23).

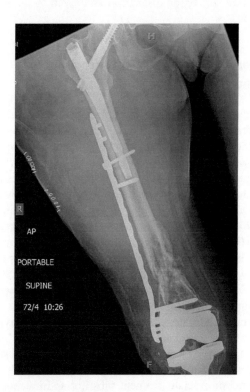

Figure 23.3 Postoperative radiographs of a locked plate construct in a patient with a distal femoral fracture with stable previously placed hardware both proximal and distal to the fracture site. Unicortical screws are used proximally in order to obtain fixation with previously implanted hardware already in place.

Locking plate implants can be used as well or when the femoral component does not allow passage or the appropriate starting point of a retrograde nail (Figure 23.2). In periprosthetic distal femur fractures, polyaxial plates can be very useful in regard to giving the surgeon the versatility of directing screws away from the implant at multiple sites of fixation. Unicortical locking screws can be placed if unable to avoid previously placed hardware, and cables can be incorporated in the final construct to add additional stability (Figure 23.3).

Distal femoral reconstruction strategy

In our opinion, most cases of osteoporotic distal femurs are amendable to surgical fixation and osteosynthesis. With that said, there are circumstances in which arthroplasty or distal femoral replacement need to be considered. In fracture patterns with severe comminution or bone loss, fixation may not be possible. Additionally, preexisting arthritis may indicate the need for primary arthroplasty, while a periprosthetic fracture with an unstable component may require revision arthroplasty. This would warrant a discussion with the patient about the risks and benefits of fixation versus reconstruction. If total knee arthroplasty, revision arthroplasty, or distal femoral replacement is chosen, then the expertise of an arthroplasty surgeon with a special interest in these complex injuries is often required (24,25).

TIPS AND TRICKS

Regardless of implant choice, the basic principles of length, alignment, and rotation should always be obtained. AO principles have been shown to reduce the chances of posttraumatic arthritis and allow for early knee range of motion (26,27). Thus, restoration of the congruity of the articular surface is essential for intra-articular fractures. In general, the first task is anatomical reduction and fixation of the articular block. This is then followed by fixation of the articular segment to the remainder of the femur, all while maintaining mechanical alignment of the extremity. Restoring the patient's normal mechanical alignment is crucial for normal knee joint function and to prevent altered biomechanics leading to early arthritis (28).

Reconstruction of the articular block and restoration of congruence of the articular surface can be difficult tasks, especially with osteoporotic bone. The use of reduction clamps and K-wires can help hold fragments in place with subsequent interfragmentary screw placement. Addressing intercondylar fractures initially can be helpful when first reconstructing the articular block (Figure 23.4). A good general rule, especially when working with comminuted fractures, is slowly building off the largest intact fragment until the entire block is reconstructed. As previously mentioned, keep the position of interfragmentary screw insertion in mind so as to not interfere with subsequent plate or nail placement (Figure 23.5).

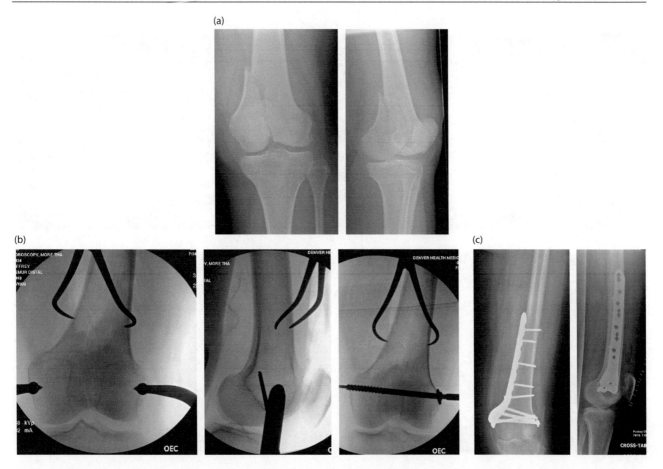

Figure 23.4 (a) Anteroposterior (AP) and lateral radiographs of an intercondylar split distal femur fracture. (b) Reduction technique for reducing fracture is shown. Clamps are used to reduce the fracture in anatomical alignment. A cannulated, partially threaded screw is placed to hold reduction after a guidewire is placed and confirmed to be in the appropriate position. (c) AP and lateral radiographs of the final construct.

Initially restoring length, even before articular surface reduction, can have several advantages. The surgeon can often better appreciate fracture patterns or comminution both clinically and with the use of fluoroscopy once the fracture is back out to length. Traction of the distal fragment can help improve overall alignment and initiate fracture reduction via ligamentotaxis. Additionally, restoring length usually eases the reduction of articular fragments during an open reduction. Complete skeletal paralysis in combination with manual traction can be used. If help in the operating room is limited, proximal tibia traction pin placement with the weight hanging at the end of the bed is a useful trick (Figure 23.6). Finally, the universal distractor device is a very powerful tool when help is limited or restoring length is difficult.

Since no varus malalignment is acceptable, coronal alignment is considered the most important to restore and also the most difficult to overcome (6,29). Manual traction with good skeletal paralysis can once again be useful techniques. If tibial skeletal traction is placed, the surgeon can adjust the angle of the weight hanging off the bed as needed. Percutaneous clamps and bone hooks can

be used to manipulate fragments while trying to maintain biology.

Anatomically precontoured distal femoral plates can help assist in coronal plane deformity as well. These plates can be used with extra-articular fractures or intra-articular fractures once the articular block has been reconstructed with an anatomically reduced articular surface. Precontoured plates often account for the valgus angle of the distal femur in regard to the mechanical axis. If this is the case, then screws placed parallel to the joint line in the distal aspect of the implant can be expected to reproduce correct coronal plan angulation when the shaft is reduced to the plate (Figure 23.7).

There is a recurvatum deformity in the sagittal plane in nearly all cases due to the deforming forces of the gastrocnemius pulling on the articular block. If there is a condylar split, then a rotational component can add to the deformity with the different heads of the gastrocnemius affecting each condyle differently. As previously stated, coronal plane fractures are commonly associated with condylar splits, which need to be identified and addressed. A radiolucent triangle, towel rolls, and small bumps can assist in

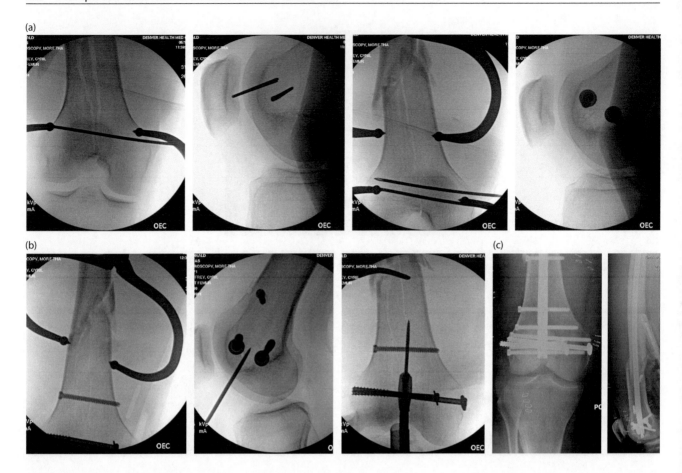

Figure 23.5 (a) Intraoperative fluoroscopy images demonstrating anatomical reduction of an intercondylar split distal femur fracture using percutaneous clamps. Reduction is then subsequently held in place with cannulated, partially threaded screws. (b) A blocking screw is placed to help prevent recurvatum deformity. The starting point for retrograde nail is then found and the opening reamer is advanced into the distal femur. Note how the interfragmentary screws were positioned to allow for reamer and nail passage. (c) Anteroposterior and lateral radiographs of final construct.

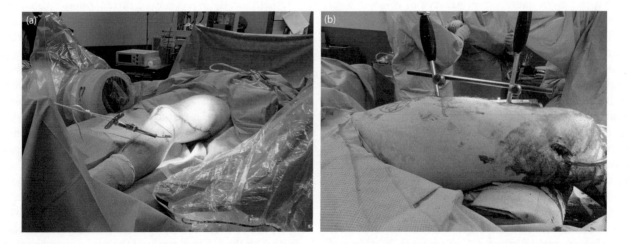

Figure 23.6 (a) Intraoperative positioning showing proximal tibia skeletal traction with weights hanging off the end of the bed. Notice that C-arm is positioned on the opposite side of where the surgeon would be standing. (b) Patient positioning once again showing skeletal traction. Note the sterile bump underneath the distal femur to help correct the sagittal deformity. Additionally, external fixation pins were placed to assist in fracture reduction and help maintain length.

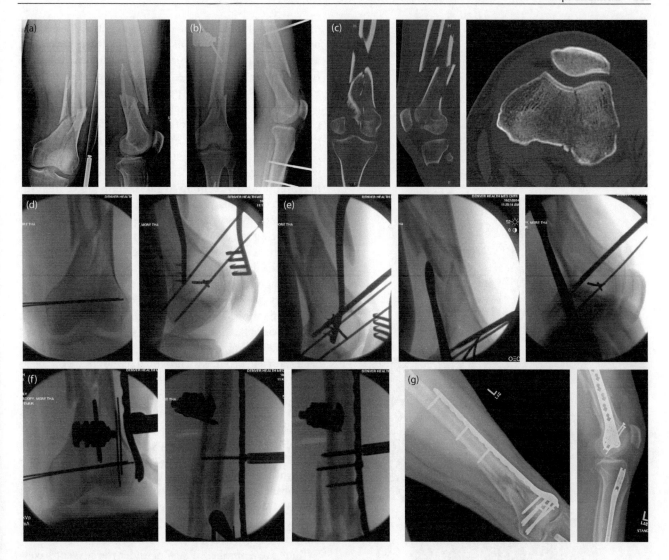

Figure 23.7 (a) Anteroposterior (AP) and lateral radiographs of a comminuted and intercondylar distal femur fracture. (b) Injury films after application of a knee-spanning external fixation device. (c) Computed tomography images of the injury post external fixation. Note the coronal plane fracture (Hoffa fragment) seen on the sagittal and axial views that is not appreciated on the plain radiographs. (d) Intraoperative fluoroscopy demonstrating anatomical reduction and provisional fixation using K-wires of the articular block. (e) Next, a Schanz pin is placed in an anterior to posterior direction into the distal, now intact, articular block. With the use of the Schanz pin and a Cobb elevator, the sagittal plane deformity can be corrected and subsequently held in place using external fixation. (f) Fluoroscopy shots demonstrating how a precontoured anatomical plate and nonlocking cortical screw can be used to help reduce the fracture in the coronal plane. After plate fixation, now the comminuted diaphyseal-metaphyseal segment is bridged to the reconstructed articular block. (g) AP and lateral radiographs displaying the final construct.

correcting sagittal deformities. Schanz pins can be placed into the articular block or individual condyles and manipulated with a T-hand chuck for reduction (Figure 23.8). If external fixation happened to be placed for provisional stabilization, consider leaving the pins in place for the same reason for placing a Schanz pin. Assess your correction using perfect fluoroscopic lateral views and correlating Blumensaat's line relative to the long axis of the femur (17). Coronal plane fractures can be provisionally held in place with K-wires after anatomical reduction. Headless screws may be needed depending on articular involvement. A Cobb elevator can also be placed posterior to the proximal end of the distal segment (under the extended segment) and lifted up toward the ceiling to correct the apex posterior deformity.

Length, alignment, and rotation must be reassessed after final reduction of the articular block has been made to the proximal aspect of the femur using plates and/or an IMN. This should be done both clinically and radiographically with perfect AP and lateral views of the femur. Rotation can be assessed comparing to the contralateral side with one or a combination of clinical exam, radiography using the lesser trochanter profile, or the direct measurement method (30–32).

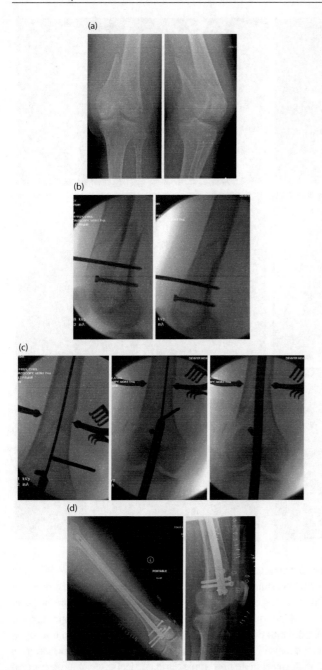

Figure 23.8 (a) Anteroposterior (AP) and lateral radiographs of an extra-articular distal femoral fracture. (b) Intraoperative fluoroscopy images displaying using a Schanz pin percutaneously to reduce the sagittal plane deformity. Reduction clamps are then used percutaneously to hold the reduction in place. Also note the placement of the blocking screw on the concave side of the coronal place deformity, distal to the fracture site. (c) Images showing introduction of the guide pin, reamer, and subsequent retrograde nail insertion. The reduction clamp remains in place during this process. (d) AP and lateral radiographs of the final construct.

Avoidable fixation pitfalls

There are many reduction and fixation pitfalls that can eventually lead to malunion or nonunion in osteoporotic

distal femoral fractures and that can potentially be avoided using good technique. Insufficient fracture reduction, a poor starting point, or eccentric reaming may lead to fracture malalignment when using a retrograde intramedullary nail. Since there is poor cortical contact in osteoporotic bone and the metaphysis of the distal femur in general, the starting point of nail insertion becomes critical in maintaining alignment. Fractures need to be adequately reduced before reaming and insertion of the nail, otherwise nail placement will cause malreduction. If choosing to ream, typically ream up to 1.0–1.5 mm larger than the anticipated nail size. Finally, blocking screws can be used in the metaphysis to help guide the nail and keep it from malreducing the articular block to the proximal segment. These screws should be applied on the concave side of the anticipated deformity.

Although the advent of improved biomechanical locking plates has provided a new frontier in fracture stability and fixation, especially in osteoporotic bone, there are still complications when these implants are not used appropriately. Failure of fixation with varus collapse has been shown to occur, with proximal screw failure or breakage of the locked screws at the plate interface frequently implicated (33,34). Causes of fixation failure include high-energy fracture with extensive metaphyseal comminution, poor reduction, poor plate position or fixation, and early weight-bearing before radiographic evidence of union (6,34). These fixed angled devices can also create an environment that is too stiff, leading to poor callous quality and subsequent delayed union and nonunion (Figure 23.9) (35–38). Higher nonunion rates have been reported after plating than previously thought since the development of this technology (17,39).

There are a number of factors under the surgeon's control that can affect construct stiffness and help avoid nonunion: implant metallurgy, choice of locking/nonlocking screws, bicortical/unicortical fixation, plate length, and screw-hole fill. For instance, a plate's working length is decreased the closer the distal most diaphyseal screw is to the fracture site, which subsequently diminishes micromotion needed for callous formation. The surgeon can modulate stiffness by using longer plates with well-spaced screws. Spreading fixation over a longer length has the advantages of increasing working length and decreasing stress concentration, all of which will reduce the risk of premature fixation failure. Locking screws are typically indicated in most osteoporotic bone fixation, but nonlocking screws can be considered in better-quality bone, such as in the femoral diaphysis. Another general rule is that no more than 50% of plate holes above the fracture site should be filled. One other caveat is that postoperative thigh pain has been correlated with stiffness at the end of the plate, possibly from using a locking screw at the most proximal screw hole. This is linked to higher risk of periprosthetic fractures as well. The surgeon should consider the use of a nonlocking screw, unicortical locking screw, or angulated locking screw at the proximal-most hole for these reasons (17,40,41).

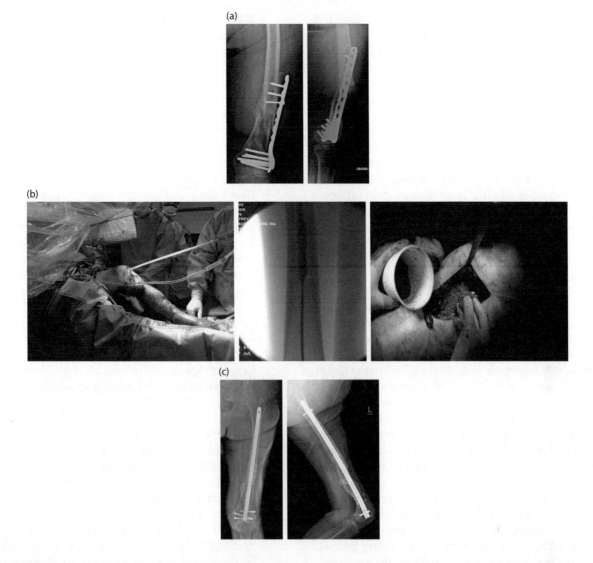

Figure 23.9 (a) Anteroposterior (AP) and lateral radiographs demonstrating a failed plate construct for a comminuted distal femur fracture. Note the relatively short plate and short working length, contributing to a stiff construct and subsequent failure of fracture healing. (b) Intraoperative images showing the use of the reamer-irrigator-aspirator device (RIA). Bone graft from the RIA is then used in a Masquelet-type technique to add additional biology to the comminuted fracture site. (c) AP and lateral radiographs revealing a healed fracture with abundant callous formation using a retrograde intramedullary nail construct.

In the setting of severe comminution or bone loss, the surgeon can consider acute bone grafting or cement augmentation. Bone cement can be placed once final reduction and fixation have been obtained. The cement can be added around already placed implants and fill defects to help add stability to the final construct. Acute bone grafting can be obtained by using a reamer-irrigator-aspirator device (RIA) on the femur of the injured side, or even the contralateral side if needed. Iliac crest bone graft or other common sources of bone autograft can be used as well (see Figure 23.9).

POSTOPERATIVE CARE

Before leaving the operating room, the femoral neck should be evaluated under fluoroscopy to rule out fracture, and a ligamentous knee exam should be performed. A hinged knee brace can be placed if there is a concern for an unstable ligamentous knee. Chemical deep venous thrombosis prophylaxis should be considered and can be started on postoperative day 1. Most importantly, physical and occupational therapy should be consulted to help with mobilization. Gait training and knee range of motion should start on postoperative day 1 at a minimum. Continuous passive motion machines can be considered if the patient is not mobilizing well.

Weight-bearing restriction and advancement is probably the most controversial topic in regard to postoperative care. Traditionally, weight-bearing is not advanced until there is radiographic evidence of callous formation. This would mean about 6–8 weeks in extra-articular fractures and 10–12 weeks in intra-articular fractures. With these restrictions, some osteoporotic patients would become nonambulatory and subsequently develop the complications that follow bedbound status. Although it was stated that early weight-bearing can lead to failure of fixation and nonunion, some evidence does show that weight-bearing as tolerated has better outcomes in the elderly (42,43). It is our opinion that early, if not immediate, weight-bearing should be encouraged in the geriatric population, especially if an intramedullary nail is used. We believe that the benefits of early weight-bearing outweigh the risks of possible fixation failure, especially since the main reason for deciding to pursue surgical fixation in this population is to avoid a nonambulatory status. Ultimately, the weight-bearing status is up to the operating surgeon's discretion, with careful thought put into the stability of the final construct and the health status of the patient.

CONCLUSION

Osteoporotic distal femoral fractures are difficult fractures to manage and treat. Reduction of these fractures can be very challenging given the poor bone quality, degree of comminution, and often insufficient implant fixation. All of these qualities put osteoporotic distal femoral fractures at higher risk of malunion and nonunion. Management and timing of surgery for osteoporotic distal femoral fractures should mirror protocols used for the elderly hip fracture population. The goal is early fixation to allow for early mobilization.

With no clear "gold standard" of fixation for distal femoral fractures, surgeons are faced with deciding on a number of treatment strategies and different implant options. These can be broken down into five basic strategies depending on fracture pattern: MIPO, ORIF with locked plating systems, retrograde intramedullary nailing, a combination of plate/screw fixation with intramedullary nailing, or arthroplasty. Regardless of the strategy, the basic principles of length, alignment, and rotation remain essential. Novel implants and materials such as PEEK locking distal femoral plates may become game changers in the field of distal femur fractures with advantages that include visualization of reduction quality in the sagittal plane and a Young modulus closer to bone allowing for more callus formation (44,45).

REFERENCES

1. Rosen AL, Strauss E. Primary total knee arthroplasty for complex distal femur fractures in elderly patients. *Clin Orthop Relat Res.* 2004;(425):101–5.
2. Court-Brown CM, Caesar B. Epidemiology of adult fractures: A review. *Injury.* 2006;37(8):691–7.
3. Martinet O, Cordey J, Harder Y, Maier A, Buhler M, Barraud GE. The epidemiology of fractures of the distal femur. *Injury.* 2000;31(Suppl 3):C62–3.
4. Arneson TJ, Melton LJ III, Lewallen DG, O'Fallon WMC. Epidemiology of diaphyseal and distal femoral fractures in Rochester, Minnesota, 1965–1984. *Clin Orthop Relat Res.* 1988;234:188–94.

5. Della Rocca GJ, Leung KS, Pape HC. Periprosthetic fractures: Epidemiology and future projections. *J Orthop Trauma.* 2011;25(Suppl 2):S66–70.
6. Gwathmey FW, Jones-Quaidoo SM, Kahler D et al. Distal femoral fractures: Current concepts. *J Am Acad Orthop Surg.* 2010;18:597–607.
7. Marsh JL, Slongo TF, Agel J et al. Fracture and dislocation classification compendium—2007: Orthopaedic Trauma Association classification, database, and outcomes committee. *J Orthop Trauma.* 2007;21(10 Suppl):S1–133.
8. Cass J, Sems SA. Operative versus nonoperative management of distal femur fracture in myelopathic, nonambulatory patients. *Orthopedics.* 2008;31(11):1091.
9. Streuble PN, Ricci WN, Wong A, Gardner MJ. Mortality after distal femur fractures in elderly patients. *Clin Orthop Relat Res.* 2011;469:1188–96.
10. Freedman EL, Hak DJ, Johnson EE, Eckardt JJ. Total knee replacement including a modular distal femoral component in elderly patients with acute fracture of nonunion. *J Orthop Trauma.* 1995;9(3):231–7.
11. Nork SE, Segina DN, Aflatoon K et al. The association between supracondylar-intercondylar distal femoral fractures and coronal plane fractures. *J Bone Joint Surg Am.* 2005;87(3):564–9.
12. Starr AJ, Jones AL, Reinert CM. The "swashbuckler": A modified anterior approach for fractures of the distal femur. *J Orthop Trauma.* 1999;13:138–40.
13. Beltran MJ, Blair JA, Huh J et al. Articular exposure with the swashbuckler vs a "Mini-swashbuckler" approach. *Injury.* 2013;44:189–93.
14. Higgins TF, Pittman G, Hines J, Bachus KN. Biomechanical analysis of distal femur fracture fixation: Fixed-angle screw-plate construct versus condylar blade plate. *J Orthop Trauma.* 2007;21(1):43–6.
15. Crist BD, Lee MA. Distal femur fractures: Open reduction, and internal fixation. In Wiss D, ed. *Master Techniques in Orthopaedic Surgery,* 3rd ed. Philadelphia, PA: Lippincott Williams and Wilkins, 2013, pp. 425–47.
16. Hak DJ, Mauffrey C, Seligson D, Lindeque B. Use of carbon-fiber-reinforced composite implants in orthopedic surgery. *Orthopedics.* 2014;37(12):825–30.
17. Beltran MJ, Gary JL, Collinge CA. Management of distal femur fractures with modern plates and nails: State of the art. *J Orthop Trauma.* 2015;29:165–72.
18. Tornetta P III, Egol KA, Jones CB et al. Locked plating versus retrograde nailing for distal femur fractures: A multicenter randomized trial. *Presented at the Annual Meeting of the Orthopaedic Trauma Association,* Phoenix, AZ, 2013.
19. Grant KD, Hatic C, Mir HR et al. Combination nail-plate fixation of osteoporotic distal metaphyseal femoral fractures. *Presented as a Poster Presentation at the Annual Meeting of the Orthopaedic Trauma Association,* San Antonio, TX, 2011.
20. Su ET, DeWal H, DiCesare PE. Periprosthetic femoral fractures above total knee replacements. *J Am Acad Orthop Surg.* 2004;12:12–20.

21. Service BC, Kang W, Turnbull N et al. Influence of femoral component design on retrograde femoral nail starting point. *J Orthop Trauma*. 2015;29:e380–4.

22. Toro-Ibarguen A, Moreno-Beamud JA, Porras-Moreno MA et al. The number of locking screws predicts the risk of nonunion and reintervention in periprosthetic total knee arthroplasty fractures treated with a nail. *Eur J Orthop Surg Traumatol*. 2015;25:661–4.

23. Tosounidis TH, Giannoudis PV. What is new in periprosthetic fracture fixation? *Injury*. 2015;46:2293–6.

24. Jassim SS, McNamara I, Hopgood P. Distal femoral replacement in periprosthetic fracture around total knee arthroplasty. *Injury*. 2014;45:550–3.

25. Calori GM, Colombo M, Malagoli E et al. Megaprosthesis in post-traumatic and periprosthetic large bone defects: Issues to consider. *Injury*. 2014;45(Suppl 6):S105–10.

26. Muller ME, Allgower M, Schneider R et al. *Manual of Internal Fixation*, 3rd ed. New York, NY: Springer-Verlag, 1991.

27. Mast J, Jakob R, Ganz R. *Planning, and Reduction Technique in Fracture Surgery*. Berlin, Germany: Springer-Verlag, 1989.

28. Pettine KA. Supracondylar fractures of the femur: Long-term follow-up of closed versus nonrigid internal fixation. *Contemp Orthop*. 1990;21(3):253–61.

29. Zehntner MK, Marchesi DG, Burch H, Ganz R. Alignment of supracondylar/intercondylar fractures of the femur after internal fixation by AO/ASIF technique. *J Orthop Trauma*. 1992;6(3):318–26.

30. Jaarsma RL, Verdonschot N, van der Venne R et al. Avoiding rotational malalignment after fractures of the femur by using the profile of the lesser trochanter: An *in vitro* study. *Arch Orthop Trauma Surg*. 2005;125:184–7.

31. Kenawey M, Krettek C, Ettinger M et al. The greater trochanter-head contact method: A cadaveric study with a new technique for intra-operative control of rotation of femoral fractures. *J Orthop Trauma*. 2011;25:549–55.

32. Krettek C, Miclau T, Grun O et al. Intraoperative control of axes, rotation and length in femoral and tibia fractures. Technical note. *Injury*. 1998; 29(Suppl 3):C29–39.

33. Kregor PJ, Stannard JA, Zlowodzki M, Cole PA. Treatment of distal femur fractures using the less invasive stabilization system: Surgical experience and early clinical results in 103 fractures. *J Orthop Trauma*. 2004;18:509–20.

34. Vallier HA, Hennessey TA, Sontich JK, Patterson BM. Failure of LCP condylar plate fixation in the distal part of the femur: A report of six cases. *J Bone and Joint Surg Am*. 2006;88(4):846–53.

35. Henderson CE, Lujan TJ, Kuhl LL et al. 2010 Mid-America Orthopedic Association Physician in Training Award: Healing complications are common after locked plating for distal femur fractures. *Clin Orthop Relat Res*. 2011;469:1757–65.

36. Lujan TJ, Henderson CE, Madey SM et al. Locked plating of distal femur fractures leads to inconsistent and asymmetric callous formation. *J Orthop Trauma*. 2010;24:156–62.

37. Harvin WH, Della Rocca GJ, Murtha YM et al. Working length and proximal screw constructs in plate osteosynthesis of distal femur fractures. *Presented as a Podium Presentation at the Annual Meeting of the Orthopaedic Trauma Association*, Tampa, FL, 2014.

38. Rodriguez EK, Zurakowski D, Herder L et al. Mechanical construct characteristics predisposing to non-union after locked lateral plating of distal femur fractures. *J Orthop Trauma*. 2016;30:403–8.

39. Ricci WM, Streubel PN, Morshed S et al. Risk factors for failure of locked plate fixation of distal femur fractures: An analysis of 355 cases. *J Orthop Trauma*. 2014;28:83–9.

40. Bottlang M, Doomink J, Byrd GD, Fitzpatrick DC, Madey SM. A nonlocking end screw can decrease fracture risk caused by locked plating in the osteoporotic diaphysis. *J Bone Joint Surg Am*. 2009;91(3):620–7.

41. Peck JB, Charpentier PM, Flanagan BP, Srivastava AK, Atkinson PJ. Reducing fracture risk adjacent to a plate with an angulated locked end screw. *J Orthop Trauma*. 2015;29(11):e431–6.

42. Criner SH, Krumrey J. Immediate weight bearing as tolerated after locked plating of fragility fractures of the distal femur. *Presented as a Podium Presentation at the Annual Meeting of the Western Orthopaedic Association*, Big Island, HI, 2014.

43. Smith WR, Stoneback JW, Morgan SJ, Stahel PF. Is immediate weight bearing safe for periprosthetic distal femur fractures treated by locked plating? A feasibility study in 52 consecutive patients. *Patient Saf Surg*. 2016;10:26.

44. Kregor PJ, Zlowodzki M. Distal femur fractures. In: Stannard JP, Schmidt AH, Kregor PJ, eds. *Surgical Treatment of Orthopaedic Trauma*. New York, NY: Thieme, 2007, p. 636.

45. Paley D. *Principles of Deformity Correction*. New York, NY: Springer-Verlag, 2005.

24

Osteoporotic distal femoral fractures

When to replace and how

RICHARD STANGE and MICHAEL J. RASCHKE

INTRODUCTION AND EPIDEMIOLOGY

Incidence of complex meta-epiphyseal knee fracture is much lower than for fracture of the femoral neck, proximal humerus, or elbow, accounting for around 1% of annual emergency admissions (1). The exact incidence of knee joint fracture is hard to determine, as it varies according to demographic and geographical factors. In a series of more than 6000 fractures, annual incidence of proximal tibia fracture was 13.3 per 100,000 in adults, and 4.5 per 100,000 for distal femoral fracture (2); there was male predominance for proximal tibia fracture and female predominance for distal femoral fracture. Approximately half of all periarticular fractures around the knee occur in osteoporotic patients older than 50 years of age as a result of low-energy trauma. A high 1-year mortality rate (22%) and significant decrease in function and quality of life have been noted in frail elderly patients who sustained supracondylar femoral fractures (3). Fractures of the distal femur in connection with osteoporosis are difficult to deal with because of poor bone quality, preexisting arthritis, high levels of comminution, and osteochondral damage at time of injury (4). Also, the often-impaired health condition of this population has to be taken in account, adding a systemic challenge to the local one. Therefore, the goal of returning a patient to prefracture level of function is often difficult to achieve.

Operative techniques that completely address problems with fixation of osteoporotic bone and articular cartilage damage still are incomplete and confront the surgeon with unforeseen challenges. To date most complex knee fractures in the elderly are still treated by internal fixation or sometimes nonoperatively (1,3,4).

Open reduction and internal fixation (ORIF) of the distal femur can be a lengthy procedure with complex fixation and high levels of blood loss. Although options are constantly evolving, poor knee function, malunion, nonunion, prolonged immobilization, implant failure, as well as high morbidity and mortality rates have been reported in several studies regardless of the fixation method. After ORIF, patients' weight-bearing is often restricted for 12 weeks or longer (5)—a protocol that is undesirable in elderly patients, especially given that the rate of mortality 1 year after these fractures has been found to be as high as 25% (6). Postoperative early mobilization and ambulation are very important to prevent complications including deep venous thrombosis (DVT), pneumonia, and decubitus ulcers. Principles of early range of motion (ROM) and weight-bearing are in sharp contradiction to the need for rigid immobilization to maintain fracture fixation for these patients. Operative as well as conservative treatment of these elderly patients continues to show consistently poor results in a clinical study. Arthritis after distal femoral fractures has been reported at rates of 36%–50% by long-term follow-up (7). However, due to improvement of different types of total knee arthroplasty (TKA) systems, as well as better training of orthopedic and trauma surgeons (higher specialization), replacement of the distal femur might play an increasingly important role in the future.

Primary arthroplasty is commonly used to treat acute fractures of the proximal femur, complex proximal humerus, or elbow fractures (8) but is less common in distal femoral fractures (1,9). However, there are good reasons, in the knee as well as for hip or shoulder fractures, for treating certain acute complex fractures using primary replacement, such as significant symptomatic osteoarthritis prior to the fracture, fracture complexity, especially of its articular part, bone fragility making fixation hazardous, and the need for early mobilization and the earliest possible resumption of walking in elderly patients, to avoid the decubitus complications and the risk of becoming bedridden (1,3,4).

Furthermore, later TKA for posttraumatic arthritis following joint fractures is more complex because of scarring, arthrofibrosis, malunion, nonunion, and the frequent need for hardware removal. In addition, these cases clearly are associated with higher incidence of infection, aseptic loosening, stiffness (10), and skin necrosis (11).

PRINCIPLES

Reliable internal fixation is difficult to achieve in diaphyseal, metaphyseal, and epiphyseal femoral fractures in severely osteoporotic patients. For these patients, partial weight-bearing is often recommended for at least 6 weeks, which greatly limits mobilization, as these patients are unable to use crutches without full weight-bearing. In case of severe joint comminution with osteoporotic bone and osteoarthritis, the benefit of internal fixation followed by prolonged non-weight-bearing is highly questionable. Moreover, when progression following internal fixation is not favorable, these patients do not always receive arthroplasty, due to their age and the risks involved in two-step or one-step material ablation and implantation (1,9).

Since relatively poor results have been reported with ORIF of complex fractures around the knee in elderly osteoporotic patients, primary TKA has been proposed as an alternative solution. Compared with ORIF, primary TKA may allow for earlier mobility and weight-bearing and thereby reduce the rates of secondary complications associated with prolonged immobilization (3,12).

For the shoulder and elbow, the objective is to restore joint function by immediate postoperative mobilization (8,12). Several authors have recommended primary TKA for patients with intra-articular distal femoral fractures and preexisting osteoarthritis or rheumatoid arthritis, severe comminution, or poor bone stock (3,11,13–16). The main objectives of arthroplasty in fractures of the distal femur are to save the patient's life, by limiting the decubitus complications, allowing instantaneous resumption of weight-bearing, and to save knee function, immediate unrestricted joint mobilization and patient autonomy (9).

INDICATIONS

The indications for first-line arthroplasty in complex epiphyseal shoulder and elbow joint fractures are well established with the same rationale as for displaced femoral neck fracture in the elderly (4,8,9). What is needed is the same, with the same contradictory requirements: it is difficult or impossible to achieve stable bone reconstruction by internal fixation, due to osteoporosis and/or fracture comminution, while rapid recovery of optimal joint function is mandatory. In the lower limb, the primary goal is to resume full weight-bearing as soon as possible.

Fortunately, the incidence of complex distal femoral fractures is much lower than for fracture of the femoral neck, proximal humerus, or elbow, accounting for around 1% of annual emergency admissions (1,9).

Most authors classify distal femoral fractures according to the AO/Orthopaedic Trauma Association (OTA) system originally described by Müller (17) (Figure 24.1).

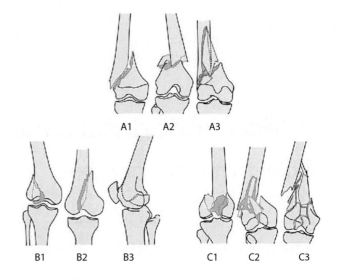

Figure 24.1 Müller AO classification for distal femoral fractures (region 33). (From AO Foundation, Müller ME. *Unfallheilkunde*. 1980;83(5):251–9.)

Type A fractures do not contain an intra-articular extension, type B are partial articular fractures, and type C are complete articular fractures with metaphyseal-diaphyseal discontinuity. Regardless of the fracture pattern, managing a distal femoral fracture with primary arthroplasty requires the surgeon to decide whether to retain or resect the distal femur.

Primary replacement in osteoporotic distal femoral fractures has to be taken into consideration in two major indications, as follows.

Osteoporotic patient with osteoarthritis prior to fracture

This is usually the most frequent situation of patients present in emergency with a complex comminuted articular fracture of the distal femur (1,3,4,9,14). Preexisting knee arthrosis is a major factor that limits the results of treatment of distal femur fractures in geriatric patients. Most patients in this age group have underlying cartilage degeneration. The recent or prior x-ray shows signs of osteoarthritis, and the patient reports that he or she was already suffering prior to trauma. In some cases, arthroplasty may even have already been scheduled before the fracture occurred.

Due to immobilization, even the most successful surgical restoration of the joint surface may result later in a stiff, painful knee. After fracture healing is complete, many of these patients will require a total joint arthroplasty. However, delayed arthroplasty in addition is technically much more demanding than a primary knee replacement and difficult with distorted anatomy, joint contracture, and internal fixation devices present. This includes the need of an extended surgical exposure, extensor mechanism reconstruction, and bulky allografts. The option of replacing the joint initially, with one surgery, is therefore a consistent solution for both the fracture and the osteoarthritis and a very attractive concept for patients with significant preexisting arthrosis (11,14,15,18).

Fracture in elderly osteoporotic patient where articular involvement and bone quality make internal fixation hazardous

This situation is frequently seen in an elderly patient with complex articular fracture of the distal femur and osteoporotic bone. The complexity of the fracture (especially C1–3 fractures, Figure 24.1), which is often very distal and with considerable articular step-off and severe bone loss, makes internal fixation uncertain. Locking plates have become popular for the treatment of complex fractures of the distal femur and proximal tibia in an osteoporotic environment.

In cases of ORIF, angular stable implants seem to be far more stable than conventional plating systems. In our experience, an additional medial or anteromedial plate offers higher load-bearing forces as well as increased rotational stability, compared to lateral fixation only, especially in a periprosthetic situation (Figure 24.2).

However, the "fatigue failure" of the osteoporotic implant–bone construct continues to be a major and so far unsolved problem in elderly patients. Nonunion and malunion of these fractures occur with all types of treatment, and there is a severe risk of inadequate reduction of the articular step-off, secondary loss of reduction, and material cut-out; therefore, functional prognosis is poor.

The postoperative treatment after fixation of these fractures demands a lengthy period of limited weight-bearing that can increase the rate of complications. First-line arthroplasty allows elimination of fracture healing issues and seems to represent a reasonable attitude, with

metaphyseal and epiphyseal femoral reconstruction, allowing immediate full weight-bearing. It might therefore be a clear alternative rather than performing internal fixation, with a high risk of failure throughout the latter course, the need for subsequent implant removal, and arthroplasty at a much less favorable time point, with the same need for reconstruction as in first-line arthroplasty (1,3,12,19).

PREOPERATIVE PLANNING AND PREPARATION

Although admitted in emergency, these patients need to be prepared and managed as meticulous as for scheduled surgery, and they require adequate preoperative management. Particularly important is a multidisciplinary approach to manage comorbidities, control of anemia and pain, and assessment and management of vascular and cutaneous conditions. Preoperative planning with appropriate special implants (revision arthroplasty systems) is crucial. Surgical technique is based on the basic principles of revision surgery. Due to the typical age and population of these patients, the complexity of care required is similar to that after hip fracture surgery; therefore, postoperative management needs to be carefully planned to address the complex situations of these patients in an interdisciplinary approach (20,21).

Analysis and management of patient´s general health condition

These patients, admitted in emergency, require rigorous orthogeriatric co-management, taking full account of comorbidities (20). Fracture-related anemia should be treated prior to surgery, pain should be controlled as of admission, and medical evaluation and optimization are

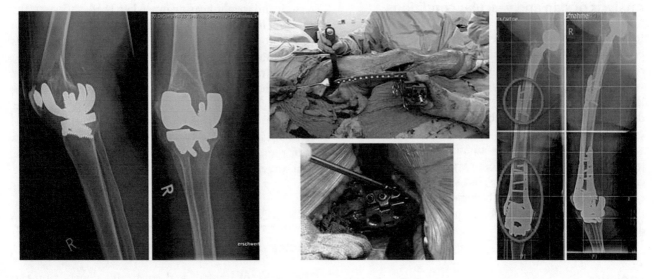

Figure 24.2 A 92-year-old female, periprosthetic distal femoral fracture with osteoporotic bone around the femoral component and ipsilateral total hip arthroplasty; open reduction and internal fixation with angular stable plating system lateral and additional medial plate.

mandatory. Adhesive traction or cast immobilization may be implemented to limit fracture site mobility. Full radiographic evaluation, including use of multiple radiographic views and computed tomography (CT) imaging, needs to be completed to accurately assess the fracture pattern.

Analysis of bone conditions and fracture morphology

Impaired bone quality and bone loss due to osteoporotic changes remain the most important challenge for the orthopedic surgeon in these patients. The combination with the complexity of the fracture makes internal fixation uncertain. Although locking plates have become an indispensable "working horse" for the treatment of complex osteoporotic fractures, the limited loading capacity of the osteoporotic implant–bone construct, due to impaired strength and stability, continues to be a problem. X-ray analysis or preexisting dual-energy x-ray absorptiometry scan will help to estimate bone quality before surgery; however, sometimes bone quality and constitution might display even worse intraoperatively. Therefore, being prepared for either internal fixation or replacement will help to manage those complex cases.

Preoperative analysis of the fracture pattern as well as previous operations in the same area (e.g., hip arthroplasty) is also crucial. Excellent preoperative scaled radiographic views are necessary in order to precisely plan the replacement procedure. CT with three-dimensional reconstruction can be helpful if good-quality x-rays are difficult to obtain due to pain, and/or to improve fracture analysis. In these contexts, it is usually impossible to obtain good-quality long-leg x-rays including the contralateral limb for length measurement.

Analysis of skin and vascular conditions

In the elderly patient, fragile soft tissue often remains a problem, with hematoma and sometimes contusions related to the trauma, for which strict preoperative surveillance is required. Open fractures luckily are rare in low-energy trauma in elderly patients. Dermal abrasions due to "corticoid skin" might be a problem in patients with concomitant diseases.

Associated vascular lesions are rare but should be systematically screened for before surgery. Some fractures could be excellent indications, but severe venous insufficiency is not unusual and may become a contraindication if there is any doubt regarding the proper healing of the skin due to poor vascular status.

Logistics

Surgical planning determines the precise needs for material. The surgical team needs to be prepared for complex fixation techniques such as double plating, strut grafting techniques, augmentation of the osteosynthesis, or conversion to revision or tumor prosthesis. Not all centers have permanent access to segmental reconstruction implants (tumoral reconstruction implants), rotating hinged implants, or revision implants with metal augmentation systems. Thus, although these patients are admitted in emergency, surgery has to be accurately planned as fast and as precisely as possible, taking account of the time needed to procure equipment. The surgical team should also be carefully chosen and experienced in trauma and reconstructive surgery as well as in arthroplasty revision surgery.

TECHNICAL SPECIFICITIES AND IMPLANT CHOICE

Surgical technique is based on the basic principles of revision surgery. The choice of implant and constraint, steps of reconstruction planning of joint-line restoration and component rotation, bone defect filling, and implant fixation are the same as in prosthetic revision or, in the case of major epiphyseal and metaphyseal destruction, the same as in segmental reconstruction following tumor resection (22,23). It is necessary to have experience in these techniques in order to keep surgical time as short as possible in these fragile elderly patients (1,9). Thus, all of the previously mentioned choices (implants, level of resection, defect filling, implant fixation, complementary internal fixation, etc.) should be anticipated and made in advance. The three main stages of TKA revision with joint reconstruction should be applied:

1. Reconstruction of the tibial base plate
2. Management of the flexion gap
3. Management of the extension gap

The main goal is to enable the patient to stand up and resume full weight-bearing immediately after surgery. The choice of fixation, modalities of the reconstruction, and the entire procedure should therefore be performed with this aim in mind.

First-line TKA for fracture should be performed by or with the help of an experienced surgeon. It is essential to be prepared for this operation, which should be performed as scheduled emergency surgery, to optimize surgical conditions (4). It should never be performed by a duty surgeon with a small team often without any training in TKA revision surgery.

SURGICAL TECHNIQUE

Choice of implant and constraint

The choice of implant and constraint depends on the fracture level and degree of metaphyseal destruction. Resecting is technically straightforward but necessitates the use of a hinged prosthesis to substitute for the collateral ligaments (13,18). Owing to the poor bone quality and typically large diaphyseal diameter associated with osteoporosis, cemented fixation is more practical than press-fit fixation in an elderly population (13). Femoral rotation and length can be maintained by provisionally reducing the fracture fragments using traction prior to resection, marking the anterior aspect of the proximal shaft fragment perpendicular to the transepicondylar axis, and then measuring the distance from the joint line to this mark. This allows the femoral component to be inserted in the correct rotation and length after resection. In order to minimize the amount of stress placed on the bone–implant interface, the least amount of constraint that is necessary should be employed, similar to that used for revision TKA surgery (24).

Unconstrained knee designs should be considered in cases in which the fracture pattern appears stable and the collateral ligaments are intact (e.g., 33A and 33BB fractures).

When the fracture involves the femoral collateral ligament insertions, a rotating-hinge implant should be used. It is usually impossible to achieve solid internal fixation of the condyles preserving a functional collateral ligament insertion. In case of severe metaphyseal destruction up to the diaphysis, a segmental megaprosthesis should be used, especially on the femoral side (Figure 24.3). In prosthetic revision in complex fractures, it is essential to obtain a pain-free, mobile, but also and above all, stable knee (9,22,23).

Mega-prostheses, which may allow for immediate weight-bearing but require considerable bone resection, would be beneficial in 33C fractures, fractures with ligamentous compromise, or periprosthetic distal femoral fractures (Figure 24.4). However, their complication rates are unclear, and comparative studies are needed to investigate whether the rates are higher for these patients than for patients treated more traditionally.

Patient positioning and management

Patient positioning is as for TKA revision, according to the surgeon's preference. Due to the fracture pattern, it is often difficult to use supports to obtain a stable knee at 90°. That makes the approach and dislocation of the patella difficult. In some cases, the surgeon should be prepared for an osteotomy of the insertion of the patella tendon in order to avoid damage to the extensors. A tourniquet is not routinely used since there frequently is a need for additional proximal release of the extensor system in order to obtain adequate exposure, especially for megaprostheses. We recommend tranexamic acid, even in these elderly patients, as contraindications are increasingly rare, as well as the use of a cell-saver (25).

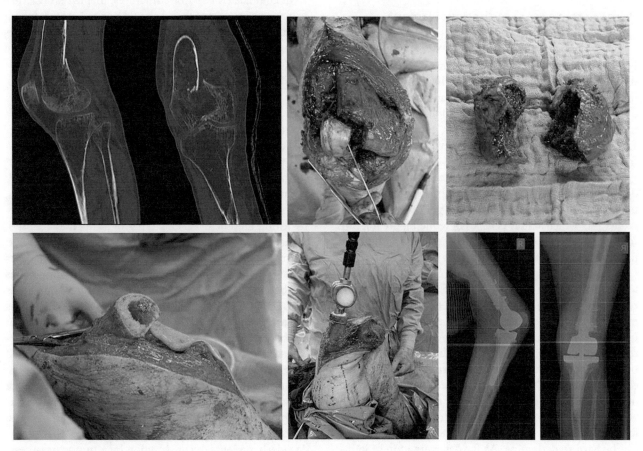

Figure 24.3 An 85-year-old female, distal femoral fracture, AO 33 C1, severe osteoporosis. Distal femoral replacement by a tumor prosthesis.

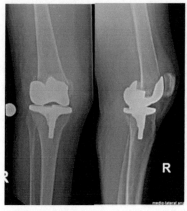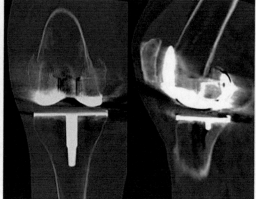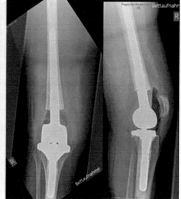

Figure 24.4 Periprosthetic distal femoral fracture with osteoporotic bone around the femoral component. Distal femur replacement by a tumor prosthesis.

Approach

The approach should be the one the surgeon adopts for revision TKA. The use of a midline incision allows for the addition of any internal fixation, if required. The surgeon may also consider using intramedullary guides for the femoral and tibial cuts, as this will simplify conversion to stemmed implants, if necessary (13).

Primary temporary reduction, implant rotation, and joint-line reconstruction

For complex fractures of the distal femur, as in prosthetic revision or reconstruction similar to the technique needed following tumor resection, two key issues comprise restoration of the joint-line and femoral rotation. Complementary internal fixation may be required in case of diaphyseal extension of the fracture and to prevent interprosthetic fractures.

In indications for TKA for acute femoral fracture, destruction is often severe, and landmarks may remain unclear. We therefore recommend "primary temporary reduction," which simply consists of reducing the fracture "as well as possible" for as long as it takes to mark the joint-line level as well as the rotation on the femur (4,9).

In revision surgery, the joint-line is classically supposed to lie about 25 mm distal to the medial epicondyle and/or 10 mm proximal to the head of the fibula (26). Primary temporary reduction, as described earlier, enables the individual native joint-line level to be restored. Once this reduction has been achieved and stabilized using reduction clamps, a mark is made on the proximal femur using electric cautery, and the distance between the mark and the native joint-line is measured using a ruler. This distance will then be used for femoral reconstruction. In complex femoral fracture, the rotation of the future femoral implant can be hard to determine. As for determination of joint-line level, taking the native femoral rotation as reference is recommended. This can be done after temporary primary reduction, marking the femoral shaft axis with an electric

cautery to indicate epiphyseal-metaphyseal rotation. This mark serves as a landmark for rotation during trials and for the definitive implantation of the prosthesis. In complex femoral fractures, the classical femoral component measurement instruments may be unusable, due to articular comminution. In such a case, it might be helpful to use the technique used for hip hemiarthroplasties: measuring one of the native condyles with a caliper and selecting the corresponding femoral implant.

In complex osteoporotic fractures, diaphyseal fracture extensions are frequent and should not be ignored during adjacent metaphyseal reconstruction. Metallic cerclages associated to cemented stem fixation allows immediate resumption of weight-bearing and reduces the risk of periprosthetic fractures.

Bone defect filling versus reconstruction implant

As in TKA revision, two types of defects can be considered: segmental defects, reconstructed using structural grafts, and cavitary defects (26), reconstructed using bone cavity filling methods. Various types of grafts may be used, depending on the surgeon's habits and availability, and should be included in the preoperative planning. In cases of severely impaired bone quality, porous tantalum cones can be specifically adapted when a conventional implant is used (Figure 24.5) (26). In these osteoporotic patients, it is important to find a reliable metaphyseal support that can be obtained with these cones or other metallic reconstruction systems (27,28). The techniques are those described for prosthetic revision with severe segmental bone defects. The ultimate stage of segmental bone defect is complete metaphyseal and epiphyseal destruction in severely comminuted fracture, in which case tumor prosthesis may be needed (23). In case of major destruction in these fragile elderly patients, reconstruction by a tumor prosthesis is more reasonable and reliable, as it allows immediate weight-bearing, than complex reconstruction using a double cone and complementary internal fixation, which is a

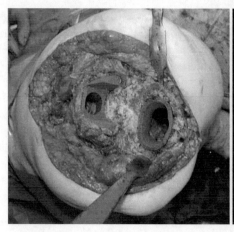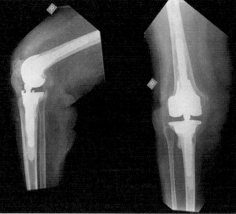

Figure 24.5 Trabecular metal distal femoral and proximal tibial cone implant to fill and reconstruct large bone deficiencies and cavitary defects in the diaphysis of the distal femur and to provide a stable platform for the support of a total knee arthroplasty femoral component.

long and hemorrhagic procedure with an uncertain outcome, as bone fragility precludes immediate postoperative full weight-bearing.

Principles of implant fixation

The principles are those of prosthetic revision (10,29). Applying the principles described by Morgan-Jones et al. (29), three zones of fixation should be considered for implant fixation: epiphyseal, metaphyseal, and diaphyseal. To achieve a reliable fixation, it should involve at least two of the three zones. The literature reports no superiority between a long uncemented stem with diaphyseal engagement and a shorter cemented stem in revision TKA (28). The current trend, however, favors fully cemented stems, but with a short stem associated to metaphyseal reconstruction. This concept optimizes the control of rotational stress and avoids pain at the end of the stem. Thus, long stems are used for trials, to control alignment, whereas the definitive stem is short and fully cemented. In TKA for acute fracture, the technique should be adapted to the status of local osteoporosis and the tubular femoral anatomy of elderly patients, which frequently is present and enables immediate resumption of weight-bearing. When a tumor prosthesis is used, the stem should be long and fully cemented to improve the stability (23).

The decision to perform complementary internal fixation is made at the end of the procedure and is also important due to sudden changes in bone elasticity caused by prosthetic implants in osteoporotic patients. It allows immediate resumption of full weight-bearing without risk of postoperative periprosthetic fracture.

It is important to check in advance of the surgery that there is no hip arthroplasty stem or other internal fixation material that would hinder the implantation of a primary knee arthroplasty. Ipsilateral hip prostheses lead to a risk of interprosthetic fractures in the bone segment

between the two stems, which could be a dramatic complication. Lehmann et al. demonstrated that the interprosthetic distance does not have a significant effect on the risk of developing an interprosthetic fracture of the femur. Furthermore, cortical thickness is a predictive factor, unlike bone mineral density. The implantation of a constrained knee prosthesis that is not loosened on the ipsilateral side does not increase the risk for a fracture (30,31).

Resurfacing the patella seems reasonable, as complications arising from cemented patellae are rare, and resurfacing the patella appears to reduce the risk of reoperation in elderly patients undergoing primary TKA (13,32). However, in our own clinical series, the percentage of retropatellar surfacing is approximately 15%.

In summary, surgical technique respecting the previously discussed reconstruction principles is crucial:

- Performing optimized metaphyseal reconstruction using tantalum cones and short cemented stems with complementary internal fixation, as for revision TKA procedures, allows immediate resumption of weight-bearing (27,28).
- Tumor prostheses also allow immediate resumption of full weight-bearing (23,33).

POSTOPERATIVE MANAGEMENT

The principles of postoperative management of elderly patients apply here: remedying blood loss, preventing decubitus complications, managing anticoagulation, and treating the comorbidities (25,34). The lessons drawn from managing elderly patients undergoing surgery for femoral neck fracture are relevant, especially including teamwork between geriatric and orthopedic surgeons (20). Pain management should be up-to-date and multimodal, avoiding morphine derivatives as far as possible. A combination of local therapeutic injections at the end of surgery and the use of an adductor canal catheter is particularly effective

(35). The main issue is resumption of full weight-bearing, which should be immediate whenever possible.

Careful consideration of each individual is necessary according to the national guidelines, as these patients are at an increased risk of venous thromboembolism. In patients at high risk of bleeding, mechanical prophylaxis, such as pneumatic compression stockings, can be used. In patients at normal risk of bleeding, chemical prophylaxis can be undertaken. We routinely use perioperative antibiotics consisting of a single intravenous dose of cephalexin within 1 hour of incision followed by further doses after 2 hours during surgery. Physiotherapy is beneficial in initiating mobilization and achieving range of movement after TKA. For patients treated with TKA, one can expect functional recovery to plateau after approximately 1 year.

COMPLICATIONS AND RESULTS

Although the literature is made up of heterogeneous groups with small sample sizes, there is some consistency in findings that permit some generalizations. Fractures around the knee in elderly osteoporotic patients are challenging, and ORIF frequently results in loss of reduction, which can result in posttraumatic arthritis and occasionally the need for TKA. Late TKA after failed fixation can be technically difficult, with modest functional outcomes and high complication rates. However, TKA as the primary method of treatment appears to have superior functional outcomes, survival, and lower complication rates, although the results certainly do not approach those of elective TKA (9,12).

In the literature, the results of primary TKA for fractures seem to be encouraging and notably better than for secondary TKA after failure of nonoperative treatment or internal fixation, with lower rates of revision and complications, earlier full weight-bearing, and better functional results. Loss of autonomy is, however, frequent, and 1-year mortality is high, especially following complex femoral fractures in the elderly (1,3,4,12,15,16,19).

One series looking specifically at the result of TKA performed for the late sequelae of distal femoral fracture reported a revision rate of 8% (4 of 48), a complication rate of 15% (7 of 48), and good outcomes in 52% (25 of 48) of patients (10). Early weight-bearing is permissible, and complication rates range from 8% to 42%, with low rates of revision, and good outcomes reported in most patients (13,18,36). Complication rates of TKAs for recent fractures range between 8% and 42%, revision rates are low, and functional results are usually satisfactory. In secondary posttraumatic TKAs, complication rates range between 20% and 48%, implant revision rates range between 8% and 20%, and functional results are satisfactory in only 75% of cases (1,9,14). In these often fragile patients, there are also general complications potentially related to three successive operations (internal fixation, hardware removal, and then TKA implantation) and a period of non-weight-bearing or protected weight-bearing following the internal fixation. In both cases, however, studies had a short follow-up, often small series, and subsequent lack of information on

the long-term survival of the implants used. Many of the authors comment on the technical difficulty of the operations, the risk of complications such as patellar tendon and collateral ligament injury, persistent deep infection, and major wound healing difficulties.

Results in first-line arthroplasty for fracture are encouraging and better than in arthroplasty secondary to failure of conservative treatment, with lower revision and complication rates, earlier resumption of weight-bearing, and better functional results.

CONCLUSION

Osteoporotic distal femoral fractures are difficult to treat because of poor bone quality, preexisting arthritis, high levels of comminution, and osteochondral damage at time of injury. The goal of returning the patient to prefracture level of function is ambitious and often difficult to achieve. The dilemma of function and fixation of distal femoral fractures is similar to issues involved in the treatment of proximal femur or proximal humerus fractures.

Reconstruction using primary arthroplasty in case of complex articular fracture of the distal femur therefore might be an interesting and promising surgical option, limiting the number of revision surgeries while addressing several main objectives:

1. Saving the patient's life by allowing early resumption of weight-bearing
2. Limiting the decubitus complications and preserving function, thanks to immediate unrestricted joint mobilization and limited loss of autonomy

A distinct algorithm for managing osteoporotic fractures above the knee might facilitate the decision for or against replacement surgery (Figure 24.6).

Recent results in the literature confirm the benefit of primary replacement strategies of distal femoral fractures.

Adjusted to this impaired population, a multidisciplinary perioperative management is crucial and essential, especially in the elderly, osteoporotic patient. The surgical technique requires profound and excellent knowledge as well as experience of the principles of prosthetic revisions and internal fixation. Since patients and fractures are complex, surgery should be performed on a delayed emergency basis to optimize planning and logistic preparation prior to operation.

Published series are as yet limited, due to the rarity of these fractures and less widespread awareness of this complex approach. However, recent demographic changes, the aging of society, and the resulting increase of osteoporosis-associated fractures requires a better definition of indications and principles in therapy of these complex and in the end, life-threatening injuries. Therefore, extensive knowledge and experience in surgical skills in the treatment of complex fractures in the distal femur, as well as knowledge in revision and tumor systems for TKA are required in order to further improve the results of distal femoral fracture treatment.

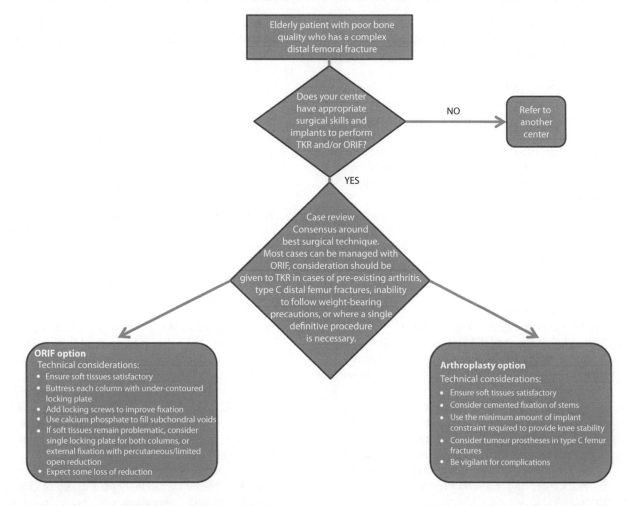

Figure 24.6 Modified algorithm for the management of osteoporotic distal femoral fractures. (According to Bohm ER et al. *J Bone Joint Surg Br.* 2012;94[9]:1160–9.)

REFERENCES

1. Ries MD. Primary arthroplasty for management of osteoporotic fractures about the knee. *Curr Osteoporos Rep.* 2012;10(4):322–7.

2. Court-Brown CM, Caesar B. Epidemiology of adult fractures: A review. *Injury.* 2006;37(8):691–7.

3. Boureau F, Benad K, Putman S, Dereudre G, Kern G, Chantelot C. Does primary total knee arthroplasty for acute knee joint fracture maintain autonomy in the elderly? A retrospective study of 21 cases. *Orthop Traumatol Surg Res.* 2015;101(8):947–51.

4. Parratte S, Ollivier M, Argenson JN. Primary total knee arthroplasty for acute fracture around the knee. *Orthop Traumatol Surg Res.* 2018;104(1S):S71–80.

5. Gwathmey FW, Jr., Jones-Quaidoo SM, Kahler D, Hurwitz S, Cui Q. Distal femoral fractures: Current concepts. *J Am Acad Orthop Surg.* 2010;18(10):597–607.

6. Streubel PN, Ricci WM, Wong A, Gardner MJ. Mortality after distal femur fractures in elderly patients. *Clin Orthop Relat Res.* 2011;469(4):1188–96.

7. Thomson AB, Driver R, Kregor PJ, Obremskey WT. Long-term functional outcomes after intra-articular distal femur fractures: ORIF versus retrograde intramedullary nailing. *Orthopedics.* 2008;1(8):748–50.

8. Obert L, Saadnia R, Tournier C et al. Four-part fractures treated with a reversed total shoulder prosthesis: Prospective and retrospective multicenter study. *Orthop Traumatol Surg Res.* 2016;102(3):279–85.

9. Bohm ER, Tufescu TV, Marsh JP. The operative management of osteoporotic fractures of the knee: To fix or replace? *J Bone Joint Surg Br.* 2012;94(9):1160–9.

10. Papadopoulos EC, Parvizi J, Lai CH, Lewallen DG. Total knee arthroplasty following prior distal femoral fracture. *Knee.* 2002;9(4):267–74.

11. Yoshino N, Takai S, Watanabe Y, Fujiwara H, Ohshima Y, Hirasawa Y. Primary total knee arthroplasty for supracondylar/condylar femoral fracture in osteoarthritic knees. *J Arthroplasty.* 2001;16(4):471–5.

12. Chen F, Li R, Lall A, Schwechter EM. Primary total knee arthroplasty for distal femur fractures: A systematic review of indications, implants, techniques, and results. *Am J Orthop.* 2017;46(3):E163–71.

13. Rosen AL, Strauss E. Primary total knee arthroplasty for complex distal femur fractures in elderly patients. *Clin Orthop Relat Res.* 2004;425:101–5.

14. Malviya A, Reed MR, Partington PF. Acute primary total knee arthroplasty for peri-articular knee fractures in patients over 65 years of age. *Injury.* 2011;42(11):1368–71.

15. Choi NY, Sohn JM, Cho SG, Kim SC, In Y. Primary total knee arthroplasty for simple distal femoral fractures in elderly patients with knee osteoarthritis. *Knee Surg Relat Res.* 2013;25(3):141–6.

16. Benazzo F, Rossi SM, Ghiara M, Zanardi A, Perticarini L, Combi A. Total knee replacement in acute and chronic traumatic events. *Injury.* 2014;45(Suppl 6):S98–104.

17. Müller ME, Nazarian SKP, Schatzker J. *The Comprehensive Classification of Fractures of Long Bones.* Berlin, Germany: Springer-Verlag, 1990.

18. Nau T, Pflegerl E, Erhart J, Vecsei V. Primary total knee arthroplasty for periarticular fractures. *J Arthroplasty.* 2003;18(8):968–71.

19. Ebied A, Zayda A, Marei S, Elsayed H. Medium term results of total knee arthroplasty as a primary treatment for knee fractures. *Sicot J.* 2018;4:6.

20. Folbert EC, Hegeman JH, Vermeer M et al. Improved 1-year mortality in elderly patients with a hip fracture following integrated orthogeriatric treatment. *Osteoporos Int.* 2017;28(1):269–77.

21. Nijmeijer WS, Folbert EC, Vermeer M, Vollenbroek-Hutten MMR, Hegeman JH. The consistency of care for older patients with a hip fracture: Are the results of the integrated orthogeriatric treatment model of the Centre of Geriatric Traumatology consistent 10 years after implementation? *Arch Osteoporos.* 2018;13(1):131.

22. Appleton P, Moran M, Houshian S, Robinson CM. Distal femoral fractures treated by hinged total knee replacement in elderly patients. *J Bone Joint Surg Br.* 2006;88(8):1065–70.

23. Pearse EO, Klass B, Bendall SP, Railton GT. Stanmore total knee replacement versus internal fixation for supracondylar fractures of the distal femur in elderly patients. *Injury.* 2005;36(1):163–8.

24. Callaghan JJ, O'Rourke MR, Liu SS. The role of implant constraint in revision total knee arthroplasty: Not too little, not too much. *J Arthroplasty.* 2005;20(4 Suppl 2):41–3.

25. Irisson E, Hemon Y, Pauly V, Parratte S, Argenson JN, Kerbaul F. Tranexamic acid reduces blood loss and financial cost in primary total hip and knee replacement surgery. *Orthop Traumatol Surg Res.* 2012;98(5):477–83.

26. Huten D. Femorotibial bone loss during revision total knee arthroplasty. *Orthop Traumatol Surg Res.* 2013;99(Suppl 1):S22–33.

27. Girerd D, Parratte S, Lunebourg A et al. Total knee arthroplasty revision with trabecular tantalum cones: Preliminary retrospective study of 51 patients from two centres with a minimal 2-year follow-up. *Orthop Traumatol Surg Res.* 2016;102(4):429–33.

28. Parratte S, Abdel MP, Lunebourg A et al. Revision total knee arthroplasty: The end of the allograft era? *Eur J Orthop Surg Traumatol.* 2015;25(4):621–2.

29. Morgan-Jones R, Oussedik SI, Graichen H, Haddad FS. Zonal fixation in revision total knee arthroplasty. *Bone Joint J.* 2015;97-B(2):147–9.

30. Lehmann W, Rupprecht M, Hellmers N et al. Biomechanical evaluation of peri- and interprosthetic fractures of the femur. *J Trauma.* 2010;68(6):1459–63.

31. Weiser L, Korecki MA, Sellenschloh K et al. The role of inter-prosthetic distance, cortical thickness and bone mineral density in the development of inter-prosthetic fractures of the femur: A biomechanical cadaver study. *Bone Joint J.* 2014;96-B(10):1378–84.

32. Abdel MP, Parratte S, Budhiparama NC. The patella in total knee arthroplasty: To resurface or not is the question. *Curr Rev Musculoskelet Med.* 2014;7(2):117–24.

33. Wakabayashi H, Naito Y, Hasegawa M, Nakamura T, Sudo A. A tumor endoprothesis is useful in elderly rheumatoid arthritis patient with acute intercondylar fracture of the distal femur. *Rheumatol Int.* 2012;32(5):1411–3.

34. Folbert EC, Hegeman JH, Gierveld R et al. Complications during hospitalization and risk factors in elderly patients with hip fracture following integrated orthogeriatric treatment. *Arch Orthop Trauma Surg.* 2017;137(4):507–15.

35. Canata GL, Casale V, Chiey A. Pain management in total knee arthroplasty: Efficacy of a multimodal opiate-free protocol. *Joints.* 2016;4(4):222–7.

36. Bell KM, Johnstone AJ, Court-Brown CM, Hughes SP. Primary knee arthroplasty for distal femoral fractures in elderly patients. *J Bone Joint Surg Br.* 1992;74(3):400–2.

37. Müller ME. Classification and international AO-documentation of femur fractures. *Unfallheilkunde.* 1980;83(5):251–9.

25

Osteoporotic long bone fractures

My preferred method of treatment

SASCHA HALVACHIZADEH and HANS-CHRISTOPH PAPE

INTRODUCTION

With constantly increasing life expectancy, the incidence of osteoporotic fractures increases (1). Life expectancy for a newborn female is 83.4 years and a newborn male 78.6 years in Germany in the year 2018, with the median age of the German population at 45.9 years in 2015, the second highest in the world after Japan (2). This leads to our societies being faced with a number of interrelated problems such as the increasing demand for adapting housing (nursing homes), pensions that cover the costs of daily life, and constant growth of medical costs. Many elderly remain healthy and active as they age, while others are in need of continuous medical or physical support. Some remain mobile, and others are completely dependent, wheelchair bound, or even bedridden. These varying groups lead to the necessity of having a treating trauma surgeon who is specially trained to treat these varying groups. Elderly persons often present with medical comorbidities that influence treatment strategies and outcomes. In the United States, more than 95% of patients older than 55 years had at least one comorbidity: hypertension, deficiency anemia, and electrolyte disorders were the most common (3). Comorbidities and the loss of physiologic reserves are considered to be independent factors that influence morbidity and mortality after trauma in the elderly (4).

Osteoporosis is defined as a systemic skeletal disease that is characterized by low bone mass and microarchitectural deterioration of bone tissue, with a consequent increase in bone fragility and susceptibility to fracture (5). This definition was established in 1993 and captures two important characteristics of the disease: its adverse effects on bone mass and microstructure and the clinical outcome of fracture. The importance of low bone mineral density (BMD) in the pathogenesis of fragility fractures is highlighted by the diagnostic criteria produced by the World Health Organization (WHO) using standard scores (SD) scores of BMD (6). Osteoporosis is a disease of the older female that can lead to visual limitations, malnutrition, hypotrophic musculature, polypharmacy, or impaired balance leading to higher risks of falls and fractures. The usual osteoporotic fractures include vertebral compression fractures, hip fractures, proximal humeral fractures, and distal radial fractures (7). The treatment of these fractures has been discussed in detail in previous studies (8–11). This chapter focuses on the treatment of osteoporotic long bone fractures and highlights benefits, indications, as well as tips and tricks of intramedullary nailing and minimally invasive plate osteosynthesis (MIPO) techniques with locking compression plates (LCPs).

PRINCIPLES OF USING LOCKING PLATES

The introduction of the locking plate has expanded the scope of internal fracture fixation. Yet, its use must be justified and optimized due to potential pitfalls and limitations. It is essential that the trauma surgeon has a good understanding of the biomechanics of the resulting constructs, as they can be completely different than those of conventional plates. The learning curve is long with these implants, and numerous failures have occurred (12). Indications and contraindications of the use of locking plates are summarized in Table 25.1.

The new biomechanical properties of locking plates follow the principles of external fixators. The stable interface of locking screws and locking plate make direct contact with the bone unnecessary. Their juxtaosseous position, however, gives them properties similar to internal fixation (13). This also leads to different bone healing with locking plates depending on the fractured part of the bone. While in the epiphyseal area, anatomical reduction of the fragments is needed, in the diaphyseal area, alignment (coronal, sagittal, and rotational) as well as bone length

Table 25.1 Indications for the use of locking plates

Indications	• Deprived bone stock (osteopenia, osteoporosis) • Periprosthetic fractures • Fractures around shoulder, knee, and ankle joints
Contraindications	• Simple fractures requiring interfragmentary compression • Need of screw angulation more than 5°

Table 25.3 Using locking plates for fracture treatment

Pitfalls	
Inadequate reduction	Malunion
Mechanical insufficiency	Impaired bone healing
Tips and tricks	
Sequential insertion	First standard screw
	Second locking screw
	Use lateral compression plate as guide for reduction if plate is anatomical

are restored without the intermediate fragments being exposed or directly reduced (14). Table 25.2 summarizes the four principle of use of locking plates as previously shown (15–18).

The positioning of locking plates is considered of great importance. As a rule of thumb, it has been shown that five holes are needed on either side of the fracture site (15). The position of the locking plate relative to the bone cortex determines the strength of the construct. They preserve the periosteum and are strongest in compression and torsion when the distance from bone to plate is less than 2 mm (19). Placement of the plate too anterior or posterior on the lateral part of the bone reduces its holding strength (12).

Features and difficulties of locking plates

Fractures cannot be reduced on a locking plate. Locking the plate with locking screws should only be performed when the fracture has adequately been reduced. One of the pitfalls in treating fractures with locking plates is the

Table 25.2 The four principles of use of a locking plate

Compression of diaphyseal fractures	• Secure one end of the plate with locking screw • Secure other end with conventional screw (off-center) in dynamic compression hole • Add locking screws to maintain initial compression
Neutralization of diaphyseal fractures	• Position locking plate after interfragmentary screws are in place to increase interfragmentary stability and maintain compression
Bridging of comminuted diaphyseal fractures	• No screws directly over the fracture site to allow bending • Leads to elastic stability
Combination	• Conventional screws in standard holes lead to compression and secure anatomical reduction • Secure epiphyseal block with bridging as needed

inadequate reduction that leads to malunion, since locking plates aim for bone union without loss of the initial correction (12,20). Further, mechanically insufficient constructs lead to higher chances of plate breaking, which subsequently increases the risk of delayed or nonunion (12). If locking plates also provide standard screw fixations, these can be placed for the initial reduction on the plate, to place the bone fragment against the plate. In this case, the plate, if anatomical, can be used as a guide to reduce the fracture. Enhanced stability is achieved by adding locking screws without altering the initial reduction (14). Table 25.3 summarizes these pitfalls and gives the preferred method of usage.

These pitfalls need to be taken into consideration, especially when the fracture is not exposed entirely, e.g., in minimally invasive plate osteosynthesis (MIPO). This technique requires traction procedures, percutaneous reduction clamps, K-wires, and so on.

Minimally invasive plate osteosynthesis

The aim of this technique is to maintain the biological environment around the fracture elementary for physiologic bone healing (21,22). This is achieved by subcutaneous and/or submuscular implantation of a plate after sliding the plate juxtaosseous through a small opening without exposing the fracture site. This small incision, distant from the fracture, preserves the integrity of the soft tissue and attempts to keep the "biology," the fracture hematoma, and the vasculature at the fracture intact (23). This procedure can be performed using locking plates with specially designed instrumentation, allowing manipulation of the plate and ease in locating the locking screw holes percutaneously. However, this technique is demanding when treating fractures with locking plates (18,19):

- The reduction of the fracture must be adequately performed prior to fixation of the plate.
- The locking plate must be properly centered along the length of the bone.
- The locking plate must follow the bone cortex anatomically and parallel.
- The locking plate should be placed as near to the bone as possible without greatly reducing the construct's stiffness.

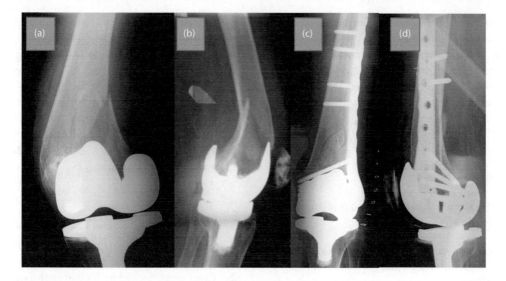

Figure 25.1   (a and b) Anteroposterior (AP) and lateral views of a periprosthetic fracture after total knee arthroplasty. (c and d) AP and lateral radiographs showing the application of a locking plate osteosynthesis.

Fracture reduction should be planned in detail prior to osteosynthesis in the MIPO technique. This includes well-planned placements of all screws and several minimally invasive reduction instruments. The elementary part is planning and performing a gentle and soft tissue-sparing reduction and internal fixation.

Summary

Using locking head screws, a secondary fracture reduction on the plate is no longer possible. The fracture must adequately be reduced prior to locking the LCP with locking screws (Figure 25.1). Using first standard screws, and the anatomical locking plate as a guide for fracture reduction and ending by adding locking head screws minimize the risk of bone healing impairment. The MIPO technique adds a special challenge and requires exact closed reduction and specific locking plate instrumentation for percutaneous fixation and fracture reduction. Treating osteoporotic long bone fractures, the biology and the integrity of the soft tissue should especially be taken into consideration to minimize the risk of delayed or nonunions.

INTRAMEDULLARY NAILING IN OSTEOPOROTIC LONG BONE FRACTURES

> Technically, marrow nailing is not effortless; it demands experience, appropriate dexterity and an imaginative mind in mechanical terms and some will not have all of these.
>
> **Gerhard Küntscher**

In principle, the modern locking and interlocking intramedullary nailing construct can be used for retrograde as well as for antegrade stabilization of diaphyseal long bone fractures (Figure 25.2) (24). A special advantage of nailing is the central stability in the medullary canal: the medullary nail can be compared to a tension band that converts tension forces into stabilizing pressure forces (25). This allows early weight-bearing and mobilization that reduces

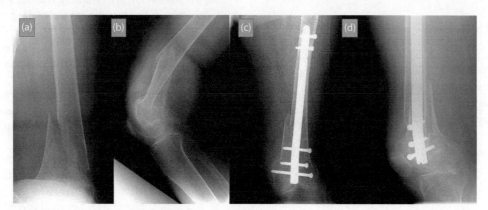

Figure 25.2   (a and b) Anteroposterior and lateral views of distal femoral shaft fractures of an osteoporotic bone. (c and d) Anteroposterior and lateral views of treatment with intramedullary nailing.

the risk of immobilization-associated complications, especially in the elderly. The intramedullary support is most effective at the isthmus; hence, the intramedullary nail should completely bridge the isthmus (26).

Intramedullary nailing shows fundamental biomechanical and biological advantages (27):

- Insertion far from the fracture through a small incision
- Efficient stabilization of the axis of long bones
- Interlocking prevents secondary loss of length, and torsional displacement

However, several complications are associated with intramedullary nailing (27):

- Malalignment/malreduction in axial, sagittal, or coronal plane (primary and secondary)
- Hardware failure
- Delayed union and nonunion
- Systemic/pulmonary/reaming

One of the difficult tasks in treating long bone fractures with intramedullary nailing is finding the correct entry point. This depends on the still controversial discussed aspect of bending. In femoral nails, a substantial variety of different curvature diameters can be found on the market that usually are adjusted to the antecurvature of the femur. Yet, this curvature changes during life and with the degree of osteoporosis: the osteoporotic femur shows more antecurvation compared to the young healthy femur (28). Since osteoporotic changes include widening of the medullary cavity, these mismatches of curvature of the nail and the femoral bone are better accepted in osteoporotic patients compared to young adults. However, ventral cortical abutment, perforation, and even fracture have been described in geriatric patients treated with less bended nails (29). When inserting the femoral nail through the piriformis fossa, special care should be taken not to damage the circumflexa artery around the femoral neck; this may lead to femoral head necrosis (30). An additional risk of this insertion is the iatrogenic femoral head fracture. To reduce this risk, a more lateral insertion point on the

greater trochanter can be chosen for a nail with an additional proximal lateral bending. Such a nail must be turned around its longitudinal axis by 90° during the process of insertion (lateral femoral nail, LFN) (Table 25.4).

Another difficult task in treating long bone fractures with intramedullary nailing is the correct reduction. The correct axis, length, and rotation are elementary to keep in mind during closed reduction of shaft fractures (14). Poorly reduced fractures increase the risk of inadequate healing, pain, and gait problems.

Summary

The surgical stabilization of long bone fractures with intramedullary nailing remains a well-established strategy. The short fragment should be locked with two to three locking screws. The compression mechanism can be used for fractures that support at least 50% of the circumference. Indications for compression nail use include use for the therapy of pseudoarthrosis and arthrodesis. Dynamization of the anterograde compression nail should always be performed through the removal of the proximal locking screw in the static holes.

REFERENCES

1. Burge R, Dawson-Hughes B, Solomon DH, Wong JB, King A, Tosteson A. Incidence and economic burden of osteoporosis-related fractures in the United States, 2005–2025. *J Bone Miner Res.* 2007;22(3):465–75.
2. Statistica. G20: Durchschnittsalter der Bevölkerung in den wichtigsten Industrie- und Schwellenländer im Jahr 2015. 2015. https://de.statista.com/statistik/daten/studie/684349/umfrage/altersmedian-der-bevoelkerung-in-g20-staaten/.
3. Nikkel LE, Fox EJ, Black KP, Davis C, Andersen L, Hollenbeak CS. Impact of comorbidities on hospitalization costs following hip fracture. *J Bone Joint Surg Am.* 2012;94(1):9–17.
4. McMahon DJ, Shapiro MB, Kauder DR. The injured elderly in the trauma intensive care unit. *Surg Clin North Am.* 2000;80(3):1005–19.
5. Consensus A. Consensus development conference: diagnosis, prophylaxis, and treatment of osteoporosis. *Am J Med.* 1993;94(6):646–50.
6. Organization WH. Assessment of fracture risk and its application to screening for postmenopausal osteoporosis: report of a WHO study group [meeting held in Rome June 22–25, 1992]. 1994.
7. Watts NB. The Fracture Risk Assessment Tool (FRAX): Applications in clinical practice. *J Womens Health (Larchmt).* 2011;20(4):525–31.
8. Stone MA, Namdari S. Surgical considerations in the treatment of osteoporotic proximal humerus fractures. *Orthop Clin North Am.* 2019;50(2):223–31.

Table 25.4 Pitfalls and tips: Insertion point for femoral nailing

Reduction of the fracture	Rotation, length, axis
Osteoporotic femur with more antecurvature	Choose appropriate nail
Circumflex artery around femoral head	Be aware of anatomical situation
Iatrogenic femoral neck fracture	Use trochanteric approach if feasible
	Insertion point more lateral than medial on the trochanter
Osteoporotic femur with wider medullary cavity	Use locking screws and/or interlocking constructs

9. Ostergaard PJ, Hall MJ, Rozental TD. Considerations in the treatment of osteoporotic distal radius fractures in elderly patients. *Curr Rev Musculoskelet Med.* 2019;12(1):50–6.

10. Bousson V, Hamze B, Odri G, Funck-Brentano T, Orcel P, Laredo JD. Percutaneous vertebral augmentation techniques in osteoporotic and traumatic fractures. *Semin Intervent Radiol.* 2018;35(4):309–23.

11. Teuber H, Tiziani S, Halvachizadeh S et al. Single-level vertebral kyphoplasty is not associated with an increased risk of symptomatic secondary adjacent osteoporotic vertebral compression fractures: A matched case-control analysis. *Arch Osteoporos.* 2018;13(1):82.

12. Kanakaris NK, Giannoudis PV. Locking plate systems and their inherent hitches. *Injury.* 2010;41(12):1213–9.

13. Egol KA, Kubiak EN, Fulkerson E, Kummer FJ, Koval KJ. Biomechanics of locked plates and screws. *J Orthop Trauma.* 2004;18(8):488–93.

14. Rüedi TP, Murphy WM. *AO Principles of Fracture Management.* Davos, Switzerland: AO Publishing and Stuttgart, Germany: Georg Thieme Verlag, 2000.

15. Gautier E, Sommer C. Guidelines for the clinical application of the LCP. *Injury.* 2003;34(Suppl 2):B63–76.

16. Stoffel K, Dieter U, Stachowiak G, Gächter A, Kuster MS. Biomechanical testing of the LCP—How can stability in locked internal fixators be controlled? *Injury.* 2003;34(Suppl 2):B11–9.

17. Au B, Groundland J, Stoops TK, Santoni BG, Sagi HC. Comparison of 3 methods for maintaining interfragmentary compression after fracture reduction and fixation. *J Orthop Trauma.* 2017;31(4):210–3.

18. Bel JC. Pitfalls and limits of locking plates. *Orthop Traumatol Surg Res.* 2019;105(1S):S103-S9.

19. Ahmad M, Nanda R, Bajwa AS, Candal-Couto J, Green S, Hui AC. Biomechanical testing of the locking compression plate: When does the distance between bone and implant significantly reduce construct stability? *Injury.* 2007;38(3):358–64.

20. Adam P, Bonnomet F, Ehlinger M. Advantage and limitations of a minimally-invasive approach and early weight bearing in the treatment of tibial shaft fractures with locking plates. *Orthop Traumatol Surg Res.* 2012;98(5):564–9.

21. Dimitriou R, Tsiridis E, Giannoudis PV. Current concepts of molecular aspects of bone healing. *Injury.* 2005;36(12):1392–404.

22. Dimitriou R, Jones E, McGonagle D, Giannoudis PV. Bone regeneration: Current concepts and future directions. *BMC Med.* 2011;9:66.

23. Wagner M. General principles for the clinical use of the LCP. *Injury.* 2003;34(Suppl 2):B31–42.

24. Mückley T, Diefenbeck M, Sorkin AT, Beimel C, Goebel M, Bühren V. Results of the T2 humeral nailing system with special focus on compression interlocking. *Injury.* 2008;39(3):299–305.

25. Blum J, Rommens PM. Komprimierte Marknagelung bei Oberarmschaftfrakturen. *Trauma und Berufskrankheit.* 2001;3(3):188–94.

26. Augat P, Penzkofer R, Nolte A et al. Interfragmentary movement in diaphyseal tibia fractures fixed with locked intramedullary nails. *J Orthop Trauma.* 2008;22(1):30–6.

27. Rommens PM, Hessmann MH. *Intramedullary Nailing: A Comprehensive Guide.* London, UK: Springer, 2015.

28. Stedtfeld H-W. *Rationale of Intramedullary Nailing. Intramedullary Nailing.* London, UK: Springer, 2015, pp. 13–25.

29. Collinge CA, Beltran CP. Does modern nail geometry affect positioning in the distal femur of elderly patients with hip fractures? A comparison of otherwise identical intramedullary nails with a 200 versus 150 cm radius of curvature. *J Orthop Trauma.* 2013;27(6):299–302.

30. Gautier E, Ganz K, Krügel N, Gill T, Ganz R. Anatomy of the medial femoral circumflex artery and its surgical implications. *J Bone Joint Surg Br.* 2000;82(5):679–83.

26

Management of osteoporotic extra-articular proximal tibial fractures

DANIELA SANCHEZ, AMRUT BORADE, and DANIEL S. HORWITZ

INTRODUCTION

As the elderly population increases, so does the prevalence of non-hip and nonvertebral osteoporotic fractures. While in the 1990s approximately 19% of tibia fractures were secondary to low-energy trauma, by 2008 33% were considered fragility fractures (1). Extra-articular fractures represent approximately 7% of the fractures involving the proximal tibia, and they can be either simple metaphyseal or complex and multifragmentary, depending on the energy of the trauma and/or the patient's bone quality (2). In most cases, these fractures require surgical treatment with the goal of restoring the length and rotation of the lower extremity, maintaining adequate anatomical and mechanical alignment to allow early range of motion, and the patient's prompt return to function (3).

In the geriatric population, the challenges in the treatment of extra-articular fractures of the proximal tibia include problems related to the fracture personality, difficulties regarding fixation in osteoporotic bone, and the patient's functional level and comorbidities.

Fracture personality: The proximal portion of the tibia has unique muscular forces acting on it that contribute to the displacement of the fragments and need to be identified and dealt with during the surgical procedure in order to avoid malalignment. These fractures usually displace with valgus angulation and an apex anterior deformity caused by the pull of the iliotibial band, the extensor mechanism and the muscles of the anterior compartment of the leg on the proximal fragment, and the hamstrings and gastrocnemius acting on the distal fragment (3). Furthermore, the anterior surface of the proximal tibia has a subcutaneous location, making soft tissues vulnerable to being damaged with either the initial trauma or the surgical procedure (4).

Extra-articular fractures involving the proximal tibia can be located in the uppermost part of the metaphysis just below the articular surface, at the junction of the metaphysis and diaphysis or somewhere between these two regions (mid-region) (Figure 26.1).

Fractures in the proximal or mid-region have a shorter proximal fragment when compared to fractures located in the metaphyseal-diaphyseal junction, and they may be stable or unstable depending on the presence of posterior or medial comminution.

Osteoporotic bone: The decrease in bone mineral density alters the bone's microstructure, especially within the metaphyseal regions of long bones, making these areas relatively weak and prone to sustain more complex and unstable fracture patterns with low-energy injuries (5). Additionally, conventional osteosynthesis techniques may not provide sufficient fixation when treating fractures in osteoporotic bone. Therefore, the challenge of fixation in osteoporotic fractures is to overcome the loss of reduction secondary to bone failure by using appropriate surgical techniques that will prevent screw migration and help create more stable implant-bone constructs (5).

Functional level and comorbidities: Geriatric patients need a prompt return to function to avoid complications related to immobility; therefore, stable fixation of proximal tibial fractures is required in order to allow them early weight-bearing (5). In addition, this group of patients must be addressed as a whole, evaluating their comorbidities as well as their prefracture activity levels with the purpose of choosing the appropriate treatment option for each patient. Metabolic illnesses can affect soft tissue and bone healing, while functional or cognitive impairments may result in a difficult postoperative rehabilitation and can affect the patient's ability to be compliant with instructions given to protect the operated extremity, thus leading to failure of fixation.

In general, the treatment of extra-articular fractures of the proximal tibia in elderly patients requires surgical reduction and internal fixation with adequate stability to

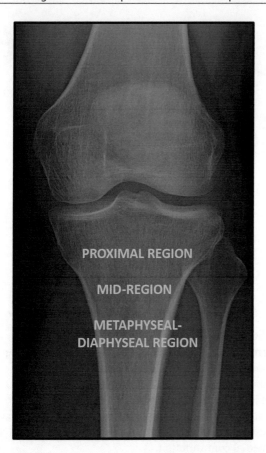

Figure 26.1 Diagram used to describe the fracture location by dividing the proximal tibia into three regions: proximal region, mid-region, and a region involving the metaphyseal-diaphyseal junction.

allow mobilization with weight-bearing and systems that allow biological fixation in order to enhance the bone healing process (6). Currently, the two most common implants used for treatment are intramedullary nails and plates.

Intramedullary nails: Nails allow for biological fixation as they are inserted at a distance from the fracture site, therefore preserving the surrounding soft tissues and extraosseous blood supply (3). In addition, they are load-sharing implants that distribute axial forces equally with the bone and consequently can tolerate weight-bearing forces faster than extramedullary implants (5). With early designs of intramedullary nails, the rate of lower limb malalignment after fixation of proximal tibial fractures was reported to be between 44% and 84% (3). This occurred because of the loss of reduction while introducing nails that had a larger proximal sagittal bend (Herzog curve) extending into the distal fragment or because the fixation of the proximal fragment was suboptimal with fewer proximal interlocking screws and no multiaxis proximal interlocks (3,7).

A new generation of intramedullary nails was designed and new surgical techniques were developed to help overcome the problem of fracture malalignment and make these implants suitable for the treatment of extra-articular fractures of the proximal tibia. Implants were designed with shorter Herzog curves, multiple proximal

interlocking screws that provide angular stability, and fixed-angle interlocks that provide a more stable fixation in short metaphyseal fragments and osteoporotic bone (7). Additionally, nailing with the knee in a semiextended position reduces the pull of the extensor mechanism on the proximal fragment, thereby decreasing the risk of an apex anterior deformity (8–10). This technique also enables the surgeon to perform the procedure with the lower limb in a fixed semiextended position, making it easier to maintain the reduction throughout the surgery and simplifying access to the appropriate starting point (medial to lateral tibial spine and proximal to the anterior edge of the articular surface), which is a major determinant for achieving adequate alignment of the lower extremity (7,11). As a result, the rates of malalignment have dropped significantly to less than 10% (7).

Different strategies, including the use of pointed reduction forceps and the use of small unilateral plates to help maintain fracture reduction while nailing, have been described (3). The use of blocking screws (Poller screws) aids reduction and fixation in osteoporotic bone as they not only narrow the medullary canal and function as a cortical substitute to maintain the nail in the correct position, but they also provide three-point fixation and hence augment the biomechanical stability of the bone-nail construct (12,13). Blocking screws should be placed in the proximal fragment (the shorter fragment), near the fracture and at the concave side of the deformity (i.e., lateral to the nail if there is a valgus angulation) (13). However, these strategies rely on the integrity and quality of the bone in order to maintain reduction and stability and therefore are less reliable in patients with severe osteoporosis or highly comminuted fractures.

CASE EXAMPLE 1

A 51-year-old female presented to the emergency department with 10/10 pain in her right leg after sustaining a fall from standing height when she was at home. She was a heavy smoker, drank alcohol on a regular basis, and had uncontrolled insulin-dependent diabetes mellitus secondary to a partial pancreatectomy. She had a history of a left humerus and left femoral shaft fracture, both surgically treated. On examination, her left lower extremity had a palpable step-off over her proximal tibia, and no gross deformity or neurovascular injuries were documented. X-rays revealed an oblique, comminuted fracture at the metaphyseal-diaphyseal junction of the proximal tibia, with varus angulation and anterior displacement of the distal fragments and a comminuted fracture of the proximal fibula (Figure 26.2a,b). The decision to proceed with surgical fixation was made, and the patient was taken to the operating room within the first 24 hours after her hospital admission for open reduction and internal fixation (ORIF) using a suprapatellar intramedullary nail.

The procedure was performed with the patient in supine position, with her right lower extremity in an extended

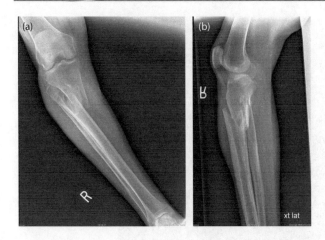

Figure 26.2 X-rays showing a complex, unstable fracture of the proximal tibia in a patient with significant osteopenia. (a) Anteroposterior view shows a significantly comminuted fracture of the metaphyseal-diaphyseal junction of the proximal tibia with varus angulation. (b) Lateral view shows a mild apex anterior deformity and anterior displacement of the distal fragment.

position. The fracture was reduced with manual traction, a 3 cm longitudinal incision above the superior pole of the patella, and dissection through the quadriceps tendon were made in order to place the protector and trocar between the trochlear groove and patella, down to the anterior-superior edge of the proximal tibia, and the starting point was checked under fluoroscopic anteroposterior (AP) and lateral views. The opening reamer was used, the guidewire passed up to the distal tibia physeal scar, and its central position confirmed under fluoroscopic views. Then, sequential reaming up to 11 mm was performed, and a 10 mm nail was placed. At this point, fracture translation, possibly due to the extent of fracture comminution, was noted on the AP view. After placing three proximal multiaxis interlocking screws, a pointed reduction clamp was used to correct malalignment; after obtaining adequate reduction, two distal interlocking screws were placed from medial to lateral, followed by removal of the reduction clamp (Figure 26.3a–d). The final reduction was again checked using fluoroscopic orthogonal views, the quadriceps tendon sutured, and surgical wounds closed. The patient was placed in a bulky splint, and no weight-bearing was allowed.

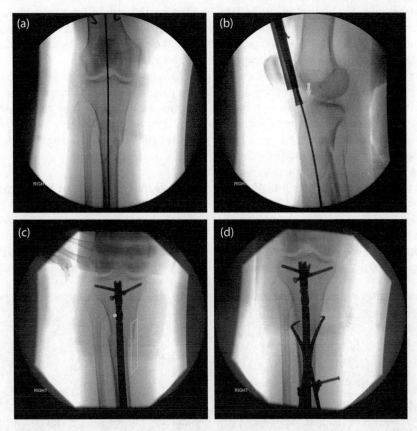

Figure 26.3 Intraoperative fluoroscopic imaging. (a) Anteroposterior (AP) view of the fracture adequately reduced. The guidewire is entering the proximal fragment medial to the lateral tibial spine and crosses the fracture site into the distal fragment. (b) Lateral view shows the guidewire being placed using a suprapatellar approach. There is an apex anterior malalignment, and the guidewire's starting point is too anterior. The arrow indicates the location of the appropriate starting point. (c) AP view of the proximal tibia showing fracture displacement after placing the intramedullary nail. The quadrilateral plate represents the potential location of a low-profile "push" plate that could have been used to reduce and help maintain fracture reduction while nailing. The white dot represents the location of a blocking screw that could have been used to correct valgus malalignment. (d) AP view of the proximal tibia showing a pointed clamp maintaining the reduction while the distal interlocking screws were being placed. Note that the proximal interlocking screws were not replaced, and no blocking screws were used.

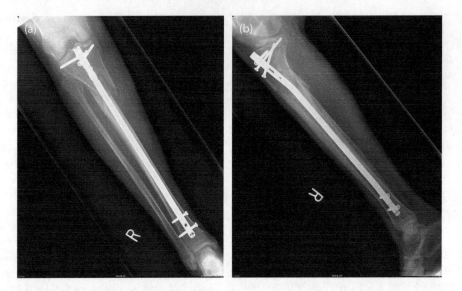

Figure 26.4 X-rays at 2 postoperative weeks showing the fracture fixed with an intramedullary nail. A slight fracture translation in the anteroposterior view (a) and apex anterior deformity (b) of the proximal fragment in the lateral view.

At 15-day follow-up, the patient reported being compliant with no weight-bearing, complained of moderate pain, and her x-rays showed a slight fracture translation in the AP view (Figure 26.4a,b). The patient was placed in a knee immobilizer and kept touch-down weight-bearing on her operated extremity. At a 6-weeks follow-up, she still complained of moderate pain. X-rays showed valgus malalignment as the fracture continued losing its reduction; therefore, the decision was made to take her back into the operating room for knee manipulation and possible revision. The patient was examined under anesthesia, and the fracture was found to be unstable with valgus stress. A reduction clamp was used to correct malalignment, and fixation was augmented using a percutaneous AP blocking screw that was placed lateral to the nail in the proximal fracture fragment. An acceptable alignment was obtained.

At 2 weeks postoperative, the patient was seen in clinic. She was asymptomatic and had maintained toe-touch weight-bearing. She therefore was allowed to start partial weight-bearing protected with a walker. At 6 weeks follow-up, x-rays showed signs of consolidation, and the patient was allowed to weight-bear as tolerated (Figure 26.5a,b).

Critical analysis: Even though the fracture healed and the patient remained asymptomatic after her second procedure, we believe that the patient's outcomes could probably have been better if problems had been identified and addressed differently during the index admission.

Problem 1: Very poor bone quality

Based on her medical and fracture history, we could anticipate this patient may have problems with bone metabolism and healing. She was an uncontrolled diabetic, a heavy smoker, and drank alcohol chronically. Also, even though

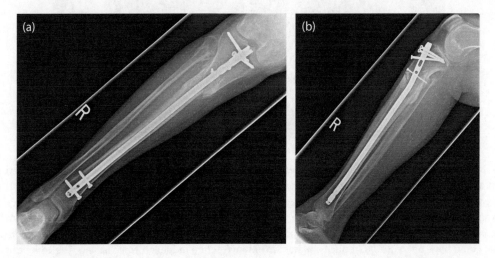

Figure 26.5 X-rays at 6 postoperative weeks after placing the blocking screw show callus formation and improved coronal alignment (a) and slight apex anterior deformity (b).

she was not a geriatric patient, she had a history of other fragility fractures, and her initial x-rays showed significant osteopenia.

Solution 1

Acknowledge all the "red flags" from the patient's medical history, consider different strategies that would help overcome problems related to poor bone quality, and be prepared to deal with them.

Problem 2: Unstable fracture pattern and inadequate fixation

The fracture was initially displaced in both sagittal and coronal planes, and the reduction was difficult to maintain during the surgical procedure. Given the patient's poor bone quality and the presence of significant comminution at the metaphyseal-diaphyseal junction, stable fixation was hard to achieve; the nail could be expected to toggle within the proximal fragment, and the extent of comminution made placing an effective blocking screw difficult. A slight loss of reduction occurred after the nail was placed, and even though the alignment was corrected using a pointed reduction clamp, the proximal interlocks were not replaced, and the final fixation was not strong enough to prevent fracture translation (Figure 26.3d).

Solution 2

It is crucial that the fracture be completely and adequately reduced before reaming (7). Recognize that there is a high risk of valgus malalignment with intramedullary nailing with this fracture pattern and be prepared to use different strategies to help maintain reduction throughout the procedure. The stability of the proximal fragment could be assessed preoperatively by flexing the knee greater than 90°; the behavior of this fragment could possibly help identify which cases could require additional methods to obtain and maintain reduction. In this case, using a reduction clamp, femoral distractor, or unicortical "push" plate would have helped maintain the reduction while reaming (3,7,14) (Figure 26.3c).

When doing your preoperative plan, include plating as an appropriate alternative for fixation and have it available in the operating room.

Problem 3: Starting point was too anterior

Identifying the correct starting point is crucial, especially when treating proximal tibial fractures. If the starting point is too anterior, the nail will be directed posterior as it engages into the distal fragment, therefore creating an apex-anterior deformity of the proximal tibia (3).

Solution 3

Intramedullary nailing using a semiextended technique allows the starting point to be located just proximal to the anterior edge of the articular surface and inserted parallel to the anterior cortex of the tibia, thus keeping the starting point aligned with the medullary canal and reducing the risk of creating an apex anterior deformity (8,10). This technique can be performed by using a suprapatellar approach or a parapatellar approach (with or without performing an arthrotomy) (15). The parapatellar approach as described by Tornetta and the suprapatellar approach, both use an arthrotomy to give access to the patellofemoral joint; therefore, they have a higher risk of damaging the cartilage of the patellofemoral joint (10,15). Also, when using the suprapatellar approach, if the anterior compartment of the knee is too tight, the angle of insertion of the nail is limited; therefore, access to the appropriate starting point may be more difficult, resulting in a starting point that is too anterior. The modified parapatellar approach is an extra-articular approach that allows for patellar subluxation; therefore, it reduces the risk of damaging articular structures inside the knee, and because the insertion angle is not restricted by the extensor mechanism, it allows an easier access to the appropriate starting point (8). This approach depends on the lateral/medial mobility of the patella, which has to be assessed prior to surgery in order to decide whether a medial or lateral incision is required to allow access to the correct starting point (8). Also, there is still a risk of iatrogenic damage to intra-articular structures, and therefore a careful dissection must be performed (15). In this case, the suprapatellar approach could have limited the insertion angle leading to an anterior starting point. It is possible that the apex anterior deformity could have been corrected by obtaining a more accurate starting point using a parapatellar approach.

Problem 4: Final alignment could be improved

At the time of the second intervention, even though the fracture was unstable and had not yet healed, the alignment obtained by using a reduction clamp and a blocking screw was better but not ideal. This is not unusual in revision situations where the percutaneous techniques used in the acute setting are not as effective.

Solution 4: Utilization of an open technique

The alignment could have been further improved by making a small incision, directly cleaning out interposed tissues, manipulating the fracture site, and using a unicortical "push" plate without further compromising the soft tissue envelope (7). This minimally invasive approach does not involve disruption of the periosteum blood supply and has potential to significantly improve stability and bony contact.

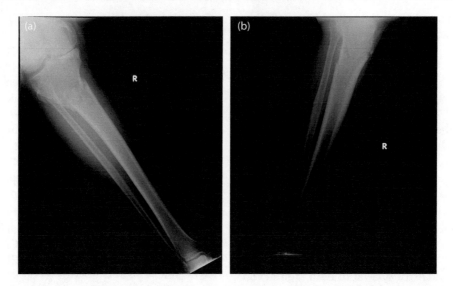

Figure 26.6 X-rays showing a short, oblique comminuted fracture at the mid-region of the proximal tibia, slightly displaced in the anteroposterior view (a) and with a fracture line that extends across the tibial tuberosity without significant displacement (b).

CASE EXAMPLE 2

A 65-year-old man with a medical history of diabetes presented to the emergency department after sustaining a fall from his standing height. He complained of 8/10 pain in his right knee and inability to weight-bear. On examination, he had tenderness and swelling over his proximal tibia, and no neurovascular deficits were documented. X-rays showed a short, oblique fracture at the mid-region of his proximal tibia, slightly displaced in the AP view. The lateral view revealed involvement of the tibial tuberosity but no significant displacement in the sagittal axis (Figure 26.6a,b). The patient was taken into the operating room for surgical fixation using an intramedullary nail.

The procedure was performed with the patient supine, and a lateral parapatellar approach to the proximal tibia was made. Reduction was maintained using a percutaneous reduction clamp. Under fluoroscopic control, the correct starting point was identified in the AP and lateral views, and the guidewire was advanced across the fracture up to the physeal scar at the distal tibia. After sequential reaming, the intramedullary nail was placed, its correct position and lower leg alignment checked under fluoroscopic views. Proximal AP and oblique interlocking screws were placed followed by an additional cancellous screw in the AP direction securing the tibial tuberosity. Then, two distal interlocking screws were placed, the reduction clamp was removed, and surgical wounds were closed. AP and lateral fluoroscopic views confirmed good alignment, and the patient was placed in a knee immobilizer in full extension without weight-bearing (Figure 26.7a,b).

The patient's postoperative course was uneventful, and he progressively gained active range of motion. At 6 postoperative weeks, he had no knee instability. His x-rays showed the fracture was healing with no limb malalignment, and the patient was allowed to initiate progressive weight-bearing.

This patient healed anatomically and without any postoperative complications. Even though he had a more proximal fracture when compared with the patient in case example 1, he seemed to have bone of better quality, and his fracture appeared more stable; its initial displacement was minimal and had significantly less metaphyseal comminution. Although these differences could explain the better outcomes seen in the second patient, there are some aspects of this patient's treatment that should be highlighted, as we believe that they positively influenced the patient's final outcomes.

1. The fracture was anatomically reduced using a pointed clamp that was not removed until the distal interlocks were placed, helping maintain the reduction throughout the procedure.
2. The tibia was nailed with the knee in a semiextended position using a lateral parapatellar approach, and this helped control the lower limb's alignment as it allowed the placement of a correct starting point.

Plates: ORIF of extra-articular fractures of the proximal tibia can also be achieved with plating, but once again, the concepts of biological fixation and the biomechanics of stabilization of osteoporotic fractures must be followed in order to obtain good clinical outcomes.

Locking plates do not rely on friction against the bone for achieving a stable fixation, but instead they shift the focus of fracture stability to the screw-plate interface, making them suitable implants for the treatment of osteoporotic fractures (5,6). Additionally, they improve proximal fixation by allowing the use of locked screws in multiple planes when the metaphyseal fragment is too short, thus providing angular stability (5).

Most commonly used implants offer jigs to assist with percutaneous application and can therefore be placed using minimally invasive plate osteosynthesis (MIPO)

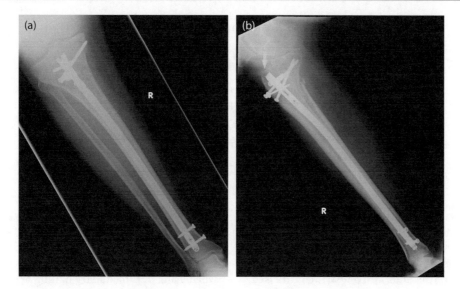

Figure 26.7 Immediate postoperative x-rays showing the fracture reduced in an anatomical position and fixed with an intramedullary nail with no malalignment in the anteroposterior (a) or lateral views (b). In this case, the starting point of the nail was in the appropriate position (white arrow).

techniques that may promote fracture healing (6,16). This biologically friendly technique may be comparable to the biological aspects of intramedullary nailing (16,17).

Stable fixation of extra-articular fractures of the proximal tibia can be achieved by using either one lateral plate or dual plating (lateral and medial plates) depending on the location and fracture pattern (16). Using a single lateral locking plate can be appropriate for more proximal stable fractures that do not involve comminution of the medial column and stable fractures in the mid-region of the proximal tibia (16). In general, single lateral locked plates should be reserved for nondisplaced fractures where reduction is not required, while dual plating should be used in all unstable fractures. Percutaneous biological techniques can be applied in this setting as well.

CASE EXAMPLE 3

A 66-year-old male presented to the emergency department with 9/10 pain in his left leg and inability to bear weight. The pain started when he twisted his right knee after being hit on his back by a tree while he was cutting wood. He denied tingling or decreased sensation. He had a history of ulcerative colitis and was currently on corticosteroid therapy. On examination, he had a palpable deformity on the anterior portion of his proximal tibia, had no evidence of compartment syndrome, and was neurovascularly intact. X-rays showed an oblique comminuted and slightly shortened fracture of the metaphyseal-diaphyseal junction of the proximal tibia and an oblique fracture of the neck of the fibula (Figure 26.8a,b). The patient was admitted to the hospital for ORIF of his fracture.

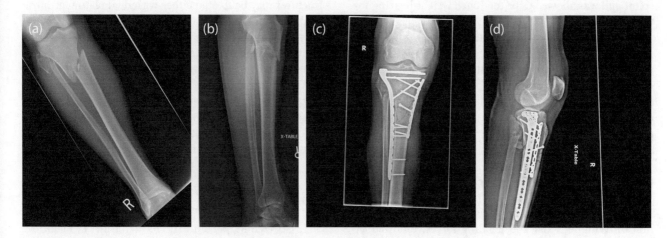

Figure 26.8 (a and b) X-rays showing a short, oblique comminuted fracture at the metaphyseal-diaphyseal junction of the proximal tibia, with valgus angulation in the anteroposterior (AP) view (a) and a slight apex anterior deformity in the lateral view (b). (c and d) Immediate postoperative x-rays showing the fracture reduced in an anatomical position and fixed with dual plating using the minimally invasive plate osteosynthesis technique. No malalignment in the AP (c) or lateral views (d).

Table 26.1 Preferred method of treatment according to fracture location and stability

	Stable nondisplaced	Unstable displaced
1. Proximal region	Single lateral locked plate	Dual plating
2. Mid-region	Single lateral locked plate or IMN ± augmentation	Dual plating
3. Metaphyseal-diaphyseal region	IMN ± augmentation	IMN ± augmentation or dual plating

Abbreviation: IMN, intramedullary nailing.

The procedure was performed with the patient in supine position. Under fluoroscopic views, reduction was obtained with longitudinal traction and a pointed reduction clamp. Then a lateral approach to the proximal tibia was performed, the fascia of the anterior compartment incised, and the iliotibial band retracted posteriorly. The fracture was exposed, and after minimal periosteal stripping, the hematoma was evacuated. The fracture was reduced under direct visualization and reduction temporarily maintained with a reduction clamp; at this point, a lag screw was placed across the fracture plane. A 12-hole locking compression plate was inserted over the lateral aspect of the proximal tibia, and its position and the quality of the reduction were assessed under fluoroscopic orthogonal views. Four cortical screws were placed in the distal fragment, six locking screws were placed in the proximal fragment, and finally a kickstand screw was placed for additional support. A small medial incision was then made, and an 8-hole 3.5 mm reconstruction plate was slid using the MIPO technique. Plate position and alignment were checked using the image intensifier, three unicortical locking screws were placed proximally, and two bicortical nonlocked screws were placed in the distal fragment. The final quality of reduction and implant position were assessed using fluoroscopic AP and lateral views, and surgical wounds were irrigated and closed (Figure 26.8c,d). The patient was placed in a bulky splint and was allowed to be toe-touch weight-bearing for the first 6 weeks.

At a 2-week follow-up, the patient had minimal pain, was placed in a hinged knee brace with 0–40° of flexion, and was allowed to start physical therapy with active range of motion out of his brace. At 6 postoperative weeks, his x-rays showed that alignment was maintained, clear evidence of fracture healing, and the patient was allowed progressive weight-bearing.

Intramedullary nailing versus locking plates

Biomechanical studies have shown that nails resist significantly higher axial and bending forces, followed by two-plate constructs, and a single lateral locking plate is the least stable method of fixation (16). As a result, single lateral locked plating is rarely advisable and when utilized should only be in the setting of a nondisplaced or non-ambulatory patient. When treating geriatric patients, it is vital to recognize that they are not always compliant with weight-bearing indications, and they benefit from stable fixations that allow earlier mobilization and return to function. Obtaining and maintaining an adequate reduction when using intramedullary nailing may be more demanding, and the fracture stability may be difficult to judge with severe osteoporosis and comminution (18). The anatomical design of plates may help achieve a better reduction, and locking screws in the proximal fragment provide rigid fixation with angular stability (17). Nevertheless, when comparing infection rates, surgical time, length of stay, range of motion, and nonunion rates, intramedullary nails and locking plates are equivalent for fractures in the mid-region and metaphyseal-diaphyseal junction, but this may not be applicable for more proximal fractures (6).

PREFERRED METHOD OF TREATMENT

We strongly suggest the use of dual plating in comminuted fractures with a short proximal segment in order to obtain stable fixation. In simple fractures with a short metaphyseal fragment and an intact medial column, a lateral locked plate may provide more stability than an intramedullary nail, and the construct may be rigid enough that no additional medial stabilization is required. Unstable distal fractures may be treated either with dual plating or intramedullary nailing with augmentation techniques. Finally, simple fractures that are located more distally can be successfully treated with intramedullary nailing, allowing the patient early weight-bearing (Table 26.1).

All treatment options rely on a careful analysis of the location and comminution, and stability should always be assessed intraoperatively. When in doubt in an osteoporotic extra-articular fracture of the proximal tibia, the use of minimally invasive dual plating is recommended.

REFERENCES

1. Goetzen M, Nicolino T, Hofmann-fliri L, Blauth M, Windolf M, Ing D. Metaphyseal screw augmentation of the LISS-PLT plate with polymethylmethacrylate improves angular stability in osteoporotic proximal third tibial fractures: A biomechanical study in human cadaveric tibiae. *J Orthop Trauma.* 2014;28(5):294–9.

2. Pape HC, Rommens PM. Tibia, proximal. In: Thomas P. Rüedi, Richard E. Buckley, Christopher G. Moran. *AO Principles of Fracture Management*. Second expanded edition 2007, pp. 814–33, New York: Thieme.

3. Hiesterman TG, Shafiq BX, Cole PA. Intramedullary nailing of extra-articular proximal tibia fractures. *J Am Acad Orthop Surg*. 2011;19:690–700.

4. Ramesh Krishna K, Ibrahim M, Shreekantha KS. Minimally invasive plate osteosynthesis in metaphyseal fractures of tibia. *Int J Med Public Health*. 2015;5(4):357–62.

5. Bogunovic L, Cherney SM, Rothermich MA, Gardner MJ. Biomechanical considerations for surgical stabilization of osteoporotic fractures. *Orthop Clin North Am*. 2013;44:183–200.

6. Naik MA, Arora G, Tripathy SK, Sujir P, Rao SK. Clinical and radiological outcome of percutaneous plating in extra-articular proximal tibia fractures: A prospective study. *Injury*. 2013;44(8):1081–6.

7. Stinner DJ, Mir H. Techniques for intramedullary nailing of proximal tibia fractures. *Orthop Clin North Am*. 2014;45(1):33–45.

8. Kubiak EN, Widmer BJ, Horwitz DS. Extra-articular technique for semiextended tibial nailing. *J Orthop Trauma*. 2010;24(11):704–8.

9. Zelle BA, Boni G, Hak DJ, Stahel PF. Advances in intramedullary nailing: Suprapatellar nailing of tibial shaft fractures in the semiextended position. *Orthopedics*. 2015;38(12):751–5.

10. Tornetta P, Collins E. Semiextended position of intramedullary nailing of the proximal tibia. *Clin Orthop Relat Res*. 1996;(328):185–9.

11. Tornetta P, Riina J, Geller J, Purban W. Intraarticular anatomic risks of tibial nailing. *J Orthop Trauma*. 1999;13(4):247–51.

12. Krettek C, Stephan C, Schandelmaier P, Richter M, Pape HC, Miclau T. The use of Poller screws as blocking screws in stabilising tibial fractures treated with small diameter intramedullary nails. *J Bone Joint Surg Br*. 1999;81(6):963–8.

13. Stedtfeld H-W, Mittlmeier T, Landgraf P, Ewert A. The logic and clinical applications of blocking screws. *J Bone Joint Surg Am*. 2004;86–A(Suppl 2):17–25.

14. Nork SE, Barei DP, Frcs C et al. Intramedullary nailing of proximal quarter tibial fractures. *J Ortho Trauma*. 2006;20(8):523–8.

15. Zamora R, Wright C, Short A, Seligson D. Comparison between suprapatellar and parapatellar approaches for intramedullary nailing of the tibia. Cadaveric study. *Injury*. 2016;47(10):2987–90.

16. Lee SM, Oh CW, Oh JK, Kim JW, Lee HJ, Chon CS, Lee BJ, Kyung HS. Biomechanical analysis of operative methods in the treatment of extra-articular fracture of the proximal tibia. *Clin Orthop Surg*. 2014;6(3):312–7.

17. Chand R, Umesh M, Gupta G, Gahlot N, Gaba S. Intramedullary nailing versus proximal plating in the management of closed extra-articular proximal tibial fracture: A randomized controlled trial. *J Orthop Traumatol*. 2015;16:203–8.

18. Lindvall E, Sanders R, Dipasquale T, Herscovici D, Haidukewych G, Sagi C. Intramedullary nailing versus percutaneous locked plating of extra-articular proximal tibial fractures: Comparison of 56 cases. *J Orthop Trauma*. 2009;23(7):485–92.

27

Osteoporotic ankle fractures
Principles of treatment

THEODOROS H. TOSOUNIDIS and MICHAEL G. KONTAKIS

INTRODUCTION

Low-energy ankle fractures constitute a significant health problem (1,2), and it is expected that in some European countries their number will increase by threefold in 2030 compared to 2000 (3). Low-energy ankle fractures occur mainly in older individuals, and the increased incidence cannot be explained only by the changing demographics of the population. In addition to the burden imposed on the individual, the cost of his or her management is also significant. In the Unites States, the cost for the inpatient care and readmission of these injuries in older individuals has been estimated to be $185 million (4).

Despite the seemingly obvious relation between osteoporosis and ankle fractures in the elderly (older than 60 years), the supporting evidence is sparse. Only recently have ankle fractures in older individuals clearly been correlated with osteoporosis. In a study investigating the osteoporotic features of ankle fractures, Lee et al. (5) documented that older patients (older than 50 years old) showed notably lower attenuation on computed tomography (CT) scan at the lateral/medial malleolus, talus, and distal tibial metaphysis compared to younger counterparts in both genders. Emerging evidence suggests that low-energy ankle fractures in older adults should be considered fractures affecting frail patients (2). In a recent study including 19,648 patients with ankle fractures older than 65 years of age, treated either operatively or nonoperatively, the 1-year mortality rate was significantly increased in both groups (2). The overall 1-year mortality rate for ankle fractures was less compared to the mortality of geriatric patients with hip fractures (6).

Monotrauma patients with a low-energy ankle fracture usually suffer a supination external rotation injury (7). However, a low-energy trauma mechanism with or without a pronation abduction injury pattern and a history of previous osteoporotic fracture are indirect signs of an osteoporotic ankle fracture (8).

In the past, high complication rates after operative management of these injuries have been documented and have led many surgeons to follow a more "conservative" approach to these injuries (9,10). Variation to the management according the geographic location of the treating surgeon has been observed (1), with surgeons of the west coast of the United States advocating more for surgical management compared to their colleagues from the east coast. Increased rates of nonunion and malunion have been documented with nonoperative management (11), while other studies have shown better functional outcomes with operative management (12). Nevertheless, the literature is still unclear as to which management provides the better outcomes. The first report of the ongoing Ankle Injury Management (AIM) trial (13,14), which is a pragmatic, multicenter, equivalence, randomized controlled trial (RCT) that has included 620 patients over 60 years of age and compared the close contact casting technique to the open reduction and internal fixation (ORIF) of unstable ankle fractures, concluded that both of these treatment options provide clinically equivalent outcome to ORIF at reduced cost to the UK National Health Service (NHS) and to society at 6 months.

In this chapter, we highlight the principles, the unique characteristics, and the technicalities of both the nonoperative and operative management of osteoporotic ankle fractures in the older population.

NONOPERATIVE MANAGEMENT

Nonoperative management of osteoporotic fractures of the ankle should strongly be considered in nonambulatory individuals, those who cannot follow postoperative weight-bearing and mobilization instructions (e.g., patients with cognitive disorders), and those who cannot tolerate an anesthetic. Nonoperative management should be applied only if the fracture is closed and stable.

The method of management is a circular fiberglass cast either placed the traditional way or with a close contact casting. As previously mentioned, the AIM trial (13,14) suggested that close contact casting offers results equivalent to those of ORIF.

The various comorbidities of an elderly individual should not be a contraindication to surgery, but the patients should be informed about the possible increased risk of postoperative complications (15). Diabetes mellitus is a disease that has to be specifically appreciated in the case of an ankle fracture of an elderly person. The presence of peripheral neuropathy at the ankle makes the nonoperative management of these injuries common for many surgeons since the surgical treatment is fraught with devastating complications (8). Nevertheless, nonoperative management is not without complications, with some studies demonstrating significant complications of the nonoperative treated patients, including malunion, loss of reduction, new-onset Charcot arthropathy, cast ulcers, deep infection, and unplanned subsequent operation (16,17).

The follow-up and the duration of immobilization with a cast should also be closely observed. Close follow-up is advisable to detect any displacements that can be corrected and also any complications such as pressure ulcers, etc. The usual regime is clinical and radiological follow-up immediately after the reduction and immobilization, and at 2 weeks, 8 weeks, and 3 months after the injury. The usual time of immobilization is a minimum of 8 weeks. During this time, non-weight-bearing is exercised, and gradual progression to weight-bearing along with gait training with active-assisted range of motion, proprioception exercises commences after the removal of the cast at 8 weeks. Strengthening exercises are initiated at about 3 months postinjury.

OPERATIVE MANAGEMENT

The operative management of osteoporotic ankle fractures should follow the principles of surgery of osteoporotic bone and take into account the need for early mobilization of the elderly individual. Preoperative planning and application of good surgical principles such as gentle handling of the soft tissues is of paramount importance. The basic methods of fixation techniques/strategies used to treat these fractures include but are not limited to the locking plating technique, the "comb" plating technique, the fibula "intramedullary" fixation, the tension band fixation technique of medial malleolus, the arthrodesis with a hindfoot nail, and the external fixation. All of the aforementioned methods of fixation are designed to provide safer fixation of the bones, and their application should be accompanied by a meticulous surgical technique to avoid additional compromise of the vulnerable soft tissues.

Internal fixation

Recent biomechanical evidence supports that locking plates offer better fixation in osteoporotic ankle fractures.

Nevertheless, in a meta-analysis of biomechanical studies on reinforced fixation of distal fibular fractures, Dingemans et al. (18) concluded that there is no superiority of locking plates to nonlocking conventional plates. Nevertheless, the authors of the study suggested that locking plates might be advantageous due to the fact that their strength is independent of the bone quality. There is conflicting evidence in regard to the rates of adverse events, mainly in terms of soft tissue complications with the use of locking and conventional plates in the treatment of osteoporotic ankle fractures. In a retrospective clinical study of 160 patients with distal fibula fractures treated either with a locking or a nonlocking plate, Moriarity et al. (19) concluded that there were no significant differences in complication rates in both groups. Also, the soft tissue complication rates were similar (3.97% for nonlocking versus 3.85% for locking plates, $P = 1.00$). On the contrary, Schepers et al. (20) in a retrospective cohort of 165 patients found a wound complication rate of 5.5% in the patient group treated with conventional plates compared to 17.5% for the wound complication rate in the locking plate group. With the cost of locking plates being significantly higher (21), the absolute need of these plates for the management of ankle fractures is not a necessity, but special consideration of this method of fixation should be given for the osteoporotic fracture management. Based on the observed complication and reoperation rates, in a retrospective study of 145 patients with ankle fractures, Lyle et al. (22) concluded that despite the cost being six times higher, bone-specific locking compression distal fibula plates are useful in the fixation of bone fractures with poor bone quality.

The "comb" technique (15) is used for the fixation of the lateral malleolus. A plate that offers a combination of locking and nonlocking screws is used, and the distal part of the plate is filled with locking screws, whereas in the proximal part, multiple fully threaded syndesmotic screws are applied. The latter screws are placed in a tri- or tetracortical fashion in order to provide multiple points of fixation and thus better fixation in the osteoporotic bone. The number of the screws placed depends on the quality of the underlying bone, but the tendency is to place as many as possible. Figure 27.1 illustrates the use of the comb technique.

Screw augmentation with bone cement is a concept that is used in the fixation of osteoporotic bone in main body areas such as the spine, the hip, the proximal humerus, and the tibial plateau (23). The rationale behind the use of polymethyl methacrylate (PMMA) or calcium phosphate cement (CPC) is to improve the anchorage of screws. In osteoporotic ankle fracture fixation, the evidence is sparse. Assal et al. (24) in a prospective nonconsecutive case series of 36 patients used augmentation of the internal fixation fixing the lateral malleolus either with a lag screw and an intramedullary wire or with only a terminally threaded wire. A nonlocking one-third tubular plate was used in all cases. Early weight-bearing at a mean of 13.5 days was initiated in all patients. The authors reported good functional results with 90% of the patients returning to the prefracture function with only two minor complications. A cadaveric study (25) comparing the biomechanical properties of

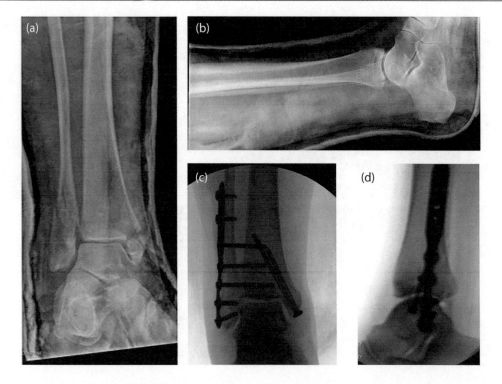

Figure 27.1 (a and b) Preoperative anteroposterior (AP) and lateral radiographs of an ankle fracture in an 84-year-old female patient. (c and d) Intraoperative AP and lateral radiographs illustrating the fixation with the "comb" technique.

different augmentation methods concluded that a locking plate and screws used for the fixation of an osteoporotic lateral malleolus had similar strength to that augmented with calcium sulfate-calcium phosphate graft and/or tibia-pro-fibula screws.

For the fixation of the medial malleolus in osteoporotic ankle fractures, the tension band technique provides a reliable and secure fixation (26,27). In small fragments, one 4.0 mm partially threaded cancellous screw placed perpendicular to the fracture line provides a safe and effective method of fixation (28).

Intramedullary fibula fixation is a method of fixation that has gained significant popularity in recent years. Intramedullary fibula fixation can be performed with either an intramedullary screw or nail, both inserted from a point distal to the tip of the lateral malleolus where the skin is usually less affected by the injury. The obvious advantage of this technique is its minimally invasive nature and the respect of the soft tissues. This is a feature specifically useful in the setting of an osteoporotic fracture in an elderly individual with compromised skin. Nevertheless, closed intramedullary nailing of the fibula can be technically demanding, especially in obese patients and in highly comminuted and/or displaced fractures. A recent systematic review (29) that included 17 eligible studies and 1008 patients concluded that this method of fixation (intramedullary device) provides excellent outcomes with few complications, yet the available evidence to date is insufficient to support its superiority to standard plating techniques. Another systematic review (30) evaluated the published data regarding intramedullary screw fixation of fibula fractures. The

review included six studies with a total of 180 patients. The authors reported that anatomical reduction was achieved in 93.3% of patients, and very few other complications were observed. They concluded that it is a safe and adequate method of fibula fixation and that more evidence is required to draw safe conclusions in regard to the functional outcome. Rehman and colleagues (31) reviewed the available literature. They found 10 different intramedullary nails that have published data, but only three of them were evaluated with RCTs. They summarized the design aspects of fibular nails and concluded that nails might be better for the fixation of the lateral malleolus in elderly patients prone to soft tissue complications. Figure 27.2 shows a patient treated with an intramedullary screw for the fixation of the fibula.

Arthrodesis

Arthrodesis for ankle and pilon fractures is a salvage fixation method that can be used in severely comminuted, unreconstructable fractures, fractures with concomitant compromised skin, and in elderly patients who need early ambulation to avoid the complications of recumbency. Every effort should be undertaken to avoid this fixation method in young patients. The fact that the subtalar joint is included in the fixation and is subsequently immobilized usually does not have a significant impact on the functional outcome of elderly osteoporotic patients, since these patients are already very frail and their preinjury mobilization status is limited. Similar to the hip fracture surgery, the goal of the operative procedure is to provide a safe and

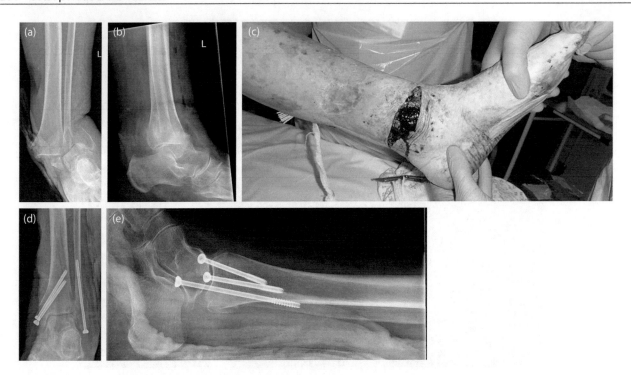

Figure 27.2 (a, b, c) Preoperative anteroposterior (AP) and lateral radiographs and clinical picture of an open fracture disloca-tion in an 80-year-old female patient. (d and e) Postoperative AP and lateral radiographs illustrating the use of intramedullary screw fixation of the fibula.

stable fixation and to mobilize the patient as soon as pos-sible after the surgery (15). When a retrograde hindfoot tibio-talar calcaneal (TCC) nail is used to treat ankle frac-tures in osteoporotic elderly patients, it is used without the intent to fuse the joints (32). In elderly patients, preparation of the joints is not necessary (33), and hardware failure has not proved to be a significant complication for nonambula-tory elderly patients (33,34).

In a retrospective review study of their practice, Taylor et al. (35) reported on the outcomes of 31 patients treated with a TTC nail for the management of ankle fragility frac-tures. The mean follow-up of the patients was 13.6 months, and the mean age of the patients was 63 years. No fusion of the ankle or subtalar joints was performed. The authors reported that decreased operative time and blood loss as well as minimal soft tissue insult and early mobilization (immediate partial or full weight-bearing according to the treating surgeon's preference) were the advantages of this fixation method. Complete union was observed in 90.3% of the patients at an average of 22.2 months after surgery. The authors concluded that the retrograde TTC nail is safe and effective in the management of fragility ankle fractures. A recent RCT (36) that included 87 patients over the age of 60 years, with closed bi- or trimalleolar ankle fractures or frac-ture dislocations randomized in either hindfoot nail fixa-tion or standard ORIF, and a mean follow-up of 14 months, concluded that the patients treated with the TTC nail had shorter hospital stays and significantly lower complica-tion rates compared to the ORIF group. The complications reported for the TTC group of patients were one superficial entry point infection, one deep venous thrombosis, and one

symptomatic pull-out of the nail. No other skin and soft tis-sue complications were reported. The return to the prein-jury level of function evaluated with the olerud-molander ankle score (OMAS) was similar in both groups. The authors advised that the TTC nail is a safe and effective method of treating ankle fractures in elderly osteoporotic patients with the major advantage being the low rate of complications.

Steinmann pin

A method of stabilization of the ankle using a Steinmann pin or multiple large-diameter wires from the calcaneus through the talus to the distal tibia (vertical transarticular pin fixation) can be used for the provisional stabilization in the setting of polytrauma in open fractures and also when internal fixation is deemed inappropriate due to a severely compromised soft tissue envelope and/or concomitant peripheral vascular disease and neuropathy. It can also be used as an adjunct to the internal fixation. Good results of this method have been reported (15,37). Figure 27.3 illustrates the management of an open ankle fracture in an older person using a combination of a Steinmann pin and internal fixation with an intramedullary fibula screw.

SUMMARY

Contemporary operative and nonoperative osteoporotic ankle fracture management should be expected to yield good results. The management should be tailored to the

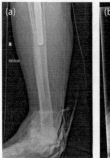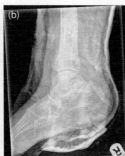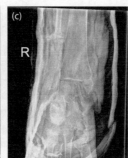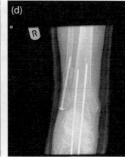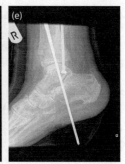

Figure 27.3 (a) Anteroposterior (AP) radiograph showing an open fracture dislocation in a 90-year-old patient. (b and c) Lateral and AP radiographs after the reduction. (d and e) Postoperative AP and lateral radiographs showing the use of an intramedullary fibular screw and a vertical transarticular pin fixation.

needs of the individual patient. Close contact casting should be strongly considered for nonoperative management. The methods of surgical treatment should respect the usually compromised soft tissue envelope and aim to achieve a stable ankle that can allow early mobilization of the patient.

REFERENCES

1. Koval KJ, Lurie J, Zhou W et al. Ankle fractures in the elderly: What you get depends on where you live and who you see. *J Orthop Trauma*. 2005;19(9):635–9.

2. Bariteau JT, Hsu RY, Mor V, Lee Y, DiGiovanni CW, Hayda R. Operative versus nonoperative treatment of geriatric ankle fractures: A Medicare Part A claims database analysis. *Foot Ankle Int*. 2015;36(6):648–55.

3. Kannus P, Palvanen M, Niemi S, Parkkari J, Jarvinen M. Increasing number and incidence of low-trauma ankle fractures in elderly people: Finnish statistics during 1970–2000 and projections for the future. *Bone*. 2002;31(3):430–3.

4. Kadakia RJ, Ahearn BM, Tenenbaum S, Bariteau JT. Costs associated with geriatric ankle fractures. *Foot Ankle Spec*. 2017;10(1):26–30.

5. Lee KM, Chung CY, Kwon SS et al. Ankle fractures have features of an osteoporotic fracture. *Osteoporos Int*. 2013;24(11):2819–25.

6. Hsu RY, Lee Y, Hayda R, DiGiovanni CW, Mor V, Bariteau JT. Morbidity and mortality associated with geriatric ankle fractures: A Medicare Part A claims database analysis. *J Bone Joint Surg Am*. 2015;97(21):1748–55.

7. Briet JP, Houwert RM, Smeeing DPJ et al. Differences in classification between mono- and polytrauma and low- and high-energy trauma patients with an ankle fracture: A retrospective cohort study. *J Foot Ankle Surg*. 2017;56(4):793–6.

8. Rammelt S. Management of ankle fractures in the elderly. *EFORT Open Rev*. 2016;1(5):239–46.

9. Beauchamp CG, Clay NR, Thexton PW. Displaced ankle fractures in patients over 50 years of age. *J Bone Joint Surg Br*. 1983;65(3):329–32.

10. Litchfield JC. The treatment of unstable fractures of the ankle in the elderly. *Injury*. 1987;18(2):128–32.

11. Anand N, Klenerman L. Ankle fractures in the elderly: MUA versus ORIF. *Injury*. 1993;24(2):116–20.

12. Makwana NK, Bhowal B, Harper WM, Hui AW. Conservative versus operative treatment for displaced ankle fractures in patients over 55 years of age. A prospective, randomised study. *J Bone Joint Surg Br*. 2001;83(4):525–9.

13. Keene DJ, Mistry D, Nam J et al. The ankle injury management (AIM) trial: A pragmatic, multicentre, equivalence randomised controlled trial and economic evaluation comparing close contact casting with open surgical reduction and internal fixation in the treatment of unstable ankle fractures in patients aged over 60 years. *Health Technol Assess*. 2016;20(75):1–158.

14. Willett K, Keene DJ, Morgan L et al. Ankle injury management (AIM): Design of a pragmatic multi-centre equivalence randomised controlled trial comparing close contact casting (CCC) to open surgical reduction and internal fixation (ORIF) in the treatment of unstable ankle fractures in patients over 60 years. *BMC Musculoskelet Disord*. 2014;15:79.

15. Olsen JR, Hunter J, Baumhauer JF. Osteoporotic ankle fractures. *Orthop Clin North Am*. 2013;44(2):225–41.

16. Lovy AJ, Dowdell J, Keswani A et al. Nonoperative versus operative treatment of displaced ankle fractures in diabetics. *Foot Ankle Int*. 2017;38(3):255–60.

17. Guyer AJ. Foot and ankle surgery in the diabetic population. *Orthop Clin North Am*. 2018;49(3):381–7.

18. Dingemans SA, Lodeizen OA, Goslings JC, Schepers T. Reinforced fixation of distal fibula fractures in elderly patients; A meta-analysis of biomechanical studies. *Clin Biomech*. 2016;36:14–20.

19. Moriarity A, Ellanti P, Mohan K, Fhoghlu CN, Fenelon C, McKenna J. A comparison of complication rates between locking and non-locking plates in distal fibular fractures. *Orthop Traumatol Surg Res*. 2018;104(4):503–6.

20. Schepers T, Van Lieshout EM, De Vries MR, Van der Elst M. Increased rates of wound complications with locking plates in distal fibular fractures. *Injury*. 2011;42(10):1125–9.

21. Moss LK, Kim-Orden MH, Ravinsky R, Hoshino CM, Zinar DM, Gold SM. Implant failure rates and cost analysis of contoured locking versus conventional plate fixation of distal fibula fractures. *Orthopedics.* 2017;40(6):e1024–e9.

22. Lyle SA, Malik C, Oddy MJ. Comparison of locking versus nonlocking plates for distal fibula fractures. *J Foot Ankle Surg.* 2018;57(4):664–7.

23. Kammerlander C, Neuerburg C, Verlaan JJ, Schmoelz W, Miclau T, Larsson S. The use of augmentation techniques in osteoporotic fracture fixation. *Injury.* 2016;47(Suppl 2):S36–43.

24. Assal M, Christofilopoulos P, Lubbeke A, Stern R. Augmented osteosynthesis of OTA 44-B fractures in older patients: A technique allowing early weight-bearing. *J Orthop Trauma.* 2011;25(12):742–7.

25. Panchbhavi VK, Vallurupalli S, Morris R. Comparison of augmentation methods for internal fixation of osteoporotic ankle fractures. *Foot Ankle Int.* 2009;30(7):696–703.

26. Ostrum RF, Litsky AS. Tension band fixation of medial malleolus fractures. *J Orthop Trauma.* 1992; 6(4):464–8.

27. Uygur E, Poyanli O, Mutlu I, Celik T, Akpinar F. Medial malleolus fractures: A biomechanical comparison of tension band wiring fixation methods. *Orthop Traumatol Surg Res.* 2018;104(8):1259–63.

28. Buckley R, Kwek E, Duffy P et al. Single screw fixation compared with double screw fixation for treatment of medial malleolar fractures: A prospective randomized trial. *J Orthop Trauma.* 2018;32(11):548–53.

29. Jain S, Haughton BA, Brew C. Intramedullary fixation of distal fibular fractures: A systematic review of clinical and functional outcomes. *J Orthop Traumatol.* 2014;15(4):245–54.

30. Loukachov VV, Birnie MFN, Dingemans SA, de Jong VM, Schepers T. Percutaneous intramedullary screw fixation of distal fibula fractures: A case series and systematic review. *J Foot Ankle Surg.* 2017;56(5): 1081–6.

31. Rehman H, Gardner WT, Rankin I, Johnstone AJ. The implants used for intramedullary fixation of distal fibula fractures: A review of literature. *Int J Surg.* 2018;56:294–300.

32. Tarkin IS, Fourman MS. Retrograde hindfoot nailing for acute trauma. *Curr Rev Musculoskelet Med.* 2018;11(3):439–44.

33. Jonas SC, Young AF, Curwen CH, McCann PA. Functional outcome following tibio-talar-calcaneal nailing for unstable osteoporotic ankle fractures. *Injury.* 2013;44(7):994–7.

34. Al-Nammari SS, Dawson-Bowling S, Amin A, Nielsen D. Fragility fractures of the ankle in the frail elderly patient: Treatment with a long calcaneotalo-tibial nail. *Bone Joint J.* 2014;96-B(6):817–22.

35. Taylor BC, Hansen DC, Harrison R, Lucas DE, Degenova D. Primary retrograde tibiotalocalcaneal nailing for fragility ankle fractures. *Iowa Orthop J.* 2016;36:75–8.

36. Georgiannos D, Lampridis V, Bisbinas I. Fragility fractures of the ankle in the elderly: Open reduction and internal fixation versus tibio-talo-calcaneal nailing: Short-term results of a prospective randomized-controlled study. *Injury.* 2017;48(2):519–24.

37. Childress HM. Vertical transarticular pin fixation for unstable ankle fractures: Impressions after 16 years of experience. *Clin Orthop Relat Res.* 1976(120): 164–71.

28

Treatment of distal intra-articular/extra-articular tibial fractures

VASILEIOS P. GIANNOUDIS and PETER V. GIANNOUDIS

INTRODUCTION

Distal tibial fractures, also known as "pilon" injuries, result when the talus, due to axial loading, is driven into the tibial articular surface causing an impaction injury. Different fracture patterns can be generated depending on the foot position during the impact and the direction of the force applied. These injuries are normally seen following high-energy trauma in the adult population with extensive soft tissue damage. In contrast, in the elderly population, pilon fractures are usually sustained following low-energy trauma (rotational force applied with trivial axial loading), resulting in less comminution with less damage to the surrounding soft tissues. In general terms, the prevalence of distal tibia fractures is approximately 9.1 per 100,000/year (1).

CLASSIFICATION

The most common fracture classification system used is the AO/Orthopaedic Trauma Association (OTA). Based on this classification, fractures are classified into extra-articular (type A), partial articular (type B), and complete articular (type C) (2). Fractures type B and type C are true intra-articular fractures and are categorized as "pilon" injuries.

DIFFERENCES BETWEEN YOUNG AND ELDERLY PATIENTS

Differences between young and elderly patients can be distinguished in terms of systemic and local issues. Systemic-related differences include the presence of comorbidities in the elderly (i.e., cardiorespiratory-related conditions, renal failure, presence of frailty, abnormal mental status, immunosuppression, etc.), whereas local-related differences include an osteoporotic bone phenotype, thinner cartilage layer, delicate soft tissues due to tissue fragility (prolonged

use of steroids), substantial degree of articular impaction, and less overall regenerative capacity. Moreover, the coexistence of peripheral vascular disease may be present complicating further the management of these elderly patients.

INITIAL ASSESSMENT

Initial assessment of the patient should follow the advanced trauma life support (ATLS) guidelines. After initial resuscitation and exclusion/management of life-threatening injuries, a detailed neurovascular examination of the injured extremity must take place. The possibility of compartment syndrome should be excluded. The state of the skin should be assessed and documented clearly in the notes (degree of swelling, presence of blisters and/or open wounds) (Figure 28.1). The presence of deformity indicates substantial fracture displacement/dislocation and should be reduced promptly to allow resuscitation of the soft tissue envelope and reduction of the painful stimuli. A back slab must be applied for maintenance of reduction. Initial plain anteroposterior (AP), lateral, and mortice view radiographs of good quality are of paramount importance to appreciate the fracture pattern and the success of fracture reduction. In cases where there is clearly intra-articular fracture involvement, a computed tomography (CT) scan with three-dimensional (3D) reconstruction can assist further in depicting the fracture pattern (Figure 28.2).

TREATMENT OPTIONS

In general terms, the management of distal tibial fractures in the elderly should follow the same principles as in young adults. Undisplaced fractures should be considered for nonoperative treatment assuming that they could remain stable in plaster. Other indications for conservative treatment include patients very frail to withstanding general or regional anesthesia, and the presence of a

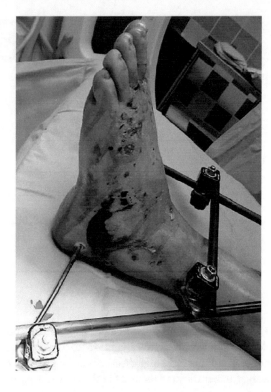

Figure 28.1 Temporary stabilization of a distal tibial fracture with an external fixator due to extensive bruising and blistering of the skin in a 72-year-old male patient.

very compromised bone stock. Following closed reduction, a well-padded plaster cast can be applied, and partial weight-bearing with the aid of two elbow crutches can be encouraged after a period of 6–8 weeks, progressing to full weight-bearing at the 12-week landmark. Patients

with intra-articular fractures with minimal displacement should avoid weight-bearing for a period of 3 months. Subsequently, physiotherapy can be initiated with the aim of improving the range of motion and strength of the affected extremity. Elderly patients and the family must be informed that protracted immobilization is associated with such risks as deep vein thrombosis, pulmonary embolism, and joint stiffness with loss of muscle power.

Displaced extra-articular fractures (AO 43A1, 43A2, 43A3) can be treated with either open reduction and internal fixation (ORIF) or intramedullary nailing (ideally three distal interlocking screws should be inserted distally providing adequate fixation of the distal segment). Options of ORIF include bridge plating and lag screw fixation of the wedge fragment where present, with the addition of a neutralization plate. Minimally invasive plate osteosynthesis (MIPO) also has a role to play here, particularly in cases where the state of the soft tissues is not optimal. Due to the osteoporotic nature of the underlying bone, different locking plate designs are available to choose for fixation.

In partial articular fractures (43B1, 43B2, 43B3), reconstruction is recommended with lag screw fixation and buttress plating. Lag screw fixation should follow the principles for optimum stability (screw inserted perpendicular to the fracture line and from smaller articular fragments to larger ones). The anatomical location of the partial articular segment would dictate the selection of the surgical incision. Such fragments have been described as Chaput (anterior lateral) and Volkmann (posterior lateral). If there is an associated articular impaction, this can be addressed with the introduction of a bony window and the appropriate technical maneuvers for elevation, reduction, and insertion of a bone graft substitute for support if required.

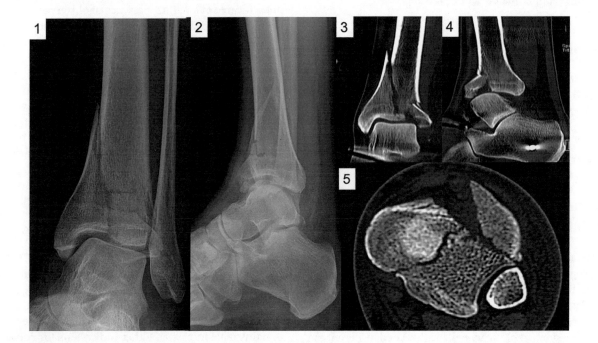

Figure 28.2 1. Anteroposterior (AP) and 2. Lateral left tibia radiographs. 3,4,5. Computed tomography scan cuts showing detailed description of the complete articular (type C injury) fracture pattern.

Complete articular fractures (43C1, 43C2, 43C3) are challenging injuries and require a good understanding of the anatomy, degree of displacement, and fracture comminution. Usually, an open reduction and anatomical fixation are essential with interfragmentary lag screws for long-term joint preservation. A plate connects the articular block to the metaphyseal segment of the tibia. Different plating systems are currently available including anatomically precontoured angular locking plates. It must be appreciated that in the elderly population, conventional nonlocking plates are not usually the choice of implant to use due to the degree of comminution and the presence of compromised osteoporotic bone.

Most of the distal tibial fractures present with an associated fibula fracture. Fixing the fibula and restoring its length facilitates improved control of the length and rotational alignment and reduction of the tibia.

It has to be appreciated that the timing of fixation of distal tibia fractures is dictated by the state of the soft tissues. It is common practice, even in low-energy trauma injuries in the elderly, to apply a staged protocol where the facture is temporarily stabilized with a splint or an external fixator until the soft tissues are amenable to operative intervention. The presence of wrinkles and epithelialization of fracture blisters are usually the clinical signs prompting the surgeon to proceed to definitive fixation of the fracture.

SURGICAL APPROACHES

Several approaches have been developed over the years to allow reconstruction of distal tibial fractures (3). It is essential for the surgical team to study carefully the CT scan findings and to do preoperative planning when deciding in advance how the existing fragments can be approached and reduced anatomically. Impaction injuries can only be visualized by the CT scan images as well as soft tissue entrapment within the fracture locations. Approaches that can be utilized include direct medial, direct lateral, anteromedial, anterolateral, direct anterior, posteromedial, and posterolateral. Each approach has its own advantages and limitations.

TECHNIQUES OF TREATMENT

Intramedullary nailing

Intramedullary (IM) nailing can be used for extra-articular and partial articular fracture patterns where there is sufficient bone distally to secure at least two distal locking screws (ideally three screws). Partial articular injuries require reconstruction of the joint prior to nailing. This can be done with anatomical reduction of the articular fragment (usually posterior malleolus) and fixation with partially threaded cannulated screws.

Standard IM nailing technique is carried out with a midline longitudinal incision from the lower pole of the patella to the tibial tuberosity. Access to the tibial entry point can be achieved using either a patellar tendon split or a parapatellar incision. The entry point for the nail is determined with fluoroscopic guidance (sweet spot: medial to the lateral tibial spine), centered on the intramedullary canal on AP fluoroscopic view, and at the top of the tibial tubercle on the lateral view (avoiding penetration of the posterior tibial cortex) (Figure 28.3). If the entry point is made too anteriorly, there is a risk of damaging the tibial tuberosity during the reaming step of the procedure. Reduction of the distal

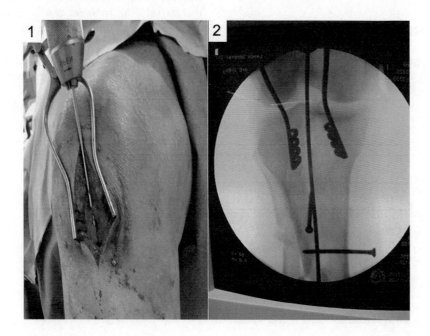

Figure 28.3 1. Intraoperative. 2. Anteroposterior fluoroscopic knee image showing identification of the entry point for tibial intramedullary nailing.

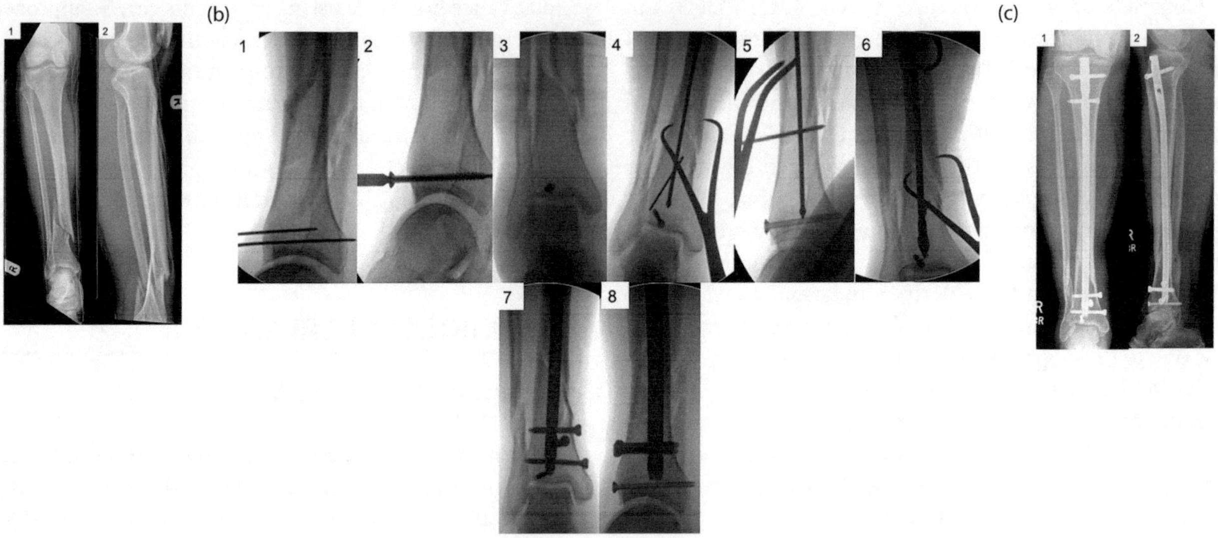

Figure 28.4 (a) 1. Anteroposterior, 2. Lateral radiograph of right tibia demonstrating a distal 1/3 tibia/fibula fracture. (b) 1. Intraoperative fluoroscopic view demonstrating insertion of k-wires for fixation of a fracture extending intraarticularly to the ankle joint, 2. Insertion of cannulated partially threated screws for fixation, 3. Anteroposterior fluoroscopic view demonstrating the screw insertion, 4. Anteroposterior fluoroscopic view showing fracture reduction with a pointed reduction forceps and advancement of the guide wire for IM nailing. Central position of guide wire achieved with the insertion of "pollar wire," 5. Lateral fluoroscopic view showing fracture reduction, 6. Anteroposterior view showing advancement distally of the reamer, 7. Anteroposterior, and 8. Lateral view showing stabilization of the tibial fracture with intramedullary nailing. (c) 1. Anteroposterior, 2. Lateral tibial radiographs 6 months after fixation showing union of the fracture.

tibial fragment can be achieved with different techniques including pointed reduction forceps, poller screws, and a unicortical external fixation frame, among others. For optimum stability and early weight-bearing, as previously stated, two proximal screws and three distal ones should be inserted (Figure 28.4).

Open reduction and internal fixation

The most common approaches used include anterolateral, medial, and lateral (4).

The anterolateral approach facilitates good exposure of the Chaput fragment, allowing good visualization of the articular surface (Figure 28.5). The lateral malleolus and the base of the fourth metatarsal represent the landmarks of this approach. The start of the incision is approximately 6 cm proximal to ankle joint and anteriorly to the lateral malleolus, extending distally to the base of the fourth metatarsal. The incision can be extended as indicated. The peroneal muscles (deep peroneal nerve) and extensor muscles (superficial peroneal nerve) constitute the internervous plane of the approach. The incision through the skin, fascia, and extensor retinacula is followed by opening

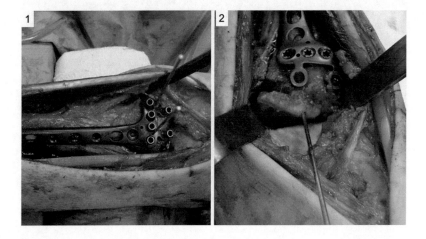

Figure 28.5 1. Anteroposterior intraoperative image of a distal tibial fracture in a 70-year-old male stabilized with a locking plate. 2. Note reduction of articular fragment with K-wiring prior to definite reconstruction.

the interval lateral to peroneus tertius and extensor digitorum longus. Subsequent retraction of them medially leads to exposure of the anterior aspect of the distal tibia and the articular surface.

For the medial approach, the palpable medial malleolus represents the landmark of the incision distally. A longitudinal curvilinear incision over the medial area of the proximal tibia is initiated, advancing it distally over the tip of the medial malleolus and then curving it forward. Identification and protection of the saphenous nerve and long saphenous vein are essential, as they run near the anterior. If required, the posterior aspect of the medial malleolus can be uncovered by dividing the flexor retinaculum and retracting posteriorly the tibialis posterior.

The anterior approach constitutes a skin incision made between the medial and lateral malleolus, starting at least 10 cm proximally and advanced distally over the ankle joint. Careful dissection and identification of the neurovascular bundle including branches of the superficial peroneal nerve is of paramount importance. The intermuscular plane between extensor hallucis longus (EHL) and extensor digitorum longus (EDL) is utilized, locating the anterior tibial artery and deep peroneal nerve distally as it crosses behind the EHL. Subsequently, safe retraction of both the EHL and neurovascular bundle medially can be carried out to expose the ankle joint, while EDL is retracted laterally. The articular surface can then be visualized by performing an anterior capsulotomy.

Finally, the posterior lateral approach allows access to the posterior aspect of the tibia.

It facilitates fixation at the same setting of distal tibial and fibula fracture fixation. Lateral malleolus and Achilles tendon represent the landmarks of the incision, while the internervous plane is located between the flexor hallucis longus (posterior tibial nerve) and the peroneus brevis (superficial peroneal nerve). In general, a

longitudinal skin incision is carried out midway among the posteromedial border of the lateral malleolus and the lateral border of the Achilles tendon. After mobilization of the skin flaps, the deep fascia is incised, and the superficial peroneal retinaculum can be incised distally in order to liberate the peroneal tendons. Identification of the flexor hallucis longus (FHL) tendon is crucial at this point, as developing a plane between the peroneal tendons and FHL tendon would allow access to the posterior tibia. Flexing and extending the great toe will allow easy identification of FHL. If fixation of the fibula is required, careful dissection should be performed to the peroneal fascia attachment on the fibula.

Reconstruction of the articular surface should follow a logical sequence. Usually, reduction and fixation start from the posterior fragment before moving onto the more anterior parts of the joint. An external fixator placed between the tibia and the calcaneus or talus would allow better exposure and visualization of the fragments prior to reduction. Disimpaction of the fragments of the articular surface can be achieved with periosteal elevator and an osteotome. Using K-wires and pointed reduction forceps, anatomical reduction can be established, which can be verified by acquisition of the appropriate fluoroscopic views. Subsequently, 3.5 mm partially threaded cancellous screws can be used to provide compression to the anatomically reduced articular fragments. When the joint has been reconstructed, a bridge plating construct can be used to connect the articular block to the proximal tibial segment (Figures 28.6–28.8). Interfragmentary lag screws applied through the distal end of the plate can be used to provide additional stability to the articular fragments. Areas of previous impaction that have a residual bone void requiring filling for subchondral support can be addressed with the injection of bone cement (bone substitute). The stability of fixation can be checked by dorsiflexion and plantarflexion of the ankle joint. Additional

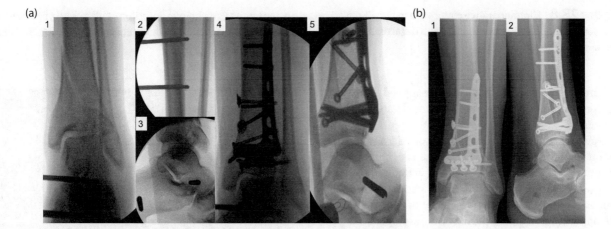

Figure 28.6 Complete articular left distal tibial fracture in a female patient 77 years of age. (a) 1. Anteroposterior (AP) ankle, 2. AP proximal tibia, and 3. lateral ankle radiographs showing initial stabilization of the fracture with an external fixator for soft tissue resuscitation and planning. 4. AP and 5. lateral radiographs of left ankle demonstrating stabilization of the fracture with a locking plate and lag screws. (b) 1. AP, and 2. Lateral radiographs at 5-month follow-up demonstrating union.

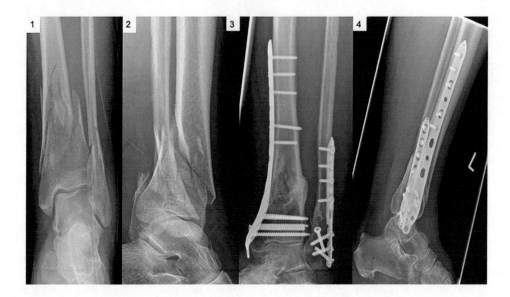

Figure 28.7 Extra-articular left distal tibial fracture in a male patient 75 years of age. 1. Anteroposterior (AP) and 2. lateral pre-operative radiographs. 3. AP and 4. lateral postoperative radiographs showing stabilization of the fracture with a locking plate at a follow-up of 6 months. (Osseous healing of fracture is demonstrated.)

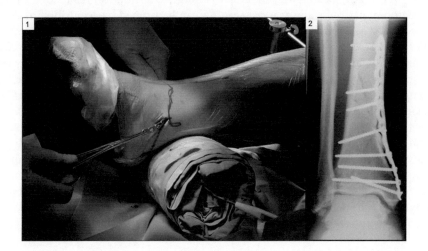

Figure 28.8 1. Intraoperative picture of a minimally invasive plate osteosynthesis technique (insertion of plate with mini-incision) for insertion of a locking plate to stabilize a distal tibial fracture. 2. Postoperative radiograph showing stabilization of right distal tibial fracture with the locking plate.

low-profile small locking plates can be applied for capturing bone fragments that require additional buttressing for optimum fixation.

Primary arthrodesis has also been considered as a good option to address injuries where there is extensive comminution and delamination of the articular cartilage (Figure 28.9), particularly in elderly patients where the bone is very fragile and not amenable to reconstruction. This approach is being supported by the argument that primary fusion of the tibiotalar joint can facilitate recovery and reduce long-term pain. Arthrodesis can be performed with hindfoot nails (Figure 28.10). A hindfoot fusion nail leads to a stiff hindfoot and inhibits movement at the ankle and subtalar joints (5). However, acute arthrodesis can be

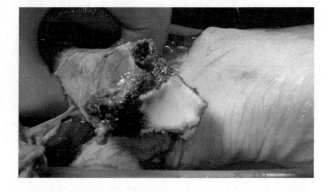

Figure 28.9 Intraoperative picture of a distal tibial fracture dislocation showing extensive loss of joint cartilage.

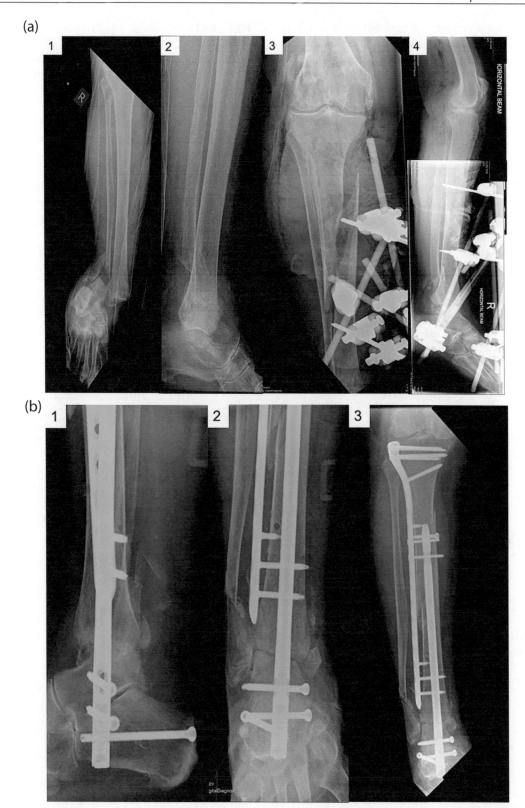

Figure 28.10 (a) Female, 92 years of age with dementia and diabetes. Fall from stairs at nursing home. Sustained open grade 3A ankle fracture/dislocation. 1. Anteroposterior (AP) and 2. lateral radiographs right tibia/ankle. Initially debrided, primary wound closure and fracture stabilized with external fixator. However, 3 days postoperatively, she fell and sustained fracture at the level of the proximal pin of the external fixator (3. AP and 4. lateral radiographs right tibia). (b) 1. Lateral ankle and 2. AP radiographs of ankle. 3. AP tibia radiographs at 6-month follow-up demonstrating stabilization of the ankle and tibial fracture with a locking plate and a hindfoot nail (fusion of ankle joint).

beneficial to elderly patients with comorbidities, such as peripheral vascular disease, diabetes, and very poor skin condition, thus reducing the risk of infectious complications. Moreover, an intraosseous load-sharing device can support early ambulation, thus facilitating early discharge to home.

CONCLUSION

The management of intra-articular distal tibial fractures in the elderly remains challenging. Delicate soft tissue envelope and bone fragility require special attention in the elderly. Extra-articular fracture patterns can be stabilized with IM nailing or plating devices. Intra-articular fractures, partial or complete articular, require anatomical reduction and early range of motion as per the AO principles of management. Staged treatment allows soft tissues to improve from the initial injury and makes surgical treatment safer.

REFERENCES

1. Wennergren D, Bergdahl C, Ekelund J, Juto H, Sundfeldt M, Möller M. Epidemiology and incidence of tibia fractures in the Swedish Fracture Register. *Injury*. 2018;49(11):2068–74.
2. Fracture and Dislocation Compendium–2018. A joint collaboration between the Orthopaedic Trauma Association and the AO Foundation. *J Orthop Trauma*. 2018;32(1 Suppl).
3. Liu J, Smith CD, White E, Ebraheim NA. A systematic review of the role of surgical approaches on the outcomes of the tibia pilon fracture. *Foot Ankle Spec*. 2016;9(2):163–8.
4. Sitnik A, Beletsky A, Schelkun S. Intra-articular fractures of the distal tibia: Current concepts of management. *EFORT Open Rev*. 2017 Aug; 2(8): 352–61.
5. Tarkin SI, Flourmann MS. Retrograde hindfoot nailing for acute trauma. *Curr Rev Musculoskelet Med*. 2018;11:439–44.

29

Osteoporotic os calcis fractures

How I manage them

ANGUS JENNINGS and RICHARD BUCKLEY

INTRODUCTION

Little has been written specifically on the plight of the osteoporotic calcaneus fracture. Osteoporosis has predominantly been implicated in calcaneal tuberosity avulsion fractures and insufficiency fractures but must also contribute to the behavior of displaced intra-articular calcaneal fractures (DIACFs) and subsequent treatment.

Rupprecht et al. (1) are the only investigators who have tried to correlate osteoporosis with fracture configuration. This was done by age and gender matching in a cohort of 182 calcaneus fractures with 60 cadaver calcanei at autopsy. The average age at the time of fracture was higher in females (46.0 ± 18.3 years) than in males (39.9 ± 13.9 years). They stated that the "relative frequency of fractures during aging shifted from males to females." The calcaneal bone mass was reduced by 19% in older females (20–40 years: 292 mg/cm [3]; 61–80 years: 237 mg/cm [3]; $P < 0.05$). They concluded that "bone mass and structure are risk factors in respect to the occurrence and severity of calcaneal fractures."

There is some literature discussing the management of DIACF fractures in the elderly population, which by virtue of age is likely to include patients with osteoporosis, but no specific discussions of the attempted diagnosis of osteoporosis or formal assessment of their bone density have been included (2,3). Essex-Lopresti (4) reported that surgery had a successful outcome in 80% of patients under the age of 50 years but only 40% of those over the age of 50 years. He also noted that elderly patients had a higher degree of satisfaction when they had been treated with extensive exercise therapy. He concluded that exercise therapy was the best treatment for displaced calcaneal fractures in patients over the age of 50 years. Buckley (5) subsequently concluded from a large randomized controlled trial (RCT) that "the best patients to treat non-operatively are those who are fifty years old or more." In contradistinction to this, Herscovici (2) concluded that "it does not appear that the age of a patient should be the primary criterion determining how a displaced calcaneal fracture should be managed," and finally, "Surgery for displaced calcaneal fractures should not be denied on the basis of age, but care should be exercised when operative management is being considered for patients with substantial pre-existing medical problems." The average age of patients in their study was 70.3 years, and all fractures resulted from a high energy mechanism. All patients had either a full-time job or participated in moderate-strenuous physical activity, which is a very select group and unlikely to represent a normal elderly population.

The calcaneus has become an important peripheral site for osteoporosis assessment (6). Significant efforts have been made to investigate the microarchitecture of the calcaneus, but much less work has focused on its function. There is little clinical evidence as to how either form or function, alone or in combination, contribute to the occurrence of calcaneal fractures.

The calcaneus displays the same characteristic changes of osteoporosis in its microarchitecture, as does the distal radius, the proximal femur, and the spine. One has to consider that calcaneal fractures occur as osteoporotic fractures, as is the case for fractures of the hip, distal radius, and spine.

The calcaneus is a complex three-dimensional shape with three subtalar articulations, a calcaneocuboid joint, and the insertions of both the Achilles tendon and plantar fascia. It has a thin cortical shell and a predominance of trabecular bone.

The trabecular composition of the calcaneus is most dense under the posterior facet (7). The trabeculae are compressive from the posterior facet to the superior tuberosity and from the middle facet to the cuboid articulation. There are tensile trabeculae from the Achilles insertion around to the inferior surface of the plantar fascia insertion and to that of the plantar ligaments (8). This configuration leaves a triangular region of low bone density beneath the angle of

Gissane. The direction of force transmission remains constant despite large changes in magnitude between walking and running (9).

During walking, biomechanical models predict the gastroc-soleus complex exerts a peak tensile load of 3.9× body weight on the calcaneus through the Achilles insertion, and 7.7× body weight during running. The actual compressive force on the calcaneus may be up to 10× body weight with running. These forces will be much higher during a fall or during forceful eccentric gastroc-soleus contraction (7).

Trabecular bone is a metabolically active tissue that shows changes in composition with aging or loading, in keeping with Wolff's law (10). The age-related changes are similar to other anatomical sites such as the distal radius, proximal femur, and vertebrae (9). There are changes in mineral composition as well as microstructure, but the structural changes are the most striking. Rupprecht showed that based on direct histomorphometric data, the calcaneus undergoes age-related loss of bone throughout, but that it is most evident beneath the posterior facet of the subtalar joint (1). Interestingly, this study also showed a higher trabecular density under the posterior facet in males but similar densities elsewhere between the sexes. The maximal rate of bone loss in females occurred between the 20–40 years and the 40–60 years age brackets, whereas in males it was between the 40–60 years and 60–80 years age groups. Other studies have demonstrated similar findings, with Ensrud noting a significant loss in the calcaneus bone mineral density after the age of 75 years in both men and women (11), and Mitchell stating that calcaneus bone mineral density loss increases with advancing age in elderly women (12).

EPIDEMIOLOGY

Calcaneus fractures account for approximately 2% of all fractures but 60% of tarsal bone injuries (13). In an epidemiological study from Edinburgh, the incidence of calcaneus fractures was 11.5 per 100,000 population per year (12). Fractures were much more common in males, with a male-to-female ratio of 2.4:1, and the mean patient age was 44 years (39 years in males, and 55 years in females) (12). Fractures were much less common in females and were rare before the age of 50 years, although there was a gradual increase in incidence with increasing age thereafter. Interestingly, 51 of 752 fractures were very low energy, following a fall from standing height or below with a mean age of 60 years and a male-to-female ratio of 1:4.1. These data would support the hypothesis that the majority of calcaneus fractures in females occur in the perimenopausal period and that decreasing bone density and/or osteoporosis is likely a contributing factor.

Rowe et al. (14) reported that the incidence of avulsion fractures is 3.8% of all calcaneal fractures. Avulsion fractures of the calcaneus are therefore uncommon but are thought to occur more commonly in patients with osteoporosis, such as the elderly or those with diabetes and autoimmune

disorders (15). Beavis et al. (16) stated that "All (avulsion fractures) occur in osteopenic or osteoporotic bone but we believe it likely that the Type I 'sleeve' fracture probably occurs in older patients with significant osteoporosis."

Calcaneal stress fractures are rare. Insufficiency fractures (normal or physiologic stress in day-to-day activities placed on bone with deficient elastic resistance [osteoporosis]) are limited to a handful of case reports (17,18), and the true incidence is not known. The majority of these are thought to be directly related to osteoporosis, whether primary or secondary.

INVESTIGATION

DIACFs require a computed tomography (CT) scan to fully appreciate the three-dimensional fracture pattern, to prognosticate, and to plan treatment and the surgical approach. Avulsion fractures are typically well visualized on plain film imaging and do not usually require advanced imaging. Insufficiency fractures can be hard to diagnose, require a high index of suspicion, and will usually require magnetic resonance imaging or nuclear medicine imaging to confirm.

CLASSIFICATION

DIACFs are most commonly classified using the Sanders classification (19). This utilizes a coronal CT image at the widest level of the posterior facet, including the sustentaculum tali, and assesses the degree of posterior facet comminution. It is prognostic, in that increased comminution has been shown to correlate with poorer results and increased rates of subtalar fusion (especially Sanders IV type).

Beavis et al. (16) proposed a classification of tuberosity avulsion fractures:

- Type 1 "sleeve" fracture
- Type 2 "beak" fracture
- Type 3 "infrabursal" fracture

They postulated that the different fracture morphologies were due to anatomical differences in Achilles tendon insertion.

Insufficiency fractures have no known classification system.

MANAGEMENT

Displaced intra-articular calcaneal fractures

Broadly speaking, the first decision is whether to manage these injuries operatively or nonoperatively. This selection process is dictated by the following:

a. Patient factors—including age, osteoporosis, medical and physical wellness
b. Limb factors and the nature of the soft tissue injury
c. Characteristics of the fracture

Patient expectations must be assessed and the patient counseled appropriately.

The management of DIACFs can be divided into the following four broad categories (20):

a. *Nonoperative management*—Older sedentary patients possibly with medical problems (>60 years old with good foot shape)

b. *Open reduction and internal fixation*—Physiologically young patients with excellent soft tissues and simple Sanders fracture patterns

c. *Minimally invasive reduction and fixation*—Significant soft tissue problems, patients with poor medical condition, bad foot shape and contour

d. *Primary open reduction and internal fixation (ORIF) and subtalar arthrodesis*—High-energy fractures (Sanders type IV), patients with significant psychiatric or social issues

Nonoperatively managed patients should be treated with rest, ice, elevation, and early range of motion. Splinting should be discontinued, if used at all, and early movement of the ankle and hind-foot should be started within 5–10 days of injury to minimize stiffness. We recommend non-weight-bearing for 6 weeks, although it is acknowledged that some authors allow partial weight-bearing earlier. After weight-bearing is started, custom orthotics are very useful for patients.

Surgical considerations in osteoporotic bone include the deleterious effect on reduction maneuvers and the maintenance of reduction. Bone that is osteoporotic does not withstand the normal open reduction maneuvers used in normal bone. Crushing and disruption of the osteoporotic fracture fragments are common with these maneuvers such that open reductions are much less accurate and satisfying. Reduction aids such as small Schantz pins and smooth wires have minimal purchase in osteoporotic bone, often rendering them ineffective. Knowledge and use of the denser areas of trabecular bone in the calcaneus may help, as might the use of multiple threaded wires and larger Steinman pins in different planes. Often, minimally invasive techniques are useful in these patients, as open reductions are unsatisfying but minimally invasive techniques can restore foot shape and alignment and "relative" joint congruity. Large Steinman pins, threaded K-wires and large cannulated screws are useful in these patients. A sawbone study (21) failed to show an increased load to failure when comparing a locked calcaneal plate and a nonlocked plate in osteoporotic bone with a Sanders 2B fracture. In another biomechanical study utilizing a different fracture pattern, Stoffel et al. showed an advantage to locked plates with a higher load to failure (22).

Joint fragments are often the only satisfactory pieces that can be reconstructed with large defects below the crucial angle of Gissane and in the tuberosity. If ORIF is performed, the use of locking plates with bicortical fixation into the periphery of the calcaneus is required. This means fixation below the posterior facet, anterior into the good

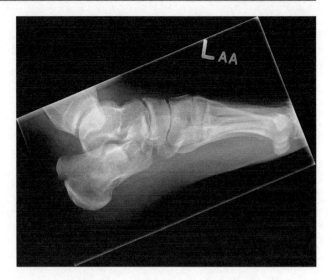

Figure 29.1 Preoperative tongue-type calcaneal fracture.

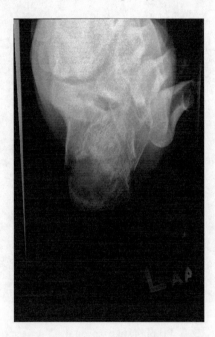

Figure 29.2 Harris axial view of same fracture as Figures 29.1.

bone near the calcaneo-cuboid joint and near the back of the posterior tuberosity of the calcaneus.

Adjuncts to help maintain reduction in the calcaneus include allograft, bone graft substitutes, and bone cement. The underlying poorer quality of cancellous bone and the volume of graft needed directs surgeons to the use of allograft or bone graft substitutes. While mechanical support makes intuitive sense, the use of graft and bone substitutes has not been specifically studied in this patient population (Figures 29.1 and 29.2).

Avulsion fractures

We recommend accurate surgical reduction and stabilization of all displaced calcaneal tuberosity fractures to allow

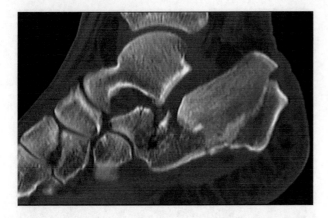

Figure 29.3 Preoperative sagittal CT of tongue type fracture.

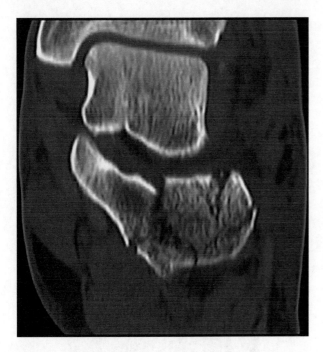

Figure 29.4 Preoperative coronal CT of tongue type fracture.

restoration of the Achilles tendon insertion as well as minimize deformity. Failure to achieve an accurate reduction could lead to loss of plantarflexion strength, skin necrosis, and severe Haglund deformities.

A number of fixation methods have been described. These include tension band wiring, screw fixation, cannulated screws with tension band wiring, suture fixation utilizing the Achilles tendon proximally and an endobutton on the plantar aspect (Figures 29.3 and 29.4) (15,16,23,24).

Insufficiency fractures

These should be managed with a 4- to 6-week period of non-weight-bearing but continuing with active motion of the ankle and hindfoot. One should attempt to identify the underlying cause of the fracture, or contributing factors, and correct any modifiable causes (17,18).

CONCLUSION

There is minimal literature specifically addressing osteoporotic calcaneal fractures, and hence little guidance for their management.

Using the outcomes of management of older patients as a proxy for osteoporotic fractures is fraught with confounding variables but is the best guidance from the literature that we have.

We believe that an algorithmic approach to the management of calcaneal fractures is justified, with osteoporosis being one important patient factor to consider.

REFERENCES

1. Rupprecht M, Pogoda P, Mumme M et al. Bone microarchitecture of the calcaneus and its changes in aging: A histomorphometric analysis of 60 human specimens. *J Orthopaed Res*. 2006;24:664–74.
2. Herscovici D, Widmaier J, Scaduto J et al. A operative treatment of calcaneal fractures in elderly patients. *J Bone Joint Surg (Am)*. 2005;87:1260.
3. Basile A. Operative versus nonoperative treatment of displaced intra-articular calcaneal fractures in elderly patients. *J Foot Ankle Surg*. 2010;49:25–32.
4. Essex-Lopresti P. The mechanism, reduction technique, and results in fractures of the OS calcis. *Br J Surg*. 1952;39:395–419.
5. Buckley R, Tough S, McCormack R et al. Operative compared with nonoperative treatment of displaced intra-articular calcaneal fractures: A prospective, randomized, controlled multicenter trial. *J Bone Joint Surg (Am)*. 2002;84-A:1733–44.
6. Khaw K-T, Reeve J, Luben R et al. Prediction of total and hip fracture risk in men and women by quantitative ultrasound of the calcaneus: EPIC-Norfolk prospective population study. *Lancet*. 2004; 363:197–202.
7. Giddings V, Beaupre G, Whalen R. Calcaneal loading during walking and running. *Med Sci Sports Exerc*. 2000;32(3):627–34.
8. Wolff J. Das gesetz der transformation der knochen. *DMW-Deutsche Medizinische Wochenschrift* 1893;19:1222–24.
9. Turunen M, Prantner V, Jurvelin J et al. Composition and microarchitecture of human trabecular bone change with age and differ between anatomical locations. *Bone*. 2013;54:118–25.
10. Cheng S, Suominen H, Sakari R et al. Calcaneal bone mineral density predicts fracture occurrence: A five-year follow-up study in elderly people. *J Bone Miner Res*. 1997;12:1075–82.

11. Ensrud KE, Palermo L, Black DM et al. Hip and calcaneal bone loss increase with advancing age: Longitudinal results from the study of osteoporotic fractures. *J Bone Miner Res.* 1995;10:1778–87.

12. Mitchell M, McKinley J, Robinson C. The epidemiology of calcaneal fractures. *Foot* 2009;19:197–200.

13. Eastwood DM. Intra-articular fractures of the calcaneum. *JBJS (Br).* 1993;75-B:183–8.

14. Rowe C, Sakellarides H, Freeman P et al. Fractures of the os calcis: A long-term follow-up study of 146 patients. *JAMA.* 1963;184:920–3.

15. Squires B, Allen P, Livingstone J et al. Fractures of the tuberosity of the calcaneus. *J Bone Joint Surg.* 2001;83:55–61.

16. Beavis C, Rourke K, Court-Brown C. Avulsion fracture of the calcaneal tuberosity: A case report and literature review. *Foot Ankle Int.* 2008; 29:863–6.

17. Ito K, Hori K, Terashima Y et al. Insufficiency fracture of the body of the calcaneus in elderly patients with osteoporosis: A report of two cases. *Clin Orthopaedics Relat Res.* 2004;422:190.

18. Lui T. Insufficiency fracture of the body of the calcaneus. *Foot.* 2013;23:93–5.

19. Sanders R, Fortin D, DiPasquale T et al. Operative treatment in 120 displaced intraarticular calcaneal fractures. Results using a prognostic computed tomography scan classification. *Clin Orthop Relat R.* 1993;290:87–95.

20. Sharr P, Mangupli M, Winson I et al. Current management options for displaced intra-articular calcaneal fractures: Non-operative, ORIF, minimally invasive reduction and fixation or primary ORIF and subtalar arthrodesis. A contemporary review. *Foot Ankle Surg.* 2016;22:1–8.

21. Richter M, Gosling T, Zech S et al. A comparison of plates with and without locking screws in a calcaneal fracture model. *Foot and Ankle Int.* 2005;26:309–19.

22. Stoffel K, Booth G, Rohrl S et al. A comparison of conventional versus locking plates in intraarticular calcaneal fractures: A biomechanical study in human cadavers. *Clin Biomech.* 2007;22:100–5.

23. Miyamura S, Ota H, Okamoto M et al. Surgical treatment of calcaneal avulsion fracture in elderly patients using cannulated cancellous screws and titanium wire. *J Foot Ankle Surg.* 2016;55:157–60.

24. Banerjee R, Chao J, Taylor R et al. Management of calcaneal tuberosity fractures. *J Am Acad Orthopaedic Surgeons* 2012;20:253–8.

30

Current trend in kyphoplasty for osteoporotic vertebral fractures

KALLIOPI ALPANTAKI, GEORGIOS VASTARDIS, and ALEXANDER G. HADJIPAVLOU

INTRODUCTION

A major complaint of 85% of patients with a radiological diagnosis of osteoporotic vertebral compression fracture (OVCF) is back pain, which may be either acute and excruciating or chronic and persistent (1,2). Acute back pain is usually caused by a recent OVCF, and in the majority of patients it is expected to subside as the fracture heals over a period of approximately 3 months (3). However, an estimated 33% (4) to 75% (5) of these patients may develop chronic back pain. Chronic pain may arise from persistent intravertebral motion as observed in cases of pseudarthrosis, which can occur with an incidence of 44% per patient or 35% per fracture (6). Deformity is another source of chronic pain following an OVCF. Furthermore, spinal deformity is a significant cause of disability resulting directly from the impairment of physical functioning, health, and quality of life (7).

Kyphotic deformity moves the center of gravity forward, resulting in increased forward bending moments, which are in turn compensated for by a contraction of the posterior spinal muscles (7) (Figure 30.1). As a result, the load within the kyphotic angle is increased, predisposing to further vertebral body (VB) fractures (8). Forward bending movement can be counterbalanced by flexing the knees to improve body posture (9). This posture causes paraspinal muscle fatigue and increases strain in the facets contributing to chronic back pain. Furthermore, the knee flexion posture requires the contraction and tightening of the thigh muscles, resulting in an impaired gait velocity, reduction of mobility, and a curtailing of most daily activities, not to mention pain (Figure 30.2). The risk of hip fractures increases 4.5-fold after a single OVCF and 7.2-fold after two or more OVCFs (10,11), independently of bone mass density (10), possibly reflecting the impaired gait. The impairment of patients' functions leads to sleep disorders, increased anxiety and depression, low self-esteem, diminished social role, and increased dependency on others (12,13). Lung function can be significantly reduced in patients with thoracic fractures. It has been reported that forced vital capacity and forced expiratory volume in 1 second can be decreased by 9% after each vertebral fracture (14,15). This may have detrimental effects in patients with preexisting lung disease and result in increased morbidity and mortality. OVCF is associated with a 23%–34% age-adjusted increase in mortality rate compared to patients without OVCF (16,17).

The treatment of OVCF is usually conservative, consisting of analgesics, bed rest, and braces. Major reconstructive surgery is recommended for crippling deformities and neurocompression. However, 75% of osteoporotic patients who are treated conservatively may continue to suffer from persistent spinal pain (18). In a systematic review (19) analyzing several reports on OVCF, it appears that osteoporosis is not innocuous as it can be complicated with serious neurological deficit, pulmonary, and social problems. Therefore, there is room for introducing more effective management of OVCF, and this can be accomplished by means of cementoplasty—percutaneous vertebroplasty (PVP) and percutaneous balloon kyphoplasty (PBK).

Since their inception, both vertebroplasty (which was introduced in the mid-1980s) (20) and balloon kyphoplasty (introduced in the late 1990s) (21) have become widespread methods for the treatment of OVCF and osteolytic tumors. However, in 2009, kyphoplasty and particularly vertebroplasty had been challenged as ineffective procedures for the treatment of OVCF, following two randomized controlled trials (RCTs) published in the *New England Journal of Medicine* (NEJM) (22,23). These two studies suggest that vertebroplasty is not significantly different than placebo. The assertions of these studies were widely accepted, reducing the practice of cementoplasty, as they compared the procedure to a sham surgery under the same operating and anesthetic conditions. Widespread debate ensued suggesting vertebroplasty as expensive and ineffectual. In September 2010, the American Academy of Orthopaedic

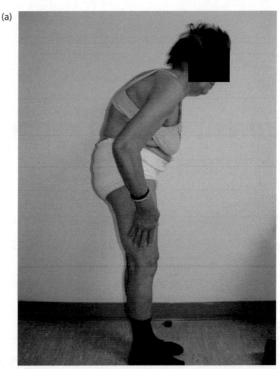

Anterior shift of compressive load path in VB adjacent to VCF

Additional flexion moments

Increased risk of new Fx

Large bending moments

Osteoporotic spine must resist these loadings

New fracture

Figure 30.1 Osteoporotic vertebral compression fracture kyphosis predisposes to future fracture. (With permission from Alpantaki K et al. *Texas Orthopaed J.* 2018. doi: 10.18600/toj.020203.)

Surgeons (AAOS) issued a strong recommendation against vertebroplasty and a weak recommendation for kyphoplasty (24). Subsequently, an editorial in the NEJM Journal Watch concluded that selective and limited use of vertebroplasty is acceptable as long as the clinician shares uncertainty about the procedure's effectiveness with the patient, and intervention should be performed neither too early nor too late (25). In a book published in 2015, *Ending Medical Reversal*, the authors extensively criticized vertebroplasty as an ineffective and harmful medical practice (26).

An extensive debate with critics has followed in the medical community raising serious concerns regarding the two RCTs and questioning their scientific integrity, including selection of patients with high patient refusal rate, lack of statistical power with high "sham group" crossover, treatment methodology, failure to analyze fracture type subgroups, and inclusion criteria with low pain scores (27–29). We analyzed these criticisms in a recent paper (30) that adds considerable scientific heft to the effectiveness of cementoplasty and, in particular, kyphoplasty. The majority of studies we reviewed support cementoplasty. Potential serious complications of OVCF (19) (Figure 30.3) and a recent RCT study (31) exonerate vertebroplasty by demonstrating its superiority over sham procedure.

CLINICAL INDICATIONS AND PATIENT SELECTION

The primary indication for a cementoplasty procedure is severe, persistent pain at the level of the fracture site refractory to conservative treatment (32) and concomitant functional physical incapacity. Pain to palpation of the spinous process at the fracture site is a reliable test indicating pain generator pathology (33).

The optimal intervention procedure time is debatable. Studies generally support earlier intervention (34) in the first 3 months, though satisfactory results have also been reported in later intervention (35). However,

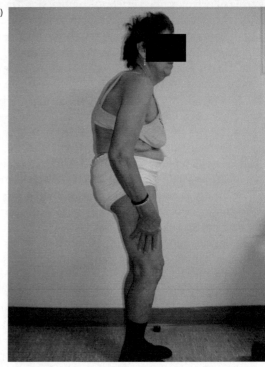

(a)

(b)

Figure 30.2 (a) This patient posture of the trunk in flexion (stooped postured) results from lumbar kyphotic deformity. (b) The patient can attain upright straight stance by bending the knees. This "flat back posture" is characterized by increased effort during ambulation and fatigue.

a late intervention may lead to an unfavorable outcome. Papanastasiou et al. proposed a therapeutic "window" of 7 weeks, with an exception of prompt intervention when progression of the wedging vertebral body is detected in the thoracic spine (36). Oh et al., in a retrospective study

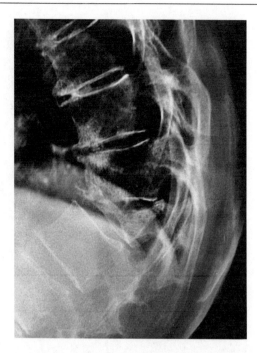

Figure 30.3 Lateral x-ray of osteoporotic vertebral compression fracture with severe kyphotic deformity and displacement of the vertebral body posteriorly compromising the cord, producing paraparesis. This could have been prevented.

evaluating the results of balloon kyphoplasty performed at different times after injury, divided 99 patients into three groups, and all three groups displayed equally significant pain relief (37).

Vertebroplasty is indicated for uncomplicated OVCF in the first 3 months and appears to be a more cost-effective procedure. In the early postfracture period, some reduction of the fracture with postural hyperextension can be accomplished. Balloon kyphoplasty is definitely advocated in older fractures, when postural reduction is not feasible, and particularly in established pseudarthrosis. In cases of indeterminate cement interdigitation in pseudarthrotic cavities, which may not prevent anterior cement migration and loss of reduction, this procedure can be augmented by a short posterior transpedicular stabilization (30).

Pseudarthrosis: Kümmel disease

Another indication for cement augmentation procedures is the presence of painful pseudarthrosis complicating OVCF as a result of osteonecrosis (38) (Figures 30.4 and 30.5). A variety of terms have been used to describe this pathology: intervertebral vacuum, cleft, delayed vertebral collapse, and vertebral nonunion (39). Herman Kümmel first described this entity in 1895 as a post-traumatic delayed collapse of the vertebral body resulting from osteonecrosis (38). Alcohol consumption, radiotherapy, and steroids have been identified as contributing factors (40). The incidence is estimated to range between 7% and 37% (41) and may be noted after 6 months of conservative treatment (42).

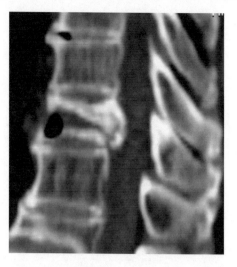

Figure 30.4 Computed tomography scan demonstrates a pseudarthrotic cleft filled with gas. Note the sclerotic margin of the pseudarthrotic cavity.

The disease may result in sequelae such as severe kyphosis and extrusion of a posterior bony fragment into the canal (Figure 30.6). This may compromise the neural elements of the spinal canal resulting in neurological deficit (42). Conservative treatment with bracing and analgesics usually is ineffective and is contraindicated in the presence of spinal cord compression (43) (see Figure 30.6).

As the majority of patients are of an advanced age, many authors have recommended minimal procedures such as cement augmentation alone (44,45) or in combination with short segmental percutaneous transpedicular fixation as safe and effective management (46). Cement augmentation alleviates pain and prevents further collapse of the vertebral body. Li and others recommend a more extended procedure if there is a severe kyphotic deformity (47,48). Patients with severe spinal stenosis and cord compression

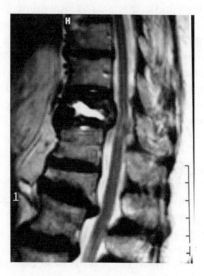

Figure 30.5 Magnetic resonance imaging demonstrates a pseudarthrotic cleft filled with fluid. The image is taken with the patient's spine in extension.

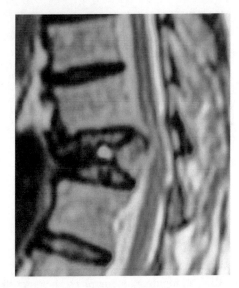

Figure 30.6 Pseudarthrotic cavity with posterior extrusion of bony fragment compromising the spinal cord. (With permission from Alpantaki K et al. *Texas Orthopaed J*. 2018. doi: 10.18600/toj.020203.)

without neurological deficit can benefit from kyphoplasty as a stand-alone procedure. In this case, the cement inserting cannula must be placed into the cleft at the anterior two-thirds of the vertebral body, dynamic monitoring during cement filling is recommended, and the cement should be infused slowly in a very doughy state (49). In a recent cohort study of one-level Kümmel disease, 12 patients, although initially displaying significant improvement of pain and deformity correction, after balloon kyphoplasty 6 months later exhibited variable degrees of kyphotic deformity and pain (50). Inadequate interdigitation of cement into the trabeculae is contributed to the insufficient outcome. These results particularly occur with vertebroplasty. This complication may be overcome by using a special kyphoplasty curette that acts as osteotome (KYPHON Latitude II Curette, 8.0 mm T-tip) to break the sclerotic margins of bone surrounding the osteonecrotic cavity in order to allow interdigitation of the cement with the trabecular bone. Following this, a KYPHON flat balloon is inserted as there is marked and uneven reduction of the vertebral body and the cement is infused slowly in a more viscous state (Figure 30.7).

Contraindications

The contraindications for these procedures include complete loss of vertebral height (vertebra plana), high-velocity burst fractures (although this was challenged by some [51]), infections, uncorrected coagulopathy or therapeutic anticoagulation, fractured pedicles, and contrast allergy (in kyphoplasty, balloons are filled with contrast that can extravasate if ruptured). Although a severely collapsed vertebra is considered as a contraindication, it has been shown that a significant percentage of these vertebrae

(a)

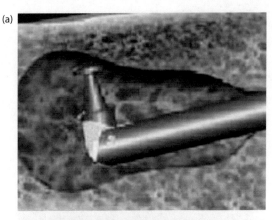

(b)

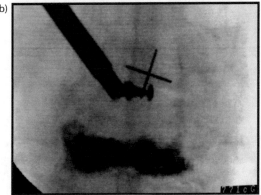

Figure 30.7 (a) The tip of a special curette (acting as osteotome) capable of breaking the sclerotic margins of pseudarthrotic cleft or creating cavities to redirect the kyphoplasty balloon. (b) Tip of the curette can be easily angulated. ([a] With permission from Kyphon Balloon Kyphoplasty UC201502590aEE. © Medtronic Inc. 2015. All rights reserved. Printed in Europe.)

can reexpand when placing the patient in hyperextension (52,53). For patients under the age of 40 years, cement vertebral augmentation should be exercised with caution.

Imaging modalities

Anteroposterior and lateral radiographs are essential for identifying radiographic landmarks for planning the trajectory of needle placement. Dynamic lateral radiographs can detect mobile fractures that are prone to reexpansion by extension of the spine. Intravertebral clefts characterizing pseudarthrosis after OVCF can be easily missed on standing lateral radiographs as they usually become evident on extension and disappear in flexion (54).

Magnetic resonance imaging (MRI) is the most useful imaging technique for the detection of edema that indicates unhealed fracture and for ruling out malignancy or infection (55). Sagittal MRI images with short tau inversion recovery (STIR) sequences better highlight the marrow edema (Figure 30.8) that is associated with acute or healing fractures (56,57). Some researchers have suggested that edema seen on MRI is predictive of a favorable response

(a) (b) (c)

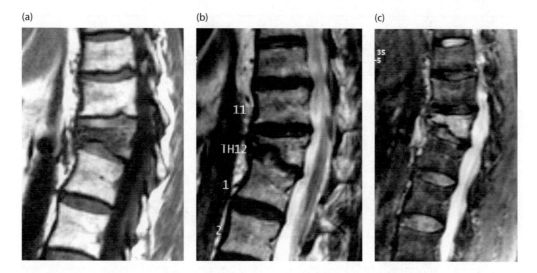

Figure 30.8 (a) T1-weighted image with low-intensity signal suggesting bone edema which is seen in (b) as high-intensity signal at T2-weighted image. (c) The high-intensity signal caused by marrow edema is better highlighted in short tau inversion recovery image.

to PVP (33,58). Others have questioned its utility, as they reported no direct correlation between symptom resolution and the presence of edema on preprocedural MRI when treating chronic OVCF with a duration of more than 1 year (59). MRI is also more sensitive than plain x-ray films in detecting intravertebral clefts. MRI appearance of intravertebral clefts can vary depending on whether they are gas or fluid filled. The contents of a cleft can vary over time in the supine position, because the gas is progressively replaced by fluid (54) (see Figures 30.4 and 30.5).

When patients are unable to tolerate MRI, CT can be helpful. Sagittal reconstructed CT images may be more sensitive than MRI in detecting intravertebral clefts (60). CT is also useful in evaluating the integrity of the posterior wall of the vertebral body and assessing posterior displacement of fragments. A 99Tc-MDP (methyldiphosphonate) bone scan can provide useful information about remodeling and thereby identify relatively fresh vertebral fractures. However, it may remain negative in cases of vertebral fractures with minimal height loss or remain positive for a prolonged period of time—as long as 2 years—after the fracture has healed, as a reflection of increased remodeling (61).

SURGICAL TECHNIQUE

PVP involves injection of polymethyl methacrylate (PMMA) into the treated vertebral body through a unilateral or bilateral percutaneous transpedicular approach or extrapedicular approach. Vertebroplasty is usually carried out under local anesthesia and conscious sedation, with constant monitoring of blood pressure, heart rate, and pulse oximetry. The technique is well described in the literature and is not detailed here (62). Gangi et al. (63) advocate a combined CT/fluoroscopic control to guide the transpedicular approach. However, Jensen et al. (62) reported that fluoroscopy is easier, safer, and less time-consuming than

CT. To minimize cement extravasation during PVP, we advocate that the cement should be of higher viscosity and should be inserted slowly using the kyphoplasty cement bone fillers.

PBK applies the principle of balloon angioplasty to vertebroplasty. In kyphoplasty a balloon is inserted into the vertebral body intended for treatment usually through a bilateral percutaneous transpedicular or extrapedicular approach, in the majority of cases under general anesthesia. A bilateral transpedicular approach is indicated for levels between T10 and L5 and the extrapedicular approach above T10 levels. The balloon device was approved as a "bone tamp" by the U.S. Food and Drug Administration (FDA) in 1998 (64). The created void is filled with bone cement.

The surgical procedure is graphically illustrated in figures from the balloon kyphoplasty manual (65). The technical guidelines are important to prevent procedural complications.

With the patient prone on a radiolucent operating table, usually under general anesthesia, the bony landmarks of the fractured vertebral body should be clearly identified with high-resolution fluoroscopy. If the resolution of the fluoroscopic images is not satisfactory, it behooves the surgeon to abort the procedure.

The cardinal landmarks for orienting and inserting the guide pin, as imaged on fluoroscopy, are the pedicle eyes, the end plates as straight lines (no contours) and parallel to each other, likewise the lateral borders of the vertebral body, and the spinous process in the center. The skin incision is made about 1.5 cm cranially and lateral to the pedicles, under fluoroscopy control a Jamshidi needle-osteointroducer is advanced through the skin incision, along an imagery trajectory toward the lateral margin of the pedicle, and should come to rest at the superolateral margin of the eye of the pedicle (between 11 and 9 o'clock on the left and between 1 and 3 o'clock on the right) as seen on anteroposterior (AP) view (Figure 30.9a). The corresponding position in the lateral image is the beginning

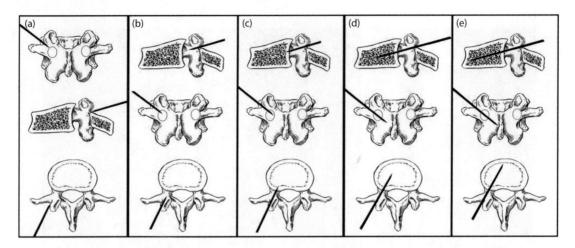

Figure 30.9 Transpendicular approach. (a) Starting position, (b) mid-pedicle, (c) junction body and pedicle, (d) mid-body position, and (e) final position. (With permission from Kyphon Balloon Kyphoplasty UC201502590aEE. © Medtronic Inc. 2015. All rights reserved. Printed in Europe.)

of the pedicle. At this stage, the instrument is gently tapped until it is seen in the middle of the eye (AP view) and the middle of the pedicle (lateral view) (Figure 30.9b). Further tapping should advance the needle to the inferomedial margin of the eye (AP view) (Figure 30.9c) and the posterior vertebral margin of the corresponding fluoroscopic view (see Figure 30.9c). No border contours should be seen; the borders should have distinct straight margins. Then the Jamshidi needle is removed from its sleeve and a blunt Kirschner guidewire is introduced into the middle of the vertebral body (the middle of the spinal process on the AP view and within 80% of the anteroposterior length anteriorly) (Figure 30.9d,e). The sleeve of the Jamshidi needle is removed and a working cannula is introduced safely over the guidewire until it penetrates the posterior vertebral wall. The correct placement of the working cannula is approximately 3 mm ventrally from the posterior vertebral body. Following this step, the trocar of the osteointroducer is removed, and a tunnel is created in the vertebral body using either a special biopsy tool that extracts an osseous core if this is deemed necessary or a special drill. At this stage, the special balloon is introduced through the working cannula in the created tunnel within the vertebral body,

then it is inflated to reduce the fracture (Figure 30.10a–c). This creates a cavity for the insertion of bone cement. Both balloons are inflated simultaneously under fluoroscopic control. Care should be taken in order for the balloon not to breach the vertebral walls (lateral cortical, superior and inferior subchondral, and anterior) (Figure 30.11). Under no circumstances should the balloon be allowed to reach the posterior wall. The balloons are then removed, and the bone fillers with bone cement are inserted through the working cannula into the void created by the balloons (Figure 30.10d). The cement should be employed slowly (Figure 30.12a–c) in a very doughy state, alternatively between the two bone fillers (not simultaneously) in order to avoid rapid rise of the intravertebral pressure.

If the confinement of the vertebral walls is violated, particularly the lateral, the balloon should be removed and reinserted more medially (likewise, it should be reinserted more inferiorly for violation of the superior subchondral bone, superiorly for the inferior, and posteriorly for the anterior wall). A special curette device that can act as an osteotome is available to achieve this action. The special curette is placed through the working cannula. This tool has a tip that can be angulated to 30°–60° and 90° (see Figure 30.7). Inside

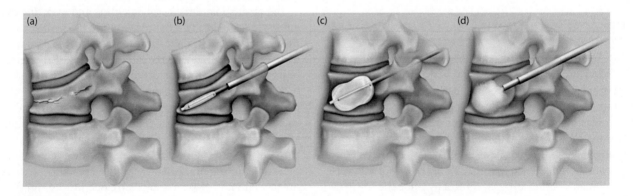

Figure 30.10 Balloon kyphoplasty. (With permission from Kyphon Balloon Kyphoplasty UC201502590aEE. © Medtronic Inc. 2015. All rights reserved. Printed in Europe.)

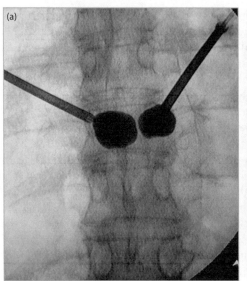
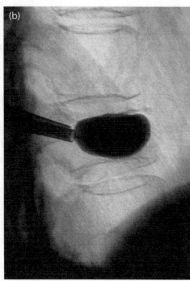

Figure 30.11   X-ray: (a) anteroposterior and (b) lateral. Balloon expansion should stay clear of the vertebral borders.

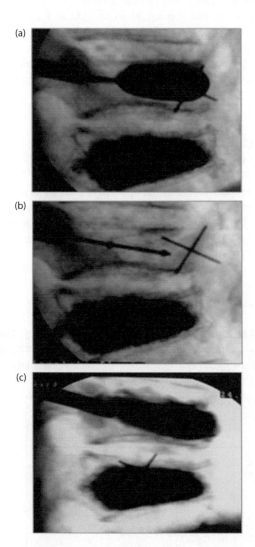

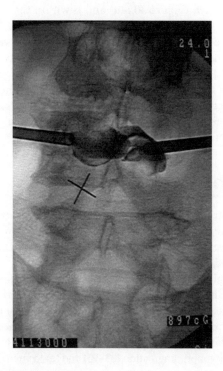

Figure 30.13   Eggshell cementoplasty. Thin shell of bone cement surrounds the expanding balloon.

Figure 30.12   (a) Fluoroscopy demonstrates reduction of osteoporotic vertebral compression fracture by an expanded balloon. (b) Deflated balloon in a cavity created by its prior expansion. (c) Cement filling the void.

the cavity, the curette is rotated to the desirable direction for scoring and scraping to open an outlet for the balloon to expand in a different direction. At this stage, a technique called "eggshell balloon cementoplasty" is employed (33). In the created cavity, 1 cc of the cement is inserted. Then the balloon is reinserted into the cement substance and reinflated. The expanding balloon carries the surrounding cement along, as a thin shell. The expanding balloon with the surrounding cement abuts the compromised vertebral wall. At this stage, the cement is allowed to harden. The balloon is removed, and a conventional cement filling is carried out in the usual fashion (Figure 30.13).

In the central and upper thoracic region, because the diameters of the pedicles are small (less than 5 mm), with a high degree of inclination in the sagittal profile and parallel in respect to the vertebral body, extrapedicular access is recommended, thus securing safe convergence of the instrumentation. The skin incision is oriented obliquely 1 cm laterally and 2 cm cranially and laterally to the pedicle eye, on a tangential imagery line that intercepts the pedicle and reaches the middle of the lower vertebral body. Usually this places the Jamshidi needle at a 45° convergence to the midline at the point of the skin incision (Figure 30.14a). Figure 30.14b depicts the needle through the skin on its way to the pedicle, at the level of the rib. When the tip of the needle comes to rest at the 10 o'clock position on the superolateral margin of the pedicle (Figure 30.14c), as seen on fluoroscopy, this should depict the tip of the needle in the lateral fluoroscopic view to reach the posterior wall of the vertebral body (see Figure 30.14c). At this stage, the Jamshidi needle is gently tapped until its tip reaches the inner lower margin of the eye of the pedicle (on AP view) (Figure 30.14d) and is within the vertebral body on the lateral fluoroscopic view (see Figure 30.14d). Then the trocar of the Jamshidi instrument is removed and a guide pin is inserted into the vertebral body (Figure 30.14e). The access instrument is then removed, and the working trocar is introduced over the K-wire. The rest of the procedure is similar to the transpedicular technique (see Figure 30.10). Figure 30.12 shows a satisfactory vertebral fracture reduction.

OUTCOMES

Based on the best available evidence in our review of the literature, it appears that both vertebroplasty and kyphoplasty are valuable procedures in the management of OVCF (30,65,66).

Several RCTs demonstrate the benefits of vertebroplasty (67–76) and kyphoplasty (34,77–80) over traditional conservative therapy. There was no statistically significant difference in pain relief or disability between vertebroplasty and kyphoplasty (81–92). Kyphoplasty demonstrated improvement of kyphotic angulation (93–95) and less cement leakage

(90). It is of interest that although some studies showed similar pain relief between vertebroplasty and kyphoplasty, the functional improvement was better in kyphoplasty (96–98).

Fracture age and outcomes

Vertebroplasty is an efficacious therapy in selected cases regardless of fracture age (58,99,100). The patient selection should not be based on the age of OVCF but rather on evidence of nonhealing on bone scans or MRI and the degree of persistent pain. Brown et al. (100) reported complete or partial relief of pain in 80% (33/41) of patients with fractures who underwent cementoplasty 1 year or more after the fracture and in 92% (45/49) of patients with fractures less than 1 year old. Patients with chronic fractures tended to have partial rather than complete relief of pain (100). When cementoplasty was performed on patients with symptoms lasting for 12 or more months, "marked to complete pain relief" was only obtained in patients with an abnormal marrow signal on an MRI and a height loss of less than 70% (100). In a prospective multicenter study, Garfin et al. (101) reported that improvements in pain and disability were independent of fracture age (greater than 60 days versus less than 60 days). The mean fracture age was 134 ± 318 days in that study.

Effect on a number of treated vertebral bodies

Vertebroplasty performed at a single fracture level and at multiple fracture levels were equally effective in bringing about long-term pain relief, increased activity level, and decreased consumption of analgesics in patients with OVCF (102).

Effect on pseudarthrotic clefts

Peh et al. reported complete pain relief in 44.4% of patients, partial pain relief in 33.3% of patients, and no change in 22.2% of patients treated for pseudarthrotic clefts (103).

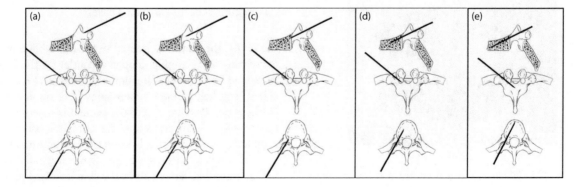

Figure 30.14 Extrapendicular approach. (a) Needle at the skin level, (b) through the skin before the pedicle, (c) starting point junction body and pedicle, (d) mid-body position, and (e) final position. (With permission from Kyphon Balloon Kyphoplasty UC201502590aEE. © Medtronic Inc. 2015. All rights reserved. Printed in Europe.)

Chen et al. (104) reported that all patients were satisfied by the procedure. According to Krauss et al. (105), patients with clefts had the same pain reduction as patients without clefts. However, Ha et al. (106) asserted that the treatment fared better in the group without clefts.

Effect on vertebral height restoration and kyphotic deformity

Failure to restore vertebral body height does not seem to compromise clinical outcomes in the immediate postoperative period after cement augmentation (34,107). But there is some evidence that in the long run, better restoration of the vertebral height might improve long-term outcomes. Grohs et al. (81), in a prospective nonrandomized study comparing vertebroplasty to kyphoplasty for OVCF, reported that although both methods resulted in a distinct decrease of pain intensity in the immediate postoperative period, in the long run the visual analogue scale (VAS) was better for the kyphoplasty group. Vertebroplasty failed to achieve any significant degree of vertebral kyphosis correction in fractures that did not show reducibility in the preoperative dynamic x-ray films (60).

Improvement of vertebral height of the OVCF with balloon kyphoplasty ranged widely: 54% (81), 58% (108), 70% (21,109–111), 84% (112), 90% (113), and 92% (33). This variation may be influenced by the age of the fracture, the degree of deformity, etc. Many authors agree that the more recent the injury, the better the chances for correction of both vertebral height and kyphotic deformity (35,108,114). Crandall et al. (35) claimed that osteoporotic fractures treated within the initial 10 weeks are more than five times as likely to be significantly reducible as compared to fractures older than 4 months. Majd et al. (110) reported that in nonhealed painful fractures, the height restoration is not related to fracture age. This observation was also corroborated by others (113,115) who agree that meaningful correction can be achieved even in older fractures, when MRI shows the typical signal changes suggesting incomplete healing (33,114). The ability to restore vertebral height can also be influenced by other parameters. Some authors reported that the more caudal the location of the fracture, the better the chances were to restore vertebral height (110,114). Others contradict this observation (113). Some observed no correlation has been found between the volume of cement injected and the degree of correction during kyphoplasty (114). Some reports fail to exhibit height restoration despite early intervention, within the first 3 months of onset of the fracture (116,117). Others failed to reveal any correlation between height restoration of the fractured vertebra and restoration of sagittal alignment of the spine (115,118). Pradhan et al. (118) reported that the majority of kyphosis correction by the PBK is limited to the treated vertebra. Therefore, it might be unrealistic to expect that a one- or two-level kyphoplasty will significantly improve the overall sagittal alignment. Global sagittal alignment is more likely to be affected by multilevel kyphoplasty (118).

In chronic fractures, reexpansion is possible in cases of progressive vertebral collapse or pseudarthrosis. Dynamic fracture mobility has been reported to range between 35% (119), 62% (115), and 68% (60) of fractured vertebral bodies. The differences probably reflect variations of the fracture age and methodology in obtaining dynamic radiographs among the studies. Similarly, the degree of height restoration that achieved some degree of correction ranged between 35% (119), 68% (60), 71.5% (120), 85% (121,122), and 92% (123). Apparently, intravertebral clefts are always present in mobile fractures and absent in immobile ones (119).

Postural correction versus balloon inflation

There is evidence that balloon inflation can have an additional beneficial effect compared to spinal hyperextension postural reduction in the correction of vertebral deformity alone (Figure 30.15) (115,124). Voggenreiter et al. (115) reported that in addition to the dynamic, position-related reduction of deformity, inflation of the balloon achieved a further 50% decrease of vertebral body kyphotic angle and 20% increase of anterior vertebral body height. However, after deflating and removing the balloon, some loss of fracture reduction can be expected (115,125). Shindle et al. (124) reported that kyphoplasty provided an additional 46.6% restoration of the lost midvertebral height over the positioning alone. With postural reduction, 51% of VCFs had over 10% restoration of the central portion of the vertebral body, whereas 91% of fractures improved at least 10% following balloon kyphoplasty. Balloon kyphoplasty enhanced the height reduction over 4.5-fold over the positioning maneuver alone and accounted for over 80% of the ultimate reduction. Boszczyk et al. (126) reported that in severe osteoporotic fractures, average correction of the kyphotic angle was 5% with balloon kyphoplasty, while vertebroplasty failed to achieve correction.

Effects of absorbable cements in maintaining correction

There is some concern that the use of absorbable cements may result in a rebound of kyphotic deformity in the long run. In a clinical study using calcium phosphate, some of the vertebral kyphosis correction achieved by vertebroplasty was lost at the 6-month follow-up (127,128). This gives rise to the hypothesis that absorption of calcium phosphate may result in a rebound of kyphotic deformity in the long run. However, these findings are not substantiated by others who claim that balloon kyphoplasty with calcium phosphate cement was safe and effective with sustained results (129).

Multilevel kyphoplasty

Balloon kyphoplasty performed under general anesthesia appears to be safe even when applied in multiple levels (up

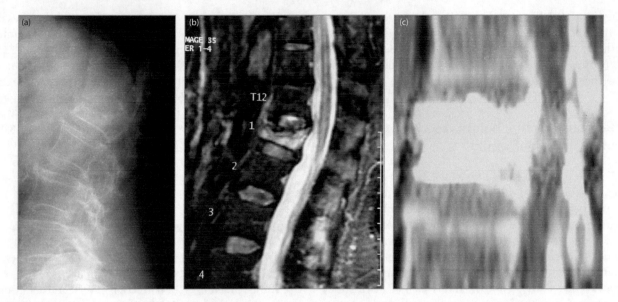

Figure 30.15 (a and b) Maximum expansion of the balloon was essential to reduce kyphotic deformity. (c) A large volume of cement was necessary to fill the created void.

to eight levels) in the same seating, provided the balloons are inflated sequentially and not simultaneously and the cement is inserted slowly in a very doughy state. Close monitoring of cardiorespiratory factors is valuable. Its rare circulatory effects are unrelated to the number of levels or the cement type (130).

COMPLICATIONS

Although vertebroplasty and kyphoplasty are generally accepted as safe procedures, there are numerous reports of complications of which the surgeon should be aware. General surgical complications such as cardiac, pulmonary, circulatory, and even mortality (17,131) are less frequent than those encountered in open conventional surgical procedures.

Procedural technical complications are more common. These include cement leakage resulting in neurological and cardiorespiratory hazards, adjacent vertebral fractures, rib fractures, and pain after the procedure. Other problems include radiation exposure and cost (66). Fracture of the pedicle during PVP has been reported by Kallmes et al. (132) in 2.4% (1/41) of patients, by Hodler et al. (133) in 0.6% (1/152) of patients, and by Voormolen et al. (134) in 0.9% (1/112) of patients. Diamond et al. (135) reported fracture of the transverse process in 3.6% (2/55) of patients who underwent vertebroplasty. Garfin et al. (64) reported three cases (0.9%) of serious neurological deficit associated with procedural technical complications from faulty tool (Jamshidi needle or filler device) placement during kyphoplasty. Among the 20 cases of neurological complications after PBK reported to the FDA during 2001–2002, at least five were caused by breakage of the pedicle, causing either the release of cement into the spinal canal or the development of an epidural hematoma at the pedicle fracture

site (136,137). Rupture of the balloon has been reported during PBK with an incidence ranging from 2.3% to 20% per treated vertebral body (21,33,35). However, other than exposure to small volumes of radiocontrast medium, this was not hazardous (64). In all instances, the ruptured tamp was easily withdrawn. This might have resulted from protruding bony spicules piercing the balloon during the procedure. This problem can be avoided by tamping the drilled channel with a bone tamping device in order to break and dispense osseous spicule (33). Other complications include hematoma formation, arterial injury, and pneumothorax. The incidence of subcutaneous, puncture site hematoma has been reported to range between 1.7% (2/117) (138) and 8.9% (10/112) (134) in patients treated with PVP. This complication has been related to decreased short-term patient satisfaction (134). Other reported complications include psoas muscle hematoma accompanied with intense pain (139), injury to a segmental branch of the L4 lumbar artery following kyphoplasty presented 10 days after surgery with pulsatile bleeding from the kyphoplasty site (140), and 1.3% asymptomatic pneumothoraces after vertebroplasty in the thoracic region (133).

Infection

Postoperative infection is a rare but devastating complication of kyphoplasty. A few cases have been reported in the literature (110,132,141–147). Ongoing back pain and/or neurological complication are the predominant presenting symptoms. *Staphylococcus aureus* is the most common pathogen (132,148). Tuberculous spondylitis has also been reported (149). Infection after cementoplasty procedure is likely related to a prior systemic infection, an immunocompromised host, or intraoperative contamination. Preoperative prophylactic antibiotic administration is recommended. Cement mixed with antibiotics has also been recommended in the cases with a previous infection or in immunocompromised patients (150). In case of concurrent infection, the procedure must be postponed until the infection is controlled. Cementoplasty infection can be treated conservatively with a course of antibiotics based on antibiotic sensitivity testing (144). Infection refractory to conservative treatment or recurrent infection should be treated with corpectomy, cement removal, and instrumented spinal reconstruction (150).

Rib and sternal fractures

Rib and sternal fractures are an infrequent complication. A systematic review cited eight studies that reported incidence ranges from 0.6% to 4.3% (66). Improper patient positioning as well as leaning over the patient's back during surgery may result in rib fractures (19,151,152). We experienced a patient with a successful kyphoplasty procedure who was seriously afflicted by severe pain from four rib fractures. This complication occurred when pressure was applied over the kyphotic deformity in order to reduce the wedged vertebra (30).

Increase in pain after procedure

On some occasions, a transient increase in pain has been described within hours or days after PVP (153–155). The reported incidence varies among authors: 1.2% (3/245 patients) (156), 4% (1/25 patients) (154), 6.2% (1/16 patients) (157), and 23.4% (4/17 patients) (158). It usually lasts less than 72 hours and may depend on the amount of cement injected (155). However, there are reports of permanent worsening of pain in 2% of patients after the PVP (102).

Cement leakage

Cement leakage is a frequent occurrence in cementoplasty. In a systematic review, the rates of cement extravasation in prospective studies for vertebroplasty range from 2% to 63% (the greater the number of patients, the higher the incidence of cement leakage), whereas for balloon kyphoplasty, they range from 2.7% to 17.8% (66). Although it is well tolerated in the majority of cases, it is also the main source of serious complications such as cement embolism or neurological problems, and even complete paraplegia. Most authors agree that in the majority of cases, the presence of cement leakage is not associated with the final clinical outcome. However, there are reports that leakage into the epidural space (159) or in the disc (99) reduces the pain relief experienced after PVP.

A postprocedural CT scan is the most sensitive way to detect cement leakage. Plain x-ray films revealed only 66% of the leaks that were identified by CT scan. On lateral radiographs, 93% of leakage that occurred via the basivertebral veins and 86% of leakage through the segmental veins were either missed or underestimated (Figure 30.16). Only 7% of the leaks into the spinal canal were correctly identified on radiographs. Therefore, cement leakage is more common than may be detected on plain radiographs (160). It seems that cement leakage occurs more frequently when cement is injected above the T7 level (159).

There is no consensus concerning the risk of cement leakage during vertebroplasty in patients with intravertebral clefts. Jang et al. (157) reported an incidence of 12.5%; similarly, Kaus et al. (105) cites an incidence of 18.2% when clefts are present versus 46% in uncomplicated OVCF. However, Ha et al. (106) observed a higher incidence of cement leak, 75% in fractures with clefts as opposed to fractures without clefts. This finding is also corroborated by Peh et al. (103) who reported an intradiscal cement leakage rate of 79% and paravertebral leaks in 42% of treated vertebrae.

The pseudarthrotic cystic cavity, which may be less permeable to injected bone cement, prevents the cement from interdigitating the microstructure of cancellous bone, rendering it more unstable. A case of anterior cement displacement 1 month after PVP for a T12 OVCF with cleft has been reported (161). The patient developed severe back pain radiating to the lower abdomen and paraparesis. Removal of the cement and reconstruction of the spine were achieved by combined anterior decompression and posterior instrumentation.

Using proper surgical technique, the incidence of cement leakage can be markedly reduced. Correct placement of the balloon, high cement viscosity, slow cement insertion, constant fluoroscopically controlled cementation, and proper cement volume minimize the risk of cement leakage. The advocated amount of cement injected per vertebral body varies in the literature from 2 to 11 mL (62,66,153,162).

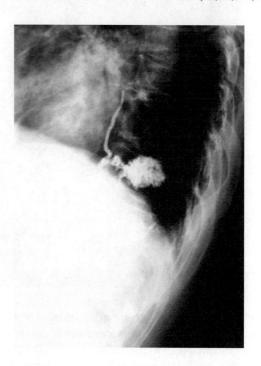

Figure 30.16 Intravascular cement leakage.

Some authors warn that attempts to inject more than 5 mL of PMMA per vertebral body should be avoided (163). Some reports advocate that sufficient cement volume to restore vertebral strength and achieve good clinical outcome should be substantial (164) as opposed to earlier reports that small cement volume is adequate (Figure 30.17) (165). A fill volume of at least 13%–16% of vertebral volume in one study and 24% in another are considered optimal for restoration of vertebral body strength (166,167). We usually insert 6–8 cc in the lumbar spine and 3–4 cc in the thoracic spine (Figure 30.18).

The eggshell balloon cementoplasty has been promoted to prevent cement leakage when the vertebral confinement is violated (33,168).

Balloon inflation during PBK creates an intervertebral cavity that allows a more viscous cement to be slowly inserted, thereby decreasing the risk of extravasation. Experimental data have shown that low cement viscosity inserted under high pressure represents the most important aspect with respect to cement extravasation (169). In addition, balloon inflation compacts the trabecular bone, which may seal potential osseous or venous leak pathways. Phillips et al. (170) reported significantly lower extravertebral leaks after injecting contrast material into the void created by the inflatable bone tamps as compared to intravertebral injection of contrast before void creation. Studies in cadavers also support the reduced leak rate with kyphoplasty (171).

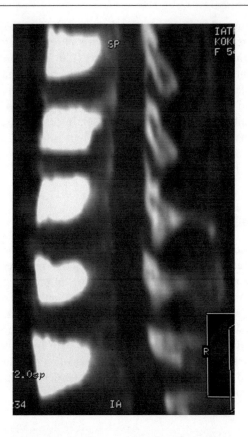

Figure 30.18 Imaging demonstrates sufficient cement volume without leakage.

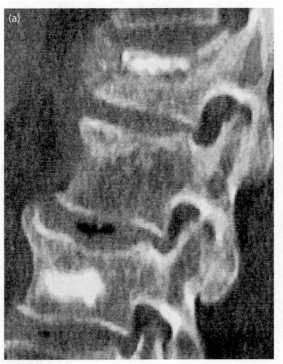
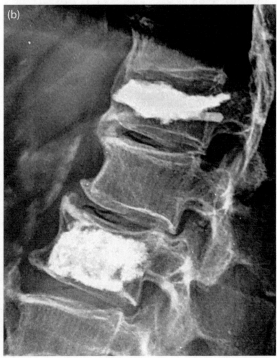

Figure 30.17 (a) A 55-year-old male patient with 3-month intractable back pain (VAS: 8/10) from osteoporotic vertebral compression fracture underwent an inadequate amount cement balloon kyphoplasty. The symptoms remained unabated and following (b) revision kyphoplasty with adequate amount of cement filling resulted in an immediate and sustained relief of pain (VAS: 0/10) at 5-year follow-up. Note the pseudarthrotic cleft of the L1 vertebra (a) and cement interdigitation in the vertebral body after revision (b). (With permission from Alpantaki K et al. *Texas Orthopaed J*. 2018. doi: 10.18600/toj.020203.)

Respiratory effects and hemodynamic changes

Hemodynamic and respiratory complications such as transient hypotension and decrease of oxygen saturation have been widely reported during cement augmentation procedures. The exact incidence is not clear. The incidence may be underestimated, as a respiratory decline during surgery in a geriatric patient may be attributed to preexisting pulmonary disease (172). Cement embolism can be asymptomatic or symptomatic and presents itself with dyspnea, tachypnea, tachycardia, cyanosis, chest pain, coughing, and hemoptysis (173).

Most cases were treated conservatively, with or without anticoagulation, resulting in satisfactory outcomes. However, in a few instances, patients required intensive care management and operative removal of the cement emboli (174), or even open heart surgery (175,176). Deaths from pulmonary embolism of bone cement have also been reported in the literature after vertebroplasty for OVCF (138,177–181). Transesophageal echocardiogram in fatal cases revealed significant showering of fat emboli resulting in complete right heart outlet obstruction (180). Some authors advise against injecting more than 30 mL or more than three levels per session (182).

Intracardial cement leakage is an extremely rare complication following kyphoplasty and vertebroplasty. There are only a few cases reported in the literature (183–185). The consequences of intracardiac cement embolism are perforation of myocardium, pericardial tamponade, or pericardial perforation, which may cause chest pain, dyspnea, and shock (184). Cardiac catheterization or open heart surgery is necessary in order to remove the cement fragment (185). Cerebral (186) and renal (187) embolisms have also been reported.

Animal studies showed that cement and fat embolism can cause serious cardiopulmonary deterioration during cement augmentation procedures (188–190). Pulmonary embolism is correlated to an increased interosseous pressure brought about by the instrumentation during the procedure, which forces fat, bone marrow, and PMMA particles into the epidural and vertebral venous system. A decline of sympathetic tone associated with this process was claimed as the probable culprit, rather than the cement toxicity itself (191). The viscosity and the amount of cement injected is a significant factor related to cement extravasation (169) as alluded to earlier.

Some methods have been advocated to minimize the risk of cardiovascular and pulmonary complications during kyphoplasty, particularly when undertaking a multiple-level procedure (eight levels) (130). There are considerations during patient positioning and anesthesia preparation. Patient prone position during surgery affects intra-abdominal (increased inferior vena cava pressure), intrathoracic, and intraosseous vertebral body venous plexus pressure (192). Higher venous pressure results in safer cement insertion by avoiding risks such as fat, bone marrow, or cement embolization (193). During general anesthesia, a transient elevation of intrathoracic and intra-abdominal pressures

should be attained when inflating the balloons or inserting the cement in order to minimize pulmonary embolism. Multilevel (over three levels) cement balloon kyphoplasty can be safely executed under proper anesthetic precautions and with the surgical technique of balloon positioning and cement handling as alluded to earlier (130). Simultaneous inflation of multiple-level balloons, and simultaneous injection of multiple levels should be discouraged (130). Close cardiorespiratory monitoring and positive pressure ventilation during balloon inflation and cement insertion are mandatory. Cement injection should be terminated in the case that cement leakage is detected during fluoroscopy (194). Under these suggested guidelines, multilevel (up to eight levels) balloon kyphoplasty can safely be performed (Figure 30.19).

A standard therapeutic protocol for pulmonary cement embolization has not been described. In general, treatment is not suggested for asymptomatic patients with small peripheral emboli. In the case of symptomatic or central embolism, the suggested recommendation consists of initiating anticoagulation treatment with heparin followed by Coumadin for 6 months (173).

Neurological complications

Leakage through the basivertebral vein leads to a distribution of cement into the epidural plexus. This type of leakage, which is relatively symmetrical, is located anterior to the thecal sac (160) and is not associated with neurological complications in the majority of cases. Epidural cement leakage through posterior cortical or pedicular defects can be distributed in the anterior and posterior epidural space,

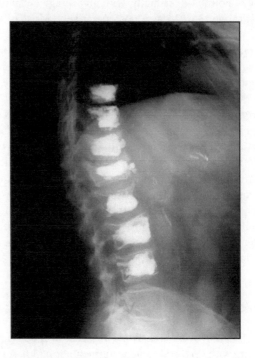

Figure 30.19 Safe and effective multiple-level balloon kyphoplasty.

resulting in circumferential constriction. A large amount of PMMA cement can extrude into the spinal canal and obliterate large cross-sectional areas of the spinal canal. This type of epidural leakage is more commonly associated with major neurological complications (151,163,195). A case of intradural leakage after dural punch that resulted in a myelographic picture in the spinal canal and severe paraparesis has also been reported (196). Cement leakage in the foramen is apparently less well tolerated than in the spinal canal. Cotten et al. (153) reported that spinal canal leakage was well tolerated by all 15 patients, while two out of eight cases of foraminal leakage were associated with radiculopathy. In most cases it causes transient radicular pain responding well to nerve root blocks, oral steroids, or nonsteroidal anti-inflammatory medication. However, severe radiculopathy with excruciating pain and nerve root palsy that required surgical decompression has also been described (4,153,197). Radiculopathy has also been reported in patients without evidence of foraminal or epidural cement leakage (138,198) suggesting that radiculopathy can also be related to needle-induced trauma (138). Although it seems that cement leakage in the paravertebral soft tissue is almost always asymptomatic, Cotten et al. (153) reported a case of transient femoral neuropathy related to PMMA leakage into the psoas muscle. Cyteval et al. (4) also reported a 5% (1/20 patients) incidence of crural pain concerning cement leakage in the psoas muscle.

Most of the cases of neurological complications after PBK are caused by faulty puncture techniques, resulting in pedicle disruption and epidural hematoma or cement leakage into the canal (64,78,199).

In the presence of pseudarthrosis, the patients may develop neurological deficit either immediately (in less than 24 hours) or gradually, with an average delay of 37.1 days (range, 3–112 days) postoperatively. Most of these patients required revision by open surgical intervention for treatment of their neurological injury (200). According to a systematic review (66), the reported incidence of neurological deficit ranges from 0, 4% to 23% for PVP, and 1%–5% for PBK.

From the published reports, it is apparent that PBK fares better than vertebroplasty in terms of neurological complications. However, according to the reported cases to the FDA, PBK is associated with a larger number of neurological complications than those reported in the literature. During 2001–2002, among 24,500 PBK procedures performed in the United States, there were 20 cases of neurological complications that required spinal decompression surgery (136,137). Six of these patients sustained permanent injury despite the surgical decompression.

Adjacent vertebral fracture

There is controversy regarding the risk of a subsequent fracture with vertebral cement augmentation (30). A number of reports indicate an increased risk of secondary fractures adjacent to the augmented vertebra. The odds ratio for a vertebral fracture in the vicinity of a cemented vertebra has been reported to be between 3.18 (201) and 2.27 (154), compared with 2.14 (201) to 1.44 (154) in the vicinity of an uncemented fracture.

The risk seems to be higher in the first 2 or 3 months after both vertebroplasty (134,202–204) and kyphoplasty. After this period, it is almost similar to the natural history of the untreated disease (205). This suggests that cement augmentation enhances the clustering phenomenon that has been reported in the natural history of OVCF.

Some authors suggest that the alteration of biomechanical balance caused by the cement filling can lead to a stress shielding phenomenon on the adjacent vertebral bodies (206). The mechanism for adjacent vertebral fracture is not clear. It is speculated that the increased stiffness of the augmented vertebra changes the biomechanics of load transfer to the adjacent vertebrae. Although it is difficult to determine the optimal amount of cement filling, it is possible that rigid augmentation may also provoke failure of the adjacent, nonaugmented level (207). The greater the degree of augmentation of the treated vertebra and the location of the adjacent vertebra at the thoracolumbar junction are considered potential risks for secondary vertebral body fractures (203).

Lin et al. showed that more than 70% of patients who sustained a subsequent fracture after vertebroplasty suffered intradiscal cement leak. Cement extravasation into the disc may increase the risk of a secondary fracture due to the alteration of disc flexibility (112,209). Also, patients with predominantly lower bone density, larger balloon or cement volume, fissure fracture, steroid use, and absence of systemic antiosteoporosis therapy run an increased risk of a contiguous vertebral compression fracture (210–212).

According to a systematic review, the rates of new fracture after cement augmentation procedures are not comparable between vertebroplasty (0%–52%), kyphoplasty (5.8%–36.8%), and conservatively treated patients (19.2%–58%) because of the poor scientific design of the studies. Most are retrospective or nonrandomized prospective reports (19).

Many authors argue that since adjacent vertebral fractures occur in untreated patients, this may suggest that this event results from preexisting osteoporosis rather than the procedure itself (213). As alluded to in the introduction, kyphotic deformity caused by untreated OVCFs is a major predisposing factor for secondary fracture development, as it transfers the center of gravity forward, resulting in an increased forward bending moment which subsequently enhances the load within the kyphotic angle (Figure 30.20). Therefore, kyphosis reduction due to kyphoplasty is expected to lessen the risk of new fracture development (214).

In a 1-year follow-up study, kyphoplasty, as an addition to medical treatment, and when performed in appropriately selected patients, showed improvement in pain and reduction in the occurrence of new vertebral fracture in individuals with primary osteoporosis (34). Similarly, after 3 years in a prospective study, the incidence of new vertebral fractures, after kyphoplasty, was significantly reduced in

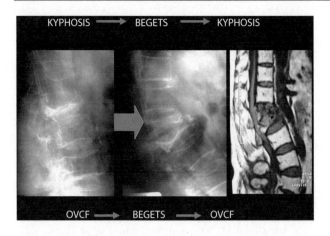

Figure 30.20 Sequelae of osteoporotic vertebral compression fracture.

the patients who received pharmacologic antiosteoporotic treatment, analgesics, and physiotherapy versus control (79). In a recent meta-analysis of 12 studies involving 1328 patients (of whom 768 underwent augmentation procedure with PMMA and 560 received nonoperative treatment) revealed that the risk of adjacent vertebral body fracture was equivalent between cementoplasty (vertebroplasty and balloon kyphoplasty) and conservative treatment (215).

Radiation exposure

Radiation exposure and associated risks during cement augmentation procedures may be considerable for the patient. Therefore, both the surgeon and the staff should exercise caution in order to minimize exposure (30,216,217). Mroz et al. (217) reported that during kyphoplasty the exposure time was 5.7 ± 2.0 minutes/vertebra for a single-level, 3.9 ± 0.8 minutes/vertebra for a two-level, and 2.9 ± 1.2 minutes/vertebra for a three-level kyphoplasty. Surgeon exposure as measured by the protected dosimeter was less than the minimum reportable dose (less than 0.010 mSv). Exposure as measured by the unprotected dosimeter, which is equivalent to deep whole-body exposure, was 0.248 ± 0.170 mSv/vertebra. Eye exposure was 0.271 ± 0.200 mSv/vertebra, and the shallow exposure (hand/skin) was 0.273 ± 0.200 mSv/vertebra. Hand exposure was 1.744 ± 1.173 mSv/vertebra. Without eye or hand protection, total radiation exposure dose to these areas would exceed the occupational exposure limit after 300 cases per year (217). Protection of the hands and the eyes of the surgeon by using proper safety equipment, including radiation safety gowns, thyroid shields, gloves, and lead glasses is strongly recommended (218). In a similar study, emphasis was given to the importance of surgeons wearing lead glove protection on their leading hands during percutaneous vertebroplasty procedures. This measure has resulted in a 75% reduction rate of exposure to radiation (219).

Measures to minimize radiation exposure during kyphoplasty involve the use of low-dose or pulsed fluoroscopy (220) and the use of simultaneous biplanar fluoroscopy.

When an optimal setting has been found, it is continued throughout the procedure, and radiation is not "wasted" by readjusting to a second plane of view (221). Patient and staff radiation exposure is closely associated with their distance from the fluoroscopy beam. The source-to-skin distance during the procedure should not be less than 35 cm (222). Unprotected staff working less than 70 cm from a fluoroscopic beam receive significant amounts of radiation, whereas those working more than 91.4 cm from the beam receive an extremely low amount of radiation (223).

COST

Cost-effectiveness is a contentious issue (30). The cost-effectiveness of vertebral augmentation techniques for OVCFs has been challenged (224,225). A drawback of balloon kyphoplasty is the high cost of the instrumentation, which has been estimated at 3500 euros per treated level, whereas for vertebroplasty the cost is approximately 500 euros per level (226,227). There is an additional cost and risk of general anesthesia with kyphoplasty, although it can be performed using local anesthesia for one or two levels. Multiple levels are often under general anesthesia. Studies have not taken into consideration patients with neurological and musculoskeletal problems associated with OVCFs. Osteoporotic compression fractures have been associated with a 15% higher mortality rate (228,229). Even for the oldest patients, both procedures are considered to be cost-effective in terms of cost per life-year gained (230). Patients have been found to require primary care services at a rate 14 times greater than the general population in the first year after a symptomatic vertebral fracture (231). Compared to conservative treatment, significant reduction in mortality and drift in social functionality in patients treated with balloon kyphoplasty was identified at 1-year follow-up in a prospective UK study (232). In US mean total cost increased for both procedures, from $10,897 per case in 2006 to $14,114 per case in 2014 for vertebroplasty, and from $12,184 per case in 2006 to $17,174 per case in 2014 for kyphoplasty (233). A cost-effectiveness analysis of OVCF treatment among 858,978 patients in the Medicare dataset (2005–2008) demonstrated kyphoplasty as a cost-effective and cost-saving procedure compared to vertebroplasty (230). Borse conducted a cost-utility analysis from a payer's perspective using a Markov model to assess the cost utility of balloon kyphoplasty compared to vertebroplasty. They found that balloon kyphoplasty is associated with a better utility and higher effectiveness compared to vertebroplasty (208).

CONCLUSION

Osteoporosis is not always a benign process of aging (19,30,66). OVCF, a common complication of osteoporosis, is frequently associated with a variety of disabling symptoms ranging from mild local back discomfort to crippling painful spinal deformity, and serious neurological deficit including paraplegia. As life expectancy continues to increase, vertebral compression fractures will become an expanding health problem. Both vertebroplasty and kyphoplasty are shown to be efficient in controlling pain and improving daily activities with sustained results.

These two procedures and particularly vertebroplasty had been challenged as ineffective procedures after two RCTs, using sham procedures as control, were published in the *New England Journal of Medicine*. The assertions of these studies were widely accepted. However, the scientific rigor and integrity of these two publications were seriously questioned by several authors (30).

Based on the best available evidence, it appears that vertebroplasty and particularly kyphoplasty are valuable procedures in the management of OVCF. However, these minimally invasive surgical procedures are not innocuous, as they can be complicated by serious neurological and cardiopulmonary problems. Strict adherence to surgical indications and meticulous surgical technique can minimize the potential risks of balloon kyphoplasty. Furthermore, available data suggest the risk of adjacent vertebral fractures after PVP and PBK ranks on a par with the natural history of untreated OVCF.

The benefit of cementoplasty and the delight in whatever pain-free life is left in elderly patients should also be considered as a strong argument for a paradigm shift in the management of OVCF.

REFERENCES

1. Lyritis GP, Mayasis B, Tsakalakos N et al. The natural history of osteoporotic vertebral fracture. *Clin Reumatol.* 1989;8(Suppl 2):66–9.
2. Sinaki M. Exercise and physical therapy. In: Riggs L, Melton L, eds. *Osteoporosis: Etiology, Diagnosis and Management.* New York, NY: Raven Press, 1988, p. 401.
3. Eck JC, Hodges SD, Humphreys SC. Vertebroplasty: A new treatment strategy for osteoporotic compression fractures. *Am J Ortop.* 2002;31(3):123–8.
4. Cyteval C, Sarrabere MP, Roux JO et al. Acute osteoporotic vertebral collapse: Open study on percutaneous injection of acrylic surgical cement in 20 patients. *Am J Roentgenol.* 1999;173(6):1685–90.
5. Old JL, Calvert M. Vertebral compression fractures in the elderly. *Am Fam Physician.* 2004;69(1):111–16.
6. McKiernan F, Faciszewski T. Intravertebral clefts in osteoporotic vertebral compression fractures. *Arthritis Rheum.* 2003;48(5):1414–19.
7. Yuan HA, Brown CW, Phillips FM. Osteoporotic spinal deformity. A biomechanical rationale for the clinical consequences and treatment of vertebral body compression fractures. *J Spinal Disord Tech.* 2004;17:236–42.
8. Lindsay R, Silverman SL, Cooper C et al. Risk of new vertebral fracture in the year following a fracture. *JAMA.* 2001;285(3):320–3.
9. Raisadeh K. Surgical management of adult kyphosis: Idiopathic, posttraumatic and osteoporotic. *Semin Spine Surg.* 1999;10:367–81.
10. Black DM, Arden NK, Palermo L et al. Prevalent vertebral deformities predict hip fractures and new vertebral fractures but not wrist fracture. Study of Osteoporotic Fractures Research Group. *J Bone Miner Res.* 1999;14(5):821–8.
11. Ismail AA, Cockerill W, Cooper C et al. Prevalent vertebral deformity predicts incident hip though not distal forearm fracture: Results from the European Prospective Osteoporosis Study. *Osteoporosis Int.* 2001;12(2):85–90.
12. Silverman SL, Minshall ME, Shen W et al. The relationship of health-related quality of life to prevalent an incident vertebral fractures in postmenopausal women with osteoporosis. *Arthritis Reum.* 2001; 44(11):2611–19.
13. Lyles KW, Gold DT, Shipp KM et al. Association of osteoporotic compression fractures with impaired functional status. *Am J Med.* 1993;94:595–601.
14. Leech JA, Dulberg C, Kellie S et al. Relationship of lung function to severity of osteoporosis in women. *Am Rev Respir Dis.* 1990;141(1):68–71.
15. Schlaich C, Minne HW, Bruckner T et al. Reduced pulmonary function in patients with spinal osteoporotic fractures. *Osteoporos Int.* 1998;8(3):261–7.
16. Cotten A, Boutry N, Cortet B et al. Percutaneous vertebroplasty: State of the art. *Radiographics.* 1998; 18(2):311–20.
17. Kado DM, Browner WS, Palermo L et al. Vertebral body fractures and mortality in older women: A prospective study. Study of Osteoporotic Fracture Research Group. *Arch Intern Med.* 1999;159(11):1215–20.
18. Young MH, Wales C. Long term consequences of stable fractures of the thoracic and lumbar vertebral bodies. *J Bone Joint Surg.* 1973;55B:295–300.
19. Hadjipavlou AG, Tzermiadianos MN, Katonis PG, Szpalski M. Percutaneous vertebroplasty and balloon kyphoplasty for the treatment of osteoporotic vertebral compression fractures and osteolytic tumours. *J Bone Joint Surg Br.* 2005;87(12): 1595–604.
20. Galibert P, Deramond H, Rosat P, Le Gars D. Preliminary note on the treatment of vertebral angioma by percutaneous acrylic vertebroplasty. *Neurochirurgie.* 1987;33(2):166–8.
21. Lieberman IH, Dudeney S, Reinhardt MK, Bell G. Initial outcome and efficacy of "kyphoplasty" in the treatment of painful osteoporotic vertebral compression fractures. *Spine.* 2001;26(14):1631–8.
22. Buchbinder R, Osborne RH, Ebeling PR et al. A randomized trial of vertebroplasty for painful osteoporotic vertebral fractures. *N Engl J Med.* 2009;361(6):557–68.
23. Kallmes DF, Comstock BA, Heagerty PJ et al. A randomized trial of vertebroplasty for osteoporotic spinal fractures. *N Engl J Med.* 2009;361(6):569–79.

24. *American Academy of Orthopaedic Surgeons*. The treatment of symptomatic osteoporotic spinal compression fractures: Guidelines and evidence report. Available from: https://www.aaos.org/research/guidelines/SCFguideline.pdf

25. Brett AS. Vertebroplasty—1 year later. NEJM Journal Watch, September 16, 2010.

26. Prasad VK, Cifu AS. *Ending Medical Reversal*. Baltimore, MD: John Hopkins University Press, 2015.

27. Noonan P. Randomized vertebroplasty trials: Bad news or sham news? *AJNR Am J Neuroradiol*. 2009; 30(10):1808–9.

28. Smith SJ, Vlahos A, Sewall LE. An objection to the *New England Journal of Medicine* vertebroplasty articles. *Can Assoc Radiol J*. 2010;61(2):121–2.

29. Aebi M. Vertebroplasty: About sense and nonsense of uncontrolled "controlled randomized prospective trials." *Eur Spine J*. 2009;18(9):1247–8.

30. Alpantaki K, Dohm M, Vastardis G, Hadjipavlou AG. Controversial issues in cementoplasty. *Texas Orthopaed J*. 2018. doi: 10.18600/toj.020203

31. Clark W, Bird P, Gonski P et al. Safety and efficacy of vertebroplasty for acute painful osteoporotic fractures (VAPOUR): A multicentre, randomized, double-blind, placebo-controlled trial. *Lancet*. 2016;388(10052):1408–16.

32. Robinson Y, Heyde CE, Försth P, Olerud C. Kyphoplasty in osteoporotic vertebral compression fractures--guidelines and technical considerations. *J Orthop Surg Res*. 2011;6:43.

33. Gaitanis IN, Hadjipavlou AG, Katonis PG, Tzermiadianos MN, Pasku DS, Patwardhan AG. Balloon kyphoplasty for the treatment of pathological vertebral compressive fractures. *Eur Spine J*. 2005;14(3):250–60.

34. Grafe IA, Da Fonseca K, Hillmeier J et al. Reduction of pain and fracture incidence after kyphoplasty: 1-year outcomes of a prospective controlled trial of patients with primary osteoporosis. *Osteoporos Int*. 2005;16(12):2005–12.

35. Crandall D, Slaughter D, Hankins PJ, Moore C, Jerman J. Acute versus chronic vertebral compression fractures treated with kyphoplasty: Early results. *Spine J*. 2004;4(4):418–24.

36. Papanastassiou ID, Filis A, Aghayev K, Kokkalis ZT, Gerochristou MA, Vrionis FD. Adverse prognostic factors and optimal intervention time for kyphoplasty/vertebroplasty in osteoporotic fractures. *Biomed Res Int*. 2014;2014:925683.

37. Oh GS, Kim HS, Ju CI, Kim SW, Lee SM, Shin H. Comparison of the results of balloon kyphoplasty performed at different times after injury. *J Korean Neurosurg Soc*. 2010;47(3):199–202.

38. Kümmel H. Die rarefizierende Ostitis der Wirbelkörper. *Deutsche Med*. 1895;21:180–1.

39. Jindal N, Sharma R, Jindal R, Garg SK. Kümmell's disease: Literature update and challenges ahead. *Hard Tissue* 2013;2(5):45.

40. Osterhouse MD, Kettner NW. Delayed posttraumatic vertebral collapse with intravertebral vacuum cleft. *J Manipulative Physiol Ther*. 2002;25(4):270–5.

41. Freedman BA, Heller JG. Kümmel disease: A not-so-rare complication of osteoporotic vertebral compression fractures. *J Am Board Fam Med*. 2009;22(1):75–8.

42. Tsujio T, Nakamura H, Terai H et al. Characteristic radiographic or magnetic resonance images of fresh osteoporotic vertebral fractures predicting potential risk for nonunion: A prospective multicenter study. *Spine (Phila Pa 1976)*. 2011;36(15):1229–35.

43. Nickell LT, Schucany WG, Opatowsky MJ. Kümmell disease. *Proc (Bayl Univ Med Cent)*. 2013;26(3):300–1.

44. Zhang GQ, Gao YZ, Chen SL, Ding S, Gao K, Wang HQ. Comparison of percutaneous vertebroplasty and percutaneous kyphoplasty for the management of Kümmell's disease: A retrospective study. *Indian J Orthop*. 2015;49(6):577–82.

45. Yang H, Gan M, Zou J, Mei X, Shen X, Wang G, Chen L. Kyphoplasty for the treatment of Kümmell's disease. *Orthopedics*. 2010;33(7):479.

46. Chen L, Dong R, Gu Y, Feng Y. Comparison between balloon kyphoplasty and short segmental fixation combined with vertebroplasty in the treatment of Kümmell's disease. Retrospective evaluation. *Pain Physician*. 2015;18:373–81.

47. Li KC, Wong TU, Kung FC, Li A, Hsieh CH. Staging of Kümmel's disease. *J Musculoskeletal Res*. 2004;8:43–55.

48. Mochida J, Toh E, Chiba M, Nishimura K. Treatment of osteoporotic late collapse of a vertebral body of thoracic and lumbar spine. *J Spinal Disord*. 2001;14(5):393–8.

49. Chen GD, Lu Q, Wang GL et al. Percutaneous kyphoplasty for Kümmell's disease with severe spinal canal stenosis retrospective study. *Pain Physician*. 2015;18:E1021–8.

50. Kim P, Kim SW. Balloon Kyphoplasty: An effective treatment for Kümmel disease? *Korean J Spine*. 2016;13(3):102–6.

51. Korovessis P, Hadjipavlou A, Repantis T. Minimal invasive short posterior instrumentation plus balloon kyphoplasty with calcium phosphate for burst and severe compression lumbar fractures. *Spine (Phila Pa 1976)*. 2008;33(6):658–67.

52. Chin DK, Kim YS, Cho YE, Shin JJ. Efficacy of postural reduction in osteoporotic vertebral compression fractures followed by percutaneous vertebroplasty. *Neurosurgery*. 2006;58(4):695–700.

53. McKiernan F, Faciszewski T, Jensen R. Latent mobility of osteoporotic vertebral compression fractures. *J Vasc Interv Radiol*. 2006;17(9):1479–87.

54. Malghem J, Maldague B, Labaisse MA et al. Intravertebral vacuum cleft: Changes in content after supine positioning. *Radiology*. 1993;187:483–7.

55. Yamato M, Nishimura G, Kuramochi E et al. MR appearance at different ages of osteoporotic compression fractures of the vertebrae. *Radiat Med*. 1998; 16(5):329–34.

56. Mayers SP, Wiener SN. Magnetic resonance imaging features of fractures using the short tau inversion recovery (STIR) sequence: Correlation with radiographic findings. *Sceletal Radiol.* 1991;20:499–501.

57. Qaiyum M, Tyrrell PN, McCall IW, Cassar-Pullicino VN. MRI detection of unsuspected vertebral injury in acute spinal trauma: Incidence and significance. *Skeletal Radiol.* 2001;30(6):299–304.

58. Kaufmann TJ, Jensen ME, Schweickert PA et al. Age of fracture and clinical outcomes of percutaneous vertebroplasty. *Am J Neuroradiol.* 2001;22:1860–3.

59. Brown DB, Glaiberman CB, Gilula LA, Shimony JS. Correlation between preprocedural MRI findings and clinical outcomes in the treatment of chronic symptomatic vertebral compression fractures with percutaneous vertebroplasty. *Am J Radiol.* 2005; 184(6):1951–5.

60. Carlier RY, Gordji H, Mompoint D et al. Osteoporotic vertebral collapse: Percutaneous vertebroplasty and local kyphosis correction. *Radiology.* 2004;233:891–8.

61. Do HM. Magnetic resonance imaging in the evaluation of patients for percutaneous vertebroplasty. *Top Magn Reson Imaging.* 2000;11:235–44.

62. Jensen ME, Evans AJ, Mathis JM et al. Percutaneous polymethylmethacrylate vertebroplasty in the treatment of osteoporotic vertebral body compression fractures: Technical aspects. *Am J Neuroradiol.* 1997; 18(10):1897–904.

63. Gangi A, Kastler BA, Dietemann JL. Percutaneous vertebroplasty guided by a combination of CT and fluoroscopy. *Am J Neuroradiol.* 1994;15:83–6.

64. Garfin SR, Yuan HA, Reiley MA. New technologies in spine: Kyphoplasty and vertebroplasty for treatment of painful osteoporotic fractures. *Spine.* 2001;26(14):1511–15.

65. Kyphon Balloon Kyphoplasty UC201502590aEE. © Medtronic Inc. 2015. All rights reserved. Printed in Europe.

66. Tzermiadianos MN, Zindrick MR, Patwardhan AG, Katonis PG, Hadjipavlou AG. The safety and effectiveness of percutaneous vertebroplasty and kyphoplasty in osteoporotic fractures and tumors. *WSJ.* 2007;2(2):64–94.

67. Chen D, An ZQ, Song S, Tang JF, Qin H. Percutaneous vertebroplasty compared with conservative treatment in patients with chronic painful osteoporotic spinal fractures. *J Clin Neurosci.* 2014;21(3):473–7.

68. Blasco J, Martinez-Ferrer A, Macho J et al. Effect of vertebroplasty on pain relief, quality of life, and the incidence of new vertebral fractures: A 12-month randomized follow-up, controlled trial. *J Bone Miner Res.* 2012;27(5):1159–66.

69. Farrokhi MR, Alibai E, Maghami Z. Randomized controlled trial of percutaneous vertebroplasty versus optimal medical management for the relief of pain and disability in acute osteoporotic vertebral compression fractures. *J Neurosurg Spine.* 2011;14(5):561–9.

70. Alvarez L, Alcaraz M, Pérez-Higueras A et al. Percutaneous vertebroplasty: Functional improvement in patients with osteoporotic compression fractures. *Spine (Phila Pa 1976).* 2006;31(10):1113–8.

71. Diamond TH, Bryant C, Browne L, Clark WA. Clinical outcomes after acute osteoporotic vertebral fractures: A 2-year non-randomised trial comparing percutaneous vertebroplasty with conservative therapy. *Med J Aust.* 2006;184(3):113–7.

72. Klazen CA, Lohle PN, de Vries J et al. Vertebroplasty versus conservative treatment in acute osteoporotic vertebral compression fractures (Vertos II): An open-label randomized trial. *Lancet.* 2010;376(9746):1085–92.

73. Rousing R, Andersen MO, Jespersen SM, Thomsen K, Lauritsen J. Percutaneous vertebroplasty compared to conservative treatment in patients with painful acute or subacute osteoporotic vertebral fractures: Three-month follow-up in a clinical randomized study. *Spine (Phila Pa 1976).* 2009;34(13):1349–54.

74. Rousing R, Hansen KL, Andersen MO, Jespersen SM, Thomsen K, Lauritsen JM. Twelve-month follow-up in forty-nine patients with acute/semiacute osteoporotic vertebral fractures treated conservatively or with percutaneous vertebroplasty: A clinical randomized study. *Spine (Phila Pa 1976).* 2010;35(5):478–82.

75. Voormolen MH, Mali WP, Lohle PN et al. Percutaneous vertebroplasty compared with optimal pain medication treatment: Short-term clinical outcome of patients with subacute or chronic painful osteoporotic vertebral compression fractures. The VERTOS study. *AJNR Am J Neuroradiol.* 2007;28(3):555–60.

76. Yang EZ, Xu JG, Huang GZ et al. Percutaneous vertebroplasty versus conservative treatment in aged patients with acute osteoporotic vertebral compression fractures: A prospective randomized controlled clinical study. *Spine (Phila Pa 1976).* 2016;41(8): 653–60.

77. Wardlaw D, Cummings SR, Van Meirhaeghe J et al. Efficacy and safety of balloon kyphoplasty compared with non-surgical care for vertebral compression fracture (FREE): A randomised controlled trial. *Lancet.* 2009;373(9668):1016–24.

78. Kasperk C, Hillmeier J, Nöldge G et al. Treatment of painful vertebral fractures by kyphoplasty in patients with primary osteoporosis: A prospective nonrandomized controlled study. *J Bone Miner Res.* 2005;20(4):604–12.

79. Kasperk C, Grafe IA, Schmitt S et al. Three-year outcomes after kyphoplasty in patients with osteoporosis with painful vertebral fractures. *J Vasc Interv Radiol.* 2010;21(5):701–9.

80. Boonen S, Van Meirhaeghe J, Bastian L et al. Balloon kyphoplasty for the treatment of acute vertebral compression fractures: 2-year results from a randomized trial. *J Bone Miner Res.* 2011;26(7):1627–37.

81. Grohs JG, Matzner M, Trieb K, Krepler P. Minimal invasive stabilization of osteoporotic vertebral fractures: A prospective nonrandomized comparison of vertebroplasty and balloon kyphoplasty. *J Spinal Disord Tech*. 2005;18(3):238–42.

82. Liu JT, Liao WJ, Tan WC et al. Balloon kyphoplasty versus vertebroplasty for treatment of osteoporotic vertebral compression fracture: A prospective, comparative, and randomized clinical study. *Osteoporos Int*. 2010;21(2):359–64.

83. Lovi A, Teli M, Ortolina A, Costa F, Fornari M, Brayda-Bruno M. Vertebroplasty and kyphoplasty: Complementary techniques for the treatment of painful osteoporotic vertebral compression fractures. A prospective non-randomised study on 154 patients. *Eur Spine J*. 2009;18(Suppl 1):95–101.

84. De Negri P, Tirri T, Paternoster G, Modano P. Treatment of painful osteoporotic or traumatic vertebral compression fractures by percutaneous vertebral augmentation procedures: A nonrandomized comparison between vertebroplasty and kyphoplasty. *Clin J Pain*. 2007;23(5):425–430.

85. Bae H, Shen M, Maurer P et al. Clinical experience using Cortoss for treating vertebral compression fractures with vertebroplasty and kyphoplasty: Twenty four-month follow-up. *Spine (Phila Pa 1976)*. 2010;35(20):E1030–6.

86. Kumar K, Nguyen R, Bishop S. A comparative analysis of the results of vertebroplasty and kyphoplasty in osteoporotic vertebral compression fractures. *Neurosurgery*. 2010;67(3 Suppl Operative):ons171–88; discussion ons188.

87. Röllinghoff M, Siewe J, Zarghooni K et al. Effectiveness, security and height restoration on fresh compression fractures—A comparative prospective study of vertebroplasty and kyphoplasty. *Minim Invasive Neurosurg*. 2009;52(5–6):233–7.

88. Santiago FR, Abela AP, Alvarez LG, Osuna RM, García Mdel M. Pain and functional outcome after vertebroplasty and kyphoplasty. A comparative study. *Eur J Radiol*. 2010;75(2):e108–13.

89. Schofer MD, Efe T, Timmesfeld N, Kortmann HR, Quante M. Comparison of kyphoplasty and vertebroplasty in the treatment of fresh vertebral compression fractures. *Arch Orthop Trauma Surg*. 2009;129(10):1391–9.

90. Dohm M, Black CM, Dacre A, Tillman JB, Fueredi G. KAVIAR investigators. A randomized trial comparing balloon kyphoplasty and vertebroplasty for vertebral compression fractures due to osteoporosis. *AJNR Am J Neuroradiol*. 2014;35(12):2227–36.

91. Omidi-Kashani F, Samini F, Hasankhani EG, Kachooei AR, Toosi KZ, Golhasani-Keshtan F. Does percutaneous kyphoplasty have better functional outcome than vertebroplasty in single level osteoporotic compression fractures? A comparative prospective study. *J Osteoporos*. 2013;2013:690329.

92. Muijs SPJ, Nieuwenhuijse MJ, van Erkel AR, Dijkstra PDS. Percutaneous vertebroplasty for the treatment of osteoporotic vertebral compression fractures: Evaluation after 36 months. *J Bone Joint Surg Br*. 2009;91(3):379–84.

93. Müller CW, Lange U, van Meirhaeghe J et al. An international multicenter randomized comparison of balloon kyphoplasty and nonsurgical care in patients with acute vertebral body compression fractures. *Eur Spine J*. 2007;16:1977.

94. Van Meirhaeghe J, Bastian L, Boonen S, Ranstam J, Tillman JB, Wardlaw D; FREE investigators. A randomized trial of balloon kyphoplasty and nonsurgical management for treating acute vertebral compression fractures: Vertebral body kyphosis correction and surgical parameters. *Spine (Phila Pa 1976)*. 2013;38(12):971–83.

95. Kim KH, Kuh SU, Chin DK et al. Kyphoplasty versus vertebroplasty: Restoration of vertebral body height and correction of kyphotic deformity with special attention to the shape of the fractured vertebrae. *J Spinal Disord Tech*. 2012;25(6):338–44.

96. Guo JB, Zhu Y, Chen BL et al. Surgical versus nonsurgical treatment for vertebral compression fracture with osteopenia: A systematic review and meta-analysis. *PLOS ONE*. 2015;10(5):e0127145.

97. Yuan WH, Hsu HC, Lai KL. Vertebroplasty and balloon kyphoplasty versus conservative treatment for osteoporotic vertebral compression fractures. *A Meta-Anal Med (Baltimore)*. 2016;95(31):e4491.

98. Papanastassiou ID, Phillips FM, Van Meirhaeghe J et al. Comparing effects of kyphoplasty, vertebroplasty, and non-surgical management in a systematic review of randomized and non-randomized controlled studies. *Eur Spine J*. 2012;21(9):1826–43.

99. Alvarez L, Perez-Higueras A, Granizo JJ et al. Predictors of outcomes of percutaneous vertebroplasty for osteoporotic vertebral fractures. *Spine*. 2004;30(1):87–92.

100. Brown DB, Gilula LA, Sehgal M, Shimony JS. Treatment of chronic symptomatic vertebral compression fractures with percutaneous vertebroplasty. *Am J Roentgenol*. 2004;182(2):319–322.

101. Garfin SR, Buckley RA, Ledlie J. Balloon Kyphoplasty Outcomes Group. Balloon kyphoplasty for symptomatic vertebral body compression fractures results in rapid, significant, and sustained improvements in back pain, function, and quality of life for elderly patients. *Spine*. 2006;31(19):2213–20.

102. Singh AK, Pilgram TK, Gilula LA. Osteoporotic compression fractures: Outcomes after single- versus multiple-level percutaneous vertebroplasty. *Radiology*. 2006;238(1):211–20.

103. Peh WC, Gelbart MS, Gilula LA, Peck DD. Percutaneous vertebroplasty: Treatment of painful vertebral compression fractures with intraosseous vacuum phenomena. *Am J Roentgenol*. 2003;180(5):1411–17.

104. Chen LH, Lai PL, Chen WJ. Unipedicle percutaneous vertebroplasty for spinal intraosseous vacuum cleft. *Clin Orthop Relat Res.* 2005;(435):148–53.

105. Krauss M, Hirschfelder H, Tomandl B et al. Kyphosis reduction and the rate of cement leaks after vertebroplasty of intravertebral clefts. *Eur Radiol.* 2006;16(5):1015–21.

106. Ha KY, Lee JS, Kim KW, Chon JS. Percutaneous vertebroplasty for vertebral compression fractures with and without intravertebral clefts. *JBJS Br.* 2006; 88B:629–633

107. McKiernan F, Faciszewski T, Jensen R. Does vertebral height restoration achieved at vertebroplasty matter? *J Vasc Interv Radiol.* 2005;16(7):973–9.

108. Phillips FM, Ho E, Campbell-Hupp M et al. Early radiographic and clinical results of balloon kyphoplasty for the treatment of osteoporotic vertebral compression fractures. *Spine.* 2003;28(19):2260–7.

109. Dudeney S, Lieberman IH, Reinhardt MK, Hussein M. Kyphoplasty in the treatment of osteolytic vertebral compression fractures as a result of multiple myeloma. *J Clin Oncol.* 2002;20(9):2382–7.

110. Majd ME, Farley S, Holt RT. Preliminary outcomes and efficacy of the first 360 consecutive kyphoplasties for the treatment of painful osteoporotic vertebral compression fractures. *Spine J.* 2005;5:244–55.

111. Theodorou DJ, Theodorou SJ, Duncan TD et al. Percutaneous balloon kyphoplasty for the correction of a spinal deformity in painful vertebral compression fractures. *J Clin Imaging.* 2002;26(1):1–5.

112. Lane JM, Hong R, Koob J et al. Kyphoplasty enhances function and structural alignment in multiple myeloma. *Clin Orthop.* 2004;(426):49–53.

113. Ledlie JT, Renfro MB. Kyphoplasty treatment of vertebral fractures: 2-year outcomes show sustained benefits. *Spine.* 2006;31(1):57–64.

114. Berlemann U, Franz T, Orler R, Heini PF. Kyphoplasty for treatment of osteoporotic vertebral fractures: A prospective non-randomized study. *Eur Spine J.* 2004;13(6):496–501.

115. Voggenreiter G. Balloon kyphoplasty is effective in deformity correction of osteoporotic vertebral compression fractures. *Spine.* 2005;30(24):2806–12.

116. Feltes C, Fountas KN, Machinis T et al. Immediate and early postoperative pain relief after kyphoplasty without significant Volume 2: Issue 2 90 restoration of vertebral body height in acute osteoporotic vertebral fractures. *Neurosurg Focu.* 2005;18(3):e5.

117. Deen HG, Aranda-Michel J, Reimer R, Putzke JD. Preliminary results of balloon kyphoplasty for vertebral compression fractures in organ transplant recipients. *Neurosurg Focus.* 2005;18(3):e6.

118. Pradhan BB, Bae HW, Kropf MA et al. Kyphoplasty reduction of osteoporotic vertebral compression fractures: Correction of local kyphosis versus overall sagittal alignment. *Spine.* 2006;31(4):435–41.

119. McKiernan F, Jensen R, Faciszewski T. Dynamic mobility of vertebral compression fractures. *J Bone Min Res.* 2003;18(1):24–9.

120. Lee ST, Chen JF. Closed reduction vertebroplasty for the treatment of osteoporotic vertebral compression fractures. Technical note. *J Neurosurg.* 2004;100(4 Suppl):392–6.

121. Hiwatashi A, Moritani T, Numaguchi Y, Westesson PL. Increase in vertebral body height after vertebroplasty. *Am J Neuroradiol.* 2003;24(2):185–9.

122. Dublin AB, Hartman J, Latchaw RE et al. The vertebral body fracture in osteoporosis: Restoration of height using percutaneous vertebroplasty. *Am J Neuroradiol.* 2005;26(3):489–92.

123. Teng MM, Wei CJ, Wei LC et al. Kyphosis correction and height restoration effects of percutaneous vertebroplasty. *Am J Neuroradiol.* 2003;24(9):1893–900.

124. Shindle MK, Gardner MJ, Koob J et al. Vertebral height restoration in osteoporotic compression fractures: Kyphoplasty balloon tamp is superior to postural correction alone. *Osteoporos Int.* 2006;17(12):1815–9.

125. Heini PF, Orler R. Kyphoplasty for treatment of osteoporotic vertebral fractures. *Eur Spine J.* 2004;13(3):184–92.

126. Boszczyk BM, Bierschneider M, Schmid K et al. Microsurgical interlaminary vertebro- and kyphoplasty for severe osteoporotic fractures. *J Neurosurg.* 2004;100(Suppl Spine):32–7.

127. Nakano M, Hirano N, Matsuura K et al. Percutaneous transpedicular vertebroplasty with calcium phosphate cement in the treatment of osteoporotic vertebral compression and burst fractures. *J Neurosurg.* 2002;97:287–93.

128. Nakano M, Hirano N, Ishihara H et al. Calcium phosphate cement-based vertebroplasty compared with conservative treatment for osteoporotic compression fractures: A match case-control study. *J Neurosurg Spine.* 2006;4:110–17.

129. Korovessis P, Repantis T, Petsinis G, Iliopoulos P, Hadjipavlou A. Direct reduction of thoracolumbar burst fractures by means of balloon kyphoplasty with calcium phosphate and stabilization with pedicle-screw instrumentation and fusion. *Spine (Phila Pa 1976).* 2008;33(4):E100–8.

130. Katonis P, Hadjipavlou A, Souvatzis X, Tzermiadianos M, Alpantaki K, Simmons JW. Respiratory effects, hemodynamic changes and cement leakage during multilevel cement balloon kyphoplasty. *Eur Spine J.* 2012;21(9):1860–6.

131. Pongchaiyakul C, Nguyen ND, Jones G et al. Asymptomatic vertebral deformity as a major risk factor for subsequent fractures and mortality: A long-term prospective study. *J Bone Miner Res.* 2005;20(8):1349–55.

132. Kallmes DF, Schweickert PA, Marx WF, Jensen ME. Vertebroplasty in the mid- and upper thoracic spine. *Am J Neuroradiol.* 2002;23(7):1117–20.

133. Hodler J, Peck D, Gilula LA. Midterm outcome after vertebroplasty: Predictive value of technical and patient-related factors. *Radiology.* 2003;227(3):662–8.

134. Voormolen MH, Lohle PN, Juttmann JR et al. The risk of new osteoporotic vertebral compression fractures in the year after percutaneous vertebroplasty. *J Vasc Interv Radiol.* 2006;17(1):71–6.

135. Diamond TH, Champion B, Clark WA. Management of acute osteoporotic vertebral fractures: A nonrandomized trial comparing percutaneous vertebroplasty with conservative therapy. *Am J Med.* 2003;114(4):257–65.

136. Nussbaum DA, Gailloud P, Murphy K. A review of complications associated with vertebroplasty and kyphoplasty as reported to the food and drug administration medical device related web site. *J Vasc Interv Radiol.* 2004;15:1185–92.

137. FDA Center for Devices and Radiological Health, Online MAUDE Database. *Clinical Trial Considerations: Vertebral Augmentation Devices to Treat Spinal Insufficiency Fractures - Guidance for Industry and FDA Staff.* Available from: https://www.fda.gov/media/71103/download

138. Barragan-Campos HM, Vallee JN, Lo D et al. Percutaneous vertebroplasty for spinal metastases: Complications. *Radiology.* 2006;238(1):354–62.

139. Bernhard J, Heini PF, Villiger PM. Asymptomatic diffuse pulmonary embolism caused by acrylic cement: An unusual complication of percutaneous vertebroplasty. *Ann Rheum Dis.* 2003;62(1):85–86.

140. Biafora SJ, Mardjetko SM, Butler JP et al. Arterial injury following percutaneous vertebral augmentation: A case report. *Spine.* 2006;31(3):E84–7.

141. Deramond H, Depriester C, Galibert P, Le Gars D. Percutaneous vertebroplasty with polymethylmethacrylate: Technique, indications, and results. *Radiol Clin North Am.* 1998;36:533–46.

142. Yu SW, Chen WJ, Lin WC et al. Serious pyogenic spondylitis following vertebroplasty: A case report. *Spine.* 2004;29(10): E209–11.

143. Walker DH, Mummaneni P, Rodts GE Jr. Infected vertebroplasty. Report of two cases and review of the literature. *Neurosurg Focus.* 2004;17(6):E6.

144. Schmid KE, Boszczyk BM, Bierschneider M et al. Spondylitis following vertebroplasty: A case report. *Eur Spine J.* 2005;14(9):895–9.

145. Vats HS, McKiernan FE. Infected vertebroplasty: Case report and review of literature. *Spine.* 2006;31(22):E859–62.

146. Alfonso Olmos M, Silva Gonzalez A, Duart Clemente J, Villas Tome C. Infected vertebroplasty due to uncommon bacteria solved surgically: A rare and threatening life complication of a common procedure: Report of a case and a review of the literature. *Spine.* 2006;31(20):E770–3.

147. Soyuncu Y, Ozdemir H, Soyuncu S et al. Posterior spinal epidural abscess: An unusual complication of vertebroplasty. *Joint Bone Spine.* 2006;73(6):753–5. (Epub ahead of print)

148. Abdelrahman H, Siam AE, Shawky A, Ezzati A, Boehm H. Infection after vertebroplasty or kyphoplasty. A series of nine cases and review of literature. *Spine J.* 2013;13(12):1809–17.

149. Kim HJ, Shin DA, Cho KG, Chung SS. Late onset tuberculous spondylitis following kyphoplasty: A case report and review of the literature. *Korean J Spine.* 2012;9(1):28–31.

150. Ha KY, Kim KW, Kim YH, Oh IS, Park SW. Revision surgery after vertebroplasty or kyphoplasty. *Clin Orthop Surg.* 2010;2(4):203–8.

151. Teng MM, Cheng H, Ho DM, Chang CY. Intraspinal leakage of bone cement after vertebroplasty: A report of 3 cases. *AJNR Am J Neuroradiol.* 2006;27(1):224–9.

152. Layton KF, Thielen KR, Koch CA et al. Vertebroplasty, first 1000 levels of a single center: Evaluation of the outcomes and complications. *AJNR Am J Neuroradiol.* 2007;28(4):683–9.

153. Cotten A, Dewatre F, Cortet B et al. Percutaneous vertebroplasty for osteolytic metastases and myeloma: Effects of the percentage of lesion filling and the leakage of methyl methacrylate at clinical follow-up. *Radiology.* 1996;200(2):525–30.

154. Grados F, Depriester C, Cayrolle G et al. Long-term observations of vertebral osteoporotic fractures treated by percutaneous vertebroplasty. *Rheumatology.* 2000;39:1410–14.

155. Weill A, Chiras J, Simon JM et al. Spinal metastases: Indications for and results of percutaneous injection of acrylic surgical cement. *Radiology.* 1996;199(1):241–7.

156. Evans AJ, Jensen ME, Kip KE et al. Vertebral compression fractures: Pain reduction and improvement in functional mobility after percutaneous polymethylmethacrylate vertebroplasty. Retrospective report of 245 cases. *Radiology.* 2003;226(2):366–72.

157. Jang JS, Kim DY, Lee SH. Efficacy of percutaneous vertebroplasty in the treatment of intravertebral pseudarthrosis associated with noninfected avascular necrosis of the vertebral body. *Spine.* 2003;28(14):1588–92.

158. Heini PF, Walchli B, Berlemann U. Percutaneous transpedicular vertebroplasty with PMMA: Operative technique and early results. A prospective study for the treatment of osteoporotic compression fractures. *Eur Spine J.* 2000;9(5):445–50.

159. Ryu KS, Park CK, Kim MC, Kang JK. Dose-dependent epidural leakage of olymethylmethacrylate after percutaneous vertebroplasty in patients with osteoporotic vertebral compression fractures. *J Neurosurg Spine.* 2002;96(1):56–61.

160. Yeom JS, Kim WJ, Choy WS et al. Leakage of cement in percutaneous vertebroplasty for painful osteoporotic compression fractures. *J Bone Joint Surg Br.* 2003;85B:83–9.

161. Tsai TT, Chen WJ, Lai PL et al. Polymethylmethacrylate cement dislodgment following percutaneous vertebroplasty: A case report. *Spine.* 2003;28(22):E457–60.

162. Heini PF, Dain Allred C. The use of a side-opening injection cannula in vertebroplasty: A technical note. *Spine.* 2002;27(1):105–9.

163. Lee B, Lee S, Yoo T. Paraplegia as a complication of percutaneous vertebroplasty with PMMA. *Spine.* 2002;27:E419–22.

164. Röder C, Boszczyk B, Perler G, Aghayev E, Külling F, Maestretti G. Cement volume is the most important modifiable predictor for pain relief in BKP: Results from SWISS spine, a nationwide registry. *Eur Spine J.* 2013;22(10):2241–8.

165. Liebschner MA, Rosenberg WS, Keaveny TM. Effects of bone cement volume and distribution on vertebral stiffness after vertebroplasty. *Spine (Phila Pa 1976)*. 2001;26(14):1547–54.

166. Boszczyk B. Volume matters: A review of procedural details of two randomized controlled vertebroplasty trials of 2009. *Eur Spine J*. 2010;19(11):1837–40.

167. Nieuwenhuijse MJ, Bollen L, van Erkel AR, Dijkstra PD. Optimal intravertebral cement volume in percutaneous vertebroplasty for painful osteoporotic vertebral compression fractures. *Spine (Phila Pa 1976)*. 2012;37(20):1747–55.

168. Greene DL, Isaac R, Neuwirth M, Bitan FD. The eggshell technique for prevention of cement leakage during kyphoplasty. *J Spinal Disord Tech*. 2007;20: 229–32.

169. Bohner M, Gasser B, Baroud G, Heini P. Theoretical and experimental model to describe the injection of a polymethylmethacrylate cement into a porous structure. *Biomaterials*. 2003;24:2721–30.

170. Phillips FM, Todd Wetzel F, Lieberman I, Campbell-Hupp M. An *in vivo* comparison of the potential for the extravertebral cement leak after vertebroplasty and kyphoplasty. *Spine*. 2002;27:2173–8.

171. Belkoff SM, Mathis JM, Fenton DC et al. An *ex vivo* biomechanical evaluation of an inflatable bone tamp used in the treatment of compression fracture. *Spine*. 2001;26:151–6.

172. Groen RJ, Toit DF, Phillips FM et al. Anatomical and pathological considerations in percutaneous vertebroplasty and kyphoplasty: A reappraisal of the vertebral venous system. *Spine (Phila Pa 1976)*. 2004;29(13):1465–71.

173. Krueger A, Bliemel C, Zettl R, Ruchholtz S. Management of pulmonary cement embolism after percutaneous vertebroplasty and kyphoplasty: A systematic review of the literature. *Eur Spine J*. 2009;18(9): 1257–65.

174. Tozzi P, Abdelmoumene Y, Corno AF et al. Management of pulmonary embolism during acrylic vertebroplasty. *Ann Thor Surg*. 2002;7:1706–8.

175. Francois K, Taeymans Y, Poffyn B, Van Nooten G. Successful management of large pulmonary cement embolus after percutaneous vertebroplasty: A case report. *Spine*. 2003;28(20):E424–5.

176. Park JH, Choo SJ, Park SW. Images in cardiovascular medicine. Acute pericarditis caused by acrylic bone cement after percutaneous vertebroplasty. *Circulation*. 2005;111(6):e98.

177. Stricker K, Orler R, Yen K et al. Severe hypercapnia due to pulmonary embolism of polymethylmethacrylate during vertebroplasty. *Anesth Analg*. 2004;98(4):1184–6.

178. Yoo KY, Jeong SW, Yoon W, Lee J. Acute respiratory distress syndrome associated with pulmonary cement embolism following percutaneous vertebroplasty with polymethylmethacrylate. *Spine*. 2004;29(14): E294–7.

179. Monticelli F, Meyer HJ, Tutsch-Bauer E. Fatal pulmonary cement embolism following percutaneous vertebroplasty (PVP). *Forensic Sci Int*. 2005;149(1): 35–8.

180. Chen HL, Wong CS, Ho ST et al. A lethal pulmonary embolism during percutaneous vertebroplasty. *Anesth Analg*. 2002;95(4):1060–2.

181. Syed MI, Jan S, Patel NA et al. Fatal fat embolism after vertebroplasty: Identification of the high-risk patient. *Am J Neuroradiol*. 2006;27(2):343–5.

182. Coumans JV, Reinhardt MK, Lieberman IH. Kyphoplasty for vertebral compression fractures: 1-year clinical outcomes from a prospective study. *J Neursurg Spine*. 2003;99:44–50

183. Audat ZA, Alfawareh MD, Darwish FT, Alomari AA. Intracardiac leakage of cement during kyphoplasty and vertebroplasty: A case report. *Am J Case Rep*. 2016;17:326–30.

184. Kim MN, Jung JS, Kim SW, Kim YH, Park SM, Shim WJ. A sword-like foreign body lodged in the ventricular septum: A rare complication of percutaneous vertebroplasty. *Eur Heart J*. 2010;31(8):1006.

185. Grifka RG, Tapio J, Lee KJ. Transcatheter retrieval of an embolized methylmethacrylate glue fragment adherent to the right atrium using bidirectional snares. *Catheter Cardiovasc Interv*. 2013;81(4):648–50.

186. Scroop R, Eskridge J, Britz GW. Paradoxical cerebral artery embolization of cement during intraoperative vertebroplasty: A case report. *Am J Neuroradiol*. 2002;23:868–70.

187. Chung SE, Lee SH, Kim TH, Yoo KH, Jo BJ. Renal cement embolism during percutaneous vertebroplasty. *Eur Spine*. 2006;15(Suppl 17):590–4.

188. Krebs J, Aebli N, Goss BG, Wilson K, Williams R, Ferguson SJ. Cardiovascular changes after pulmonary cement embolism: An experimental study in sheep. *AJNR Am J Neuroradiol*. 2007;28(6):1046–50.

189. Aebli N, Krebs J, Davis G, Walton M, Williams MJ, Theis JC. Fat embolism and acute hypotension during vertebroplasty: An experimental study in sheep. *Spine (Phila Pa 1976)*. 2002;27(5):460–6.

190. Krebs J, Aebli N, Goss BG et al. Cardiovascular changes after pulmonary embolism from injecting calcium phosphate cement. *Biomed Mater Res B Appl Biomater*. 2007;82(2):526–32.

191. Aebli N, Krebs J, Schwenke D, Davis G, Theis JC. Pressurization of vertebral bodies during vertebroplasty causes cardiovascular complications: An experimental study in sheep. *Spine (Phila Pa 1976)*. 2003;28(14):1513–20.

192. Theron J, Moret J. *Spinal Phlebography. Lumbar and Cervical Techniques*. Berlin, Germany: Springer-Verlag, 1978.

193. Vogelsang H. *Intraosseous Spinal Venography*. Amsterdam: Excerpta Medica, 1970.

194. Souvatzis X, Alpantaki K, Hadjipavlou AR et al. Re: Tran I, Gerckens U, Remig J et al. First report of a life-threatening cardiac complication after

percutaneous balloon kyphoplasty. Spine (Phila Pa 1976). 2013;38:E316–8. *Spine (Phila Pa 1976).* 2013;38(19):1709.

195. Harrington KD. Major neurological complications following percutaneous vertebroplasty with PMMA. *J Bone Joint Surg.* 2001;83-A(7):1070–3.

196. Chen YJ, Tan TS, Chen WE et al. Intradural cement leakage. A devastating rare complication of vertebroplasty. *Spine.* 2006;31(2) E379–82.

197. Schmidt R, Cakir B, Mattes T et al. Cement leakage during vertebroplasty: An underestimated problem? *Eur Spine J.* 2005;14:466–73.

198. Perez-Higueras A, Alvarez L, Rossi R et al. Percutaneous vertebroplasty: Long-term clinical and radiological outcome. *Neuroradiology.* 2002;44(11): 950–4.

199. Hillmeier J, Grafe I, Da Fonseca K et al. (The evaluation of balloon kyphoplasty for osteoporotic vertebral fractures. An interdisciplinary concept). *Orthopade.* 2004;33(8):893–904.

200. Patel AA, Vaccaro AR, Martyak GG et al. Neurologic deficit following percutaneous vertebral stabilization. *Spine (Phila Pa 1976).* 2007;32(16):1728–34.

201. Legroux-Gerot I, Lormeau C, Boutry N et al. Long-term follow-up of vertebral osteoporotic fractures treated by percutaneous vertebroplasty. *Clin Rheumatol.* 2004;23:310–7.

202. Uppin A, Hirsch J, Centenera L et al. Occurrence of new vertebral fracture after percutaneous vertebroplasty in patients with osteoporosis. *Radiology.* 2003;226(1):119–24.

203. Kim SH, Kang HS, Choi JA, Ahn JM. Risk factors of new compression fractures in adjacent vertebrae after percutaneous vertebroplasty. *Acta Radiol.* 2004;45(4):440–5.

204. Trout AT, Kallmes DF, Kaufmann TJ. New fractures after vertebroplasty: Adjacent fractures occur significantly sooner. *Am J Neuroradiol.* 2006;27(1): 217–23.

205. Fribourg D, Tang C, Sra P, Delamarter R, Bae H. Incidence of subsequent vertebral fracture after kyphoplasty. *Spine.* 2004;29(20):2270–7.

206. Robinson Y, Tschöke SK, Stahel PF, Kayser R, Heyde CE. Complications and safety aspects of kyphoplasty for osteoporotic vertebral fractures: A prospective follow-up study in 102 consecutive patients. *Patient Saf Surg.* 2008;2:2.

207. Berlemann U, Ferguson SJ, Nolte LP, Heini PF. Adjacent vertebral failure after vertebroplasty. *J Bone Joint Surg B.* 2002;84(5):748–52.

208. Borse MS. Cost utility analysis of balloon kyphoplasty and vertebroplasty in the treatment of vertebral compression fractures in the United States (2013). *Theses and Dissertations.* Paper 33.

209. Lin EP, Ekholm S, Hiwatashi A, Westesson PL. Vertebroplasty: Cement leakage into the disc increases the risk of new fracture of adjacent vertebral body. *Am J Neuroradiol.* 2004;25:175–80.

210. Yang S, Liu Y, Yang H, Zou J. Risk factors and correlation of secondary adjacent vertebral compression fracture in percutaneous kyphoplasty. *Int J Surg.* 2016;36(Pt A):138–42.

211. Wu J, Guan Y, Fan S. Analysis of risk factors of secondary adjacent vertebral fracture after percutaneous kyphoplasty. *Biomed Res.* 2017;28(5):1956–61.

212. Harrop JS, Prpa B, Reinhardt MK, Lieberman I. Primary and secondary osteoporosis' incidence of subsequent vertebral compression fractures after kyphoplasty. *Spine (Phila Pa 1976).* 2004;29(19):2120–5.

213. Mukherjee S, Lee Y-P. Current concepts in the management of vertebral compression fractures. *Oper Techn Orthop.* 2011;21(3):251–60.

214. Gaitanis IN, Carandang G, Phillips FM et al. Restoring geometric and loading alignment of the thoracic spine with a vertebral compression fracture: Effects of balloon (bone tamp) inflation and spinal extension. *Spine J.* 2005;5(1):45–54.

215. Zhang H, Xu C, Zhang T, Gao Z, Zhang T. Does Percutaneous vertebroplasty or balloon kyphoplasty for osteoporotic vertebral compression fractures increase the incidence of new vertebral fractures? A *Meta-Analysis Pain Physician.* 2017;20(1):E13–28.

216. Boszczyk BM, Bierschneider M, Panzer S et al. Fluoroscopic radiation exposure of the kyphoplasty patient. *Eur Spine J.* 2006;15(3):347–55.

217. Mroz TE, Yamashita T, Davros WJ, Lieberman IH. Radiation exposure to the surgeon and the patient during kyphoplasty. *Spinal Disord Tech.* 2008;21(2):96–100.

218. Fabricant PD, Berkes MB, Dy CJ, Bogner EA. Diagnostic medical imaging radiation exposure and risk of development of solid and hematologic malignancy. *Orthopedics.* 2012;35(5):415–20.

219. Synowitz M, Kiwit J. Surgeon's radiation exposure during percutaneous vertebroplasty. *J Neurosurg Spine.* 2006;4(2):106–9.

220. Goodman BS, Carnel CT, Mallempati S, Agarwal P. Reduction in average fluoroscopic exposure times for interventional spinal procedures through the use of pulsed and low-dose image settings. *Am J Phys Med Rehabil.* 2011;90(11):908–12.

221. Boszcayk BM, Bierschneider M, Panzer S et al. Fluoroscopic radiation exposure of the kyphoplasty patient. *Eur Spine J.* 2006;15(3):347–55.

222. Perisinakis K, Damilakis J, Theocharopoulos N, Papadokostakis G, Hadjipavlou A, Gourtsoyiannis N. Patient exposure and associated radiation risks from fluoroscopically guided vertebroplasty or kyphoplasty. *Radiology.* 2004;232(3):701–7.

223. *National Council on Radiation Protection and Measurements.* Ionizing Radiation Exposure of the Population of the United States, NCRP Report 160, Bethesda, MD; 2009.

224. Borgström F, Beall DP, Berven S et al. Health economic aspects of vertebral augmentation procedures. *Osteoporos Int.* 2015;26(4):1239–49.

225. McCullough BJ, Comstock BA, Deyo RA, Kreuter W, Jarvik JG. Major medical outcomes with spinal augmentation vs conservative therapy. *JAMA Intern Med.* 2013;173(16):1514–21.

226. Hillmeier J, Meeder PJ, Nöldge G et al. Minimal invasive Reposition und innere Stabilisierung osteoporotischer Wirbelkörperfrakturen (Ballonikyphoplastie). In: *Operative Orthopädie und Traumatologie.* 2003;15:343–62.

227. Fisher A. *Percutaneous Vertebroplasty: A Bone Cement Procedure for Spinal Pain Relief.* Ottawa: Canadian Coordinating Office for Health Technology Assessment (CCOHTA), 2002. Available from: http://www.ccohta.ca

228. Wong CC, McGirt MJ. Vertebral compression fractures: A review of current management and multimodal therapy. *J Multidiscip Healthc.* 2013;6:205–14.

229. Cooper C, Atkinson EJ, Jacobsen SJ, O'Fallon WM, Melton LJ 3rd. Population-based study of survival after osteoporotic fractures. *Am J Epidemiol.* 1993;137(9):1001–5.

230. Edidin AA, Ong KL, Lau E, Schmier JK, Kemner JE, Kurtz SM. Cost-effectiveness analysis of treatments for vertebral compression fractures. *Appl Health Econ Health Policy.* 2012;10(4):273–84.

231. McGirt MJ, Parker SL, Wolinsky JP, Witham TF, Bydon A, Gokaslan ZL. Vertebroplasty and kyphoplasty for the treatment of vertebral compression fractures: An evidenced-based review of the literature. *Spine J.* 2009;9(6):501–8.

232. Klezl Z, Bhangoo N, Phillips J, Swamy G, Calthorpe D, Bommireddy R. Social implications of balloon kyphoplasty: Prospective study from a single UK centre. *Eur Spine J.* 2012;21(9):1880–6.

233. Laratta JL, Shillingford JN, Lombardi JM, Mueller JD, Reddy H, Saifi C, Fischer CR, Ludwig SC, Lenke LG, Lehman RA. Utilization of vertebroplasty and kyphoplasty procedures throughout the United States over a recent decade: An analysis of the Nationwide Inpatient Sample. *J Spine Surg.* 2017; Sep3(3):364–70 doi: 10.21037/jss.2017.08.02PMCID: PMC5637187 PMID: 29057344.

31

Osteoporotic thoracolumbar fractures
My preferred method of nonoperative treatment

TERENCE ONG and OPINDER SAHOTA

INTRODUCTION

Symptomatic vertebral fragility fractures are predominantly managed nonoperatively. With advancing age, loss of bone density in the cortex and trabeculae of the vertebra occurs mostly in the anterior, middle, and superior portions of the vertebra (1). In the event of either a low-trauma injury or repetitive compression loading, these fractures affect this particular area of the vertebra. Therefore, vertebral fragility fractures, of which osteoporosis is the most prevalent underlying cause, are usually stable without involvement of the posterior vertebral arch. This means that injury to the spinal cord is uncommon, and these fractures can be managed conservatively.

The goals of vertebral fragility fracture management are to control pain, encourage early mobilization, limit disability, and restore function. In the longer term, the aim is to reduce the risk of future vertebral fractures and prevent irreversible spinal deformity (kyphosis). Unfortunately, pain and disability can persist months after the fracture (2,3). The chronic pain at this stage is no longer just due to the fracture but would now include a combination of the bony injury, kyphosis, muscle spasm, and facet arthropathy. Hence, treatment of these fractures need a multicomponent approach involving pharmacologic and nonpharmacologic approaches covering the acute and potentially chronic symptomatic stage of the fracture. In this chapter, we discuss the nonoperative treatment options available to date for the management of vertebral fragility fractures due to osteoporosis.

OPIOID AND NONOPIOID ANALGESIA

High-quality clinical trials of pain medication use and its effectiveness in this particular cohort are limited. In practice, paracetamol (acetaminophen) and nonsteroidal anti-inflammatory drugs (NSAIDs) are the first analgesics of choice. The inflammatory process that occurs at the periosteum and fracture site contributes to the pain, and NSAIDs are hypothesized to have a role in addressing this. However, this same inflammatory process has been recognized to be crucial in fracture healing, and recent studies have reported an association between NSAID use and fracture nonunion (4). This has led to a number of clinicians becoming cautious on its use in patients with acute fractures. To date, high-quality clinical trials on this is lacking, and pooled analysis of a small number of existing higher-quality studies has not reported on the risk of nonunion (4). It is also uncertain if the risk of nonunion is dependent on the type of bone fractured, as different rates of nonunion have been reported in long bones and vertebral bones (4). Further studies are clearly needed to fully address this particular area of uncertainty. NSAIDs also have to be used with caution due to the risk of gastrointestinal bleeding, kidney injury, and cardiovascular risk. This is even more of a concern in the older population, and any use of NSAIDs has to be for the shortest possible duration.

Stronger analgesia such as opioids are usually indicated, especially in the acute stages of the fracture, to provide pain relief and aid mobilization. Oral and topical opioids have demonstrated effectiveness in reducing pain at rest and on movement due to acute vertebral fractures (5,6). Being able to get on top of the pain was associated with improved participation in physical therapy and better reported quality of life (6). However, opioids have significant side effects such as cardiorespiratory depression, gastrointestinal disturbance, cognitive impairment, and increased risk of falls (7). As vertebral fragility fractures are more prevalent in older people, they are also most susceptible to these adverse effects. Use of opioids needs to be balanced between its potential benefits and risk (8). The duration the opioid is prescribed also needs to be considered and exposure to it must be kept to the least possible time frame. The effectiveness of opioids in improving pain and disability has not robustly been demonstrated in chronic low back pain due to vertebral fractures (9). This is unsurprising as chronic pain, unlike acute pain, has an unpredictable and nonlinear trajectory that is complicated by the patient's mood, perception of pain, experience, circumstances, and fear (10). Increasing or decreasing opioid doses has not shown to correlate with changes in pain scores (11). Hence, there are dangers in increasing opioid doses in the pursuit of improving chronic pain including overuse and dependency and the associated untoward adverse effects (10).

Paravertebral muscle spasms can occur as a consequence of vertebral fractures. This may benefit from muscle relaxants to break the cycle of pain and muscle spasm (7). Again, their potential benefit needs to be balanced with the likely side effects that such a class of medication can bring, e.g., drowsiness and long-term dependency. Besides that, pain can also occur due to the fracture compressing the nerve root. The radicular pain may need specific pharmacologic pain relief such as tricyclic antidepressants, anticonvulsants, or neuropathic pain analgesics, e.g., gabapentin or pregabalin (12).

OSTEOPOROSIS MEDICATION

The ability to use osteoporosis medication to provide pain relief is an attractive option as this group of medication is able to improve bone mineral density and reduce future fracture risk at the same time. Besides that, use of these medications may reduce the opioid burden and the risk of adverse effects among this particular cohort. A number of osteoporosis medications have been studied to evaluate their analgesic effects. Here we present data on the most studied osteoporosis medication used in the context of managing pain in the event of a vertebral fracture.

Calcitonin

Calcitonin is a 32 amino acid peptide that is produced by the C cells of the thyroid gland (13). It acts on the bone by inhibiting osteoclast activity to decrease bone resorption. Calcitonin is indicated for the prevention of acute bone loss due to sudden immobilization, treatment of Paget disease, and treatment of hypercalcemia of malignancy. A number of trials have studied the analgesic effect of intranasal, intramuscular, and subcutaneous calcitonin. However, the exact mechanism of how calcitonin provides pain relief has not been conclusively demonstrated (14). In animal models, the injection of salmon calcitonin into the intracerebroventricular area reduced pain, which points toward a central mode of action. Its mechanism of action has also been demonstrated to not depend on opioid receptors. The analgesic effect of calcitonin in these studies was seen as early as within 20 minutes of injection (14). Animal studies have also reported on the anti-inflammatory properties of calcitonin by demonstrating suppression of edema, inhibition of prostaglandin and thromboxane synthesis, and reduction in histamine-induced vascular leakage (15–17).

Compared to placebo, calcitonin improved pain both at rest and on movement in patients presenting with a history of back pain in the last 2–4 weeks due to a vertebral fracture (18). Patients were able to be mobilized much earlier (19,20), and there was also a reduction in the use of other systemic analgesia (19–22). This improvement was seen within the first week of administration (18,23). Depending on the route of administration, the effective daily doses used in clinical trials were 200 IU intranasally, 200 IU via the rectal route, and 100 IU intramuscularly and subcutaneously given over a period ranging from 2 to 4 weeks (18). There is no consensus on the most effective method of administration, as clinical trials comparing the different routes have reported different results (14). The reduction in pain was not as consistently demonstrated in patients with chronic pain where symptoms have persisted for more than 3 months (18). Common side effects associated with calcitonin include gastrointestinal disturbance, flushing, headache, and musculoskeletal pain. However, it was well tolerated in clinical trials where similar numbers of withdrawals were reported when it was compared to a placebo group (18). To date, there has not been any clinical trial that has compared calcitonin with conventional analgesia, which is still the treatment option in vertebral fracture management.

Concerns about calcitonin have been raised in relation to its associated increased risk of cancer (24). Meta-analysis of this association has reported a possible small increased risk of developing cancer in recipients of calcitonin delivered by nasal spray compared to placebo in clinical trials (24). Although basal cell carcinoma was the most frequently reported cancer, different cancers have been reported in scientific literature (24). However, in postmarketing data, the U.S. Food and Drug Administration did not identify any significant association on this (24). To date, there has also not been any experimental data to establish the oncogenic properties of calcitonin (24). In light of this, regulatory authorities such as the UK Medicines and Healthcare products Regulatory Agency have withdrawn nasal salmon calcitonin, and calcitonin in general is no longer recommended for the treatment of osteoporosis in the guidance provided by the European Medicines Agency. Other forms of calcitonin are still available and if used should be for the shortest time possible.

Bisphosphonate

Bisphosphonates are the most prescribed drugs to treat osteoporosis (25). They are also widely used to treat pain arising from metastatic cancer involving the skeletal sites and bone pain from Paget disease. Similar to calcitonin, the exact analgesic mechanism of bisphosphonate is unclear. Bisphosphonates work by inhibiting osteoclast activity and resorption of bone (26). It also has anti-interleukin (IL)-1, IL-6, and anti-tumor necrosis factor alpha (anti-TNF-α) properties that dampen the inflammatory process (26,27). Hence, it is hypothesized that the reduction in osteoclast activity, i.e., the rate of osteolysis, and local anti-inflammatory effect result in pain relief (27). Besides that, the analgesic response seen in animal models after intracerebroventricular injection of clodronate also points toward a central nociceptive effect (27). Not all bisphosphonates have demonstrated the same degree of pain relief, as trials in animal studies reported varying degrees of pain-relieving response with different bisphosphonates (27,28).

However, there have been concerns regarding giving bisphosphonates during the period of the acute fracture. Osteoclastic resorption is an important component of bone remodeling after a fracture, and the theoretical possibility of bisphosphonates delaying fracture healing has been proposed (29–31). However, in animal models, although remodeling was affected by the introduction of bisphosphonates, it did not translate into delayed formation of the fracture callus (32). Clinical trials to date have not demonstrated an increased risk of delayed fracture healing with bisphosphonates administered within 2 weeks of an acute fracture (33–35).

The analgesic effects of bisphosphonates have been reported with both intravenous and oral bisphosphonates. Many of these trials have been either nonrandomized, open-labeled, observational, or limited to a small number of study participants. Intravenous pamidronate has been the most studied, and its therapeutic effects were first reported in an observational study of 26 patients with vertebral fragility fractures related to back pain for at least 2 months (36). These patients were given 30 mg pamidronate over 2 consecutive days, and repeated every 3 months for 1 year, reported pain relief and improved mobility within 48 hours of the first treatment (36). The analgesic effect of pamidronate was further supported by a case series of five patients who were prescribed 15 mg daily for 3 days where a significant reduction in pain and ability to mobilize was seen as early as day 3 (37). A subsequent randomized double-blind controlled clinical trial of 32 patients comparing 30 mg pamidronate given daily for 3 consecutive days and a placebo infusion demonstrated at least a 50% reduction in pain at days 7 and 30 (26). Fever and transient myalgia were reported infrequently in those receiving pamidronate (26,36).

Other intravenous bisphosphonates have also reported analgesic benefits. Clodronate administered in a dose of 300 mg daily for 5 days for 2 weeks to patients with acute vertebral fractures with pain for less than 1 week has shown a reduction in pain, with the benefits seen up to 30 days postadministration (39,40). The clinical trials involving zoledronate, alendronate, and risedronate also demonstrated improvement in pain after treatment was initiated. However, it recruited participants with osteoporosis where a significant proportion of them had vertebral fractures (41–43). An annual infusion of 15 mg zoledronate administered to women with postmenopausal osteoporosis where 63% of them had vertebral fractures demonstrated that the incidence of back pain and days of limited activity were less in the zoledronate group (43): 18 and 11 fewer days of back pain and days of limited activity, respectively, were reported (43). There were also less days of bed rest in the event of a vertebral fracture (43). The oral bisphosphonates risedronate and alendronate have also demonstrated improvement in back pain (41,42).

Overall, the fact that improvement in pain was reported within a short period of initiation of the bisphosphonates, especially pamidronate and clodronate, reaffirms a mechanism of action other than pain reduction by reducing subsequent vertebral fractures. In studies where there was longer-term follow-up, reduction in back pain was independent of incident fracture (43).

Teriparatide

Teriparatide is a recombinant human N-terminal fragment of parathyroid hormone (rhPTH 1–34) (44). It is a bone anabolic agent used in osteoporosis to increase bone density, mass, and strength (44). The pivotal randomized controlled trial of teriparatide in fracture prevention reported less participants with new or worsening back pain in the intervention group compared to placebo (45). Since then, two multicenter observational studies of teriparatide have shown a reduction in back pain and severity of back pain during 18–24 months of treatment (44,46). This was also associated with less days in bed, limitation of activities, and analgesic requirement (44,46). This improvement was seen within 3 months of initiating treatment (44,46). As these were observational studies, it is challenging to say with certainty if the pain would have improved without teriparatide.

A meta-analysis of randomized trials of teriparatide compared to placebo or another osteoporosis drug (alendronate or hormone replacement therapy) in reducing back pain reported that the pooled teriparatide group had a lower rate of back pain compared to the pooled comparator group (47). The teriparatide group was 27% less likely to develop back pain and 61% less likely to have severe back pain (47).

There is no evidence that teriparatide has direct analgesic effect, and its benefit in back pain reduction may be related to its potential to stabilize the fracture and the microdamage within it, promote fracture healing, and reduce further vertebral fractures (47). When patients with vertebral fractures were prescribed teriparatide, risedronate (an oral bisphosphonate), or no medication, the percentage of vertebral collapse and change in kyphotic angle was less in the teriparatide group at 8 and 12 weeks after treatment initiation (48). This lower rate of back pain was seen even after discontinuation of teriparatide up to 30 months posttreatment (44,47). This reduction in back pain was also seen to accompany a reduction in subsequent vertebral fractures (44), which again points toward its action of fracture stabilization and preventing further fractures, as opposed to a direct analgesic effect. Teriparatide appears to be well tolerated with about 80% completing the prescribed course (44,46,49).

MINIMALLY INVASIVE PROCEDURES

Pain from vertebral fragility fractures can persist and be difficult to manage, at times leading to high doses of analgesia, opioids in particular. Increasing systemic analgesia doses are associated with adverse effects, especially in vulnerable groups of patients such as older multimorbid persons. Hence, minimally invasive procedures could potentially provide an alternative to increasing doses of analgesia.

In patients with degeneration of the facet joint, sustaining an acute vertebral fracture could lead to mechanical loading and compression of the joint resulting in pain. Besides that, subluxation of facet joints and periosteal irritation due to the altered spinal biomechanics post fracture can be painful (50). Diagnosing facet joint arthropathy pain can be difficult, as there are no distinguishing clinical features from other sources of back pain. Imaging of the spine is not entirely helpful and is usually done to exclude other pathology, e.g., skeletal malignancy, and correlation between symptoms and degeneration detected radiologically is poor (51). Injecting local anesthetic or steroid under fluoroscopic guidance to the facet joint (52,53) or to the nerves adjacent to the joint space, called the medial branch (54,55), has been shown to provide pain relief in a selected group patients with vertebral fractures. Most of these studies focused on patients with chronic back pain where symptoms have persisted for at least 3 months, and magnetic resonance imaging (MRI) of the spine has not been diagnostic of an acute vertebral fracture (52,54,55). An observational study of patients with acute vertebral fracture reported that a third of patients referred for percutaneous vertebroplasty no longer required it after fluoroscopic facet joint injection (53).

Gray ramus communicans nerve block is another minimally invasive procedure that has demonstrated a role in managing symptoms in patients with chronic back pain due to their vertebral fractures. The gray ramus nerve was observed to course around the midvertebral body and into the anterior intervertebral disc (56,57). This provides sensory input for painful vertebral fractures (56). A number of small observational studies have reported pain reduction postprocedure in patients with chronic vertebral fracture pain (56–58). Radicular pain can also feature as a consequence of a vertebral fragility fracture. Nerve root injections, similar to the other minimally invasive procedures described so far, also involve injecting local anesthetic and/or steroid under fluoroscopic guidance to the nerve root at the level of the affected vertebra. In this particular cohort, it has also demonstrated improvement in pain, although over half needed repeated injections over the course of a year (59,60).

Although these procedures offer an alternative to conservative treatment, there are technical and operative challenges that will determine the success of such interventions. At this point in time, there is still a lack of robust clinical evidence with studies so far restricted to observational studies with a small number of participants. Hence, there is a need for high-quality clinical trials before advocating its use in routine clinical care.

ELECTROTHERAPY MODALITIES

Electrotherapy has been advocated by some researchers as a potential treatment option in relieving pain in those with vertebral fractures. One study reported that capacitively coupled electric field (CCEF) improved pain, reduced the need for analgesia, and also improved quality of life scores in older women with multiple vertebral fractures of at least 6 months' duration (61). Although the exact underlying mechanism is unclear, this particular technique of inducing an electrical field may increase new bone formation by upregulating osteoblast function (61). This is supported by *in vitro* studies that demonstrate it was able to accelerate bone cell proliferation and differentiation and enhance synthesis of cells, leading to promoted matrix formation and maturation (62), which points toward a role in promoting fracture healing. However, the scientific literature presenting clinical studies in accelerating fracture healing in long bone fractures is still restricted to small-scale randomized and nonrandomized studies, and further evidence is clearly required before implementation in clinical practice (63,64). Another treatment option utilized interferential therapy, and horizontal therapy reported improvement in pain scores after 2 weeks of treatment, with the analgesic effects lasting after that for another 12 weeks (65). However, the evidence behind such treatment modalities, and therapies such as laser therapy, therapeutic ultrasound, and transcutaneous electrical nerve stimulation are still lacking. Therefore, it has been neither widely adopted in clinical practice nor formed as part of vertebral fracture care guidelines.

EXTERNAL SUPPORT DEVICES

External support devices, i.e., orthosis or braces, have been used to stabilize the spine that has sustained a fracture. The majority of studies that have evaluated its effectiveness were done in acute traumatic burst fractures (66). Hence, spinal stabilization with such devices is routinely employed in nonoperative and postoperative management of traumatic fractures. These devices aim to maintain neutral spinal alignment, limit flexion to reduce axial loading on the fractured vertebra, prevent further kyphotic collapse, and facilitate mobilization (66,67). They also encourage hyperextension and biofeedback of spinal alignment (68,69). Besides that, supporting the spine allows for less fatigue of the paraspinal muscles and provides relief from muscle spasms (7,66). However, as described earlier, vertebral fragility fractures due to osteoporosis, especially the ones without neurological involvement, are relatively stable fractures, as they usually involve the anterior column of the vertebra (67). Hence, extrapolating data and findings from support devices in traumatic fractures to a vertebral fragility fracture cohort where the underlying cause is likely osteoporosis may not be ideal.

A number of orthoses made from different materials with differing mechanisms of action are available and have been evaluated in vertebral fractures. Orthotic devices can be grouped into either rigid supports (thoracolumbosacral orthosis, plaster corset), semirigid supports (Spinomed, Spinomed Active), and flexible supports (soft brace). Only the rigid and semirigid orthoses have been studied in vertebral fragility fracture management. The current practice appears to point toward rigid supports such as thoracolumbosacral orthosis used in the acute stage, and the semirigid supports in the postacute phase (70). However, none of these orthoses have been studied under standardized conditions; studies to date use different devices and have very different trial methods, outcome measures, and metrics used (71,72). Most of these studies were conducted in an outpatient or community setting in patients with chronic back pain. There does appear to be general improvement in back extensor strength (68,73,74) and kyphotic angle (73–75). However, this has not conclusively translated into improvement in pain, postural stability, or improved quality of life and well-being (71,72).

In an acute vertebral fragility fracture setting, a randomized trial of patients presenting to medical attention within 3 days of their injury were allocated into either a rigid, soft brace or no brace (67). The group without a brace was no worse in terms of pain and disability compared to the group prescribed an orthosis (67). Another study with a relatively younger cohort with stable thoracolumbar fractures demonstrated no difference in developing neurological complications whether patients were using an orthosis or not (76).

Compliance with wearing such devices can be challenging, as the devices can be uncomfortable when worn for long periods of time. Prolonged bracing may lead to deconditioning and atrophy of the trunk and paraspinal muscles. There is also the risk of skin breakdown in the older frail patient. Too restrictive a brace may impede lung function (70). Hence, some clinicians have advocated that orthosis should be discontinued as soon as the pain subsides (77).

EXERCISE AND REHABILITATION

Once pain from the acute fracture is manageable, it is important for the patient to start mobilizing with a formal rehabilitation exercise program (7). Prolonged bed rest is associated with bone density reduction and increased bone turnover (78), which may worsen bone fragility, expose the patient to the adverse effects of physical inactivity (79), and possibly lead to the development of pressure sores. The goals of rehabilitation are prevention of falls and subsequent fractures, reduction of kyphosis, enhanced axial muscle strength, and correct spinal alignment to improve posture. However, there is no consensus on what to include or how best to deliver this form of rehabilitation exercise program. Trials so far have been limited to small randomized studies of varied interventional programs delivered in the community to generally less-frail patients with vertebral fragility fracture (80). Programs varied in duration from 10 weeks to 2 years and were delivered in either the participants' home or as part of group exercise. Exercise programs ranged from ones that focused only on back strengthening exercises, to programs incorporating manual spinal mobilization and postural taping, to multi-component exercise programs, and they had varying levels of supervision (77,81–87). Findings have not been consistent, with no conclusive reduction in pain, improvement in markers of quality of life, and improvement in levels of disability (80,88,89). However, there was a clear increase in muscle strength as part of the prescribed exercise programs (80).

Pain from vertebral fragility fractures can eventually lead to abnormal flexion of the spine to compensate for the discomfort. The overuse of spinal flexors will further aggravate the kyphotic spine. This overall imbalance between the use of back extensors and flexors will worsen the pain already present from the bony injury, subsequently leading to chronic pain. The degree of kyphosis has also been associated with increasing risk of vertebral fractures (90). Therefore, exercise programs focused on strengthening the spinal extensor muscles and correcting posture with the aim of reducing the degree of kyphosis to relieve pressure on the anterior aspect of the vertebral body has been recommended (77). The extensor muscles are considered the main supportive muscles of the spine, and in an erect posture, they resist the effects of gravity (77). A study comparing participants allocated to spinal extension, flexion, or extension and flexion programs reported statistically significant less vertebral fractures in the spinal extension group, where the focus is on strengthening the spinal erector muscles (91). Therefore, rehabilitation exercise programs for vertebral fragility fractures have incorporated this into their prescribed programs.

As no overall consensus can be sought from current scientific literature, expert opinion has recommended that patients with vertebral fragility fractures participate in a multicomponent exercise program that includes resistance training and balance training (92). It needs to be progressive, structured, and frequent enough (2 days a week for resistance training, and 15–20 minutes a day of balance training), with a component specifically targeted at the muscles responsible for maintaining posture, e.g., spinal extensor muscles (92). Resistance training has a more potent impact on bone density (93). Resistance training and weight-bearing exercise decrease the rate of bone loss, although not significantly enough to be measured on bone densitometry assessment (89). Exercises also need to be individualized to the patients' ability (66). Aerobic exercise, although not specific to osteoporosis or vertebral fractures, is recommended as part of improving overall health status (92). The biggest challenge with any exercise rehabilitation program is maintaining compliance, which has been reported to range from 50% to 80% (84–86,94). As the most significant gains in muscle strength appear to be in the first

3 months with fewer gains after that, short-term intensive exercises with good compliance is favored over longer-term programs (77).

The rehabilitation program also needs to include elements aimed at falls prevention. Two-thirds of vertebral fragility fractures that are admitted to hospital present with a fall (95). An older person presenting with a fall is two-thirds more likely to fall again in the subsequent year, with half of those who fall at risk of sustaining an injury (96). Those with a kyphotic spine as a consequence of multiple vertebral fractures are even more at risk of falls. A structured exercise program has robustly demonstrated improvement in muscle strength and balance and fall prevention (97). Hence, an effective falls prevention program as part of rehabilitation after a fracture is crucial in reducing the risk of further injury and fractures.

Besides exercises aimed at reducing falls, an effective falls prevention program needs to have a multifactorial falls risk assessment with a multicomponent intervention targeted at it (98). This includes assessment of vision, cognition, neurological problems, continence, cardiovascular issues, medication, and environmental risks. Patients also need to be educated regarding their condition, osteoporosis; their management plan; ways to avoid pain in activities of daily living and mobility; and the importance of maintaining spinal biomechanics and posture (12,92).

SECONDARY PREVENTION

Sustaining a vertebral fragility fracture increases the risk of another vertebral fracture fourfold and any other fracture twofold (99). Therefore, effective secondary prevention is needed to minimize this risk. With each subsequent fracture, there tends to be an associated increase in morbidity (100). An effective exercise program to reduce the risk of falls and fractures will minimize this risk. Other nonpharmacologic strategies to improve bone mineral density and minimize future fracture risk include stopping smoking and excessive consumption of alcohol; maintaining a well-balanced diet that is rich in calcium and vitamin D; ensuring adequate sunlight exposure; and promoting regular exercise with a focus on exercises that promote weight-bearing (101).

There are robust data that have reported effective fracture risk reduction and improvement in bone mineral density with pharmacologic osteoporosis treatment (102). In recent years, both alendronate and risedronate, the oral bisphosphonates, have become the two most prescribed treatments for osteoporosis (25). Both reduce the risk of a subsequent vertebral and nonvertebral fracture. The annual intravenous zoledronate and 6-monthly denosumab subcutaneous injections are parenteral antiresorptive options that are also clinically effective in fracture risk reduction and provide an option where gastrointestinal side effects and compliance or adherence are an issue. The daily anabolic agent, teriparatide, which offers a different fracture reduction mechanism, is licensed for up to 2 years and has demonstrated effective fracture reduction.

However, persistence with oral bisphosphonates is poor and can be as low as 30% at 1 year, and even less 3 and 5 years later (25,104). Although not as well-studied as the oral treatments, patients on parenteral treatments for osteoporosis appear to have better compliance, with over 80% of those prescribed denosumab and teriparatide persisting with treatment at 1 year and throughout the whole treatment duration, respectively (49,105). The poor persistence with osteoporosis medication has been shown to be associated with an increased risk of further fractures and hospitalization (107,108). This emphasizes the importance of ensuring treatment for osteoporosis as an effective means of preventing a subsequent fracture.

Therefore, effective secondary prevention needs to include an effective system of ensuring compliance and persistence with treatment. Regular follow-ups have been shown to improve compliance (109). Any issues around medication compliance can be addressed during any of these follow-ups, and a switch to a parenteral option may be more appropriate. Just like any other chronic disease management, the monitoring of osteoporosis and the patient's treatment helps determine whether persistent treatment is appropriate. Caution has been raised with long-term bisphosphonates and atypical fractures of the femur and bisphosphonate-induced osteonecrosis of the jaw. Although the incidences of these complications are low, unnecessary exposure to bisphosphonates needs to be avoided. Therefore, it is recommended that treatment be reviewed every 3–5 years (106).

COMORBID MANAGEMENT

Vertebral fragility fractures are more prevalent in older people, and accompanying their fracture is their underlying comorbid burden and frailty (3,103). On top of all of this, there may be prevailing cognitive impairment, sensory impairment, and limited physiologic reserve, which will not only affect how they respond to treatment but also make them vulnerable to the adverse effects of their treatment. Medication for pain relief could potentially interact with existing medication causing further problems. Their rehabilitation postfracture will also need to be personalized with their own rehabilitation goals.

Therefore, management of their fracture needs to also include management of their fracture symptoms, optimizing comorbid conditions, rehabilitation, and falls and fracture risk reduction. The heterogenous presentation of an older person with a vertebral fracture means that treatment needs to be individualized and directed to his or her specific health needs. Hence, a multidisciplinary approach incorporating a comprehensive geriatric assessment may have a role in this cohort of patients (3,38).

CONCLUSION AND RECOMMENDATIONS

Vertebral fragility fractures are mostly managed nonoperatively. The aim of treatment is to control pain, encourage early mobilization, limit disability, and restore function. To achieve this, opioids and nonopioids are needed, with adjunct treatment to address muscle spasms, facet arthropathy pain, or nerve root pain. Individualizing treatment is required. A multidisciplinary rehabilitation exercise program is needed to aid recovery. Exercises prescribed need to include aspects of restrictive and balance training that are structured and progressive. In the longer term, the aim is to reduce the risk of future vertebral and nonvertebral fractures with nonpharmacologic and pharmacologic strategies. Nonpharmacologic approaches need to include effective multicomponent falls prevention strategies. All pharmacologic treatment for osteoporosis has demonstrated future fracture risk reduction. Therefore, regular review of the condition and treatment is crucial to ensure compliance and persistence.

REFERENCES

1. Adam MA, Dolan P. Biomechanics of vertebral compression fractures and clinical application. *Arch Orthop Trauma Surg.* 2011;131(12):1703–10.
2. Suzuki N, Ogikubo O, Hansson T. The course of the acute vertebral body fragility fracture: Its effect on pain, disability and quality of life during 12 months. *Eur Spine J.* 2007;17(10):1380–90.
3. Ong T, Sahota O, Gladman JRF. The Nottingham Spinal Health (NoSH) Study: A cohort study of patients hospitalised with vertebral fragility fractures. *Osteoporos Int.* 2019. https://doi.org/10.1007/s00198-019-05198-x
4. Dodwell ER, Latorre JG, Parisini E et al. NSAID exposure and risk of nonunion: A meta-analysis of case-control and cohort studies. *Calcif Tissue Int.* 2010;87(3):193–302.
5. Vorsanger GJ, Farrell, J, Xiang J, Chow W, Moskovitz BL, Rosenthal NR. Tapentadol, oxycodone or placebo for acute pain of vertebral compression fractures: A randomized phase IIIb study. *Pain Manag.* 2013; 3(2):109–18.
6. Ringe JD, Faber H, Bock O et al. Transdermal fentanyl for the treatment of back pain caused by vertebral osteoporosis. *Rheumatol Int.* 2002;22(5):199–203.
7. Longo UG, Loppini M, Denaro L, Maffulli N, Denaro V. Osteoporotic vertebral fractures: Current concepts of conservative care. *Br Med Bull.* 2012;102:171–89.
8. Cherasse A, Muller G, Ornetti P, Piroth C, Tavernier C, Maillefert JF. Tolerability of opioids in patients with acute pain due to non-malignant musculoskeletal disease. A hospital-based observational study. *Joint Bone Spine.* 2004;71(6):572–6.
9. Deyo RA, Von Korff M, Duhrkoop D. Opioids for low back pain. *BMJ.* 2015;350:g6380.
10. Ballantyne JC, Kalso E, Stannard C. WHO analgesic ladder: A good concept gone astray. *BMJ.* 2016;352:i20.
11. Chen L, Vo T, Seefeld L et al. Lack of correlation between opioid dose adjustment and pain score change in a group of chronic pain patients. *J Pain.* 2013;14(4):384–92.
12. Prather H, Hunt D, Watson JO, Gilula LA. Conservative care for patients with osteoporotic vertebral compression fractures. *Phys Med Rehabil Clin N Am.* 2007;18(3):577–91.
13. Eastell R. Treatment of postmenopausal osteoporosis. *N Engl J Med.* 1998;338(11):736–46.
14. Silverman SL, Azria M. The analgesic role of calcitonin following osteoporotic fracture. *Osteoporos Int.* 2002;13(11):858–67.
15. Abdullahi SE, Bastiani GD, Nogarin L, Velo GP. Effect of calcitonin on carrageenan foot oedema. *Agents Actions.* 1975;5(4):371–3.
16. Ceserani R, Colombo M, Olgiati VR, Pecile A. Calcitonin and prostaglandin system. *Life Sci.* 1979;25(21):1851–5.
17. Strettle RJ, Bates RFL, Buckley GA. Evidence for a direct anti-inflammatory action of calcitonin: Inhibition of histamine-induced mouse pinnal oedema by porcine calcitonin. *J Pharm Pharmacol.* 1980;32(1):192–5.
18. Knopp-Sihota JA, Newburn-Cook CV, Homik J, Cummings GG, Voaklander D. Calcitonin for treating acute and chronic pain of recent and remote osteoporotic vertebral compression fractures: A systematic review and meta-analysis. *Osteoporos Int.* 2012;23(1):17–38.
19. Lyritis GP, Tsakalakos N, Magiasis B, Krachalios T, Yiatzides A, Tsekoura M. Analgesic effect of salmon calcitonin in osteoporotic vertebral fractures: A double-blind placebo-controlled clinical study. *Calcif Tissue Int.* 1991;49(6):369–72.
20. Lyritis GP, Paspati I, Karachalios T, Ioakimidis D, Skarantavos G, Lyritis PG. Pain relief from nasal salmon calcitonin in osteoporotic vertebral crush fractures. A double blind, placebo-controlled clinical study. *Acta Orthop Scand Suppl.* 1997;275: 112–4.
21. Pun KK, Chan LWL. Analgesic effect of intranasal salmon calcitonin in the treatment of osteoporotic vertebral fractures. *Clin Ther.* 1989;11(2):205–9.
22. Lyritis GP, Ionnidis GV, Karachalios T et al. Analgesic effect of salmon calcitonin suppositories in patients with acute pain due to recent osteoporotic vertebral crush fractures: A prospective double-blind, randomized, placebo controlled clinical study. *Clin J Pain.* 1999;15(4):284–9.
23. Blau LA, Hoehns JD. Analgesic efficacy of calcitonin for vertebral fracture pain. *Ann Pharmacother.* 2003;37(4):564–70.
24. Wells G, Chernoff J, Gilligan JP, Krause DS. Does salmon calcitonin cause cancer? A review and meta-analysis. *Osteoporos Int.* 2016;27(1):13–9.
25. Li L, Roddam A, Gitlin M et al. Persistence with osteoporosis medications among postmenopausal women in the UK General Practice Research Database. *Menopause.* 2012;19(1): 33–40.

26. Armingeat T, Brondino R, Pham T, Legre V, Laafforgue P. Intravenous pamidronate for pain relief in recent osteoporotic vertebral compression fracture: A randomized double-blind controlled study. *Osteoporos Int.* 2016;17(11):1659–65.

27. Bonabello A, Galmozzi MR, Bruzzese T, Zara GP. Analgesic effect of bisphosphonates in mice. *Pain.* 2001;91(3):269–75.

28. Kim S, Seiryu M, Okada S et al. Analgesic effects of the non-nitrogen-containing bisphosphonates etidronate and clodronate, independent of anti-resorptive effects on bone. *Eur J Pharmacol.* 2013;699: 14–22.

29. Goldhahn J, Feron JM, Kanis J et al. Implications for fracture healing of current and new osteoporosis treatments: An ESCEO consensus paper. *Calcif Tissue Int.* 2013;90(5):343–53.

30. Ng AJ, Yue B, Joseph S, Richardson M. Delayed/nonunion of upper limb fractures with bisphosphonates: Systematic review and recommendations. *ANZ J Surg.* 2014;84(4):218–24.

31. Molvik H, Khan W. Bisphosphonates and their influence on fracture healing: A systematic review. *Osteoporos Int.* 2015;26(4):1251–60.

32. Kates SL, Ackert-Bicknell CL. How do bisphosphonates affect fracture healing? *Injury.* 2016;47(Suppl 1):S65–8.

33. Colon-Emeric C, Nordsletten L, Olson S et al. Association between timing of zoledronic acid infusion and hip fracture healing. *Osteoporos Int.* 2011;22(8):2329–36.

34. Kim TY, Ha YC, Kang BJ, Lee YK, Koo KH. Does early administration of bisphosphonate affect fracture healing in patients with intertrochanteric fractures? *J Bone Joint Surg Br.* 2012;94(7):956–60.

35. Li YT, Cai HF, Zhang ZL. Timing of the initiation of bisphosphonates after surgery for fracture healing: A systematic review and meta-analysis of randomized controlled trials. *Osteoporos Int.* 2015;26(2):431–41.

36. Gangji V, Appelboom T. Analgesic effect of intravenous pamidronate on chronic back pain due to osteoporotic vertebral fractures. *Clin Rheumatol.* 1999;18(3):266–7.

37. Abdulla A. Use of pamidronate for acute pain relief following osteoporotic vertebral fractures. *Rheumatology.* 2007;39:567–8.

38. Kammerlander C, Zegg M, Schmid R, Gosch M, Luger TJ, Blauth M. Fragility fractures requiring special consideration. Vertebral fractures. *Clin Geriatr Med.* 2014;30:361–72.

39. Rovetta G, Monteforte P, Balestra V. Intravenous clodronate for acute pain induced by osteoporotic vertebral fracture. *Drugs Exptl Clin Res.* 2000;26(1):25–30.

40. Rovetta G, Maggiani G, Molfetta L, Monteforte P. One-month follow up of patients treated by intravenous clodronate for acute pain induced by osteoporotic vertebral fracture. *Drugs Exptl Clin Res.* 2001;27(2):77–81.

41. Nevitt MC, Thompson DE, Black DM et al. Effect of alendronate on limited activity days and bed disability days caused by back pain in postmenopausal women with existing vertebral fractures. *Arch Intern Med.* 2000;160(1):77–85.

42. Majima T, Shimatsu A, Komatsu Y et al. Effect of risedronate or alfacalcidol on bone mineral density, bone turnover, back pain, and fractures in Japanese men with primary osteoporosis: Results of a two-year struct observational study. *J Bone Miner Metab.* 2009;27(2):168–74.

43. Cauley JA, Black D, Boonen S et al. Once-yearly zoledronic acid and days of disability, bed rest, and back pain: Randomized, controlled HORIZON Pivotal Fracture Trial. *J Bone Miner Res.* 2011;26(5):984–92.

44. Fahrleitner-Pammer A, Langdahl B, Marin F et al. Fracture rate and back pain during and after discontinuation of teriparatide: 36-month data from the European Forsteo Observational Study (EFOS). *Osteoporos Int.* 2011;22(10):2709–19.

45. Neer RM, Arnaud CD, Zanchetta JR et al. Effect of parathyroid hormone (1–34) on fractures and bone mineral density in postmenopausal women with osteoporosis. *N Engl J Med.* 2001;344(19):1434–41.

46. Langdahl BL, Ljunggren O, Benhamou CL et al. Fracture rate, quality of life and back pain in patients with osteoporosis treated with teriparatide: 24-month results from the Extended Forsteo Observational Study (ExFOS). *Calcif Tissue Int.* 2016;99(3):259–71.

47. Nevitt MC, Chen P, Kiel DP et al. Reduction in the risk of developing back pain persists at least 30 months after discontinuation of teriparatide treatment: A meta-analysis. *Osteoporos Int.* 2006;17(2):1630–7.

48. Tsuchie H, Miyakoshi N, Kasukawa Y et al. The effect of teriparatide to alleviate pain and to prevent vertebral collapse after fresh osteoporotic vertebral fracture. *J Bone Miner Metab.* 2016;34(1):86–91.

49. Thorsteinsson AL, Vestergaard P, Eiken P. Compliance and persistence with treatment with parathyroid hormone for osteoporosis. A Danish national register-based cohort study. *Arch Osteoporos.* 2015;10:35.

50. Bogduk N, MacVicar J, Borowczyk J. The pain of vertebral compression fractures can arise in the posterior elements. *Pain Med.* 2010;11(11):1666–73.

51. Eno JJT, Boone CR, Bellino MJ, Bishop JA. The prevalence of sacroiliac joint degeneration in asymptomatic adults. *J Bone Joint Surg Am.* 2015;97(11):932–6.

52. Mitra R, Do H, Alamin T, Cheng I. Facet pain in thoracic compression fractures. *Pain Med.* 2010;11(11):1674–7.

53. Wilson DJ, Owen S, Corkill RA. Facet joint injections as a means of reducing the need for vertebroplasty in insufficiency fractures of the spine. *Eur Radiol.* 2011;21(8):1772–8.

54. Park KD, Jee H, Nam HS et al. Effect of medial branch block in chronic facet joint pain for osteoporotic compression fracture: One year retrospective study. *Ann Rehabil Med.* 2013;37(2):191–201.

55. Lee HS, Park SB, Lee SH, Chung YS, Yang HJ, Son YJ. The effect of medial branch block for low back pain in elderly patients. *Nerve*. 2015;1(1):15–9.

56. Chandler G, Dalley G, Hemmer Jr J, Seely T. Gray ramus communicans nerve block: Novel treatment approach for painful osteoporotic vertebral compression fracture. *South Med J*. 2001;94(4):387–93.

57. Tae HS, Kim SD, Park JY, Kim SH, Lim DJ, Suh K. Gray ramus communicans nerve block: A useful therapeutic adjuvant for painful osteoporotic vertebral compression fracture. *J Korean Neurosurg Soc*. 2003;34(6):505–8.

58. Kim SW, Ju CI, Lee SM, Shin H. Radiofrequency neurotomy of the gray ramus communicans for lumbar osteoporotic compression fracture. *J Korean Neurosurg Soci*. 2007;41(1):7–10.

59. Kim DJ, Yun YH, Wang JM. Nerve-root injections for the relief of pain in patients with osteoporotic vertebral fractures. *J Bone Joint Surg Br*. 2005;85(2):250–3.

60. Ohtori S, Yamashita M, Inoue G et al. L2 spinal nerve-block effects on acute low back pain from osteoporotic vertebral fracture. *J Pain*. 2009;10(8):870–5.

61. Rossini M, Viapiana O, Gatti D, de Terlizzi F, Adami S. Capacitively coupled electric field for pain relief in patients with vertebral fractures and chronic pain. *Clin Orthop Relat Res*. 2010;468(3):735–40.

62. Hartig M, Joos U, Wiesmann HP. Capacitively coupled electric fields accelerate proliferation of osteoblast-like primary cells and increase bone extracellular matrix formation *in vitro*. *Eur Biophys J*. 2000;29(7):499–506.

63. Griffin XL, Warner F, Costa M. The role of electro-magnetic stimulation in the management of established non-union of long bone fractures: What is the evidence? *Injury*. 2008;39(4):419–29.

64. Griffin XL, Costa ML, Parsons N, Smith N. Electromagnetic field stimulation for treating delayed union or non-union of long bone fractures in adults. *Cochrane Database Syst Rev*. 2011;13(4):CD008471.

65. Zambito A, Bianchini D, Gatti D, Rossini M, Adami S, Viapiana O. Interferential and horizontal therapies in chronic low back pain due to multiple vertebral fractures: A randomized, double blind, clinical study. *Osteoporos Int*. 2007;18(11):1541–5.

66. Wong CC, McGirt MJ. Vertebral compression fractures: A review of current management and multimodal therapy. *J Multidiscip Healthc*. 2013;6:205–14.

67. Kim HJ, Yi JM, Cho HG et al. Comparative study of the treatment outcomes of osteoporotic compression fractures without neurologic injury using a rigid brace, a soft brace, and no brace. *J Bone Joint Surg Am*. 2014;96(23):1959–66.

68. Valentin GH, Pedersen LN, Maribo T. Wearing an active spinal orthosis improves back extensor strength in women with osteoporotic vertebral fractures. *Prosthet Orthot Int*. 2014;38(3):232–8.

69. Dionyssiotis Y, Trovas G, Thoma S, Lyritis G, Papaioannou N. Prospective study of spinal orthoses in women. *Prosthet Orthot Int*. 2015;39(6):487–95.

70. Li M, Law SW, Cheng J, Kee HM, Wong MS. A comparison study on the efficacy of Spinomed and soft lumbar orthosis for osteoporotic vertebral fracture. *Prosthet Orthot Int*. 2015;39(4):270–6.

71. Goodwin VA, Hall AJ, Rogers E, Bethel A. Orthotics and taping in the management of vertebral fractures in people with osteoporosis: A systematic review. *BMJ Open*. 2016;6:e010657.

72. Newman M, Lowe CM, Barker K. Spinal orthoses for vertebral osteoporosis and osteoporotic vertebral fracture: A systematic review. *Arch Phys Med Rehabil*. 2016;97(6):1013–25.

73. Pfeifer M, Begerow B, Minne HW. Effects of a new spinal orthosis on posture, trunk strength and quality of life in women with postmenopausal osteoporosis. *Am J Phys Med Rehabil*. 2004;83(3):177–86.

74. Pfeifer M, Kohlwey L, Begerow B, Minne HW. Effects of two newly developed spinal orthoses on trunk muscle strength, posture, and quality-of-life in women with postmenopausal osteoporosis. A randomized trial. *Am J Phys Med Rehabil*. 2011;90(10):805–15.

75. Grejg AM, Bennell KL, Briggs AM, Hodges PW. Postural taping decreases thoracic kyphosis but does not influence trunk muscle electromyographic activity or balance in women with osteoporosis. *Man Ther*. 2008;13(3):249–57.

76. Ohana N, Sheinis D, Rah E, Sasson A, Atar D. Is there a need for lumbar orthosis in mild compression fractures of the thoracolumbar spine? A retrospective study comparing the radiographic results between early ambulation with and without lumbar orthosis. *J Spinal Disord*. 2000;13(4):305–8.

77. Sinaki M. Critical appraisal of physical rehabilitation measures after osteoporotic vertebral fracture. *Osteoporos Int*. 2003;14(9):773–9.

78. Zerwekh JE, Ruml LA, Gottschalk F, Pak CYC. The effects of twelve weeks of bed rest on bone histology, biochemical markers of bone turnover, and calcium homeostasis in eleven normal subjects. *J Bone Miner Res*. 1998;13(10):1594–601.

79. Inouye SK, Wagner DR, Acampora D et al. A predictive index for functional decline in hospitalized elderly medical patients. *J Gen Intern Med*. 1993;8(12):645–52.

80. Dusdal K, Grundmanis J, Luttin K et al. Effects of therapeutic exercise for persons with osteoporotic vertebral fractures: A systematic review. *Osteoporos Int*. 2011;22(3):755–69.

81. Malmros B, Mortensen L, Jensen MB, Charles P. Positive effects of physiotherapy on chronic pain and performance in osteoporosis. *Osteoporos Int*. 1998;8(3):215–21.

82. Gold DT, Shipp KM, Pieper CF, Duncan PW, Martinez S, Lyles KW. Group treatment improves trunk strength and psychological status in older women with vertebral fractures: Results of a randomized, clinical trial. *J Am Geriatr Soc*. 2004;52(9):1471–8.

83. Hongo M, Itoi E, Sinaki M et al. Effect of low-intensity back exercise on quality of life and back extensor strength in patients with osteoporosis: A randomized controlled trial. *Osteoporos Int.* 2007;18(10):1389–95.

84. Bennell KL, Matthews B, Greig A et al. Effects of an exercise and manual therapy program on physical impairments, function and quality-of-life in people with osteoporotic vertebral fracture: A randomised, single-blind controlled pilot trial. *BMC Musculoskelet Disord.* 2010;11:36.

85. Bautmans I, van Arken J, van Mackelenberg M, Mets T. Rehabilitation using manual mobilization for thoracic kyphosis in elderly postmenopausal patients with osteoporosis. *J Rehabil Med.* 2010;42(2):129–35.

86. Bergland A, Thorsen H, Karesen R. Effect of exercise on mobility, balance and health-related quality of life in osteoporotic women with a history of vertebral fracture: A randomized, controlled trial. *Osteoporos Int.* 2011;22(6):1863–71.

87. Papaioannou A, Adachi JD, Winegard K et al. Efficacy of home-based exercise for improving quality of life among elderly women with symptomatic osteoporosis-related vertebral fractures. *Osteoporos Int.* 2003;14(8):677–82.

88. Ensrud KE, Schousboe JT. Vertebral fractures. *N Engl J Med.* 2011;364:1634–42.

89. Giangregorio LM, MacIntyre NJ, Thabane L, Skidmore CJ, Papaioannou A. Exercise for improving outcomes after osteoporotic vertebral fracture. *Cochrane Database Syst Rev.* 2013;(1):CD008618.

90. Huang MH, Barrett-Connor E, Greendale GA, Kado DM. Hyperkyphotic posture and risk of future osteoporotic fractures: The Rancho Bernado Study. *J Bone Miner Res.* 2006;21(3):419–23.

91. Sinaki M, Mikkelsen BA. Postmenopausal spinal osteoporosis: Flexion versus extension exercises. *Arch Phys Med Rehabil.* 1984;65(10):593–6.

92. Giangregorio LM, Papaioannou A, MacIntyre NJ et al. Too fit to fracture: Exercise recommendations for individuals with osteoporosis or osteoporotic vertebral fractures. *Osteoporos Int.* 2014;25(3):821–35.

93. Layne JE, Nelson ME. The effects of progressive resistance training on bone density: A review. *Med Sci Sports Exerc.* 1999;31(1):25–30.

94. Nelson DA, Bouxsein ML. Exercise maintains bone mass, but do people maintain exercise. *J Bone Miner Res.* 2001;14(2):202–5.

95. Ong T, Kantachuvesiri P, Sahota O, Gladman JRF. Characteristics and outcomes of hospitalised patients with vertebral fragility fractures: A systematic review. *Age Ageing.* 2018;47:17–25.

96. Masud T, Morris RO. Epidemiology of falls. *Age Ageing.* 2001;30(S4):3–7.

97. Sherrington C, Tiedemann A, Fairhall N, Close JCT, Lord SR. Exercise to prevent falls in older adults: An updated meta-analysis and best practice recommendations. *NSW Public Health Bull.* 2011;22(3–4): 78–83.

98. Oliver D, Connelly JB, Victor CR et al. Strategies to prevent falls and fractures in hospitals and care homes and effect of cognitive impairment: Systematic review and meta-analyses. *BMJ.* 2007;334(7584):82.

99. Klotzbuecher CM, Ross PD, Landsman PB, Abbott III TA, Berger M. Patients with prior fractures have an increased risk of future fractures: A summary of the literature and statistical synthesis. *J Bone Miner Res.* 2000;15(4):721–39.

100. Kanis JA, Johnell O. The burden of osteoporosis. *J Endocrinol Invest.* 1999;22(8):583–8.

101. Body JJ, Bergmann P, Boonen S et al. Non-pharmacological management of osteoporosis: A consensus of the Belgian Bone Club. *Osteoporos Int.* 2011;22(11):2769–88.

102. Khosla S, Hofbauer LC. Osteoporosis treatment: Recent developments and ongoing challenges. *Lancet Diabetes Endocrinol.* 2017;5(11):898–907.

103. Walters S, Chan S, Goh L, Ong T, Sahota O. The prevalence of frailty in patients admitted to hospital with vertebral fragility fractures. *Curr Rheumatol Rev.* 2016;12(3):244–7.

104. Cramer JA, Gold DT, Silverman SL, Lewiecki EM. A systematic review of persistence and compliance with bisphosphonates for osteoporosis. *Osteoporos Int.* 2007;18(8):1023–31.

105. Karlson L, Lundkvist J, Psachoulia E, Intorcia M, Strom O. Persistence with denosumab and persistence with oral bisphosphonates for the treatment of postmenopausal osteoporosis: A retrospective, observational study, and a meta-analysis. *Osteoporos Int.* 2015;26(10):2401–11.

106. McClung M, Harris ST, Miller PD et al. Bisphosphonate therapy for osteoporosis: Benefits, risks, and drug holiday. *Am J Med.* 2013;126(1):13–20.

107. McCombs JS, Thiebaud P, McLaughlin-Miley C, Shi J. Compliance with drug therapies for the treatment and prevention of osteoporosis. *Maturitas.* 2004;48(3):271–87.

108. Huybrechts KF, Ishak KJ, Caro JJ. Assessment of compliance with osteoporosis treatment and its consequences in a managed care population. *Bone.* 2006;38(6):922–8.

109. Naranjo A, Ojeda-Bruno S, Bilbao-Cantarero A, Quevedo-Abeledo JC, Diaz-Gonzalez BV, Rodriguez-Lozano C. Two-year adherence to treatment and associated factors in a fracture liaison service in Spain. *Osteoporos Int.* 2015;26(11):2579–85.

32

Augmentation of fracture fixation

An update

PETER V. GIANNOUDIS and PANAGIOTIS DOURAS

INTRODUCTION

One of the challenges in the elderly population that clinicians are facing is to adequately stabilize fractures for a sufficient period of time until fracture union occurs. However, due to the underlying compromised bone stock, adequate fixation to withstand the weight-bearing load is difficult, and not infrequently, failure of fixation takes place prior to bony union. Noteworthy, such complications have been reported in the literature as metalwork failure (1%−10%), malalignment (4%−40%), nonunion (2%−10%), and reoperation rates of 3%−23% (1).

Overall, the characteristics of osteoporotic bone can be summarized as follows: (a) increased bone porosity and decreased cortical thickness, (b) reduced connectivity in the trabecular network, (c) imbalanced bone resorption and formation, (d) reduced bone strength and volume, and (e) altered bone matrix resorption.

Failure of fixation in this elderly frail patient cohort is associated with increased incidence of mortality, morbidity, and health-care costs. Interestingly, several years ago, the introduction of locked plating provided a good solution to this clinical problem, allowing patients to ambulate early. However, despite this advancement in fracture management, failure of fixation and nonunion continues to be an issue in the elderly population (2). Of interest, the number of patients with osteoporotic/fragile bone will continue to increase in the years to come. According to the National Osteoporosis Foundation, it has been estimated that there is an incidence of approximately 2 million osteoporosis-related fractures in the United States each year. Further studies suggest that the worldwide incidence is almost 9 million. A conservative estimation is that by 2050 the numbers will have doubled in Europe and tripled on a worldwide scale.

Clinicians therefore have been seeking other options/techniques to improve the outcome of fracture stabilization in the elderly population. One technique that has gained popularity during the past decade is "bone augmentation." Bone augmentation refers to the surgical modification of cancellous periarticular bone after injury or disease with a bone substitute material in conjunction with fracture reduction and internal fixation. This procedure is relevant to the management of fragility fractures aiming to enhance the mechanical environment of the fixation. In general terms, aims of augmentation include retardation of migration of implant and bone, provision of an environment for bone remodeling, and limitation of intrusion of synovial fluid into intra-articular fractures. However, one may argue that there are a number of questions that need to be answered regarding the role of bone augmentation, including the following: (a) In which cases is augmentation necessary, important, or beneficial?; (b) What are the types and methods of augmentation?; (c) What biomaterials should be used?; and (d) Are there any potential disadvantages?

Ideally, biomaterials to be used must possess certain properties such as being biocompatible, having void-filling capacity, providing structural support and osteoconductivity, being cost-effective, and having unlimited availability. Naturally, if they also possess osteoinductivity and osteogenicity, that would be ideal (3).

In regard to how augmentation can be applied, one can consider three options:

1. Open packing of the defect area (apply cement, fracture reduction and fixation)
2. Spot augmentation (cement is injected, setting is awaited, drilling and definitive fixation take place)
3. Fixation of fracture with implant and subsequent delivery of the cement (fracture is reduced and is fixed, and then cement is delivered)

MATERIALS FOR AUGMENTATION

The most common biological materials that have been used for augmentation include polymethyl methacrylate

(PMMA) cement and calcium-based materials. Of note, bone cements vary in biological properties.

Polymethyl methacrylate

PMMA is a substance that can harden *in situ*. It has been used to fill subchondral bone void, such as in vertebroplasty, kyphoplasty, and metastatic fractures. In pathologic fractures related to bone tumors, routine use of cement augmentation in addition to internal stabilization has been advocated. For instance, PMMA has been used for prophylactic treatment of long bone metastatic lesions with improved pain and function scores (4). In periacetabular tumors (percutaneous cement augmentation following tumor), it has been used with very good pain control and clinical outcomes (5,6). Interestingly, PMMA has also been used for the treatment of benign cystic bony lesions following curettage with good results (7).

Despite the successful use of PMMA as an augmentation material, concerns have been raised regarding the potential damaging effect of its exothermic reaction, the inability of remodeling, the potential nonunion if cement is interposed between the fracture edges, and the difficulty of its removal during revision surgery. Several studies have examined the exothermic reaction of PMMA polymerization. In one of them, focusing on augmentation of a humeral head fracture treated with screws and PMMA, it was reported that the highest temperature measured at the tips of the screws was 43.5°C in the subchondral area and 38.3°C in the articular surface. The authors concluded that the temperature increase was not sufficient to lead to thermal necrosis of cartilage and bone tissue (8).

In spite of this finding, PMMA cement is mostly used for augmentation of metastatic fractures rather than acute fractures in elderly patients due to its lack of osteoconductive properties and resorption (9).

Calcium phosphate cement

Calcium phosphate cement is another material that hardens *in situ*. This usually consists of two components: a fluid that is a sodium phosphate solution, and a powder that is a mixture of monocalcium, monohydrate, and tricalcium phosphate. These are mixed together, either by hand or with a mixing device with or without vacuum. The mixture is then applied in the area of interest. It takes 10–15 minutes to harden, depending on the temperature of the storage area, the temperature of the operating room, and other parameters. The cement hardens creating a mechanically stable component along with the surrounding cancellous bone. Several studies have been performed where the solution was used to fill voids of subchondral bone in tibia plateau fractures. Calcium phosphate cement has osteoconductive capabilities. After osteoclastic activity and neovascularization, a remodeling procedure begins, and new bone formation takes place. Studies have shown,

particularly for tibial plateau fractures, that calcium phosphate cement has less capability to subside compared to autologous bone graft (10).

Calcium sulfate cement

This type of cement has been used to fill subchondral defects. It is associated with rapid degradation leading to a potential loss of strength capability. Recent research has led to the development of different types known as α- and β-hemihydrate with differentiation as far as load strength is concerned. Overall, one can argue that it is not the ideal material to be used for subchondral support or enhancement of fixation.

SPECIFIC ANATOMICAL INDICATIONS

Anatomical sites where augmentation can be useful include proximal femoral fractures (extracapsular), distal femur, pelvic ring and acetabulum, spine, tibial plateau, distal tibia, proximal humerus, distal radius, and os calcis.

Proximal femoral fractures

Surgical treatment is the method of choice in managing proximal femoral fractures except when certain reasons or comorbidities recommend a different approach. When dealing with trochanteric hip fracture, certain parameters have to be taken into consideration: age of patient, mobility status, integrity of lateral and medial proximal femoral cortex, and degree of comminution. The goal of treatment is to give the patient the chance to mobilize as quickly as possible, avoiding risks of prolonged bed rest, or deterioration of comorbidities. Stable fracture patterns do not usually present any difficulties, whereas multifragmentary or unstable fractures remain a challenging task. When the lateral cortex is intact, fixation can be performed with the use of a dynamic hip screw (DHS).

Sermon et al. investigated the effect of different localizations and amounts of bone cement in a polyurethane foam model where the specimens were instrumented with a proximal femoral nail antirotation (PFNA) blade and subsequently augmented with PMMA bone cement. Eight study groups were formed based on localization and amount of cement volume related to the blade. All specimens underwent cyclic loading with physiologic orientation of the force vector until construct failure. Interestingly, the groups were compared between each other and to a cadaveric control group. The experiments revealed a significant dependency of implant purchase on localization and amount of cement. Biomechanically favorable cement positions were noted at the implant tip and at the cranial side (11).

In a clinical prospective study regarding 64 patients with 31-A2 and 31-A3 type fractures, treatment with a

PMMA-augmented DHS depicted good fracture consolidation without complications such as avascular necrosis (12).

The use of PMMA cement in order to augment intramedullary nailing of proximal femur fractures led to the evolution of implants such as a perforated head screws or blade (Perforated PFNA) (13). The new implant can achieve better distribution of the cement in the femoral head. The use of a dissolved contrast agent under fluoroscopy is paramount in this technique in order to avoid leakage of the cement into the hip joint. After a high-viscosity bone cement is mixed as mentioned before, it is injected into the blade using a trauma needle under fluoroscopy. Then 3–5 mL of cement may be injected via the blade. Hardening of the cement may take about 10–15 minutes with the aim to have a mantle of bone cement surrounding the tip of the blade (13).

Overall, cement augmentation for plate and screw fixation constructs (Figure 32.1) as well as intramedullary fixation constructs of geriatric proximal femur fractures has been reported with good outcomes. Nonetheless, taking into consideration the cost to the health-care system, such a technique is not necessary for every patient with a proximal femur fracture. Cement augmentation for proximal femoral fractures should be reserved for unstable fracture patterns (31A2, 31A3) and profound osteoporosis.

In intracapsular neck of femur fractures, the findings are not so optimistic.

There have been several randomized clinical studies. However, augmentation of intracapsular fractures of the neck of the femur with calcium phosphate cement was associated with poor long-term results. This was secondary to the development of nonunion, avascular necrosis of the femoral head, and failure of fixation (14).

Humeral head fractures

At the first stage, there were attempts to improve screw fixation in the humeral head with the use of fibular grafts in order to enhance the trabecular bone quality of the humeral head. Later, biomechanical and clinical studies were performed investigating the strength of implant fixation that was augmented with calcium phosphate cements.

In an experimental study performed by Scola et al., a three-part fracture model of the proximal humerus was

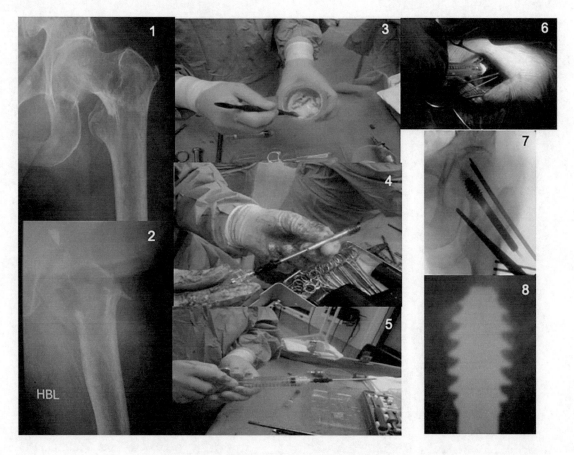

Figure 32.1 1. Anteroposterior and 2. Lateral radiographs of an extracapsular neck of femur fracture in a female patient 89 years of age. 3. Mixing of tricalcium phosphate cement. 4. Insertion of delivery needle of cement material in the canal of dynamic hip screw (DHS) demonstrating route of cement delivery. 5. Preparation of syringe containing cement with injection needle. 6. Intraoperative picture showing injection of calcium phosphate bone cement through canal of DHS after withdrawal of three turns of DHS, then immediate advancement of DHS in liquid cement. 7. Fluoroscopic image showing cement delivery out of the head of DHS. 8. Postoperative lateral radiograph demonstrating cement around the threads of the DHS.

simulated by a 10 mm horizontal gap just below the anatomical neck and a greater tuberosity osteotomy using an oscillating saw with a blade thickness of 0.4 mm (15). The fracture was fixed with standard locking plate (PHILOS, Synthes). The plate was fixed to the humeral shaft using three bicortical locking screws. For fixation of the head fragment, locking screws were placed in the six most proximal plate holes following the direction as provided by the aiming block of the PHILOS plate. One group was augmented using biological cement, and the other group was not. Both groups were tested under cyclic loading. The augmented group depicted greater strength. As the bone quality in the humeral head is not homogenously distributed, there is a question as to which and how many screws should be augmented. After determining the breakdown of each screw, it was suggested that the screws in the anteromedial and anteroinferior aspects of the humeral head had to be selected for augmentation with 0.5 mL of PMMA cement. In a varus bending test, the results of augmentation of two screws with the lowest breakaway torque achieved almost the same stability as augmentation of the four most proximal screws (15).

In the clinical setting, it has been demonstrated that cement augmentation enhances the filling of voids (Figure 32.2), improves fixation, and reduces the incidence of screw penetration into the shoulder joint following stabilization (16,17).

Nonetheless, the location and amount of cement augmentation in proximal humeral osteoporotic fractures remain a subject of debate.

Tibial plateau fractures

Tibial plateau fractures are categorized into certain types. As described, often a depression of the articular surface is involved, with collapse of subchondral bone. This is the result of axial loading combined with valgus force. In order to restore the articular surface, the depression area needs to be elevated, and the void created underneath has

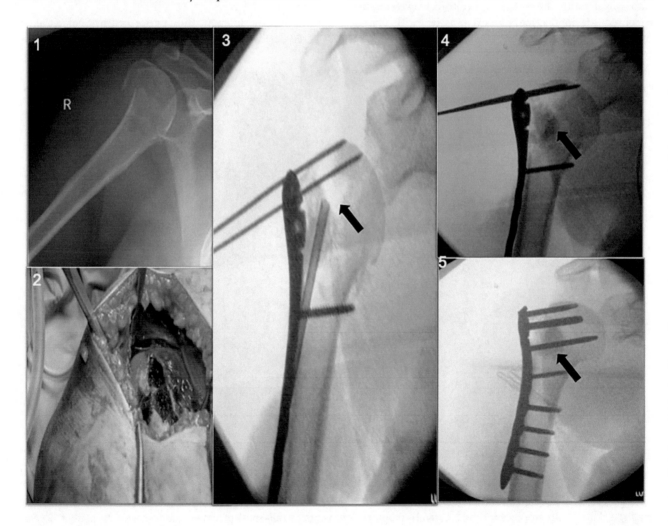

Figure 32.2 1. Proximal humerus radiograph in a female patient 70 years old showing a three-part head fracture with valgus impaction. 2. Intraoperative picture showing degree of comminution. 3. Intraoperative fluoroscopic image showing temporary stabilization of fracture with K-wires, locking plate position, and cancellous void in humeral head (arrow) with syringe tip inferior to the void prior to cement injection. 4. Intraoperative fluoroscopic image showing void occupied by cement (arrow). 5. Postoperative picture with fixation of the fracture with locking plate and previous bone void filled with cement.

to be managed (Figure 32.3a–c). The material to be used has to withstand compression forces, with the capacity to address shearing and bending forces as well. The void is usually filled with tricalcium phosphate cement or other types of autologous bone or allograft. After the graft is applied, the fracture is supported with metalwork. In the postoperative period, weight-bearing is restricted for 6–12 weeks so that the fixation stability and the restored congruency are not jeopardized. In a study involving 49 patients with an isolated tibial plateau fracture, Keating et al. fixed the void using biological cement Norian SRS. Postoperatively, the patients began weight-bearing after 6 weeks. No loss of reduction and collapse were reported (18).

Goff et al. carried out a review of the literature in terms of the application of cement augmentation in the management of tibial plateau fractures (19). Nineteen studies were analyzed reporting on 672 patients (674 fractures), with a mean age of 50.35 years (range 15–89 years), and a gender ratio of 3/2 males/females. The graft substitutes assessed were calcium phosphate cement, hydroxyapatite granules, calcium sulfate, bioactive glass, tricalcium phosphate, demineralized bone matrix (DBM), allografts, and xenograft. Fracture healing was uneventful in over 90% of the cases over a variant period of time. Secondary collapse of the knee joint surface 2 mm or greater was reported in 8.6% in the biological substitutes (allograft, DBM, and xenograft), 5.4% in the hydroxyapatite, 3.7% in the calcium phosphate cement, and 11.1% in the calcium sulfate cases. Shorter total operative time, greater tolerance of early weight-bearing, and improved early functional outcomes within the first year postsurgery were also recorded in the studies reporting on the use of injectable calcium phosphate cement (Norian SRS) (19).

Despite a lack of good-quality randomized controlled trials, there is arguably sufficient evidence supporting the use of bone graft substitutes at the clinical setting of depressed plateau fractures.

Spinal compressive fractures

VERTEBROPLASTY

During the 1980s, a new method that consisted of injecting PMMA cement in the spinal vertebrae under fluoroscopy was introduced. The aim of the method was to address the hemangioma that was discovered in the spine. Thereafter, due to its successful results, this treatment was further used to address compression fractures of the spinal column. The results were remarkable as far as quick pain alleviation was concerned. However, the potential cement leakage toward the soft tissues, nerves, vessels, and spinal canal and the potential exothermic reaction, raised concerns. With the use of high-viscosity cement, large-diameter needles, and fluoroscopic guidance, this issue was somewhat addressed.

KYPHOPLASTY

As an evolution of vertebroplasty, kyphoplasty was introduced. The difference of the method is that before cement

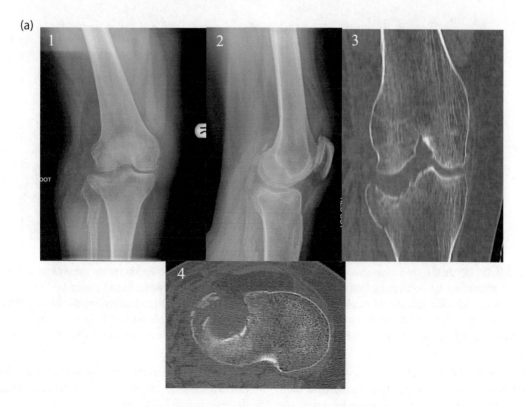

Figure 32.3 (a) 1. Anteroposterior (AP) and 2. Lateral radiographs of lateral depressed tibial plateau fracture in a 70-year-old male. 3 and 4. CT scan images demonstrating the extent of articular impaction. *(Continued)*

(b)

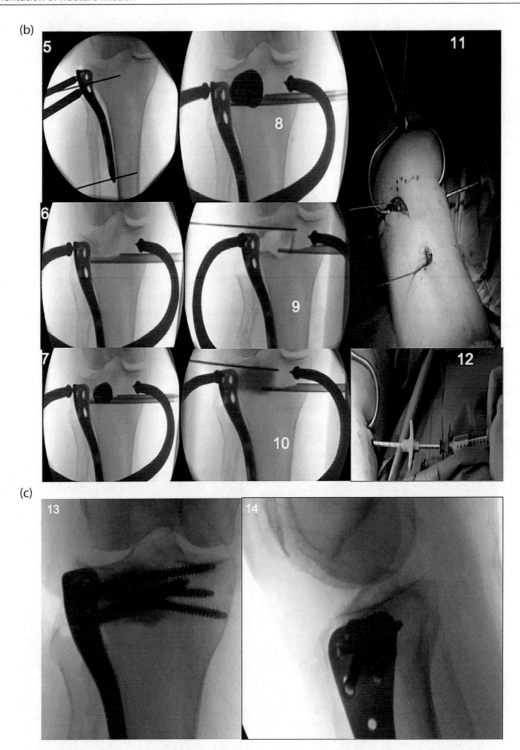

(c)

Figure 32.3 (Continued) (b) 5. Fluoroscopic image demonstrating application of locking plate over lateral border of proximal tibia. 6. Support of locking plate with reduction forceps. Insertion of cannula from medial side to be used for indirection reduction of depressed segment with the inflation of a balloon. 7. Inflammation of balloon. 8. Further balloon inflation and indirect reduction of depressed fragment. 9. Removal of balloon and visualization of bone void created. Reduction help with K-wire. 10–12. Delivery of cement with syringe into the subchondral void. (c) 13. AP and 14. Lateral fluoroscopic image after completion of reconstruction.

injection, the shape of the vertebrae is restored with the use of an inflatable balloon. The gap that is created is then filled with the cement. With this method, further vertebrae collapse, and kyphotic deformity of the spine is inhibited. The optimum cement volume required to avoid any risks is 15% of the vertebra that is addressed. Furthermore, cement-filled cages are introduced when addressing larger defects such as in malignancies. Recently, augmentation of pedicle screws with cement in order to improve mechanical stability has been suggested (20).

Distal radius fractures

Distal radius is one of the most common types of osteoporotic fractures in the elderly population. The majority of them are treated conservatively with manipulation under anesthesia and application of plaster for 6 weeks. In the case of marked comminution, severe collapse, and secondary displacement, surgical management with open reduction and internal fixation (ORIF) or application of external fixation is suggested. In order to address the issue of articular impaction and enhanced fixation, the use of augmentation techniques was introduced. Several studies have been performed, either with percutaneous injection of cement or with an open application after good results with hematoma evacuation.

Hedge et al. used synthetic hydroxyapatite (HA) in unstable fractures of the distal radius in 31 elderly patients. Twenty-seven patients were available for follow-up. All subjects underwent closed reduction with K-wire fixation and HA augmentation. They were followed up at 8- and 16-week intervals postoperatively to assess the functional outcome using patient-related wrist evaluation (PRWE), clinical outcome, and radiological outcome. At a mean of 16 weeks, there was no metaphyseal defect, no collapse, and satisfactory clinical outcomes were observed. The authors concluded that fixation with hydroxyapatite augmentation for fractures of the distal radius in elderly patients is an attractive therapeutic option (21).

Kainz et al. used human fresh-frozen cadaver pairs of radii to simulate an AO/Orthopaedic Trauma Association (OTA) 23-A3 fracture. In four groups ($n = 7$ for each group), two volar fixed-angle plates (Aptus 2.5 mm locking fracture plate, Medartis, Switzerland, and VA-LCP two-column distal radius plate 2.4, volar, Synthes, Switzerland) with or without an additional injection of a biomaterial (Hydroset Injectable HA Bone Substitute, Stryker, Switzerland) into the dorsal comminution zone were used to fix the distal metaphyseal fragment. Each specimen was load-controlled tested under cyclic loading with a servohydraulic material testing machine. Displacement, stiffness, dissipated work, and failure mode were recorded. The authors reported improved mechanical properties (decreased displacement, increased stiffness, decreased dissipated work) in both plates if the biomaterial was additionally injected. Improvement of mechanical parameters after biomaterial injection was more evident in the Synthes plate compared to the Aptus plate. Pushing out of the screws was noticed as a failure mode only in samples lacking supplementary biomaterial. They concluded that injection of a biomaterial into the dorsal comminution zone increases stability after volar locking plating of distal radius fractures *in vitro* (22).

In contrast, Kim et al. studied 48 patients with 50 unstable distal radial fractures with a mean age of 73 years. Surgical procedures were randomized between volar locking plate fixation alone (group 1) and volar locking plate fixation with injection of calcium phosphate bone cement (group 2). The patients were assessed clinically at 3 and 12 months postoperatively. Clinical assessments included determinations of grip strength, wrist motion, wrist pain, modified Mayo wrist scores, and DASH (disabilities of the arm, shoulder, and hand) scores. Radiographic evaluations were performed immediately postoperatively and at 1 year following surgery. The adequacy of the reduction was assessed by measuring radial inclination, volar angulation, and ulnar variance. The authors reported that the two groups were comparable with regard to age, sex, fracture type, injury mechanism, and bone mineral density. No significant differences were observed between the groups with regard to the clinical outcomes at the 3- or 12-month follow-up examinations. No significant intergroup differences in radiographic outcomes were observed immediately after surgery or at the 1-year follow-up visit. Furthermore, no complication-related differences were observed, and there were no nonunions. They concluded that augmentation of metaphyseal defects with calcium phosphate bone cement after volar locking plate fixation offered no benefit over volar locking plate fixation alone in elderly patients with an unstable distal radial fracture (23).

Further studies are needed to elucidate the role of augmentation of distal radius fractures.

Calcaneal fractures

Surgical management of calcaneal fractures is a challenging effort taking into consideration the complex anatomy of this bone along with the peculiar orientation of the subtalar joint. Furthermore, when addressing a severe comminution, it is somehow difficult to maintain congruency. Even though anatomical plating has evolved, this is not enough to achieve and maintain the appropriate restoration of the anatomy. The use of biological cement in calcaneal fracture treatment was introduced with the aim to support the crushed cancellous bone. Previously, restricted weight-bearing for 8–12 weeks was suggested. With the cement use, this time frame could be reduced, providing the ability for earlier mobilization without compromising the reduction and fixation.

Schildhauer assessed 36 joint depression–type calcaneal fractures in 32 patients who were augmented with the calcium phosphate cement after standard open reduction with internal fixation. Postoperative full weight-bearing was allowed progressively earlier, and as the study progressed, the last patients were bearing full weight as early as 3 weeks postoperatively. Biopsies for histologic analysis were performed at the time of hardware removal after 1 year (seven biopsies) or in case of infection at time of debridement (five biopsies). The authors reported that cement injection averaged 10 cc and could easily be performed under fluoroscopic control. Progressively earlier full weight-bearing was achieved without loss of reduction. There was no statistical difference in clinical outcome scores in patients with full weight-bearing before or after 6 weeks postoperatively. The infection rate was 11%, possibly related to the skin incisions. The biopsies from clinically satisfactory cases showed nearly complete bone apposition, areas of vascular penetration, and reversal lines illustrating progressive cycles of resorption and new bone formation. They concluded that calcium phosphate cement augmentation of standard open reduction with internal fixation in joint depression–type calcaneal fractures allows postoperative full weight-bearing as early as 3 weeks postoperatively. The injectable bone cement can easily be handled surgically under fluoroscopic control and is able to be remodeled (24).

Vicenti et al. retrospectively examined 42 patients treated operatively having sustained Sander type II, III, and IV calcaneal fractures with a minimally invasive reduction technique using an inflatable bone tamp filled with tricalcium phosphate (calcaneoplasty). Conventional x-rays and computed tomography scan were performed preoperatively, at 3 and 12 months postoperatively, and at the last-follow-up. At the last follow-up, the mean AOFAS score was 82.1 (good), and the mean Maryland Foot Score (MFS) was 80.8 (good). The mean Böhler angle improved from 1.29° preoperatively to 27.8° at the last follow-up. No cases of adverse reaction or deep infection were observed. The authors reported that calcaneoplasty appears to be a valid option for treatment for calcaneal fractures and a reliable alternative to ORIF. This technique allows stable fracture reduction and early weight-bearing combined with good clinical and radiological results and few complications (25).

Elsner et al. studied 18 patients with intra-articular calcaneal fractures treated with open reduction and internal fixation and augmentation with an injectable carbonated apatite cement. Functional follow-up studies using the Zwipp Foot Score and densitometry were performed at 6-month intervals postoperatively. Histological samples of biopsies obtained at the time of hardware removal (6 months postoperatively) were also analyzed. The use of bone cement led to intermediate-term functional outcomes that were no better than those reported with conventional surgical procedures using bone graft. Patients demonstrated postoperative difficulties similar to those seen in other studies of this fracture, including pain, subtalar motion restrictions, peroneal impingement, and difficulties on uneven terrain and with toe- and heel-walking. However, compared to patients treated surgically without injectable carbonated apatite cement, full weight-bearing on the affected extremity was regained at an average of 4 weeks postoperatively. In addition, autogenous bone graft was not required to fill the osseous defect using this technique, minimizing morbidity and discomfort (26).

Overall, further studies are welcome to provide further evidence on the role of augmentation in displaced intra-articular calcaneal fractures.

Other anatomical locations

The bone augmentation technique can be used for other cases and circumstances, as in pelvic ring injures (27) and acetabular fractures, where the need to restore the impacted articular surface leads to the use of a bone substitute (Figure 32.4).

(a)

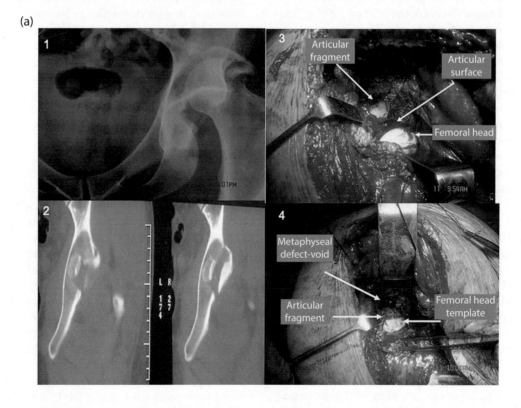

Figure 32.4 (a) 1. Anteroposterior (AP) radiograph demonstrating a right hip fracture dislocation in a 54-year-old male. 2. Computed tomography images showing articular impaction. 3. Intraoperative images demonstrating area of impaction. 4. Intraoperative images showing creation of cancellous void after reduction of depressed segment using the femoral head as a template. *(Continued)*

(b)

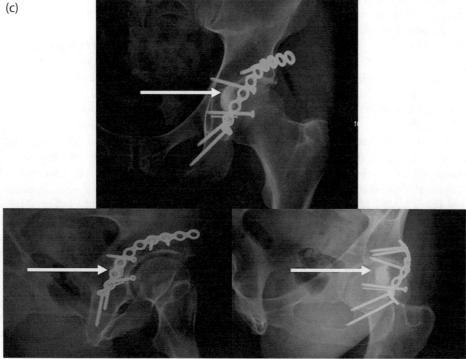

(c)

Figure 32.4 (Continued) (b) Intraoperative picture showing injection of bone substitute in the area of the bone void created due to impaction. (c) Postoperative AP, iliac oblique, and obturator oblique views of right acetabulum showing reduction and fixation of fracture with posterior wall buttress plating and lag screw fixation.

CONCLUSION

Taking into consideration the upcoming changes in the aging population, there is a need for early ambulation of patients to minimize the risk of functional impairment.

The use of bone augmentation techniques can provide a new weapon in orthopedic trauma surgery to improve the management of a variety of osteoporotic-/fragility-related fractures. Different materials can be used for reconstruction of osseous voids in different anatomical locations.

PMMA implantation has been associated with improving the implant–bone fixation interface, particularly in pathologic fractures. Similarly, calcium cements provide subchondral support in articular impaction injuries. However, the predictability and reliability of the strengthening effect of augmentation materials are rather moderate.

We need to understand the ideal area of application of these cements in order to expect the best outcomes. Further studies need to be carried out regarding substances and their use. For instance, none of the hip studies have investigated if strengthening of the proximal femur would lead to distal femoral or acetabular fractures. Moreover, careful surgical planning and appropriate instrumentation and execution are essential for a successful outcome.

REFERENCES

1. Kammerlander C, Neuerburg C, Verlaan JJ, Schmoelz W, Miclau T, Larsson S. The use of augmentation techniques in osteoporotic fracture fixation. *Injury*. 2016;47(Suppl 2):S36–43.
2. von Rüden C, Augat P. Failure of fracture fixation in osteoporotic bone. *Injury*. 2016;47(Suppl 2):S3–S10.
3. Larsson S, Hannink G. Injectable bone-graft substitutes: Current products, their characteristics and indications, and new developments. *Injury*. 2011;42(Suppl 2):S30–4.
4. Park JW, Kim Y-I, Kang HG, Kim JH, Kim HS. Preliminary results: Use of multi-hole injection nails for intramedullary nailing with simultaneous bone cement injection in long-bone metastasis. *Skeletal Radiol*. 2019 Feb;48(2):219–25.
5. Hartung MP, Tutton SM, Hohenwalter EJ, King DM, Neilson JC. Safety and efficacy of minimally invasive acetabular stabilization for periacetabular metastatic disease with thermal ablation and augmented screw fixation. *J Vasc Interv Radiol*. 2016;27(5):682–8.
6. Guzik G. Treatment of metastatic lesions localized in the acetabulum. *J Orthop Surg Res*. 2016;11(1):54.
7. Gupta SP, Garg G. Curettage with cement augmentation of large bone defects in giant cell tumors with pathological fractures in lower-extremity long bones. *J Orthop Traumatol*. 2016;17(3):239–47.
8. Blazejak M, Hofmann-Fliri L, Büchler L, Gueorguiev B, Windolf M. *In vitro* temperature during cement augmentation of proximal humerus plate screw tips. *Injury*. 2013;44(10):1321–6.
9. DeGroot H, Donati D, Di Liddo M, Gozzi E, Mercuri M. The use of cement in osteoarticular allografts for proximal humeral bone tumors. *Clin Orthop Relat Res*. 2004;(427):190–7.
10. Russell TA, Leighton RK. Alpha-BSM Tibial Plateau Fracture Study Group. Comparison of autogenous bone graft and endothermic calcium phosphate cement for defect augmentation in tibial plateau fractures. A multicenter, prospective, randomized study. *J Bone Joint Surg Am*. 2008;90(10):2057–61.
11. Sermon A, Hofmann-Fliri L, Richards RG, Flamaing J, Windolf M. Cement augmentation of hip implants in osteoporotic bone: How much cement is needed and where should it go? *J Orthop Res*. 2014;32(3):362–8.
12. Gupta RK, Gupta V, Gupta N. Outcomes of osteoporotic trochanteric fractures treated with cement-augmented dynamic hip screw. *Indian J Orthop*. 2012;46(6):640–5.
13. Kammerlander C, Gebhard F, Meier C et al. Standardised cement augmentation of the PFNA using a perforated blade: A new technique and preliminary clinical results. A prospective multicentre trial. *Injury*. 2011;42(12):1484–90.
14. Lindner T, Kanakaris NK, Marx B, Cockbain A, Kontakis G, Giannoudis PV. Fractures of the hip and osteoporosis: The role of bone substitutes. *J Bone Joint Surg Br*. 2009;91(3):294–303.
15. Scola A, Gebhard F, Röderer G. Augmentation technique on the proximal humerus. *Unfallchirurg*. 2015;118(9):749–54.
16. Egol KA, Sugi MT, Ong CC, Montero N, Davidovitch R, Zuckerman JD. Fracture site augmentation with calcium phosphate cement reduces screw penetration after open reduction-internal fixation of proximal humeral fractures. *J Shoulder Elbow Surg*. 2012;21:741–8.
17. Unger S, Erhart S, Kralinger F, Blauth M, Schmoelz W. The effect of *in situ* augmentation on implant anchorage in proximal humeral head fractures. *Injury*. 2012;43:1759–63.
18. Keating JF, Hajducka CL, Harper J. Minimal internal fixation and calcium-phosphate cement in the treatment of fractures of the tibial plateau. A pilot study. *J Bone Joint Surg Br*. 2003;85(1):68–73.
19. Goff T, Kanakaris NK, Giannoudis PV. Use of bone graft substitutes in the management of tibial plateau fractures. *Injury*. 2013;44(Suppl 1):S86–94.
20. Ghermandi R, Pipola V, Colangeli S et al. Polymethylmethacrylate-augmented fenestrated pedicle-screw fixation in low bone quality patients: A case series and literature review. *J Biol Regul Homeost Agents*. 2018;32(6 Suppl 1):71–6.
21. Hegde C, Shetty V, Wasnik S, Ahammed I, Shetty V. Use of bone graft substitute in the treatment for distal radius fractures in elderly. *Eur J Orthop Surg Traumatol*. 2013;23(6):651–6.
22. Kainz H, Dall'Ara E, Antoni A, Redl H, Zysset P, Weninger P. Calcium phosphate cement augmentation after volar locking plating of distal radius fracture significantly increases stability. *Eur J Orthop Surg Traumatol*. 2014;24(6):869–75.
23. Kim JK, Koh YD, Kook SH. Effect of calcium phosphate bone cement augmentation on volar plate fixation of unstable distal radial fractures in the elderly. *J Bone Joint Surg Am*. 2011;93(7):609–14.
24. Schildhauer TA, Bauer TW, Josten C, Muhr G. Open reduction and augmentation of internal fixation

with an injectable skeletal cement for the treatment of complex calcaneal fractures. *J Orthop Trauma.* 2000;14(5):309–17.

25. Vicenti G, Solarino G, Caizzi G et al. Balloon-assisted reduction, pin fixation and tricalcium phosphate augmentation for calcaneal fracture: A retrospective analysis of 42 patients. *Injury.* 2018;49(Suppl 3):S94–9.

26. Elsner A, Jubel A, Prokop A, Koebke J, Rehm KE, Andermahr J. Augmentation of intraarticular calcaneal fractures with injectable calcium phosphate cement: Densitometry, histology, and functional outcome of 18 patients. *J Foot Ankle Surg.* 2005;44(5):390–5.

27. Hopf JC, Krieglstein CF, Müller LP, Koslowsky TC. Percutaneous iliosacral screw fixation after osteoporotic posterior ring fractures of the pelvis reduces pain significantly in elderly patients. *Injury.* 2015;46(8):1631–6.

33

Complications of surgical treatment for osteoporotic fractures

PAUL C. BALDWIN III and CHRISTIAN KRETTEK

INTRODUCTION

Osteoporotic fragility fractures are becoming a major health issue in all regions of the world. As the world's population ages, the rate of osteoporotic fractures will increase, and caring for osteoporotic fractures will become more routine in day-to-day practice. Currently in the United States, osteoporotic fragility fractures occur more frequently than heart attacks, strokes, and breast cancer combined (1). Trends like this are not isolated to the United States, and it is estimated that nearly half of the world's hip fractures will occur in Asia by 2050 (2). The increase in osteoporotic fractures also necessitates increased need for surgical interventions.

The risk for potential complications exists with any surgical intervention, and it is no different with the surgical treatment of osteoporotic fragility fractures. In addition to the baseline risks of anesthesia, infection, wound complications, and medical complications, patients with osteoporotic fractures have additional risks that are less common in patients with normal bone density. These include fixation failure, hardware failure, and nonunions. This chapter focuses on the complications associated with surgical treatment of the most common osteoporotic fractures of the upper and lower extremities, the spine, as well as potential perioperative medical complications.

UPPER EXTREMITY FRACTURES

Proximal humerus fractures

Fractures of the proximal humerus account for between 4% and 5% of all fractures (3). The majority of these fractures are osteoporotic fractures, with 71% of these fractures occurring in patients older than 60 years of age, making fixation challenging (4). As the world's population ages, a threefold increase in the incidence of osteoporotic proximal humerus fractures is predicted over the next 30 years (5). Minimally displaced or valgus impacted proximal humerus fractures are often amendable to nonoperative treatment. However, displaced two-part, three-part, and four-part proximal humerus fractures can meet the criteria for surgical intervention. Surgical treatment of these displaced fractures includes percutaneous fracture fixation, open reduction and internal fixation (ORIF), and arthroplasty procedures. Each of these procedures carries unique complication profiles.

With percutaneous pinning, malunion rates have been reported as high as 28% (6).

Patients with osteoporotic bone and highly comminuted fractures are at highest risk for malunions with the most common deformity being varus angulation of the humeral head and posterior-superior displacement of the greater tuberosity (7). Pin migration is a second complication that can develop with the use of percutaneous pinning and is more commonly observed in patients with osteoporosis. Pin migration can lead to loss of fixation, malunion, or more serious complications such as migration into the vascular system or other major organ systems. Even with the use of terminally threaded pins, pin migration has been reported to occur in up to one-third of patients (6). An early study by Lyons and Rockwood reviewed 47 reports of pin migration when used for fixation around the shoulder girdle. In this study, 17 of the pins were found to have migrated into major vascular structures including the subclavian artery, ascending aorta, pulmonary artery, and the heart. Ten pins migrated into the mediastinum, eight to the lungs, and five to the cervical spine. One pin was reported to have migrated to the trachea where it was subsequently coughed up by the patient. Eight patients died, and six of these patients died of sudden catastrophic cardiovascular events (8). Most of the pin migration events occurred at 8 months postoperatively; however, pin migration can occur earlier (7). It is therefore recommended that patients treated with percutaneous pinning of proximal humerus fractures be followed closely after surgery with radiographs to detect pin loosening early and prior to potential catastrophic pin migration. Early intervention with pin removal or revision of pin placement should be considered if loosening is present. In addition, counseling of the patient and caretakers regarding the importance of compliance with postoperative instructions and concerning symptoms should take place after surgery.

With the development of fixed-angle locked plates, there was an increase in the frequency of surgical intervention for proximal humerus fractures. In the United States alone, Bell et al. reported a 29% increase in the treatment of proximal humerus fractures with ORIF from 1999 to 2005 (3). The use of fixed-angle locking plates has significantly improved the fixation in osteoporotic bone and osteoporotic fractures; however, it is not without complications. This can be seen with a significantly increased rate of reoperation after ORIF between 1999 and 2005 that correlates with the increased frequency of ORIF previously described during this time frame. In addition, a meta-analysis of 514 proximal humerus fractures treated with fixed-angle locked plating demonstrated a 13.8% rate of reoperation and a 49% overall complication rate (9). Reduced humeral head bone density and quality increase the risk of fixation failure, resultant fracture displacement, and poor functional outcomes. Patients with osteoporotic proximal humerus fractures are at increased risk for fixation failure when treated with fixed-angle plate constructs (10). The commonly described modes of fixation failure in osteoporotic proximal humerus fractures include screw cut-out, intra-articular screw penetration, postoperative fracture displacement, and avascular necrosis (AVN) (11–14). In the meta-analysis by Sproul et al., the rates of complications were reported as varus malunion (16%), AVN (10%), intra-articular screw penetration (8%), subacromial impingement (6%), and infection (4%) (9). Of these complications, the most common reason for reoperation was intra-articular screw perforation and cut-out.

These findings have been supported in subsequent studies evaluating the outcomes of fixed-angle locking plate fixation in osteoporotic proximal humerus fractures. Micic et al. analyzed early failure (less than 4 weeks) of fixed-angle locking plate constructs in eight osteoporotic patients and found that varus collapse and screw cut-out was the cause of failure (14). In all eight patients, medial calcar support was absent. In three of the eight patients, initial malreduction of the fracture was observed. In a second study, Oswley et al. retrospectively reviewed 53 patients treated with fixed-angle locking plates for displaced proximal humerus fractures. Of these 53 patients, 36% developed postoperative complications including screw cut-out (23%), varus displacement (25%), and AVN (4%). Revision surgery was performed in 13% of the 53 patients. When secondary analysis was performed, the observed complications disproportionately occurred in patients older than 60 years of age and with osteoporosis (57%) (15).

Given the increased rates of fixation failure with locked plates in osteoporotic proximal humerus fractures, attention has been focused on developing methods to augment fixation.

One such augmentation technique is the use of rotator cuff sutures. Often utilized to aid in reduction and neutralization of deforming forces, these heavy, nonabsorbable sutures are placed through the junction of tendon and tuberosity and tied after being passed through the locking plate. These sutures can prove helpful in reducing the initial varus deformity as well as maintaining tuberosity reduction postoperatively, an essential step for achieving satisfactory functional outcomes. In addition, the rotator cuff sutures may neutralize the deforming forces on fracture fragments that are not sufficiently stabilized with screws, such as a comminuted greater tuberosity fragment often seen in osteoporotic proximal humerus fractures.

The use of bone void fillers is a technique utilized to augment fixation of osteoporotic proximal humerus fractures. Allograft in the form of corticocancellous chips and cortical strut grafts is commonly used to supplement fixation in osteoporotic fractures. Corticocancellous chips provide osteoconductive filler for humeral head and metaphyseal defects or voids. In theory, the osteoconductive properties of the corticocancellous graft allow for the host bone to integrate and form new native bone, but it provides little mechanical support. When mechanical support is required, as in the setting of a comminuted medial calcar, a cortical strut graft can be utilized. The use of a fibular strut allograft to support and restore the medial calcar has been described in both biomechanical and clinical studies. In multiple cadaveric studies comparing the biomechanical properties of proximal humerus locking plates in isolation and proximal humerus locking plates in conjunction with the use of fibular strut allograft, the use of both a locking plate and strut allograft demonstrated superior biomechanical properties. In a study of 14 cadavers, Bae et al. showed that with the use of a locking plate and fibular strut, there was significantly less displacement and significantly increased load to failure and stiffness when compared to the use of a locking plate in isolation (16). Chow et al. supported these results in a subsequent biomechanical cadaveric study where none of the eight cadaveric fractures treated with locking plate and fibular strut allograft demonstrated varus collapse compared to varus collapse of six of the eight fractures treated without augmentation (17).

Clinical studies have also demonstrated the efficacy of fibular strut allograft augmentation in the treatment of proximal humerus fractures. In a small study of seven patients, Gardner et al. demonstrated a 100% union rate and no loss of fixation stability or reduction at 3–6 months and no loss of reduction with the use of a fibular strut graft to augment the locking plate fixation (18). A more recent retrospective study by Nevaiser et al. evaluated 38 patients treated for proximal humerus fractures with a locking plate and fibular strut augmentation (19). At a mean follow-up of 75 weeks, no cases of intra-articular screw penetration or cut-out were observed. Loss of reduction was reported in one patient, and one patient demonstrated partial AVN. With promising biomechanical and clinical results such as these, the use of fibular strut allograft augmentation should be considered in osteoporotic fractures to restore or support the medial calcar.

The use of bone cement to augment fixation of proximal humerus fractures has also been described. Calcium phosphate cement demonstrates osteoconductive properties and can increase screw purchase in cancellous bone. Given its relatively viscous nature during application, it can be injected or molded into bone defects to provide enhanced strength in compression. Resorption of calcium phosphate cement occurs via a cell-mediated process that mirrors bone remodeling; therefore, it does not disappear until new native bone has formed, allowing for increased duration of benefit. The clinical efficacy of calcium phosphate cement augmentation in the setting of proximal humerus fractures was evaluated by Egol et al. in a retrospective review (20). In this study, 92 patients with two-part, three-part, and four-part proximal humerus fractures were treated with a proximal humerus locking plate. The metaphyseal defects were treated with augmentation using corticocancellous chip allograft, calcium phosphate cement, or no augmentation. The addition of calcium phosphate cement was found to be associated with a lower incidence of intra-articular screw penetration and cut-out as well as humeral head subsidence. These clinical findings were supported in a biomechanical study utilizing a cadaveric two-part proximal humerus fracture model with metaphyseal comminution. In this study, calcium phosphate cement augmentation demonstrated increased axial stiffness, reduced screw cutout, and increased load to failure (21).

Augmentation of proximal humerus fracture fixation with calcium sulfate bone cement has demonstrated similar results to calcium phosphate cement augmentation. In a study by Somasundaram et al., 82% of patients treated with proximal humerus locking plates and calcium sulfate cement augmentation of metaphyseal voids demonstrated good clinical outcomes (22). A 100% union rate was reported without infection, malunion, AVN, or loss of fixation or reduction. Based on these results, cement augmentation can be a useful adjunct to fixation in the setting of osteoporotic fractures with metaphyseal defects and voids.

While augmentation of proximal humeral locking plates can improve fixation and reduce the risk of complications, proper technique and screw placement are essential regardless of the selected augmentation. In an effort to optimize mechanical stability and medial calcar support, screws should be directed in the posterior-medial-inferior aspect of the humeral head (23). Humeral head trabecular density significantly affects pullout strength of cancellous screws; therefore, screws should be placed into the region of the humeral head with the highest trabecular densities (24). Cadaveric studies have shown that the highest cancellous bone density in the proximal humerus is found in the proximal, posterior, and medial portions of the humeral head (24–28). Additional cadaveric studies have shown increased screw purchase and pullout strength when a screw was placed in the center of the humeral head within subchondral bone. The trabecular density is lowest in the superior and anterior portions of the head, which correlates to poor screw purchase and lower pullout strength (24–28).

The majority of modern proximal humerus locking plates designs allow for a medial column support screw to be placed along the medial calcar. In a study by Zhang et al., patients with two-part, three-part, and four-part proximal humerus fractures were treated with a proximal humerus locking plate (23). These patients were randomized to treatment using a locking plate with or without a medial calcar support screw. While no difference in outcomes was noted for two-part fractures, the three-part and four-part fractures treated with a medial calcar support screw demonstrated a significantly higher final neck-shaft angle and reduced loss of angulation when compared to the fractures treated without a calcar support screw. In a cadaveric study of a proximal humerus fracture model, Erhardt et al. analyzed different fixation methods using a polyaxial locking plate (28). This study revealed that five screws in the head fragment and an inferior-medial calcar support screw significantly decreased the risk of screw cutout and perforation.

Proximal humerus fractures are the third most common osteoporotic fracture. When the fracture pattern and patient health meet surgical criteria, multiple surgical fixation pathways exist. Each treatment brings with it its own unique complication profile. Strategies have been developed to improve fixation and reduce complications. Regardless of what technique, implant, and augment is utilized, special care to minimize disruption of blood flow to the humeral head and restoration of the medial calcar are essential to a successful outcome.

Distal humerus fractures

Fractures of the distal humerus in an elderly person can present a challenging treatment dilemma to orthopedic surgeons. These fractures are often comminuted and intra-articular, which, when combined with the limited subchondral bone in this anatomical region, increases the complexity level in surgical fixation. The difficulty level is increased in elderly patients who often have low bone mineral density and osteoporosis. In the setting of osteoporosis, traditional principles of ORIF of distal humerus fractures have been prone to failure, with some studies reporting complication rates up to 30% (29–35). Given the high reported complication rates with ORIF, total elbow arthroplasty has been advocated as an alternative primary treatment for these challenging fractures (36–41).

Various fixation constructs have been discussed for treatment of distal humerus fractures, including bicolumnar parallel plating and bicolumnar 90–90 plating (42–44). An olecranon osteotomy can be performed at the discretion of the surgeon if deemed necessary to address and appropriately reduce the articular surface of the distal humerus. With osteoporosis and comminution, careful analysis of the articular surface reduction is necessary to avoid narrowing the trochlear notch with overcompression if using a lag screw (45). Following reduction of the articular surface, the articular block is reconstructed to the medial and lateral columns. Fixation of the lateral and medial columns can be achieved with 3.5 mm pelvic reconstruction plates or 3.5 mm low-contact dynamic compression plates contoured to the lateral and medial columns. Anatomically precontoured locking plates can also be utilized. However, the cost of these plates has been reported to average 348% more than the standard 3.5 mm pelvic reconstruction plate (46). While locking plates are more costly, they have been shown to provide more biomechanical stability, especially in osteoporotic bone. Schuster et al. reported that locking 3.5 mm reconstruction plates applied in a 90–90 plate orientation demonstrated superior cyclic load to failure properties when compared to traditional nonlocking plates in cadaveric specimens with low bone mineral density (47). With respect to anatomically precontoured distal humerus locking plates, Stofell et al. reported significantly higher stability in compression and external rotation, and an increased resistance to axial plastic deformity when applied in a parallel orientation compared to a 90–90 orientation (48). While controversy exists over utilization of nonlocking versus locking plates, the use of one-third tubular plates is not recommended, as they have been shown to convey insufficient strength and are susceptible to breakage and failure when used as the primary two-plate construct in distal humerus fractures (49–51). The potential complications of using a one-third tubular plate as a primary plate construct were demonstrated in a retrospective study of 45 distal humerus fractures in patients over 60 years of age. In this study by Korner et al., there was a 29% postoperative complication rate with 12 cases of implant failure or screw loosening, and 58% of the cases required revision surgery. In cases where a one-third tubular plate was used for fixation of the medial column, three of the eight cases had failure and breakage of the medial plate (32).

While a one-third tubular plate is often insufficient to use independently as medial or lateral column fixation, it can be used to augment fixation as a third plate when used in conjunction with 3.5 mm reconstruction or locking plates (52–54). Kirchner wires (K-wire) have also been utilized to augment fixation of distal humerus fractures in osteoporotic bone. Molloy et al. analyzed the biomechanical properties of K-wire augmentation in cadaveric distal humerus fractures (cadavers of persons aged 75–87 years) (53). In this biomechanical study, two 2 mm K-wires were placed into the medial and lateral columns prior to applying two 3.5 mm reconstruction plates in a 90–90 orientation. The K-wire augmented fixation demonstrated significantly increased cyclic loading survival compared to controls without K-wire augmentation.

In elderly patients, distal humerus fractures with extensive comminution and poor bone quality make ORIF a less than desirable treatment option in some patients. In these instances, treatment with primary total elbow arthroplasty has been advocated (17,37,40,55,56). The results of total elbow arthroplasty for distal humerus fractures have demonstrated reproducibly satisfactory short- and mid-term outcomes. In a retrospective study by Frankle et al., 24 female patients over the age of 65 years with comminuted intra-articular distal humerus fractures were treated with either ORIF or primary total elbow arthroplasty (57). At short-term follow-up, patients in the arthroplasty group demonstrated improved outcomes compared to the ORIF group. In a more recent prospective, randomized, multicenter trial, McKee et al. also compared ORIF versus primary total elbow arthroplasty in comminuted, intra-articular distal humerus fractures in 40 patients over the age of 65 years (58). At 2-year follow-up, the patients in the total elbow arthroplasty group demonstrated improved functional outcomes based on the DASH (disabilities of the arm, shoulder, and hand) and Mayo Elbow Performance (MEPS) scores when compared to patients treated with ORIF. Analysis of short-term follow-up function scores also showed improved DASH and MEPS scores at 6 weeks and 3 months, indicating an earlier return to function in the patients who had total elbow arthroplasty. Of the 15 patients treated with ORIF, four patients required reoperation. One patient required conversion to total elbow arthroplasty for a symptomatic nonunion, two patients required reoperation for stiffness, and a single patient required ulnar neurolysis for ulnar neuropathy. Three of the 25 patients treated with total elbow arthroplasty required reoperation. The reasons for reoperation in patients treated by total elbow arthroplasty were stiffness, deep infection, and heterotopic ossification with ulnar neuropathy. Based on these findings, the authors concluded that total elbow arthroplasty for the treatment of comminuted, intra-articular distal humerus fractures is a valid and effective surgical option.

Distal radius fractures

Surgical treatment of distal radius fractures in elderly patients is controversial. Traditional treatment of distal radius fractures in elderly patients consisted of nonoperative casting; however, with the development of fixed-angle volar locking plates, there has been an increase in surgical fixation of these fractures (59). Surgical treatment of these fractures is not without potential complications. In a study comparing nonoperative to operative treatment of distal radius fractures, Egol et al. found that surgical treatment yielded equivalent functional scores to nonoperative treatment but with a higher number of complications (60). In this study, 7 surgical patients had complications, and 4 out of the 44 patients who were treated surgically required reoperations. The indications for reoperations included carpal tunnel syndrome, stiffness, prominent hardware, or persistent ulnar-sided wrist pain. Of the 4 complications reported in the 45 patients treated nonoperatively, none required surgical intervention.

A subsequent study by Lutz et al. also demonstrated the potential complications of surgical treatment of distal radius fractures in patients aged 65 years or older (61). In this study, there was a statistically significant difference in the number of patients who experienced complications after distal radius operative treatment ($n = 37/129$; 29%) when compared to patients treated nonoperatively ($n = 22/129$; 22%). Median neuropathy was the most common complication across both groups, and the second most common complication was surgical site infection. The need for surgical intervention due to a complication was also higher in the patients treated operatively when compared to the nonoperative patients.

LOWER EXTREMITY FRACTURES

Hip fractures

Hip fractures in elderly patients are one of the most common osteoporotic fractures encountered in clinical practice. The majority of these fractures are caused by low-energy trauma due to low bone mineral density in the proximal femur. Early operative intervention (less than 24 hours) is recommended for patients with hip fractures, as it has been shown to reduce the potential risk for adverse events (62,63). One of the goals of surgical treatment of hip fractures is to restore the patient to a weight-bearing as tolerated status immediately postoperatively, as this has been shown to improve patient outcomes (64,65). Based on this principle, it is recommended that surgeons select a procedure that will allow for restoration of weight-bearing status in a single surgery (66). When elderly patients require multiple procedures or revision surgeries, they often suffer significant loss of function, and the risk for complication increases.

Fortunately, many fixation options exist in the treatment of hip fractures dependent on fracture characteristics and location. With femoral neck fractures, the majority of patients are treated with either fixation or arthroplasty. Nondisplaced femoral neck fracture can be treated with multiple cancellous screws or sliding hip screw constructs. While the majority of surgeons treat these nondisplaced fractures with cancellous screws, some studies have indicated a reduction in failure and complications with the use of a sliding hip screw (67). In a randomized controlled trial by Kuokkanen et al., 33 patients with nondisplaced femoral neck fractures were treated with either cancellous screws ($n = 16$) or a sliding hip screw ($n = 17$) (68). Three of the 16 patients (19%) treated with cancellous screws had failure that required revision surgery, while none of the patients treated with a sliding hip screw required revision. Ma et al. supported this finding in a more recent systematic review where treatment with a sliding hip screw demonstrated fewer complications and faster time to union (69).

Nonunion following internal fixation of femoral neck fractures is a costly and devastating complication to both the health-care system and the patient. Numerous studies have identified fracture displacement and poor fracture reduction as the two most common factors predictive of femoral neck nonunion (70). Internal fixation in osteoporotic femoral neck fractures should be reserved for valgus impacted or minimally displaced fractures, Garden I and Garden II, respectively. Even in Garden I and Garden II

fractures, the risk for nonunion is not negligible. Kain et al. reported a 6.4% incidence of nonunion in nondisplaced osteoporotic femoral neck fractures treated with *in situ* fixation using cannulated screws, with 10% undergoing revision to total hip arthroplasty (71). This finding was supported in a second retrospective study of 52 elderly patients greater than 70 years of age treated with internal fixation for nondisplaced and impacted femoral neck fractures (72). In this study by Han et al., major complications were reported in 34.6% of patients with nonunion occurring in 15.38% of patients. Based on this study, Han and colleagues advised caution when treating Garden II femoral neck fractures with internal fixation and recommended arthroplasty be considered for elderly patients (70). An additional retrospective study by Yang et al. analyzed 202 patients with a mean age of 64 years treated with internal fixation using cannulated screws for femoral neck fractures. Nonunion was reported in 21.3% of patients treated with cannulated screws in a triangular configuration. Poor reduction and fracture displacement were identified as risk factors for nonunion.

Displaced femoral neck fractures are often treated with arthroplasty procedures given the increased rate of AVN due to disruption of blood flow to the femoral head. Treatment with internal fixation has been reported to have a failure rate above 40% at 80 years (73–76). The high rate of failure with internal fixation of displaced femoral neck fractures is most commonly attributable to nonunion and AVN (77–79). Revision surgery of failed internal fixation to arthroplasty procedures place the patient at a significantly increased risk of complications including infection, dislocation, and loosening when compared to patients treated with primary arthroplasty procedures (80).

When compared to treatment with internal fixation, primary arthroplasty procedures have been reported to be cost-effective and have a lower rate of complications (81). Hemiarthroplasty or total hip arthroplasty procedures can be performed based on patient characteristics such as health, independent activity level, functional level and cognitive level, as well as surgeon preference. Literature suggests that patients treated with total hip arthroplasty have better functional outcomes and health-quality of life when compared to patients treated with hemiarthroplasty (82).

When performing hemiarthroplasty for displaced femoral neck fractures, the surgeon can utilize either a cemented or press-fit uncemented femoral component. The use of cemented stems has been advocated in patients with osteoporosis due to poor bone quality, decreased ability for the bone-implant in-growth needed in press-fit stems, and reduced risk for intraoperative fracture. However, the use of cemented stems is not without complication. Cementing of the femoral canal is often done in a pressurized manner leading to fat embolization and potential catastrophic cardiopulmonary collapse (83). In a randomized study, DeAngelis et al. analyzed the use of cemented and uncemented stems for hemiarthroplasty in the treatment of displaced femoral neck fractures in elderly patients (84). In this study of 130 patients, cemented stems were used in

66 patients, and 64 were treated with uncemented stems. The patients treated with uncemented stems had a slightly increased rate of intraoperative fracture (4.7%) in comparison to patients treated with cemented stems (3.0%), but this difference did not reach statistical significance. Overall, there was no statistically significant difference in complication rate, mortality rate, or functional status between the two groups at 1-year follow-up. The authors concluded that the use of cemented or uncemented stems was equivocal in the setting of hemiarthroplasty for displaced femoral neck fractures in elderly patients.

Extracapsular hip fractures are among the most common hip fractures observed in elderly patients. Intertrochanteric or pertrochanteric hip fractures account for nearly half of all hip fractures observed in elderly patients (85). The most commonly used implants in the treatment of intertrochanteric hip fractures are cephalomedullary nails and compression dynamic hip screws (86). In the treatment of osteoporotic intertrochanteric hip fractures, complication rates have been estimated at 6.9%, with the most frequently encountered complications being mechanical failure and infections (87). With respect to mechanical failure and fixation failure requiring reoperation, the most commonly reported complications include nonunion, AVN of the femoral head, implant cut-out, the "Z-effect," implant fracture, detachment of the implant from the femur, as well as intraoperative and postoperative fracture. In a review by Broderick et al., the overall failure rate for osteoporotic hip fractures was reported at 41% with a reoperation rate of 45.5% for patients older than 60 years (88). While initial fracture displacement and fracture pattern stability were felt to correlate to fixation failure rates, some technical factors during surgery can help to minimize potential failure of fixation.

Lag screw cut-out is one of the most common complications and modes of failure reported with the treatment of intracapsular and extracapsular hip fractures in osteoporotic fractures. It occurs with both extramedullary and intramedullary implants. The rate of cut-out has been correlated to the tip-apex distance (TAD), which is a sum of the distances from the tip of the lag screw to the center of the femoral head as measured on anterior-posterior and lateral radiographs (89). When placed correctly, the lag-screw TAD should be less than 25 mm, as TAD higher than 25 mm has been shown to correlate with cut-out and fixation failure. Patients with TAD greater than 45 mm have been shown to have a 60% risk of cut-out (89). In a recent systematic review, Rubio-Avila et al. further analyzed the correlation between TAD and lag screw cut-out in intertrochanteric hip fractures. They concluded that the relative risk of cut-out in patients with TAD greater than 25 mm was 12.71, and the mean difference between patients with cut-out and those without cut-out was at TAD of 5.54 mm (90). In addition, a more inferior lag screw position has been reported to reduce the risk of cut-out failure. When compared to a central lag screw position, the inferior lag screw position has been suggested to confer higher axial and torsional stiffness. In a study by Kashigar et al., 77 patients

treated with cephalomedullary nails for hip fractures demonstrated no cut-out failure when the calcar-referenced tip-apex distance (CalTAD) of less than 20.98 mm was used (91). The authors concluded that a more inferior-central position was the optimal position for the lag screw.

The Z-effect and reverse Z-effect are modes of fixation failure observed in cephalomedullary nails that utilize two proximal lag screws crossing the femoral neck into the femoral head. Under physiologic loading, the inferior lag screw migrates laterally and the superior lag screw migrates medially, leading to the characteristic Z-effect. The biomechanics of this failure are not fully understood; however, it is likely due to the vertical loading of the hip causing a varus moment as well as rotational and torsional motion of the proximal fracture fragment (92). Medial cortical and calcar comminution, as well as poor bone quality, are risk factors for Z-effect failures. In an attempt to prevent this mode of failure, implants designed with static locking mechanisms of the proximal lag screws have been developed.

Nonunion of proximal femur fractures mainly occurs with femoral neck fractures and subtrochanteric femur fractures, as the excellent vascular supply of the metaphyseal cancellous bone in the intertrochanteric region provides an ideal environment for bony healing. Given its rich blood supply, nonunions of intertrochanteric hip fractures are rare, with an incidence reported between 1% and 4% (93).

Subtrochanteric hip fractures present a complex injury in elderly patients. Relatively poor vascularity and resultant decreased healing potential, increased stress concentration, and strong deforming muscular forces that can lead to malreduction are risk factors that lead to increased potential complications in elderly patients with subtrochanteric femur fractures. Collectively, the incidence of delayed union or malunion with subsequent failure of fixation has been reported to range from 7% to 20% (94–96). Similar to femoral neck fractures, additional risk factors for subtrochanteric hip fracture fixation failure include medial cortical comminution and poor fracture reduction (97).

While limited high-level evidence in research is available on subtrochanteric femur fracture complications, Gianoudis et al. reported on a small cohort of patients (14 patients) with subtrochanteric femur fracture nonunions and implant failure treated with implementation of the diamond concept (98). In this study, 11 of the 14 patients were older than 63 years. Giannoudis and colleagues identified varus malalignment as a consistent finding that predisposed patients to delayed union and implant failure. The mode of failure most commonly observed was distal screw breakage followed by breakage of the nail at the nail-lag screw junction. Based on their findings, the authors concluded that anatomical reduction is an important surgeon-dependent factor that can reduce the risk of nonunion and implant failure. They also highlighted the importance of close follow-up and early identification of distal screw breakage, as this could indicate an unstable fixation construct and prompt the surgeon to modify weight-bearing or possibly perform revision surgery (98).

Osteoporotic patients are often treated with bisphosphonate therapy for medical management of their condition. In some patients treated with long-term bisphosphonate therapy, atypical subtrochanteric femur fractures may occur. These fractures present a unique challenge to surgeons given the suppression of bone remodeling by bisphosphonates, and they differ from typical femur fractures in at least three ways: mechanism of injury, fracture location, and radiographic appearance (99,100). When compared to patients with typical femur fractures, patients with atypical femur fractures have similar postoperative outcomes including mobility, reoperation rate, postoperative complication rates, hospital length of stay, changes in independent living status, readmission rate at 4 weeks, and mortality rate at 1 year (101). While this study showed similar outcomes between patients with atypical and typical femur fractures, other studies have reported patients with atypical femur fractures have slower union rates and increased periods of immobility (102). Given the reports of slower union rates and increased periods of limited mobility, consideration of medical augmentation of fracture healing with teriparatide has been evaluated. In a study by Yeh et al., the effect of teriparatide on surgical outcomes of bisphosphonate-related atypical subtrochanteric femur fractures in osteoporotic patients was analyzed (103). Although the sample size was small (13 patients), when compared to ORIF without teriparatide, patients treated with teriparatide demonstrated more rapid time to union as well as significantly higher Harris Hip Scores and Numerical Rating Scale scores at 6 months postoperatively. The authors concluded that teriparatide treatment in patients with bisphosphonate-related atypical femur fractures aids in healing, recovery of hip function, and pain relief. After a bisphosphonate-related atypical femur fracture, medical treatment should be modified in order to discontinue the bisphosphonate therapy. In addition, this patient population should be treated with calcium and vitamin D supplementation (104).

As demonstrated by multiple studies, decreased bone density increases the risk for potential complications in the treatment of hip fractures. Augmentation of fracture fixation in the setting of hip fractures aims to reduce the risk for loss of reduction and fixation failure. The use of polymethyl methacrylate (PMMA) has gained popularity for augmentation of hip fracture fixation. Biomechanical studies have demonstrated increased bone-implant interface, improved implant anchorage, reduced screw cut-out, and improved early full weight-bearing when augmenting fracture fixation with PMMA (105,106). In a clinical study by Mattsson et al., the outcomes following the treatment of intertrochanteric hip fractures with a dynamic hip screw (DHS) augmented with either PMMA or resorbable calcium phosphate cement were compared to patients treated with DHS alone. The patients treated with cement augmentation showed greater biomechanical strength, more rapid reduction in pain, and improved healing when

compared to the control group (106). In a separate prospective analysis of 64 patients with proximal femur fractures, Gupta et al. demonstrated that DHS fixation augmented with PMMA showed good fracture consolidation without adverse complications such as avascular necrosis. The use of cement augmentation in the treatment of proximal femur fractures with intramedullary nailing has also been investigated. When compared to extramedullary fixation augmented with bone cement, PMMA-augmented intramedullary nail fixation shows increased biomechanical stability (107). Recently designed implants are incorporating cement augmentation into instrumentation. Newer implants with fenestrated lag screw designs allow for a surgeon to augment fixation with injection of bone cement into the femoral neck and head via a cannulated system. While this has been shown to offer increased biomechanical stability, future prospective randomized trials are necessary to determine if this will correlate to improved clinical outcomes.

Ankle fractures

In general, unstable ankle fractures are treated with ORIF with overall good surgical outcomes (108). In the case of an elderly patient with ankle fracture with osteoporotic bone, ankle fractures can prove challenging to treat with standard ORIF techniques due to decreased bone density and poor implant bone interface (109). Studies have demonstrated that the risk and complication profile for the surgical treatment of ankle fractures is higher in elderly patients with osteoporotic fractures (110,111). The most commonly observed complications include soft tissue and wound complications in addition to implant failure (89,112,113). More recent studies have identified medical comorbidities such as diabetes, peripheral vascular disease, and smoking as predictive factors that correlated to the development of postoperative complications after surgical treatment of ankle fractures in elderly persons (111,114,115). The increased potential for complications in elderly patients with ankle fractures was demonstrated in a large retrospective review by Aigner et al. (116). In this study, 237 patients over the age of 65 years were treated with ORIF of unstable ankle fractures. Seventy-four complications were reported for a total complication rate of 28.7%. The most common complications observed were impaired wound healing and surgical site infections. Multivariate analysis identified that the operative time was the only independent and modifiable risk factor for the development of a complication. Increased operative time as well the fracture being open increased the risk for requiring revision surgery. In this study, the presence of medical comorbidities did not directly increase the risk for complications.

Biomechanical studies have been carried out to evaluate the strongest biomechanical method of fixation and most stable implant in an attempt to optimize outcomes in the treatment of osteoporotic ankle fractures in elderly patients. One such biomechanical study was performed by

Switaj et al. using an osteoporotic cadaveric distal fibula fracture model. In this study, the authors compared modern lateral distal fibular locking plates to antiglide plates in 16 paired fresh cadavers (117). The ankle fractures were treated with either an independent lag screw and lateral distal fibular locking plate or a posterior antiglide plate with a lag screw through the plate. The lateral locking plate construct demonstrated a higher torque to failure and construct stiffness when compared to the antiglide plate construct. In the lateral locking plate group, seven of the eight failures occurred through the distal locking screws. The antiglide group failed without pullout of the distal screws and fracture displacement in six of the eight specimens. The authors concluded that the modern lateral locking plates provided a biomechanically stronger construct than a one-third tubular posterior antiglide plate construct in the setting of osteoporotic distal fibular fractures.

Given the unpredictable outcomes and the poor bone quality available for fixation in the surgical treatment of osteoporotic ankle fractures, alternative treatment options have been discussed such as tibio-talar-calcaneal (TTC) nailing. Normally utilized in ankle arthrodesis procedures resulting from ankle arthritis or Charcot arthropathy, TTC nailing is a somewhat novel technique in the treatment of osteoporotic ankle fractures. The efficacy of TTC nailing of osteoporotic ankle fractures was recently compared to that of standard ORIF in a prospective randomized controlled study by Georgiannos et al. (118). Over 6 years, 43 elderly patients (mean age 78 years) with unstable ankle fractures underwent treatment with TTC nailing, and 44 patients were treated with ORIF. The mean follow-up was 14 months, and the only statistically significant difference noted was a shorter hospital length of stay in the TTC nailing group. No intraoperative complications were reported in either group. While the differences did not reach statistical significance, the patients treated with TTC nailing trended toward a lower complication rate, lower reoperation rate, and higher rate of return to preoperative functional status. The patients in the TTC nailing group were also permitted to return to weight-bearing as tolerated status earlier than the ORIF patients. The authors concluded that TTC nailing is a safe and effective treatment alternative to ORIF in the treatment of unstable osteoporotic ankle fractures.

SPINE FRACTURES

Different from osteoporotic fractures of the upper extremity and hip, spine fragility fractures often occur without a history of fall or trauma. Studies have estimated that only 30% of osteoporotic vertebral fractures are reported, and many are found incidentally during routine imaging studies (119–122). Osteoporotic vertebral fractures, while often not diagnosed at the time of injury, are a cause of significant back pain and disability in elderly patients. Even after the initial pain from the acute vertebral fracture subsides, many patients will develop an irreversible progressive kyphotic deformity that is associated with significant decline in health (121,123–125). In addition, patients with one or more vertebral fragility fracture at baseline have a five-time increased risk for subsequent spinal fragility fractures compared to patients without vertebral fragility fractures (126). Osteoporotic spinal fractures have also been correlated with an increased risk of mortality (127–130). Using a review of U.S. Medicare claims from 1997 to 2004, Lau et al. found the overall mortality rate following a vertebral fracture was double that of matched individuals without a vertebral fracture and higher for men than women (131).

While the majority of osteoporotic vertebral fractures are initially treated nonoperatively, select groups of patients are candidates for surgical intervention. These patients often demonstrate radiculopathy, myelopathy, recalcitrant back pain, progressive spinal deformity, neurogenic claudication, and failure of conservative treatment methods (132). Several surgical treatment options exist for the treatment of osteoporotic vertebral fractures including cement augmentation procedures as well as decompression and fusion.

Cement augmentation procedures for osteoporotic vertebral lumbar and thoracic compression fractures include vertebroplasty and kyphoplasty. With both techniques, cement is injected into the fracture site to provide stability and improved pain and function. The safety and efficacy of these procedures are well documented, with nearly 90% of patients reporting at least some pain relief (133). However, as with any invasive procedure, vertebroplasty and kyphoplasty are not without potential complications. These complications include pedicle fracture during trochar insertion, dural tear, and cement leakage. Of these potential complications, PMMA cement leakage accounts for the majority of reported major complications (134,135). The complications related to cement leakage are embolism, new fractures, and neurological injury. The most common sites of cement leakage are the vertebral endplate or disc, lateral recess, paraspinal venous system, and epidural space. In a retrospective review of 292 patients treated with percutaneous vertebroplasty for osteoporotic vertebral compression fractures, Ding et al. reported cement leakage occurred in 77.7% of patients (136). No clinically significant complications related to cement leakage were reported. The authors found a strong correlation between fracture severity, cement viscosity, fracture type, cortical disruption, and the presence of a cleft on magnetic resonance imaging with the occurrence of cement leakage. In the appropriate setting, some authors advocate for early vertebroplasty intervention, as it was shown to improve pain relief and reduce the duration of bed rest (137). This in turn reduces potential complications associated with prolonged bed rest including pneumonia, deep vein thrombosis, urinary tract infection, worsening osteopenia, and deterioration of musculoskeletal function. In addition, early intervention with vertebroplasty has been shown to have a lower rate of cement leakage when compared to late vertebroplasty (137).

Embolization of cement particles can also occur with percutaneous vertebroplasty or kyphoplasty. This often occurs as a result of when small cement fragments or the cement monomer, which can polymerize in distant locations, enter into the vascular system. While rare, cases of fatal pulmonary embolism, embolization into the heart, and embolization into the brain have been reported. In a systematic review, the incidence of cardiopulmonary embolism following percutaneous cement augmentation of osteoporotic vertebral compression fractures ranged from 2% to 26% depending on the diagnostic screening method utilized (138). The majority of the emboli in this study were symptomatic, causing obstruction in the pulmonary arterial circulation as well as the right heart. Embolization of bone marrow fat can also occur during vertebroplasty causing transient hemodynamic changes.

Adjacent level fracture is also a complication related to cement augmentation of osteoporotic vertebral compression fractures. Following cement augmentation of a fracture, the increased stiffness at the level of augmentation leads to increased loads at the adjacent vertebral levels. This increases the risk for adjacent level vertebral fractures.

When indicated, open decompression and fusion of osteoporotic spine pathology present a challenge to surgeons. Obtaining optimal hardware fixation in the spine of osteoporotic patients is technically demanding. In addition, elderly patients with osteoporosis have been reported to have higher complication rates and decreased ability to fuse, with fusion rates reported as low as 56% (139). These findings were supported in a 2016 study by Fromby et al. (140). In this study, Fromby and colleagues compared clinical outcomes following transforaminal lumbar interbody fusion (TLIF) in patients with and without osteoporosis ($n = 18$ patients with osteoporosis, $n = 70$ patients without osteoporosis). The complication rate was significantly higher in the patients with osteoporosis when compared to those without osteoporosis. The patients with osteoporosis had a 72.2% rate of subsidence compared to a 45.7% rate of subsidence in patients without osteoporosis. The patients with osteoporosis also demonstrated a higher rate of iatrogenic fracture when compared to the patients without osteoporosis, 16.7% and 1.4%, respectively. Last, the rate of radiographic complication was higher in the osteoporotic patients (77.8%) when compared to the patients without osteoporosis (48.6%). While the overall rate of complications was higher in patients with osteoporosis, there was no significant difference in the need for revision surgery between the two patient groups.

Surgical complications in the treatment of the osteoporotic spine are not isolated to the lumbar or thoracic spine. Complications of surgical interventions on the cervical spine have also been reported to be higher in patients with osteoporosis when compared to patients without osteoporosis. In a 2016 retrospective database analysis by Guzman et al., the effects of osteoporosis on complications and patient outcomes following cervical spine surgery were evaluated (141). The analysis of 1,602,129 patients found 2% (32,557 patients) had osteoporosis. This cohort of osteoporotic patients was more likely to undergo posterior cervical spine fusion than patients without osteoporosis and three times more likely to undergo circumferential fusion. Adjusted complication rates showed that osteoporotic patients were at increased risk for postoperative hemorrhage, increased length of hospital stay, and a 30% increased cost of hospitalization. In addition, patients with osteoporosis demonstrated significantly increased odds of requiring revision surgery compared to patients without osteoporosis.

Surgical treatment of osteoporotic spine fractures is associated with a higher complication rate when compared to patients without osteoporosis. These complications include medical-related issues such as pneumonia, urinary tract infections, as well as the side effects related to narcotic pain medication usage. In addition, the disadvantageous biomechanical environment of osteoporotic bone increases the risk for fixation and instrumentation failure, implant and graft subsidence, and adjacent level fracture. Complications such as these have been reported in up to 70% of patients (142). Cement augmentation can potentially increase the biomechanical stability of pedicle screw fixation, resulting in a decreased rate of instrumentation failure. While this technique may provide improved outcomes in the treatment of osteoporotic vertebral fractures, additional studies of cement augmentation of pedicle screws is necessary to further evaluate the efficacy of this technique.

MEDICAL COMPLICATIONS

Complications of surgical treatment of patients with osteoporotic fractures are not all related to surgical technique or specific to the surgical procedure. Often complications occur after surgery from medical illness or preexisting medical comorbidities, with 1-year mortality rates after hip fracture reported as high as 36% (143,144). A systematic review by Ali et al. analyzed predictors of 30-day hospital readmission after hip fractures. In this study, they demonstrated that readmissions for medical causes were significantly more common than surgical complications, with pneumonia being the most common reason for readmission. Older age, preexisting respiratory disease, and neurological disorders such as dementia were also strong risk factors for complications and 30-day hospital readmission (145).

Preexisting medical comorbidities are predictive of postoperative complications and potential mortality in patients undergoing surgical treatment for osteoporotic fractures such as hip fractures. In a 2017 prospective study by Bliemel et al., preexisting medical comorbidities including renal disease, neurological disease, gastrointestinal disease, cardiovascular disease, and respiratory disease were all found to increase the risk of postoperative complications and mortality (146). In the acute setting and during medium-duration follow-up, preexisting renal and neurological diseases demonstrated the most significant impact on functional outcomes and mortality rates. Increased mortality rates during medium-term follow-up were also correlated to preexisting neurological, renal, pulmonary, and gastrointestinal disease (146).

Postoperative delirium is a common and costly life-threatening complication observed after both elective and emergent surgeries in older patients. The incidence of postoperative delirium has been estimated to occur in 7%–10% of older patients undergoing elective surgery and up to 50% of patients undergoing unplanned urgent and emergent surgeries (147–151). Patients with delirium have been shown to have increased hospital length of stay, increased disability, a higher need for skilled nursing care, and increased mortality within 1 year of surgery (152–154). Given the significant risk for complications that delirium presents to patients, minimizing potential risk factors for delirium is instrumental in care. When possible, reducing risk factors for delirium such as sensory impairment, polypharmacy, alcohol consumption, the use of psychoactive drugs, and poor baseline function will reduce the likelihood of postoperative delirium (155). In addition, screening patients for delirium risk factors will help care providers identify patients at increased risk for this potentially devastating postoperative complication.

CONCLUSION

Osteoporotic fractures present a unique and challenging problem for orthopedic surgeons. Given the decreased bone quality and bone metabolism, the risk for fixation failure is higher than in patients with normal bone density. In addition, patients with osteoporotic fractures often have preexisting medical comorbidities that increase the risk for both surgical and nonsurgical medically related complications and mortality. Given these factors, surgical treatment of these fractures must be performed in a time-efficient and technically sound manner that accounts for patient comorbidities over the entire spectrum of care to reduce potential complications.

REFERENCES

1. Burge R, Dawson-Hughes B, Solomon DH, Wong JB, King A, Tosteson A. Incidence and economic burden of osteoporosis-related fractures in the United States, 2005–2025. *J Bone Miner Res.* 2007;22(3):465–75.
2. Cooper C, Campion G, Melton LJ 3rd,. Hip fractures in the elderly: A world-wide projection. *Osteoporos Int.* 1992;2(6):285–9.
3. Bell JE, Leung BC, Spratt KF, Koval KJ, Weinstein JD, Goodman DC, Tosteson AN. Trends and variation in incidence, surgical treatment, and repeat surgery of proximal humeral fractures in the elderly. *J Bone Joint Surg Am.* 2011;93(2):121–31.
4. Aaron D, Shatsky J, Paredes JC, Jiang C, Parsons BO, Flatow EL. Proximal humeral fractures: Internal fixation. *J Bone Joint Surg Am.* 2012;94(24):2280–8.
5. Kannus P, Palvanen M, Niemi S, Parkkari J, Jarvinen M, Vuori I. Increasing number and incidence of osteoporotic fractures of the proximal humerus in elderly people. *BMJ.* 1996;313(7064):1051–2.
6. Calvo E, de Miguel I, de la Cruz JJ, Lopez-Martin N. Percutaneous fixation of displaced proximal humeral fractures: Indications based on the correlation between clinical and radiographic results. *J Shoulder Elbow Surg.* 2007;16(6):774–81.
7. Magovern B, Ramsey ML. Percutaneous fixation of proximal humerus fractures. *Orthop Clin North Am.* 2008;39(4):405–16, v.
8. Lyons FA, Rockwood CA Jr,. Migration of pins used in operations on the shoulder. *J Bone Joint Surg Am.* 1990;72(8):1262–7.
9. Sproul RC, Iyengar JJ, Devcic Z, Feeley BT. A systematic review of locking plate fixation of proximal humerus fractures. *Injury.* 2011;42(4):408–13.
10. Namdari S, Voleti PB, Mehta S. Evaluation of the osteoporotic proximal humeral fracture and strategies for structural augmentation during surgical treatment. *J Shoulder Elbow Surg.* 2012;21(12):1787–95.
11. Agudelo J, Schurmann M, Stahel P et al. Analysis of efficacy and failure in proximal humerus fractures treated with locking plates. *J Orthop Trauma.* 2007;21(10):676–81.
12. Schliemann B, Siemoneit J, Theisen C, Kosters C, Weimann A, Raschke MJ. Complex fractures of the proximal humerus in the elderly—Outcome and complications after locking plate fixation. *Musculoskelet Surg.* 2012;96(Suppl 1):S3–11.
13. Thanasas C, Kontakis G, Angoules A, Limb D, Giannoudis P. Treatment of proximal humerus fractures with locking plates: A systematic review. *J Shoulder Elbow Surg.* 2009;18(6):837–44.
14. Micic ID, Kim KC, Shin DJ et al. Analysis of early failure of the locking compression plate in osteoporotic proximal humerus fractures. *J Orthop Sci.* 2009;14(5):596–601.
15. Owsley KC, Gorczyca JT. Fracture displacement and screw cutout after open reduction and locked plate fixation of proximal humeral fractures [corrected]. *J Bone Joint Surg Am.* 2008;90(2):233–40.
16. Bae JH, Oh JK, Chon CS, Oh CW, Hwang JH, Yoon YC. The biomechanical performance of locking plate fixation with intramedullary fibular strut graft augmentation in the treatment of unstable fractures of the proximal humerus. *J Bone Joint Surg Br.* 2011;93(7):937–41.
17. Chow RM, Begum F, Beaupre LA, Carey JP, Adeeb S, Bouliane MJ. Proximal humeral fracture fixation: Locking plate construct ± intramedullary fibular allograft. *J Shoulder Elbow Surg.* 2012;21(7):894–901.
18. Gardner MJ, Collinge C. Management principles of osteoporotic fractures. *Injury.* 2016;47(Suppl 2):S33–5.
19. Neviaser AS, Hettrich CM, Beamer BS, Dines JS, Lorich DG. Endosteal strut augment reduces complications

associated with proximal humeral locking plates. *Clin Orthop Relat Res.* 2011;469(12):3300–6.

20. Egol KA, Sugi MT, Ong CC, Montero N, Davidovitch R, Zuckerman JD. Fracture site augmentation with calcium phosphate cement reduces screw penetration after open reduction-internal fixation of proximal humeral fractures. *J Shoulder Elbow Surg.* 2012;21(6):741–8.

21. Gradl G, Knobe M, Stoffel M, Prescher A, Dirrichs T, Pape HC. Biomechanical evaluation of locking plate fixation of proximal humeral fractures augmented with calcium phosphate cement. *J Orthop Trauma.* 2013;27(7):399–404.

22. Somasundaram K, Huber CP, Babu V, Zadeh H. Proximal humeral fractures: The role of calcium sulphate augmentation and extended deltoid splitting approach in internal fixation using locking plates. *Injury.* 2013;44(4):481–7.

23. Zhang L, Zheng J, Wang W et al. The clinical benefit of medial support screws in locking plating of proximal humerus fractures: A prospective randomized study. *Int Orthop.* 2011;35(11):1655–61.

24. Tingart MJ, Lehtinen J, Zurakowski D, Warner JJ, Apreleva M. Proximal humeral fractures: Regional differences in bone mineral density of the humeral head affect the fixation strength of cancellous screws. *J Shoulder Elbow Surg.* 2006;15(5):620–4.

25. Brianza S, Roderer G, Schiuma D et al. Where do locking screws purchase in the humeral head? *Injury.* 2012;43(6):850–5.

26. Hepp P, Lill H, Bail H et al. Where should implants be anchored in the humeral head? *Clin Orthop Relat Res.* 2003; (415):139–47.

27. Liew AS, Johnson JA, Patterson SD, King GJ, Chess DG. Effect of screw placement on fixation in the humeral head. *J Shoulder Elbow Surg.* 2000;9(5):423–6.

28. Erhardt JB, Stoffel K, Kampshoff J, Badur N, Yates P, Kuster MS. The position and number of screws influence screw perforation of the humeral head in modern locking plates: A cadaver study. *J Orthop Trauma.* 2012;26(10):e188–92.

29. Hausman M, Panozzo A. Treatment of distal humerus fractures in the elderly. *Clin Orthop Relat Res.* 2004; 425:55–63.

30. Huang TL, Chiu FY, Chuang TY, Chen TH. The results of open reduction and internal fixation in elderly patients with severe fractures of the distal humerus: A critical analysis of the results. *J Trauma.* 2005;58(1):62–9.

31. John H, Rosso R, Neff U, Bodoky A, Regazzoni P, Harder F. [Distal humerus fractures in patients over 75 years of age. Long-term results of osteosynthesis]. *Helv Chir Acta.* 1993;60(1–2):219–24.

32. Korner J, Lill H, Muller LP et al. Distal humerus fractures in elderly patients: Results after open reduction and internal fixation. *Osteoporos Int.* 2005;16 Suppl 2:S73–9.

33. Letsch R, Schmit-Neuerburg KP, Sturmer KM, Walz M. Intraarticular fractures of the distal humerus. Surgical treatment and results. *Clin Orthop Relat Res.* 1989 (241):238–44.

34. O'Driscoll SW, Sanchez-Sotelo J, Torchia ME. Management of the smashed distal humerus. *Orthop Clin North Am.* 2002;33(1):19–33, vii.

35. Pereles TR, Koval KJ, Gallagher M, Rosen H. Open reduction and internal fixation of the distal humerus: Functional outcome in the elderly. *J Trauma.* 1997; 43(4):578–84.

36. Cobb TK, Morrey BF. Total elbow arthroplasty as primary treatment for distal humeral fractures in elderly patients. *J Bone Joint Surg Am.* 1997;79(6):826–32.

37. Kamineni S, Morrey BF. Distal humeral fractures treated with noncustom total elbow replacement. *J Bone Joint Surg Am.* 2004;86-A(5):940–7.

38. Kamineni S, Morrey BF. Distal humeral fractures treated with noncustom total elbow replacement. Surgical technique. *J Bone Joint Surg Am.* 2005;87(Suppl 1, Pt 1):41–50.

39. Morrey BF. Fractures of the distal humerus: Role of elbow replacement. *Orthop Clin North Am.* 2000;31(1):145–54.

40. Muller LP, Kamineni S, Rommens PM, Morrey BF. Primary total elbow replacement for fractures of the distal humerus. *Oper Orthop Traumatol.* 2005;17(2):119–42.

41. Ray PS, Kakarlapudi K, Rajsekhar C, Bhamra MS. Total elbow arthroplasty as primary treatment for distal humeral fractures in elderly patients. *Injury.* 2000;31(9):687–92.

42. Helfet DL, Hotchkiss RN. Internal fixation of the distal humerus: A biomechanical comparison of methods. *J Orthop Trauma.* 1990;4(3):260–4.

43. Schemitsch EH, Tencer AF, Henley MB. Biomechanical evaluation of methods of internal fixation of the distal humerus. *J Orthop Trauma.* 1994;8(6):468–75.

44. Self J, Viegas SF, Buford WL, Jr., Patterson RM. A comparison of double-plate fixation methods for complex distal humerus fractures. *J Shoulder Elbow Surg.* 1995;4(1 Pt 1):10–6.

45. Strauss EJ, Alaia M, Egol KA. Management of distal humeral fractures in the elderly. *Injury.* 2007;38(Suppl 3):S10–6.

46. Berkes M, Garrigues G, Solic J et al. Locking and nonlocking constructs achieve similar radiographic and clinical outcomes for internal fixation of intra-articular distal humerus fractures. *HSS J.* 2011;7(3):244–50.

47. Schuster I, Korner J, Arzdorf M, Schwieger K, Diederichs G, Linke B. Mechanical comparison in cadaver specimens of three different 90-degree double-plate osteosyntheses for simulated C2-type distal humerus fractures with varying bone densities. *J Orthop Trauma.* 2008;22(2):113–20.

48. Stoffel K, Cunneen S, Morgan R, Nicholls R, Stachowiak G. Comparative stability of perpendicular versus parallel double-locking plating systems in osteoporotic comminuted distal humerus fractures. *J Orthop Res.* 2008;26(6):778–84.

49. O'Driscoll SW. Optimizing stability in distal humeral fracture fixation. *J Shoulder Elbow Surg.* 2005;14(1 Suppl S):186S–94S.

50. O'Driscoll SW. Supracondylar fractures of the elbow: Open reduction, internal fixation. *Hand Clin.* 2004;20(4):465–74.

51. Tyllianakis M, Panagopoulos A, Papadopoulos AX, Kaisidis A, Zouboulis P. Functional evaluation of comminuted intra-articular fractures of the distal humerus (AO type C). Long term results in twenty-six patients. *Acta Orthop Belg.* 2004;70(2):123–30.

52. Korner J, Lill H, Muller LP, Rommens PM, Schneider E, Linke B. The LCP-concept in the operative treatment of distal humerus fractures—Biological, biomechanical and surgical aspects. *Injury.* 2003;34(Suppl 2):B20–30.

53. Molloy S, Jasper LE, Burkhart BG, Brumback RJ, Belkoff SM. Interference Kirschner wires augment distal humeral fracture fixation in the elderly. *J Orthop Trauma.* 2005;19(6):377–9.

54. Ring D, Jupiter JB. Complex fractures of the distal humerus and their complications. *J Shoulder Elbow Surg.* 1999;8(1):85–97.

55. Caja VL, Moroni A, Vendemia V, Sabato C, Zinghi G. Surgical treatment of bicondylar fractures of the distal humerus. *Injury.* 1994;25(7):433–8.

56. Garcia JA, Mykula R, Stanley D. Complex fractures of the distal humerus in the elderly. The role of total elbow replacement as primary treatment. *J Bone Joint Surg Br.* 2002;84(6):812–6.

57. Frankle MA, Herscovici D, Jr., DiPasquale TG, Vasey MB, Sanders RW. A comparison of open reduction and internal fixation and primary total elbow arthroplasty in the treatment of intraarticular distal humerus fractures in women older than age 65. *J Orthop Trauma.* 2003;17(7):473–80.

58. McKee MD, Veillette CJ, Hall JA et al. A multicenter, prospective, randomized, controlled trial of open reduction—Internal fixation versus total elbow arthroplasty for displaced intra-articular distal humeral fractures in elderly patients. *J Shoulder Elbow Surg.* 2009;18(1):3–12.

59. Chung KC, Shauver MJ, Birkmeyer JD. Trends in the United States in the treatment of distal radial fractures in the elderly. *J Bone Joint Surg Am.* 2009;91(8):1868–73.

60. Egol KA, Walsh M, Romo-Cardoso S, Dorsky S, Paksima N. Distal radial fractures in the elderly: Operative compared with nonoperative treatment. *J Bone Joint Surg Am.* 2010;92(9):1851–7.

61. Lutz K, Yeoh KM, MacDermid JC, Symonette C, Grewal R. Complications associated with operative versus nonsurgical treatment of distal radius fractures in patients aged 65 years and older. *J Hand Surg Am.* 2014;39(7):1280–6.

62. Friedman SM, Mendelson DA, Bingham KW, Kates SL. Impact of a comanaged Geriatric Fracture Center on short-term hip fracture outcomes. *Arch Intern Med.* 2009;169(18):1712–7.

63. Simunovic N, Devereaux PJ, Sprague S et al. Effect of early surgery after hip fracture on mortality and complications: Systematic review and meta-analysis. *CMAJ.* 2010;182(15):1609–16.

64. Koval KJ, Friend KD, Aharonoff GB, Zukerman JD. Weight bearing after hip fracture: A prospective series of 596 geriatric hip fracture patients. *J Orthop Trauma.* 1996;10(8):526–30.

65. Koval KJ, Sala DA, Kummer FJ, Zuckerman JD. Postoperative weight-bearing after a fracture of the femoral neck or an intertrochanteric fracture. *J Bone Joint Surg Am.* 1998;80(3):352–6.

66. Bukata SV, Kates SL, O'Keefe RJ. Short-term and long-term orthopaedic issues in patients with fragility fractures. *Clin Orthop Relat Res.* 2011;469(8):2225–36.

67. Bhandari M, Tornetta P, 3rd, Hanson B, Swiontkowski MF. Optimal internal fixation for femoral neck fractures: Multiple screws or sliding hip screws? *J Orthop Trauma.* 2009;23(6):403–7.

68. Kuokkanen H, Korkala O, Antti-Poika I, Tolonen J, Lehtimaki MY, Silvennoinen T. Three cancellous bone screws versus a screw-angle plate in the treatment of Garden I and II fractures of the femoral neck. *Acta Orthop Belg.* 1991;57(1):53–7.

69. Ma JX, Kuang MJ, Xing F et al. Sliding hip screw versus cannulated cancellous screws for fixation of femoral neck fracture in adults: A systematic review. *Int J Surg.* 2018;52:89–97.

70. Yang JJ, Lin LC, Chao KH et al. Risk factors for nonunion in patients with intracapsular femoral neck fractures treated with three cannulated screws placed in either a triangle or an inverted triangle configuration. *J Bone Joint Surg Am.* 2013;95(1):61–9.

71. Kain MS, Marcantonio AJ, Iorio R. Revision surgery occurs frequently after percutaneous fixation of stable femoral neck fractures in elderly patients. *Clin Orthop Relat Res.* 2014;472(12):4010–4.

72. Han SK, Song HS, Kim R, Kang SH. Clinical results of treatment of garden type 1 and 2 femoral neck fractures in patients over 70-year old. *Eur J Trauma Emerg Surg.* 2016;42(2):191–6.

73. Rogmark C, Carlsson A, Johnell O, Sernbo I. A prospective randomised trial of internal fixation versus arthroplasty for displaced fractures of the neck of the femur. Functional outcome for 450 patients at two years. *J Bone Joint Surg Br.* 2002;84(2):183–8.

74. Keating JF, Grant A, Masson M, Scott NW, Forbes JF. Randomized comparison of reduction and fixation, bipolar hemiarthroplasty, and total hip arthroplasty. Treatment of displaced intracapsular hip fractures in healthy older patients. *J Bone Joint Surg Am.* 2006;88(2):249–60.

75. Barnes R, Brown JT, Garden RS, Nicoll EA. Subcapital fractures of the femur. A prospective review. *J Bone Joint Surg Br.* 1976;58(1):2–4.

76. Heetveld MJ, Raaymakers EL, Luitse JS, Nijhof M, Gouma DJ. Femoral neck fractures: Can physiologic status determine treatment choice? *Clin Orthop Relat Res.* 2007;461:203–12.

77. Bhandari M, Devereaux PJ, Swiontkowski MF et al. Internal fixation compared with arthroplasty for displaced fractures of the femoral neck. A meta-analysis. *J Bone Joint Surg Am*. 2003;85-A(9):1673–81.

78. Masson M, Parker MJ, Fleischer S. Internal fixation versus arthroplasty for intracapsular proximal femoral fractures in adults. *Cochrane Database Syst Rev*. 2003(2):CD001708.

79. Lu-Yao GL, Keller RB, Littenberg B, Wennberg JE. Outcomes after displaced fractures of the femoral neck. A meta-analysis of one hundred and six published reports. *J Bone Joint Surg Am*. 1994;76(1):15–25.

80. McKinley JC, Robinson CM. Treatment of displaced intracapsular hip fractures with total hip arthroplasty: Comparison of primary arthroplasty with early salvage arthroplasty after failed internal fixation. *J Bone Joint Surg Am*. 2002;84-A(11):2010–5.

81. Heetveld MJ, Rogmark C, Frihagen F, Keating J. Internal fixation versus arthroplasty for displaced femoral neck fractures: What is the evidence? *J Orthop Trauma*. 2009;23(6):395–402.

82. Blomfeldt R, Tornkvist H, Eriksson K, Soderqvist A, Ponzer S, Tidermark J. A randomised controlled trial comparing bipolar hemiarthroplasty with total hip replacement for displaced intracapsular fractures of the femoral neck in elderly patients. *J Bone Joint Surg Br*. 2007;89(2):160–5.

83. Pitto RP, Blunk J, Kossler M. Transesophageal echocardiography and clinical features of fat embolism during cemented total hip arthroplasty. A randomized study in patients with a femoral neck fracture. *Arch Orthop Trauma Surg*. 2000;120(1–2):53–8.

84. Deangelis JP, Ademi A, Staff I, Lewis CG. Cemented versus uncemented hemiarthroplasty for displaced femoral neck fractures: A prospective randomized trial with early follow-up. *J Orthop Trauma*. 2012;26(3):135–40.

85. Koval KJ, Aharonoff GB, Rokito AS, Lyon T, Zuckerman JD. Patients with femoral neck and intertrochanteric fractures. Are they the same? *Clin Orthop Relat Res*. 1996;330:166–72.

86. Aros B, Tosteson AN, Gottlieb DJ, Koval KJ. Is a sliding hip screw or im nail the preferred implant for intertrochanteric fracture fixation? *Clin Orthop Relat Res*. 2008;466(11):2827–32.

87. Tsang ST, Aitken SA, Golay SK, Silverwood RK, Biant LC. When does hip fracture surgery fail? *Injury*. 2014;45(7):1059–65.

88. Broderick JM, Bruce-Brand R, Stanley E, Mulhall KJ. Osteoporotic hip fractures: The burden of fixation failure. *Sci World J*. 2013;2013:515197.

89. Baumgaertner MR, Curtin SL, Lindskog DM, Keggi JM. The value of the tip-apex distance in predicting failure of fixation of peritrochanteric fractures of the hip. *J Bone Joint Surg Am*. 1995;77(7):1058–64.

90. Rubio-Avila J, Madden K, Simunovic N, Bhandari M. Tip to apex distance in femoral intertrochanteric fractures: A systematic review. *J Orthop Sci*. 2013;18(4):592–8.

91. Kuzyk PR, Zdero R, Shah S, Olsen M, Waddell JP, Schemitsch EH. Femoral head lag screw position for cephalomedullary nails: A biomechanical analysis. *J Orthop Trauma*. 2012;26(7):414–21.

92. Strauss EJ, Kummer FJ, Koval KJ, Egol KA. The "Z-effect" phenomenon defined: A laboratory study. *J Orthop Res*. 2007;25(12):1568–73.

93. Talmo CT, Bono JV. Treatment of intertrochanteric nonunion of the proximal femur using the S-ROM prosthesis. *Orthopedics*. 2008;31(2):125.

94. Craig NJ, Sivaji C, Maffulli N. Subtrochanteric fractures. A review of treatment options. *Bull Hosp Jt Dis*. 2001;60(1):35–46.

95. Sims SH. Subtrochanteric femur fractures. *Orthop Clin North Am*. 2002;33(1):113–26, viii.

96. de Vries JS, Kloen P, Borens O, Marti RK, Helfet DL. Treatment of subtrochanteric nonunions. *Injury*. 2006;37(2):203–11.

97. Yoon RS, Donegan DJ, Liporace FA. Reducing subtrochanteric femur fractures: Tips and tricks, do's and don'ts. *J Orthop Trauma*. 2015;29(Suppl 4):S28–33.

98. Giannoudis PV, Ahmad MA, Mineo GV, Tosounidis TI, Calori GM, Kanakaris NK. Subtrochanteric fracture non-unions with implant failure managed with the "Diamond" concept. *Injury*. 2013;44(Suppl 1):S76–81.

99. Shane E, Burr D, Ebeling PR et al. Atypical subtrochanteric and diaphyseal femoral fractures: Report of a task force of the American Society for Bone and Mineral Research. *J Bone Miner Res*. 2010;25(11):2267–94.

100. Shane E, Burr D, Abrahamsen B et al. Atypical subtrochanteric and diaphyseal femoral fractures: Second report of a task force of the American Society for Bone and Mineral Research. *J Bone Miner Res*. 2014;29(1):1–23.

101. Khow KS, Paterson F, Shibu P, Yu SC, Chehade MJ, Visvanathan R. Outcomes between older adults with atypical and typical femoral fractures are comparable. *Injury*. 2017;48(2):394–8.

102. Teo BJ, Koh JS, Goh SK, Png MA, Chua DT, Howe TS. Post-operative outcomes of atypical femoral subtrochanteric fracture in patients on bisphosphonate therapy. *Bone Joint J*. 2014;96-B(5):658–64.

103. Yeh WL, Su CY, Chang CW et al. Surgical outcome of atypical subtrochanteric and femoral fracture related to bisphosphonates use in osteoporotic patients with or without teriparatide treatment. *BMC Musculoskelet Disord*. 2017;18(1):527.

104. Feron JM, Cambon-Binder A. Medication management after intramedullary nailing of atypical fractures. *Injury*. 2017;48(Suppl 1):S15–7.

105. Kammerlander C, Erhart S, Doshi H, Gosch M, Blauth M. Principles of osteoporotic fracture treatment. *Best Pract Res Clin Rheumatol*. 2013;27(6):757–69.

106. Mattsson P, Alberts A, Dahlberg G, Sohlman M, Hyldahl HC, Larsson S. Resorbable cement for the augmentation of internally-fixed unstable trochanteric fractures. A prospective, randomised multicentre study. *J Bone Joint Surg Br*. 2005;87(9):1203–9.

107. Moroni A, Larsson S, Hoang Kim A, Gelsomini L, Giannoudis PV. Can we improve fixation and outcomes? Use of bone substitutes. *J Orthop Trauma*. 2009;23(6):422–5.

108. Ali MS, McLaren CA, Rouholamin E, O'Connor BT. Ankle fractures in the elderly: Nonoperative or operative treatment. *J Orthop Trauma*. 1987;1(4): 275–80.

109. Michelson JD. Fractures about the ankle. *J Bone Joint Surg Am*. 1995;77(1):142–52.

110. Carragee EJ, Csongradi JJ, Bleck EE. Early complications in the operative treatment of ankle fractures. Influence of delay before operation. *J Bone Joint Surg Br*. 1991;73(1):79–82.

111. Zaghloul A, Haddad B, Barksfield R, Davis B. Early complications of surgery in operative treatment of ankle fractures in those over 60: A review of 186 cases. *Injury*. 2014;45(4):780–3.

112. Crist BD, Ferguson T, Murtha YM, Lee MA. Surgical timing of treating injured extremities. *J Bone Joint Surg Am*. 2012;94(16):1514–24.

113. Barquet A, Mayora G, Guimaraes JM, Suarez R, Giannoudis PV. Avascular necrosis of the femoral head following trochanteric fractures in adults: A systematic review. *Injury*. 2014;45(12):1848–58.

114. Costigan W, Thordarson DB, Debnath UK. Operative management of ankle fractures in patients with diabetes mellitus. *Foot Ankle Int*. 2007;28(1):32–7.

115. Ovaska MT, Makinen TJ, Madanat R et al. Risk factors for deep surgical site infection following operative treatment of ankle fractures. *J Bone Joint Surg Am*. 2013;95(4):348–53.

116. Aigner R, Salomia C, Lechler P, Pahl R, Frink M. Relationship of prolonged operative time and comorbidities with complications after geriatric ankle fractures. *Foot Ankle Int*. 2017;38(1):41–8.

117. Switaj PJ, Wetzel RJ, Jain NP et al. Comparison of modern locked plating and antiglide plating for fixation of osteoporotic distal fibular fractures. *Foot Ankle Surg*. 2016;22(3):158–63.

118. Georgiannos D, Lampridis V, Bisbinas I. Fragility fractures of the ankle in the elderly: Open reduction and internal fixation versus tibio-talo-calcaneal nailing: Short-term results of a prospective randomized-controlled study. *Injury*. 2017;48(2):519–24.

119. Cooper C, Atkinson EJ, O'Fallon WM, Melton LJ 3rd,. Incidence of clinically diagnosed vertebral fractures: A population-based study in Rochester, Minnesota, 1985–1989. *J Bone Miner Res*. 1992;7(2):221–7.

120. Svedbom A, Alvares L, Cooper C, Marsh D, Strom O. Balloon kyphoplasty compared to vertebroplasty and nonsurgical management in patients hospitalised with acute osteoporotic vertebral compression fracture: A UK cost-effectiveness analysis. *Osteoporos Int*. 2013;24(1):355–67.

121. Nevitt MC, Ettinger B, Black DM et al. The association of radiographically detected vertebral fractures with back pain and function: A prospective study. *Ann Intern Med*. 1998;128(10):793–800.

122. Black DM, Cummings SR, Karpf DB et al. Randomised trial of effect of alendronate on risk of fracture in women with existing vertebral fractures. Fracture Intervention Trial Research Group. *Lancet*. 1996;348(9041):1535–41.

123. Hallberg I, Rosenqvist AM, Kartous L, Lofman O, Wahlstrom O, Toss G. Health-related quality of life after osteoporotic fractures. *Osteoporos Int*. 2004;15(10):834–41.

124. Silverman SL, Minshall ME, Shen W, Harper KD, Xie S, Health-Related Quality of Life Subgroup of the Multiple Outcomes of Raloxifene Evaluation S. The relationship of health-related quality of life to prevalent and incident vertebral fractures in postmenopausal women with osteoporosis: Results from the Multiple Outcomes of Raloxifene Evaluation Study. *Arthritis Rheum*. 2001;44(11):2611–9.

125. Sinaki M, Brey RH, Hughes CA, Larson DR, Kaufman KR. Balance disorder and increased risk of falls in osteoporosis and kyphosis: Significance of kyphotic posture and muscle strength. *Osteoporos Int*. 2005;16(8):1004–10.

126. Lindsay R, Burge RT, Strauss DM. One year outcomes and costs following a vertebral fracture. *Osteoporos Int*. 2005;16(1):78–85.

127. Edidin AA, Ong KL, Lau E, Kurtz SM. Mortality risk for operated and nonoperated vertebral fracture patients in the medicare population. *J Bone Miner Res*. 2011;26(7):1617–26.

128. Hasserius R, Karlsson MK, Nilsson BE, Redlund-Johnell I, Johnell O, European Vertebral Osteoporosis S. Prevalent vertebral deformities predict increased mortality and increased fracture rate in both men and women: A 10-year population-based study of 598 individuals from the Swedish cohort in the European Vertebral Osteoporosis Study. *Osteoporos Int*. 2003;14(1):61–8.

129. Ross PD, Davis JW, Epstein RS, Wasnich RD. Pre-existing fractures and bone mass predict vertebral fracture incidence in women. *Ann Intern Med*. 1991;114(11):919–23.

130. Pongchaiyakul C, Nguyen ND, Jones G, Center JR, Eisman JA, Nguyen TV. Asymptomatic vertebral deformity as a major risk factor for subsequent fractures and mortality: A long-term prospective study. *J Bone Miner Res*. 2005;20(8):1349–55.

131. Lau E, Ong K, Kurtz S, Schmier J, Edidin A. Mortality following the diagnosis of a vertebral compression fracture in the Medicare population. *J Bone Joint Surg Am*. 2008;90(7):1479–86.

132. Lehman RA, Jr., Kang DG, Wagner SC. Management of osteoporosis in spine surgery. *J Am Acad Orthop Surg*. 2015;23(4):253–63.

133. Hulme PA, Krebs J, Ferguson SJ, Berlemann U. Vertebroplasty and kyphoplasty: A systematic review of 69 clinical studies. *Spine (Phila Pa 1976)*. 2006;31(17):1983–2001.

134. Murphy KJ, Deramond H. Percutaneous vertebroplasty in benign and malignant disease. *Neuroimaging Clin N Am*. 2000;10(3):535–45.

135. Cotten A, Boutry N, Cortet B et al. Percutaneous vertebroplasty: State of the art. *Radiographics.* 1998;18(2):311–20; discussion 320–3.

136. Ding J, Zhang Q, Zhu J et al. Risk factors for predicting cement leakage following percutaneous vertebroplasty for osteoporotic vertebral compression fractures. *Eur Spine J.* 2016;25(11):3411–7.

137. Yang EZ, Xu JG, Huang GZ et al. Percutaneous vertebroplasty versus conservative treatment in aged patients with acute osteoporotic vertebral compression fractures: A prospective randomized controlled clinical study. *Spine (Phila Pa 1976).* 2016;41(8):653–60.

138. Wang LJ, Yang HL, Shi YX, Jiang WM, Chen L. Pulmonary cement embolism associated with percutaneous vertebroplasty or kyphoplasty: A systematic review. *Orthop Surg.* 2012;4(3):182–9.

139. Park SB, Chung CK. Strategies of spinal fusion on osteoporotic spine. *J Korean Neurosurg Soc.* 2011;49(6):317–22.

140. Formby PM, Kang DG, Helgeson MD, Wagner SC. Clinical and radiographic outcomes of transforaminal lumbar interbody fusion in patients with osteoporosis. *Global Spine J.* 2016;6(7):660–4.

141. Guzman JZ, Feldman ZM, McAnany S, Hecht AC, Qureshi SA, Cho SK. Osteoporosis in cervical spine surgery. *Spine (Phila Pa 1976).* 2016;41(8):662–8.

142. Okuda S, Oda T, Yamasaki R, Haku T, Maeno T, Iwasaki M. Surgical outcomes of osteoporotic vertebral collapse: A retrospective study of anterior spinal fusion and pedicle subtraction osteotomy. *Global Spine J.* 2012;2(4):221–6.

143. Roche JJ, Wenn RT, Sahota O, Moran CG. Effect of comorbidities and postoperative complications on mortality after hip fracture in elderly people: Prospective observational cohort study. *BMJ.* 2005;331(7529):1374.

144. Abrahamsen B, van Staa T, Ariely R, Olson M, Cooper C. Excess mortality following hip fracture: A systematic epidemiological review. *Osteoporos Int.* 2009;20(10):1633–50.

145. Ali AM, Gibbons CE. Predictors of 30-day hospital readmission after hip fracture: A systematic review. *Injury.* 2017;48(2):243–52.

146. Bliemel C, Buecking B, Oberkircher L, Knobe M, Ruchholtz S, Eschbach D. The impact of pre-existing conditions on functional outcome and mortality in geriatric hip fracture patients. *Int Orthop.* 2017;41(10):1995–2000.

147. Canet J, Raeder J, Rasmussen LS et al. Cognitive dysfunction after minor surgery in the elderly. *Acta Anaesthesiol Scand.* 2003;47(10):1204–10.

148. Neufeld KJ, Leoutsakos JS, Sieber FE et al. Evaluation of two delirium screening tools for detecting postoperative delirium in the elderly. *Br J Anaesth.* 2013;111(4):612–8.

149. Ansaloni L, Catena F, Chattat R et al. Risk factors and incidence of postoperative delirium in elderly patients after elective and emergency surgery. *Br J Surg.* 2010;97(2):273–80.

150. Williams-Russo P, Urquhart BL, Sharrock NE, Charlson ME. Post-operative delirium: Predictors and prognosis in elderly orthopedic patients. *J Am Geriatr Soc.* 1992;40(8):759–67.

151. Fong HK, Sands LP, Leung JM. The role of postoperative analgesia in delirium and cognitive decline in elderly patients: A systematic review. *Anesth Analg.* 2006;102(4):1255–66.

152. Leslie DL, Zhang Y, Holford TR, Bogardus ST, Leo-Summers LS, Inouye SK. Premature death associated with delirium at 1-year follow-up. *Arch Intern Med.* 2005;165(14):1657–62.

153. McAvay GJ, Van Ness PH, Bogardus ST, Jr. et al. Older adults discharged from the hospital with delirium: 1-year outcomes. *J Am Geriatr Soc.* 2006;54(8):1245–50.

154. McCusker J, Cole M, Abrahamowicz M, Primeau F, Belzile E. Delirium predicts 12-month mortality. *Arch Intern Med.* 2002;162(4):457–63.

155. Dworkin A, Lee DS, An AR, Goodlin SJ. A simple tool to predict development of delirium after elective surgery. *J Am Geriatr Soc.* 2016;64(11):e149–53.

34

Total shoulder replacement and osteoporosis
An Update

DAVID LIMB

INTRODUCTION

Involvement of the proximal humerus in the osteoporotic process is significant, making the occurrence of a proximal humeral fracture a marker to instigate the investigation of bone mineral density. The prevalence of further fractures in patients who sustain a proximal humeral fracture is approximately double that seen in age- and sex-matched controls (1). Surgical management of the fractured proximal humerus by open reduction and internal fixation creates challenges, discussed elsewhere in this book, and the use of locking plates, strut grafts, bone substitutes, and a variety of other approaches are invoked. The degree of fracture displacement increases overall with age and, for fracture dislocations in particular, joint replacement becomes increasingly used, especially in elderly patients. In these patients, it is often performed as a "once and for all" operation designed to last the remainder of the patient's lifetime, but revision rates for hemiarthroplasty carried out for trauma are around 10% (although this is approximately half the failure rate for internal fixation with locking plates or intramedullary devices) (2).

Total shoulder replacement is an effective treatment for painful arthritis of the shoulder, most commonly osteoarthrosis and inflammatory arthrosis. The number of procedures being performed is increasing substantially—in 2012 the UK National Joint Registry documented around 2500 shoulder replacements, and by 2017 more than 6500 procedures were reported. It is estimated that in the United States around 53,000 shoulder replacements are performed each year. However, that compares with more than 91,000 hip replacements in the United Kingdom and a million in the United States during 2017.

The link between osteoporosis and osteoarthritis, the most common reason for performing a total shoulder replacement, has been investigated, and the majority of studies have demonstrated an inverse relationship—that osteoporosis is actually less common in patients with osteoarthrosis (3). It may be that there are genetic factors common to the etiology of both osteoarthritis and high bone mass. However, there is sufficient experience in performing total shoulder replacement in patients with osteoporosis, particularly in those with inflammatory joint disease and fracture sequelae who tend to share a tendency to low bone mass, that lessons can be drawn from the experience.

SHOULDER REPLACEMENT IN TRAUMA

Shoulder replacement was developed into a successful procedure in the 1950s, notably by Charles Neer, and his early publications focused on humeral head replacement for trauma using a stemmed prosthesis (4). This became the standard operation for head splitting fractures and three- and four-part fracture dislocations in the elderly population: cases in which internal fixation would be predicted to be followed by avascular necrosis and/or posttraumatic osteoarthrosis in a high proportion of individuals. Humeral head replacement relies on the successful reconstruction of the tuberosities around the prosthesis, which in turn restores proper rotator cuff function, centering the humeral head on the glenoid during movement and minimizing shear forces across the glenoid. In trauma, the glenoid is often unaffected by the trauma process, however, and hemiarthroplasty was shown to have durable good results. Development of a glenoid component was a natural next step, particularly in the wake of the success of total hip replacement. While this proved useful in cases of arthritis with affected glenoids, however, the results in trauma were in fact worse, with early loosening of the glenoid a particular problem. It became apparent that for "anatomical" joint replacements, deviation from anatomical conditions had significant implications. Thus, inserting a glenoid component that is 5–6 mm thick without removing a similar thickness of normal glenoid (in cases

343

of trauma) moved the articulation laterally and increased tension in the rotator cuff. More problematically, any mal-reduction of the tuberosities, any loss of position, or any damage to the rotator cuff led to loss of the centering ability of the rotator cuff and the generation of abnormal shear forces on the glenoid during shoulder movement. Total anatomical shoulder replacement in cases of trauma was observed to be associated with early and frequent glenoid component loosening such that it was largely abandoned in favor of hemiarthroplasty.

Thus it was that for decades hemiarthroplasty was used in acute trauma and posttrauma sequelae, though it was increasingly recognized that compared to total shoulder replacement, the functional results were poorer for post-trauma sequelae, and indeed that overall the functional results for hemiarthroplasty fell short of what was being seen with total shoulder replacement (5). Efforts were put into developing trauma-specific stems for shoulder replace-ment, which allowed more room for the attachment and bone grafting of tuberosities to increase the chance of restoring rotator cuff function. Although promising case series were published from a number of expert centers, the results seemed to be difficult to achieve in the day-to-day practice of the average trauma or shoulder surgeon.

A field change occurred throughout the 1990s and 2000s with the refinement of the reverse shoulder arthroplasty. This achieved something rarely seen in prosthetic surgery—the biomechanics of the natural joint were transformed by the prosthesis rather than replicated, totally altering the distribution of forces generated by the musculoskeletal system on the components of the total joint arthroplasty. While this is observed in tendon transfers across a natural joint, for example, the effect has not been deliberately and successfully used in any other large joint replacement. The hemispherical humeral head is removed and replaced by a socket attached to a stem fixed in the humeral canal. The shallow socket of the shoulder against which the humeral head hemisphere normally articulates is then replaced by a prosthetic metallic hemisphere, against which the new socket fixed into the humeral shaft is allowed to articulate.

The effect is biomechanically dramatic—the natural humeral head on the humerus creates a center of rotation at its own geometric center, which is effectively sitting within the proximal humeral metaphysis about 2.5 cm from the glenoid. The line of action of the deltoid is about 3 cm from the center of rotation and pulls vertically, creat-ing a tendency for superior migration of the humeral head that is resisted by the rotator cuff. Any deficiency in the rotator cuff, be it a degenerative tear, tuberosity malunion, posttraumatic stiffness, or whatever, and the normal force couple becomes unbalanced. The effect is a tendency to superior movement of the humeral head as the arm is ele-vated and a shear force at the glenoid surface. This is the "rocking horse effect" responsible for early glenoid compo-nent failure in total shoulder replacement with anything other than a normally functioning rotator cuff.

In the reverse shoulder, the center of rotation—the geo-metric center of the glenosphere attached to the glenoid itself—is approximately on the surface of the glenoid. Thus, the humerus in elevation is rotating around a point on the surface of the glenoid, and this dramatically reduces shear forces and to all intents and purposes solves the problem of early glenoid loosening, while still permitting glenohu-meral movement. The tendency to superior migration of the natural humeral head against the shallow dish of the glenoid is counteracted by the deep humeral component concavity articulating against a hemisphere, meaning the humerus would have to move a substantial distance later-ally in order to move upward only a few millimeters, so instead the glenosphere becomes a fulcrum for rotation. This means that a rotator cuff is no longer essential to neu-tralize the forces of the deltoid in arm elevation, so reverse total shoulder replacement can be carried out even if the rotator cuff is totally absent.

Reverse shoulder replacement was developed to address the problem of glenoid component loosening in the rota-tor cuff–deficient shoulder. The problems experienced by patients with shoulder replacement after trauma in large part are a result of rotator cuff insufficiency. The success of reverse shoulder replacement in the cuff-deficient shoulder was soon, therefore, followed by use of this design of pros-thesis in elderly patients with shoulder fractures that would previously have been treated by hemiarthroplasty. The fail-ure mechanism of anatomical shoulder replacement has long been recognized in many patients to be promoted by failure of the rotator cuff, so reverse shoulder replacement soon became used for revision procedures after cuff failure following hemiarthroplasty or total shoulder replacement. Shortly thereafter, reverse shoulder replacement became the design of choice in elderly patients who were felt to be at risk of rotator cuff failure—and given that the incidence of degenerative cuff tears in asymptomatic individuals in their 70s is about one in three, this may be taken to be any elderly patient. The result is that reverse shoulder replace-ment is now carried out more commonly worldwide than anatomical total shoulder replacement or hemiarthro-plasty. Its specific use in the very elderly patient also means that any consideration of the impact of osteoporosis on arthroplasty surgery applies at least as much, if not more so, than for anatomical shoulder replacement.

OSTEOPOROSIS AND HUMERAL ANATOMY

The pursuit of maintaining proper rotator cuff function in anatomical shoulder replacement meant that, unlike the hip, considerable work was done in attempting to replicate "normal" proximal humeral anatomy with the prosthesis, so many studies examined the morphology, and varia-tion thereof, of the proximal humerus, and such interest continues as novel stem designs and fixation methods are contemplated (6,7). Although considerable variation has been identified in humeral head shape, inclination, offset (in multiple planes), etc., there is no description of varia-tion in the external shape occurring as a consequence (or cause) of osteoporosis. However, the internal anatomy of the proximal humerus is affected by this metabolic process. In common with observations elsewhere, the osteoporotic proximal humerus has a thinner cortex and thinner, sparser, trabeculae within the head. Compared to the proximal femur, the absolute values for bone density and therefore the ability to maintain fixation with screws and stems is such that only 50% of the energy is required to indent the bone of the proximal humerus compared to the proximal femur (8).

Thinning of the cortex, without a change in external dimensions, means that the canal of the osteoporotic proximal humerus becomes wider. As elsewhere, the cortical thickness of the proximal humerus has been shown to decrease with age and to be correlated with bone mineral density (9).

Unlike its effect on the proximal humerus, there seems to be little alteration of the glenoid fossa by osteoporosis. The vast literature on dealing with bone loss in the glenoid results from destruction by erosion from the humeral head or by the loosening process of a glenoid component, which is outside the scope of this chapter.

STEM FIXATION IN THE HUMERUS

The humeral head replacement designed by Charles Neer was held in place by a stem designed to fit down the humeral canal and, in keeping with developments in hip arthroplasty at that time, was thinner than the canal to accommodate a cement mantle, cement fixation being the norm.

However, it was earlier described that the humeral head has a center of rotation that is situated in the proximal humeral metaphysis. The rotator cuff attaches to the tuberosities surrounding the center of rotation, and this neutralizes the force of the deltoid and other muscles acting on the shoulder to allow rotation about this center of rotation. The result of this is that in fact there is very little force transmitted down the humeral stem, provided that the metaphysis and tuberosities are intact and functioning. For this reason, there is little to drive humeral stem loosening in these circumstances. Although cement fixation and hydroxyapatite coatings were developed, they are not strictly necessary unless there is a problem other than articular surface damage. A number of successful anatomical total shoulder systems therefore allow the press-fit insertion of a humeral stem, with fins to provide stability in rotation, without the need for cement or a hydroxyapatite coating (Figure 34.1).

In trauma, however, the initial placement of the stem into the humeral shaft has to leave the metaphyseal segment standing straight to allow the tuberosities to be reconstructed around the prosthesis (Figure 34.2). The tuberosities need to unite to each other and to the shaft for function to return to normal, and the humeral head is often used as bone graft to stimulate this union. The metaphyseal segment is therefore relatively unsupported, and there is no resistance to rotation such as would be afforded by fins engaging the metaphysis in a primary shoulder

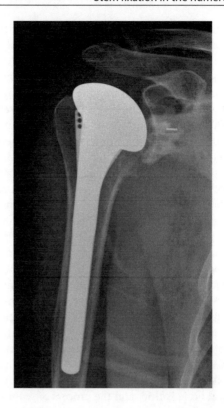

Figure 34.1 An anatomical shoulder replacement—the tuberosities and rotator cuff are intact, so although this prosthesis is not cemented and has no surface coating such as hydroxyapatite, the mechanical environment of the stem means that minimal force is transmitted through it, and loosening of the humeral component is not a significant worry.

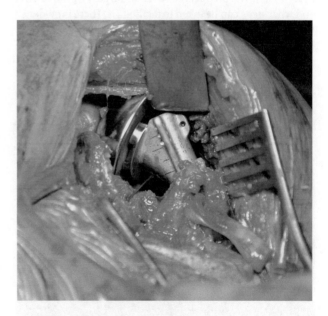

Figure 34.2 During shoulder hemiarthroplasty for trauma, the initial stem fixation has to leave room for the tuberosities to be reconstructed in the metaphyseal region. The stem therefore has no support to prevent it sinking into the shaft or rotating, so fixation of the stem, either by cement or a bioactive coating, is essential.

replacement, nor any resistance to subsidence of the stem into the canal. In trauma, therefore, it is essential to provide initial stability for the prosthesis in order to allow the tuberosities to heal and rotator cuff function to return. This is achieved either by cementing the stem or using a tight press-fit with a bioactive coating such as hydroxyapatite.

The effect of osteoporosis on humeral anatomy is, as discussed, to widen the medullary canal. Consequently, a broader stem is needed to fill the canal and provide a press-fit in the case of uncemented stems. This may create some problems with some shoulder replacement systems, in which a broader stem is linked to a bulkier metaphyseal section. This is obviated in later modular systems but could be a problem in systems that provide the stem and metaphyseal segment as one component. Although the frail, osteoporotic individual may have a capacious canal, their metaphyseal segment is related in dimensions to their general body habitus; therefore, a large stem may be accompanied by an overly large metaphyseal segment. In these circumstances, the problem is overcome by choosing a smaller stem size and cementing the components.

Bulky stems that are not cemented require a press-fit, and this brings its own problems in osteoporosis. The diaphyseal bone is thin, and the process of reaming then impacting a bulky prosthesis can lead to humeral shaft fracture. These are often undetected at the time of surgery, minimally displaced (Figure 34.3), and may unite with a period of restricted rehabilitation, but this interferes with the postoperative progress and is best avoided.

One further issue to consider when conducting a primary anatomical shoulder replacement in an osteoporotic individual is the prospect of revision surgery in the future, and what steps can be taken to facilitate it. There is evidence that the already thin cortex of the osteoporotic individual becomes thinner due to stress shielding (10). Clearly the aim is to provide a prosthesis that will last a patient's lifetime, and this is achieved in the majority. When revision is needed, it is often because of either glenoid loosening or rotator cuff failure, and both are dealt with most effectively by reverse shoulder replacement. In any individual, the use

of a platform system facilitates this—a modular system that subsequently, at revision surgery, allows the head of an anatomical replacement to be removed and, on the same stem, a reverse replacement can be inserted.

The broad canal of an osteoporotic individual also means that if a cemented primary is to be carried out with a standard (nonplatform) system, then choosing a large stem may be beneficial. This means that if revision is required and the cement mantle is stable, the broad stem can be removed and a "cement in cement" revision carried out, inserting a narrower reverse shoulder stem into the cement mantle previously occupied by an anatomical stem of a different design.

METAPHYSEAL FIXATION IN THE HUMERUS

The poor quality of trabeculae in the metaphyseal region in osteoporosis means that rotational stability, normally provided by fins on the prosthesis engaging in the dense trabeculae, is less effective. This is a significant contributor to the observation that humeral stem fixation in rheumatoid patients is best achieved by cement fixation rather than relying on press-fit (11). The observation that initial fixation in osteoporotic bone is diminished is better researched in dental surgery than orthopedics (12,13), but the shoulder bears some resemblance to the problems of resistance to subsidence and rotation faced by dental implants. It has been suggested that computed tomography (CT) scans may provide a useful measure of bone density (in both dental and shoulder cases), and although routine CT scanning may not be justified for all shoulder replacements, if a scan is obtained to study glenoid bone stock, for example, then useful information may be gleaned on the bone mineral density of the proximal humerus and the components needed to deal with the width of the humeral canal and the confines and quality of the metaphyseal region (14). If the metaphyseal bone is of poor quality, then the solution is to use an alternative form of fixation such as cement, or a tight press-fit providing more than just rotational stability through fins. The risk of periprosthetic fracture with the latter strategy has already been mentioned and is not uncommon, such fractures being reported at 0.5%–2.4% in total (15) with the majority occurring as the implant is seated into the humerus. Periprosthetic fractures occurring after surgery are rarer than perioperative fractures, more common in osteoporotic individuals, and usually occur after a fall from standing height (15).

There is a trend toward short stems and even metaphyseal fixation (stemless) shoulder replacement. While resurfacing of the osteoporotic humeral head does not pose a problem, since the subchondral bone is preserved, the use of a stemless prosthesis is best avoided in the osteoporotic individuals because the support provided by metaphyseal cancellous bone after removal of the humeral head will be inadequate.

In clinical practice, the assessment of metaphyseal bone quality is a judgement call made at the time of surgery. It is

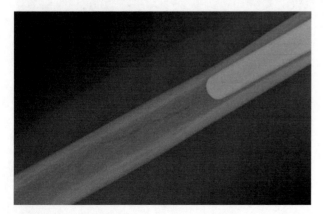

Figure 34.3 A minimally displaced humeral shaft fracture that occurred during insertion of a press-fit humeral component in an osteoporotic individual.

almost irrelevant if a cemented or hydroxyapatite-coated, stemmed prosthesis is being used. If an uncoated prosthesis is being used, then it is inserted without cement if the process of reaming and cutting with metaphyseal jigs produces a seating for the prosthesis in cancellous bone with clean-cut spaces to accommodate the body and fins of the prosthesis. If the cancellous structure collapses during preparation and the seating slots for the fins in the cancellous bone are no longer well delineated, then the prosthesis is cemented. As noted earlier, stemless prostheses are best avoided in these circumstances.

SUMMARY

Total shoulder replacement is being increasingly used, and the advent of reverse shoulder replacement means that it is now being used in older patients and those with rotator cuff deficiency and therefore inevitably in more osteoporotic individuals. The three main issues arising in osteoporosis are the capacious canal with thin walls, poor-quality metaphyseal cancellous bone, and the risk of periprosthetic fracture. The capacious canal means that large-diameter stems should be available. Poor metaphyseal bone may mean converting the operative plan to use a press-fit prosthesis to choosing a cemented component. Periprosthetic fractures are more commonly seen during the insertion of a press-fit humeral stem than at any time after surgery. Although the majority are minimally displaced and heal with short-term modification of rehabilitation, it may still be necessary to consider plate fixation or revision to a long-stem prosthesis, much as described for other forms of arthroplasty.

REFERENCES

1. Horak J, Nilsson BE. Epidemiology of fracture at the upper end of the humerus. *Clin Orthop Rel Res.* 1975;(112):250–3.
2. Katthagen JC, Huber M, Grabovski S, Ellwein A, Jensen G, Lill H. Failure and revision rates of proximal humeral fracture treatment with the use of a standardized treatment algorithm at a level-1 trauma center. *J Orthop Traumatol.* 2017;18(3):265–74.
3. Antonaides L, MacGregor AJ, Matson M, Spector TD. A cotwin control study of the relationship between hip osteoarthritis and bone mineral density. *Arthritis Rheum.* 2000;43(7):1450–5.
4. Neer CS 2nd. Articular replacement for the humeral head. *J Bone Joint Surg Am.* 1955;37-A:215–8.
5. Sowa B, Thierjung H, Bülhoff M et al. Functional results of hemi- and total shoulder arthroplasty according to diagnosis and patient age at surgery. *Acta Orthop.* 2017;88(3):310–4.
6. Wataru S, Kazuomi S, Yoshikazu N, Hiroaki I, Takaharu Y, Hideki Y. Three-dimensional morphological analysis of humeral heads. *Acta Orthop.* 2005;76(3):392–6.
7. Reeves JM, Johnson JA, Athwal JS. An analysis of proximal humerus morphology with special interest in stemless shoulder arthroplasty. *J Shoulder Elbow Surg.* 2018:27(4);650–8.
8. Saitoh S, Nakatsuchi Y. Osteoporosis of the proximal humerus: Comparison of bone-mineral density and mechanical strength with the proximal femur. *J Shoulder Elbow Surg.* 1993:2(2);78–84.
9. Tingart MJ, Apreleva M, von Stechow D, Zurakowski D, Warner JJ. The cortical thickness of the proximal humeral diaphysis predicts bone mineral density of the proximal humerus. *J Bone Joint Surgery Br.* 2003:85(4);611–7.
10. Nagels J, Stokdijk M, Rozing PM. Stress shielding and bone resorption in shoulder arthroplasty. *J Shoulder Elbow Surg.* 2003;12(1):35–9.
11. Stewart MP, Kelly IG. Total shoulder replacement in rheumatoid disease: 7- to 13-year follow-up of 37 joints. *J Bone Joint Surgery Br.* 1997:79(1);68–72.
12. Turkyllmaz I, Sennerby L, McGlumphy EA, Tözüm TF. Biomechanical aspects of primary implant stability: A human cadaver study. *Clin Implant Dent Relat Res.* 2009;11(12):113–9.
13. Turkyllmaz I, Turner C, Ozbeck EN, Tözüm TF. Relations between the bone density values for CT, and implant stability parameters: A clinical study of 230 regular platform implants. *J Clin Periodontol.* 2007;34(8):716–22.
14. Pervaiz K, Cabezas A, Downes K, Santoni BG, Frankle MA. Osteoporosis and shoulder osteoarthritis: Incidence, risk factors, and surgical implications. *J Shoulder Elbow Surg.* 2013;22:e1–8.
15. Kirchoff C, Brunner U, Biberhalter P. Periprosthetic humeral fractures: Strategies and techniques for osteosynthesis. *Unfallchirurg.* 2016;119(4):275–80.

Total hip replacement and osteoporosis
Current trends

ANTONIOS KOUTALOS, GEORGIOS KOMNOS, and THEOFILOS KARACHALIOS

INTRODUCTION

Osteoarthritis (OA) and osteoporosis (OP) are two chronic, debilitating diseases whose prevalence increases with age. It is widely accepted that they have an inverse relationship, meaning that OA protects a person from OP, and vice versa (1). More than 40 years ago, it was noted in a retrospective study that osteoporotic fractured hips lacked osteoarthritic changes (2). This led to the assumption that osteoarthritic hips were protected from osteoporotic fractures. However, a clinical study found that almost 75% of female patients listed for cementless total hip arthroplasty (THA) had osteopenia or OP (Figure 35.1) (3). Bone mineral density (BMD) of osteoarthritic hips was lower in the trochanteric region and greater in the neck compared to control hips. The authors concluded that OA did not protect patients from generalized OP (3). Another study found an OP prevalence of 26% in patients undergoing THA, which was at least similar to the OP prevalence of the general population (4).

There are several important clinical issues related to the implantation of THA in osteoporotic patients: the initial osseointegration of the prosthesis, especially when cementless THA is used; the incidence of intraoperative fractures; the incidence of late periprosthetic fractures (0.9% after primary THA and 4.2% after revision THA), and the long-term survival of THA, since reports comparing cemented to cementless hips are scarce (Figure 35.2). In this chapter, we present a critical review of all of these issues and try to draw practical conclusions.

EFFICACY OF TOTAL HIP ARTHROPLASTY

The question of the efficacy of THA in osteoporotic bones revolves around the fact that the bone-implant interface is active (high bone turnover) and that there is an age-related medullary expansion, especially in women after menopause (BMD correlates with medullary width) (5). In a case-control study, it was reported that hips with aseptic loosening had four times higher medullary expansion compared to stable hips (6). Medullary expansion may be more clinically relevant in women undergoing THA under the age of 60 years, since the postmenopausal period is characterized by accelerated bone loss and medullary expansion (5).

Early subsidence, indicating failure of osseointegration, is a major concern when cementless implants are used in osteoporotic hips. Basic science studies have tried to clarify this controversy (Figure 35.3). It has been reported that poor-quality cancellous bone in the intertrochanteric region did not affect distal migration or early osseointegration of anatomically shaped femoral components with proximal hydroxyapatite (HA) coating, measured by radiostereometric analysis (RSA) (7), even though earlier biomechanical studies showed that these stems are associated with axial migration when implanted in osteoporotic bones (8). Osseointegration depends more on the presence or recruitment of mesenchymal stem cells than on the bone quality of the intertrochanteric region. Other studies have confirmed the notion that host bone quality is not a critical factor for establishing primary stability or osseointegration in anatomical cementless hip stems (9,10). However, there is still a concern about the stress shielding that a large-size cementless stem can produce on thin cortical bone.

Bone loss after THA is a concern, especially in osteoporotic or osteopenic patients. Bone loss occurs immediately after THA during the first year but is later restored up to a degree. Some bone loss, especially in Gruen zone 7, persists as a result of stress shielding. In the long term, bone stock is compromised due to osteolysis. The hypothesis that improvement in bone mineral density may have a clinically important effect on long-term implant fixation and the incidence of periprosthetic fractures after total joint arthroplasty has been tested in both experimental and clinical studies (11). For this reason, bisphosphonates have been tried as a pharmaceutical approach to prevent bone

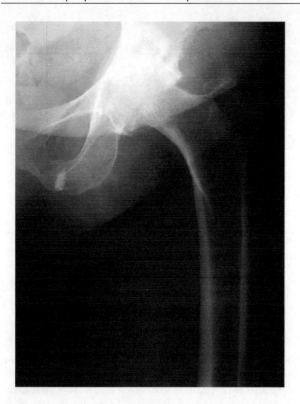

Figure 35.1 Radiograph shows an atrophic osteoarthritic hip. Radiographic signs of advanced osteoporosis are also shown.

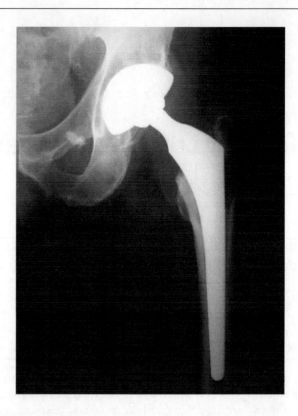

Figure 35.2 A 16-year follow-up anteroposterior radiograph of a left total hip arthroplasty, performed in an osteoporotic female patient.

loss. Several quality studies (including systematic reviews and meta-analyses) have been performed in humans showing the early (up to 2 years) positive effect of the administration of mainly bisphosphonates on the preservation of periprosthetic bone stock, especially in cementless THAs at short- to mid-term follow-up (12–20). A retrospective cohort study revealed that bisphosphonates users had lower revision rates (21). Similar conclusions were reached by a registry-based study. Older patients with osteopenia or OP who were on bisphosphonate treatment had a hazard ratio of 0.51 and 0.11 for revision, respectively, while young patients (younger than 65 years) with normal BMD values had an increased risk (22). In this study, the indications for taking bisphosphonates were not reported (probably as a protection against concomitant use of steroids), and the number of periprosthetic fractures was small. Moreover, these periprosthetic fractures may represent atypical fractures that are associated with the long-term use of bisphosphonates (22). However, another study reported that besides a lower revision rate, the use of bisphosphonates was associated with an increased infection rate (23). Bisphosphonates are generally thought to decrease the risk of periprosthetic fracture.

Data from large nationwide population studies do not suggest inferior results for THA in patients with osteoporosis. The 10-year revision rate of a large cohort of osteoporosis patients in Denmark was 8.3%, which was similar to the 8.9% revision rate of all patients from the Danish Registry (24). However, the authors noted that either surgeons or osteoporotic patients may be unwilling to perform revision surgery due to fears of increased morbidity and mortality, which would skew the results in favor of OP.

Cemented implants are considered the gold standard for osteoporotic hips. They can provide immediate stability and allow full weight-bearing from day 1. Sometimes, however, in wide osteoporotic femoral canals, even the largest cemented stem cannot fill the canal. Cementation of osteoporotic femurs may result in an increased cement mantle beyond 1–2 mm or in undersized components that predispose to aseptic loosening (25,26). In addition, there is slight increased mortality during cement application and a risk of cardiovascular compromise (27,28). This has led the authors to use cementless stems and to advise patients about protected weight-bearing in the immediate postoperative period. The use of collared cementless stems is also an option, but their implantation is technically challenging depending on proximal femoral morphology (Figure 35.4). Other options include the use of hydroxyapatite cementless stems in order to enhance ingrowth, and the use of double-tapered stems (29). Unfortunately, the insertion of a cementless proximally coated press-fit stem into an osteoporotic femur is technically demanding due to the development of increased hoop stress and the increased risk of intraoperative fracture (30). Moreover, the insertion of a large-size cementless stem into a wide osteoporotic canal can lead to leg-length discrepancy if appropriate measures (like low neck cut) are not taken into account. Another concern with large-size stems in the osteoporotic femur is

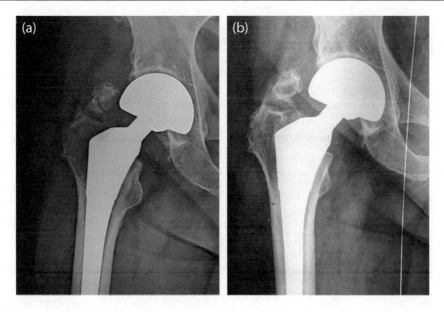

Figure 35.3 Radiographs of a cementless hemiarthroplasty, performed in a 78-year-old female osteoporotic patient with a femoral head fracture at (a) 6 months and the (b) 10-year follow-up.

stress shielding. Stress shielding is more prominent with larger sizes of femoral stems. Fully porous coated stems have been shown to produce stress shielding in 26% of the stems at 2 years (31). This effect has also been observed with proximally coated stems (32). The long-term result of stress shielding is, however, unknown. In a study of 228 patients over 75 years old, Healy et al. found that cemented hips had 2.6% loosening compared to no loosening in the cementless group. It was suggested that surgical technique was more important than the method of implant fixation (33). Rhyu et al. did not find any difference in short-term complications when utilizing cementless stems in osteoporotic femurs (34). All patients were allowed immediate weight-bearing. Neither femur fracture nor subsidence was different between osteoporotic and control hips when using a wedge-shaped press-fit stem. In addition, subsidence

was similar to all Dorr types of femoral morphology. The authors concluded that OP was not a contraindication for using a cementless double-tapered wedge-shaped stem with early full weight-bearing. A limitation of this study was the small sample size. Long-term outcomes were not available in terms of periprosthetic fractures in osteoporotic hips with thin cortices and mismatching larger stems (34). Kligman reported similar functional outcomes and no revisions for aseptic loosening between osteoporotic and nonosteoporotic patients with hydroxyapatite-coated THA at a mean follow-up of 5 years (35).

Long-term results of the use of cementless stems in osteoporotic hips are also encouraging (Table 35.1) (24,34–41). After mean follow-up of 6 years, 100% survival of 127 Dorr type C femurs was reported in a retrospective study (36). These authors used a double-tapered

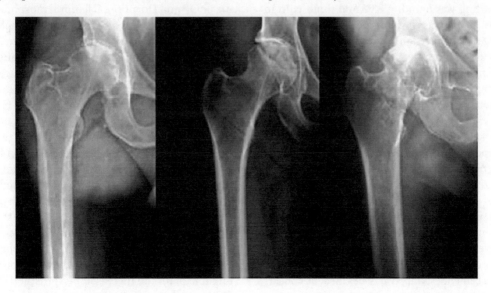

Figure 35.4 Proximal femoral morphology according to Dorr.

Table 35.1 Details of published papers on cementless total hip arthroplasty in patients with osteoporosis

Study	Number of hips	Follow-up (years)	Survival	Comments
Thilleman et al., 2010			91.7% at 10 years	Various implants, Danish Registry
Rhyu et al., 2012	40 hips	Mean 2.2 (1.4–3.25)	No revision. 100% at 2 years	Accolade TMZF (Stryker, Mahwah, NJ); tapered proximal coated stem
Kligman and Kirsh, 2000	22 osteoporotic	Mean 5 (2–7)	100% at 5 years	Hydroxyapatite-coated stem
Kelly et al., 2007	16 hips Dorr type C	Mean 11.5 (9–14)	100% at 10 years	Omnifit HA (Stryker Or- thopaedics, Mahwah, NJ); straight titanium alloy stem with a proximal double-wedge design; proximal HA coating
Meding et al., 2010	127 Dorr type C	Mean 5.9 (2–19.5)	100% survival at 15 years	Bi-Metric (Biomet, Inc, Warsaw, IN); tapered proximally porous coated stem
McLaughlin and Lee, 2016	60 Dorr type C	Mean 16.6 (10–29)	One revision for late sepsis	Taperloc (Zimmer Biomet, Warsaw, IN); tapered proximally porous coated stem
Kim et al., 2013	92 Dorr type C	Mean 5.6 (5–7)	98.2% survival; one stem revised due to stem migration	Stubby stem: metaphyseal- fitting anatomical cementless femoral stem (Proxima; DePuy, Leeds, UK)
Reitman et al., 2003	72 Dorr type C	Mean 13.2 (minimum 10 years)	Revision of one stem due to infection	Mallory-Head press-fit stem; tapered proximally porous coated stem
Dalury et al., 2012	60 Dorr type C	Mean 6 (4–9)	No revisions	Summit (Depuy Orthopaedics, Inc.); proximally porous coated stem

proximal plasma sprayed stem and found no difference in survival or in functional outcomes between different Dorr-type femurs. Likewise, the use of a titanium alloy double-wedge proximal stem with hydroxyapatite coating in 15 patients resulted in excellent mid- to long-term (9–11.5 years) survival and function (37). A more recent study also found excellent outcomes after a mean follow-up of 16.6 years in 60 Dorr C type hips (38). The authors used a single wedge proximal-coated stem and reported similar survival between Dorr type C and type B or A femur. No intraoperative fractures were encountered. In the long term, no periprosthetic fractures were recorded, but proximal stress shielding was found in 83% and thigh pain in 5% of the hips. Nonetheless, the implant achieved 98% survival at 20 years for revision for any reason as an endpoint (38). The use of short metaphyseal fitting anatomical cementless stems has been successfully utilized in osteoporotic Dorr type C femoral bones. The authors did not find any difference in the osseointegration of short stems between different Dorr type femurs. At 7-year follow-up, there was no osteolysis or aseptic loosening. Despite the fear that osteoporotic metaphysis may not be suitable for the osseointegration of "stubby" stems, this was not the case in this study.

The effect of osteoporosis on acetabular cup fixation and long-term survivorship has not been studied in depth. Studies with control groups (not osteoporotic patients) are lacking. However, cemented and cementless cups perform equally well in osteoporotic patients. When the surgeon chooses to use a cementless cup, two issues must be considered to avoid intraoperative fractures. First, under-reaming

during acetabulum preparation must be limited to 1 mm or line-to-line to safely impact the cup. Second, for more initial stability, screw placement is suggested (40). Cup designs with increased risk of intraoperative fracture, like elliptical monoblock cups, should be avoided (42).

While cementless stems have shown good results in elective THA in patients with osteoporosis, this may not be true for trauma patients undergoing THA for fractures with an osteoporotic neck of the femur. Pentlow et al. compared the subsidence of cementless press-fit hydroxyapatite-coated stems in matched elective and trauma patients (29). Most trauma patients had osteopenia or OP and Dorr type C femoral morphology. Revision and dislocation rates at 6 months were higher in trauma patients (both 8.7% compared to 0%). Three of the four revisions were carried out due to dislocation secondary to femoral subsidence. The authors concluded that in trauma patients who have increased incidence of osteoporosis, the use of cementless collarless THA may not be appropriate and suggested the utilization of cemented or collared cementless THA (29). In a similar study, with a mean follow-up of 5 years, using RSA and dual-energy x-ray absorptiometry (DEXA) scans, cementless stems (double-tapered collared HA coated used for femoral neck fractures) were associated with a high number of late periprosthetic fractures (12%) (43). RSA studies showed stable fixation and no migration after 2 years, but DEXA showed increasing bone loss in all Gruen zones (especially in zones 1 and 7) throughout the study period, and this might explain the increased periprosthetic fracture rate. The lower the initial BMD values, the greater was the bone loss. The authors recommended against the use of this cementless stem in THAs for the treatment of osteoporotic femoral neck in elderly patients.

Periprosthetic fractures seem to be associated with the degree of femoral OP and are reported to have an incidence of 4% after THR, and age, cementless stems, female gender, and revision surgery are risk factors. Periprosthetic fractures can occur either intraoperatively or later. Intraoperative fractures usually occur in the calcar region during the insertion of a cementless stem in a brittle osteoporotic femur. This is one of the reasons why cemented stems, which produce lower hoop stress during insertion, are preferred to cementless stems. Registry data support the view that cementless stems and increased age with poor bone quality are the main predisposing factors for periprosthetic fractures (44). The relative risk of revision due to periprosthetic fracture was 8.72 for cementless stems (45). Cemented stems have a lower risk of late periprosthetic fractures, and this has been supported by biomechanical studies. However, not all cemented stems have the same periprosthetic fracture rate. In a recent study, shape closed stem designs (Charnley cemented stem) were found to have lower periprosthetic fracture rates compared to the force closed design stem (Exeter stem, polished tapered stem). A polished tapered implant with a small radius of the shoulder (CPT stem) had the greater periprosthetic fracture rate (46). It was also found that polished tapered stems (Exeter V40) had a higher risk for revision due to periprosthetic fracture compared to anatomically designed stems (anatomic Lubinus SPII) (45). Various designs of cementless stems offer the same low periprosthetic fracture rates (30). In a registry-based study, the cementless, fully HA-coated stem (Corail) outperforms a more anatomically designed stem (ABG II) (45). The early osteointegration of the HA-coated stem might have contributed to the decreased periprosthetic fracture rate.

CONCLUSION

Bone health should be evaluated and improved before patients undergo THA in order to ensure the most successful outcome. Patients undergoing THA should be counseled on calcium and vitamin D intake and should be advised to quit smoking and to reduce the dose of medications known to be harmful to bone quality (e.g., cortisone). Measurement of BMD values in high-risk patients can help diagnose those with osteopenia or OP. In OP, a cemented stem can be chosen, while for osteopenic hips the utilization of bisphosphonates may improve implant osseointegration and reduce periprosthetic fractures (46). A cementless stem can be chosen as well, if bone geometry is suitable. The surgical technique of stem fixation is of paramount importance, since poor bone quality is an adverse risk factor for implant loosening regardless of the fixation method.

REFERENCES

1. Dequeker J, Aerssens J, Luyten FP. Osteoarthritis and osteoporosis: Clinical and research evidence of inverse relationship. *Aging Clin Exp Res.* 2003;15:426–39.
2. Foss MV, Byers PD. Bone density, osteoarthrosis of the hip, and fracture of the upper end of the femur. *Ann Rheum Dis.* 1972;31:259–64.
3. Mäkinen TJ, Alm JJ, Laine H, Svedström E, Aro HT. The incidence of osteopenia and osteoporosis in women with hip osteoarthritis scheduled for cementless total joint replacement. *Bone.* 2007;40(4):1041–7.
4. Labuda A, Papaioannou A, Pritchard J, Kennedy C, DeBeer J, Adachi JD. Prevalence of osteoporosis in osteoarthritic patients undergoing total hip or total knee arthroplasty. *Arch Phys Med Rehabil.* 2008;89(12):2373–4.
5. Ahlborg HG, Johnell O, Karlsson MK. An age-related medullary expansion can have implications for the long-term fixation of hip prostheses. *Acta Orthop Scand.* 2004;75(2):154–9.
6. Hofmann AA, Wyatt RW, France EP, Bigler GT, Daniels AU, Hess WE. Endosteal bone loss after total hip arthroplasty. *Clin Orthop Relat Res.* 1989;245:138–44.
7. Moritz N, Alm JJ, Lankinen P, Mäkinen TJ, Mattila K, Aro HT. Quality of intertrochanteric cancellous bone as predictor of femoral stem RSA migration in cementless total hip arthroplasty. *J Biomech.* 2011;44(2):221–7.
8. Mears SC, Richards AM, Knight TA, Belkoff SM. Subsidence of uncemented stems in osteoporotic and non-osteoporotic cadaveric femora. *Proc Inst Mech Eng H.* 2009;223:189–94.
9. Viceconti M, Brusi G, Pancanti A, Cristofolini L. Primary stability of an anatomical cementless hip stem: A statistical analysis. *J Biomech.* 2006;39: 1169–79.
10. Dutton A, Rubash HE. Hot topics and controversies in arthroplasty: Cementless femoral fixation in elderly patients. *Instr Course Lect AAOS.* 2008;57:255–9.
11. Mori H, Manabe M, Kurachi Y, Nagumo M. Osseointegration of dental implants in rabbit bone with low mineral density. *J Oral Maxillofac Surg.* 1997;55(4):351–61.
12. Fujimoto T, Niimi A, Sawai T, Ueda M. Effects of steroid-induced osteoporosis on osseointegration of titanium implants. *Int J Oral Maxillofac Implants.* 1998;13(2):183–9.
13. Jakobsen T, Kold S, Bechtold JE, Elmengaard B, Søballe K. Effect of topical alendronate treatment on fixation of implants inserted with bone compaction. *Clin Orthop Relat Res.* 2006;444:229–34.
14. Jakobsen T, Kold S, Bechtold JE, Elmengaard B, Søballe K. Local alendronate increases fixation of implants inserted with bone compaction: 12-week canine study. *J Orthop Rec.* 2007;25(4):432–41.

15. Kajiwara H, Yamaza T, Yoshinari M et al. The bisphosphonate pamidronate on the surface of titanium stimulates bone formation around tibial implants in rats. *Biomaterials.* 2005;26(6):581–7.

16. Tanzer M, Karabasz D, Krygier JJ, Cohen R, Bobyn JD. The Otto Aufranc Award: Bone augmentation around and within porous implants by local bisphosphonate elution. *Clin Orthop Relat Res.* 2005;441:30–9.

17. Bobyn JD, Hacking SA, Krygier JJ, Harvey EJ, Little DG, Tanzer M. Zoledronic acid causes enhancement of bone growth into porous implants. *J Bone Joint Surg Br.* 2005;87(3):416–20.

18. Eberhardt C, Habermann B, Müller S, Schwarz M, Bauss F, Kurth AH. The bisphosphonate ibandronate accelerates osseointegration of hydroxyapatite-coated cementless implants in an animal model. *J Orthop Sci.* 2007;12(1):61–6.

19. Bobyn JD, Thompson R, Lim L, Pura JA, Bobyn K, Tanzer M. Local alendronic acid elution increases net periimplant bone formation: A micro-CT analysis. *Clin Orthop Relat Res.* 2014;472(2):687–94.

20. Zeng Y, Lai O, Shen B et al. A systematic review assessing the effectiveness of alendronate in reducing periprosthetic bone loss after cementless primary THA. *Orthopedics.* 2011;34(4) doi: 10.3928/01477447-20110228-09.

21. Prieto-Alhambra D, Javaid MK et al. Association between bisphosphonate use and implant survival after primary total arthroplasty of the knee or hip: Population based retrospective cohort study. *BMJ.* 2011;343:d7222.

22. Khatod M, Inacio MC, Dell RM, Bini SA, Paxton EW, Namba RS. Association of bisphosphonate use and risk of revision After THA: Outcomes from a US total joint replacement registry. *Clin Orthop Relat Res.* 2015;473(11):3412–20.

23. Russell LA. Osteoporosis and orthopedic surgery: Effect of bone health on total joint arthroplasty outcome. *Curr Rheumatol Rep.* 2013;15(11):371.

24. Thillemann TM, Pedersen AB, Mehnert F, Johnsen SP, Søballe K. Postoperative use of bisphosphonates and risk of revision after primary total hip arthroplasty: A nationwide population-based study. *Bone.* 2010;46(4):946–51.

25. Cristofolini L, Erani P, Bialoblocka-Juszczyk E et al. Effect of undersizing on the long-term stability of the Exeter hip stem: A comparative *in vitro* study. *Clin Biomech (Bristol Avon).* 2010;25(9):899–908.

26. Ramos A, Simoes JA. The influence of cement mantle thickness and stem geometry on fatigue damage in two different cemented hip femoral prostheses. *J Biomech.* 2009;42(15):2602–10.

27. Parvizi J, Holiday AD, Ereth MH, Lewallen DG. The Frank Stinchfield Award. Sudden death during primary hip arthroplasty. *Clin Orthop Relat Res.* 1999;369:39–48.

28. Issack PS, Lauerman MH, Helfet DL et al. Fat embolism and respiratory distress associated with cemented femoral arthroplasty. *Am J Orthop (Belle Mead NJ).* 2009;38:72.

29. Pentlow AK, Heal JS. Subsidence of collarless uncemented femoral stems in total hips replacements performed for trauma. *Injury.* 2012;43(6):882–5.

30. Mears CS. Management of severe osteoporosis in primary total hip arthroplasty. *Curr Transl Geriatr Exp Gerontol Rep.* 2013;2:99–104.

31. Engh Jr CA, Mohan V, Nagowski JP et al. Influence of stem size on clinical outcome of primary total hip arthroplasty with cementless extensively porous-coated femoral components. *J Arthroplasty.* 2009;24(4):554–9.

32. Nishino T, Mishima H, Miyakawa S et al. Midterm results of the synergy cementless tapered stem: Stress shielding and bone quality. *J Orthop Sci.* 2008;13(6):498–503.

33. Healy WL. Hip implant selection for total hip arthroplasty in elderly patients. *Clin Orthop Relat Res.* 2002;405:54–64.

34. Rhyu KH, Lee SM, Chun YS, Kim KI, Cho YJ, Yoo MC. Does osteoporosis increase early subsidence of cementless double-tapered femoral stem in hip arthroplasty? *J Arthroplasty.* 2012;27(7):1305–9.

35. Kligman M, Kirsh G. Hydroxyapatite-coated total hip arthroplasty in osteoporotic patients. *Bull Hosp Jt Dis.* 2000;59(3):136–9.

36. Meding JB, Galley MR, Ritter MA. High survival of uncemented proximally porous-coated titanium alloy femoral stems in osteoporotic bone. *Clin Orthop Relat Res.* 2010;468(2):441–7.

37. Kelly SJ, Robbins CE, Bierbaum BE, Bono JV, Ward DM. Use of a hydroxyapatite-coated stem in patients with class C femoral bone. *Clin Orthop Relat Res.* 2007;465:112–6.

38. McLaughlin JR, Lee KR. Long-term results of uncemented total hip arthroplasty with the Taperloc femoral component in patients with Dorr type C proximal femoral morphology. *Bone Joint J.* 2016;98(5):595–600.

39. Reitman RD, Emerson R, Higgins L, Head W. Thirteen year results of total hip arthroplasty using a tapered titanium femoral component inserted without cement in patients with type C bone. *J Arthroplasty.* 2003;18(S1):116–21.

40. Dalury DF, Kelley TC, Adams MJ. Modern proximally tapered uncemented stems can be safely used in Dorr type C femoral bone. *J Arthroplasty.* 2012;27:1014–8.

41. Kim YH, Park JW, Kim JS. Is diaphyseal stem fixation necessary for primary total hip arthroplasty in patients with osteoporotic bone (Class C bone)? *J Arthroplasty.* 2013;28(1):139–46.

42. Haidukewych GJ, Jacofsky DJ, Hanssen AD, Lewallen DG. Intraoperative fractures of the acetabulum during primary total hip arthroplasty. *J Bone Joint Surg Am.* 2006;88(9):1952–6.

43. Sköldenberg OG, Sjöö H, Kelly-Pettersson P et al. Good stability but high periprosthetic bone mineral loss and late-occurring periprosthetic fractures with use of uncemented tapered femoral stems in patients with a femoral neck fracture. *Acta Orthop Scand.* 2014;85(4):396–402.

44. Hailer NP, Garellick G, Karrholm J. Uncemented and cemented primary total hip arthroplasty in the Swedish Hip Arthroplasty Register. Evaluation of 170,413 operations. *Acta Orthop Scand.* 2010;81(1):34–41.

45. Thien TM, Chatziagorou G, Garellick G et al. Periprosthetic femoral fracture within two years after total hip replacement. analysis of 437,629 operations in the Nordic Arthroplasty Register Association database. *J Bone Joint Surg Am.* 2014;96(19):e167.

46. Palan J, Smith MC, Gregg P et al. The influence of cemented femoral stem choice on the incidence of revision for periprosthetic fracture after primary total hip arthroplasty: An analysis of national joint registry data. *Bone Joint J.* 2016;98(10):1347–54.

Total knee replacement and osteoporosis

An overview

EDWARD S. HOLLOWAY and VEYSI T. VEYSI

INTRODUCTION

According to the National Joint Registry (NJR) (1), there were 102,177 knee replacement procedures performed in England, Wales, Northern Ireland, and the Isle of Man in 2017. Most of these (89%) were total knee replacements (TKRs) with smaller numbers of unicondylar knee replacements (UKRs) (10%), and patella-femoral (1%) joint (PFJ) replacements. The vast majority of these (97%) are performed for osteoarthritis (OA), and the average age of a patient is 68.9 years. For most patients who have their primary surgery around this average age of implantation, we expect that no further future surgery will be required. Currently, the Kaplan-Meier estimate of revision rate at 14 years for all cemented TKRs in the NJR is 4.47% (1). A recent meta-analysis of worldwide arthroplasty registries with a minimum of 15 years of follow-up showed that approximately 82% of TKRs last 25 years (2).

The number of primary TKRs being performed is expected to rise. Estimates vary significantly as to the magnitude of this rise (3–6). However, there is greater consensus regarding the predicted rise in the number of patients who will outlive their TKRs and therefore require complex revision surgery (6–9). This is attributable to an increasing number of patients having their primary surgery earlier in life, the increasing incidence of obesity, and patients demanding more from their implants as they pursue active lifestyles and continued employment into later life.

The functional outcomes and patient satisfaction scores are generally very good for TKR (10,11) but not as predictable as for total hip replacement (THR) (12). Other than subdividing knee replacements into total or partial (unicondylar or patella-femoral) joint replacements, they are also distinguished according to whether they leave the posterior cruciate ligament (PCL) intact or not. Those implants designed to replace the function of the PCL are referred to as posterior stabilized and those which leave the PCL intact, unconstrained. According to the NJR,

86.5% of TKRs in 2017 were implanted using bone cement. Uncemented implants are generally reserved for younger, more active patients (13).

OP is of particular significance in the context of a TKR as it increases the risk of implant failure (14), impaired function (15), and periprosthetic fracture (16).

RELATIONSHIP BETWEEN OSTEOPOROSIS AND OSTEOARTHRITIS OF THE KNEE

The relationship between osteoarthritis (OA) and osteoporosis (OP) is complex and controversial. Many studies have found an inverse relationship between the two diseases, in that the presence of OA is associated with higher bone mineral density (BMD) (17–19). The inference is that OA may infer a protective effect against OP, the two diseases being separate entities and not the consequence of a normal aging process. How OA is defined affects the strength of this association. Studies that define knee OA according to Kellgren-Laurence grade (20) or the presence of osteophytes (21,22) show a stronger association than those that define knee OA according to loss of joint space (23,24). However, in contrast to these studies, high rates (25%, 17/68) of occult OP have been found in patients awaiting THR for OA (25).

The findings of longitudinal studies do not offer further clarity as to the relationship between the diseases. Findings from the Framingham Study (26) suggest that while high BMD and a rise in BMD may be associated with a risk of incident OA of the knee, both of these factors also protect against the risk of radiographic progression of the OA. The authors concluded that their insight into the influence of bone quality on OA may offer potential therapeutic options.

Lingard et al. (27) used dual-energy x-ray absorptiometry (DEXA) to calculate the BMD at the femur, lumbar spine, and radius of 199 patients awaiting THR or TKR. Their aims were to estimate the prevalence of OP in this patient group between the ages of 65 and 80 years, and to examine the association between OP at these sites with each other and other potential risk factors for low BMD. They found that the overall rate of OP at any anatomical site was 23%, and that according to World Health Organization (WHO) guidelines, a further 43% would be diagnosed as osteopenic. Of interest, and diagnostic importance, was that OP was more likely to be diagnosed from DEXA of the forearm (14%) than the lumbar spine (8.5%) and proximal femur on the index side (8.2%). In agreement with the findings of Goerres et al. (28), it was found that patients had lower BMD at the symptomatic hip compared to the contralateral side. Given that patients with OA of sufficient severity to merit arthroplasty are likely to also have OA at the other hip or knee, or lumbar spine, there is an argument that OP may be underdiagnosed if DEXA is not performed at a site distant to the osteoarthritic joint.

Im and Kim (29) sought to explain the difference of the inverse relationship between OA and OP seen in cross-sectional studies compared to the more complex relationship seen in longitudinal studies. They conclude that the subchondral sclerosis and bone formation seen in OA results in increased BMD but that this can accelerate the onset of OA. Once OA progresses and the patient develops symptoms, the resultant reduction causes a decrease in BMD. However, the extra bone already formed in the early stages of the disease will result in higher measured BMD compared to control patients without OA.

Many patients who are to undergo knee arthroplasty will not have been assessed or investigated for OP. Ishii et al. (30) investigated the relationship between BMD as measured by DEXA and various radiographic knee parameters. To account for the confounding variables of sex and age, they looked at the ratio of medial-to-lateral BMD (M/L-BMD) rather than absolute values. Looking at 178 consecutive medial, or varus pattern, OA knees, they found a significant association between the tibio-femoral angle and the femoral M/L-BMD ratio and between the mechanical axis angle and the tibial M/L-BMD ratio. As well as supporting the relationship between end-stage OA and increased BMD, this study has identified two parameters that may provide *in vivo* data to evaluate preoperative M/L-BMD ratios in the femur and tibia without DEXA in patients with advanced medial OA of the knee.

BONE MINERAL DENSITY CHANGES AFTER TOTAL KNEE REPLACEMENT

Multiple studies have reported a loss of BMD post-TKR. This may occur around the femoral component because of "stress-shielding" or more proximally as a result of disuse porosis. This may lead to an increased fracture risk or compromise of component fixation.

Hopkins et al. (31) looked at DEXA results in 19 postmenopausal Caucasian patients following TKR comparing to 43 controls. Neck of femur (NOF) and total femur BMD losses were significantly higher in those who had undergone

TKR. This combined with relatively decreased muscle mass, impaired weight-bearing, and poorer function led to their conclusion of a likely increased risk of NOF fracture 1-year postsurgery. Similar findings have been reported in a Korean population (32). Kim et al. found that BMD of the trochanteric region, the femoral neck, and total femur was significantly lower compared to pre-TKR in the 96 hips evaluated at 1 and 3 months post arthroplasty. However, at each time measurement, there was no significant difference between the operative and nonoperative sides. At 12 months, the difference compared to preoperative BMD in each of the studied areas was not significantly different.

Changes in BMD of the distal femur have been studied by van Loon et al. (33). In patients ranging from 41 to 80 years, the BMD in the distal femur around 12 cemented TKRs, the femoral necks, and lumbar spine was measured and compared preoperatively and at 1 year. There was a nonsignificant change of 1% in BMD at the femoral necks and lumbar spine. The differences around the region deep to the anterior flange of the femoral component (22%) and the region just proximal to the femoral component (8%) were significantly different.

The polyethylene bearing found in a TKR is most commonly fixed, but there are designs in which the bearing is mobile and allowed some freedom to rotate as the knee moves. The aim of this is to allow self-correction of rotational mismatch during the complex movements that the knee makes during the gait cycle. This maximizes congruency of the TKR components throughout the range of motion and potentially decreases stresses at the implant-bone or implant-cement interface. Potential disadvantages are increased polyethylene wear from a greater surface-area of mobile surfaces, dislocation of mobile bearings, and increased cost.

Minoda (34) compared BMD changes seen around 28 knees receiving a cemented fixed-bearing TKR with 28 receiving a cemented mobile-bearing TKR. The BMD of the femur decreased postoperatively in the fixed-bearing group, but not the mobile-bearing group. At 24 months postsurgery, the difference in the postoperative BMD change between the two groups was statistically significant ($P < 0.05$). The authors concluded that a mobile-bearing TKR has a favorable effect on the BMD versus a fixed-bearing design.

The BMD changes seen around PFJ replacements have been studied by van Jonbergen (35) et al. They hypothesized that given the relatively small size of a PFJ replacement compared to a TKR, there would be no significant change in the distal femur BMD after a PFJ arthroplasty. However, they found that 1-year postsurgery there was a 15% reduction in BMD behind the femoral component and 2% in the supracondylar region compared to baseline readings taken 2 weeks before the operation. In the unoperated limb, there was a 2% reduction in both sites.

A TKR is most commonly inserted with a polymethyl methacrylate bone cement, but uncemented designs are available. Hybrid fixations are also possible. Uncemented have a high-friction porous or grit-blasted surface finish that affords initial fixation. The goal is for bone to grow into the implant, and bioactive coatings such as hydroxyapatite accelerate this process. The theoretical advantage of uncemented implants is that once osteointegration has taken place, it is highly unlikely to loosen unless there is infection or lysis. The disadvantages associated with bone cement, debris causing third-body wear, and cardiovascular instability at the time of implantation, are also avoided.

There are concerns that osteoporotic bone is less likely to offer sufficient initial stability to allow osteointegration. Petersen et al. (36) examined 22 knees with uncemented TKRs using DEXA scans and radiographs to evaluate implant stability and migration up to 3 years. There was a positive correlation between BMD and migration, leading to the conclusion that the tibias of patients with higher BMD preoperatively showed less continuous implant migration. There was no correlation between inducible displacement as measured by stress radiograph at 1 year and BMD.

UKR can be performed when OA predominantly affects either the medial or, less commonly, the lateral side of the knee. Hooper et al. (37) reviewed BMD changes in 79 patients with a mean age of 65 years after uncemented UKR with a minimum 2-year follow-up. They focused on changes seen in the proximal tibia. No significant differences were seen in BMD comparing operated versus non-operated limbs. The authors conclude that these findings suggest that this implant acts more physiologically than a TKR. Blaty et al. (38) correlated BMD losses post-TKR with cortical width in 30 patients with a TKR implanted within 2–5 years. Measurements were taken at 15%, 25%, and 60% of the femur length as measured from the distance from the distal femoral notch. They concluded that the distal femur BMD can be reproducibly measured using DEXA and was approximately 10% lower on the operated side. The cortical width measurements taken at 25% of the femur length were found to be significantly lower on the operated side.

Recognizing that future work is required to further understand how BMD changes after TKR in larger samples, Thomas et al. (39) have performed a pilot study building toward a standardized method of assessing distal femur BMD in patients with a TKR by defining the regional distribution of BMD in 30 volunteers with a TKR implanted 2–5 years previously. Both these authors and Blaty et al. (38) discuss the potential to use DEXA as a preoperative assessment tool to identify those at particular risk of periprosthetic fracture and aid surgical planning and implant selection. It could also be used to monitor the impact of therapies implemented to reduce postoperative BMD losses.

PHARMACOLOGIC MODULATION OF BMD LOSS FOLLOWING TKR

The reduction in BMD seen after TKR may lead to increased risk of fracture, worse function, implant migration, and aseptic loosening. To mitigate against these complications, there has been much interest in the use of bisphosphonates (BP) following TKR with the aim of decreasing BMD loss through the inhibition of bone resorption.

In a retrospective cohort study, Prieto-Alhambra et al. (40) studied the association between BP use and implant survival after primary TKR or THR. Utilizing the UK General Practice Research Database, 1912 BP users were identified. This group had a lower rate of revision at 5 years than nonusers 0.93% (95% confidence interval 0.52%–1.68%) versus 1.96% (1.80%–2.14%). Implant survival was also significantly longer in the BP users than in nonusers with a hazard ratio of 0.54 (0.29–0.99; $P = 0.047$). The time to revision was almost twice as long. It was calculated that assuming a 2% failure over 5 years, the number needed to treat to avoid one revision was 107 for oral BPs.

The same group from Oxford, UK (41), undertook a propensity score analysis to examine the association between BP use and risk of periprosthetic fracture in TKR patients using the same database as previously mentioned. Their results suggest that BP use as primary prevention could reduce postoperative risk of fracture by 50% and by 55% in secondary prevention.

An American group (42) looked at the same endpoints in a cohort of 34,116 primary TKR patients (6692 BP users). Bone quality (normal, osteopenia, osteoporosis) and age (younger than 65 years versus older than 65 years) were used as risk modifiers. Among BP users, 0.5% underwent an aseptic revision and 0.6% a periprosthetic fracture. In non-BP users, 1.6% underwent aseptic revision and 0.1% a periprosthetic fracture. This is the first study to identify BPs as a risk factor for periprosthetic fracture in TKA, but the authors acknowledge that the numbers are small and some factors that may contribute to fracture risk (smoking, activity levels, steroid use) are not known. This study is also unique in including DEXA findings as a variable. Twenty-six percent of those taking BPs had an unremarkable DEXA scan. Reasons given in the study for prescription in this group of patients included prophylaxis in high-risk groups, or empiric treatment after osteoporotic hip or vertebral fracture in postmenopausal women. This allowed the authors to conclude that regardless of BMD in patients older than 65 years, there was a lower revision risk with BP usage. In those younger than 65 years, BP use was associated with lower revision risk in osteopenic and osteoporotic patients.

A meta-analysis of five randomized controlled trials (RCTs) with a total of 188 patients was published by Shi et al. (43) to analyze the effect of BPs (all used alendronate) on periprosthetic bone loss after TKR. None of the studies reported severe or fatal adverse effects of BP use. In the proximal part of the tibia, the BP group had significantly higher total BMD versus control at 3 and 6 months, but not at 12 months. In the distal aspect of the femur, the anterior, central, and posterior aspects of the femoral metaphysis, and the medial and lateral aspects of the tibial metaphysis, the difference was maintained at 3, 6, and 12 months. No significant difference was seen at any time point between the groups at the tibial diaphysis. The conclusion of the meta-analysis is that BPs have a short-term effect on reducing periprosthetic bone loss after TKR and that this effect is more effective in the metaphysis compared to the diaphysis. The authors called for more clinical trials to characterize the longer-term outcomes.

The effect of teriparatide for this indication has also been studied (44). Twenty-two knees in 17 patients received teriparatide and were compared to controls. The teriparatide group had significant BMD increases in the posterior condyles and lateral aspect of the tibia at 6 months. At 12 months, the differences between groups was significant at the anterior condyle, posterior condyle, and tibial diaphysis. At 6 and 12 months, the teriparatide had higher adjusted mean BMD in all regions than did the control group. It was concluded that teriparatide may be a reasonable treatment option to preserve or improve BMD post-TKR in osteoporotic patients.

Any benefits of reduced BMD loss must be balanced against potential risks associated with BP use including osteonecrosis of the jaw, infection, and atypical femoral fractures, as discussed earlier in this book.

RELATIONSHIP BETWEEN BONE QUALITY AND FUNCTION POST-TKR

Huang et al. (15) investigated the relationship between bone quality, as measured by DEXA and microcomputed tomography, and functional endpoints rather than more simply the endpoints of fracture or revision for aseptic loosening. They argue that bone microarchitecture parameters, including the structural model index, bone volume fracture, and Euler number, are more strongly correlated with bone strength than areal BMD. During surgery in 43 postmenopausal patients, the intercondylar box of bone removed to make way for the femoral component of the TKR was retained. These specimens were imaged using a high-resolution microcomputed tomography scanner. Volumetric BMD, trabecular separation, and a structural model index were all significantly associated with postoperative pain scores and improvement in the patient-reported Knee Injury and Osteoarthritis Outcome Scores (KOOS). The authors hypothesize that those scores that indicate greater porosity of trabecular bone might allow better penetration of cement into the bone during implantation. Deterioration of the local bone architecture in combination with better cement interdigitation in the affected bone may affect local nociception resulting in lower reported postoperative pain scores and a greater improvement in functional scores.

SUMMARY

The relationship between OP and OA as it relates to TKR is complex and controversial. It is likely that OP and those who may have a suboptimal outcome because of poor function, implant loosening, or periprosthetic fracture are underdiagnosed. Further research to enable improved

preoperative diagnosis of OP, to identify those whose outcome may be compromised by peri-implant BMD loss, and to clarify whether pharmacologic intervention would improve outcomes is required.

REFERENCES

1. National Joint Registry for England W. *Northern Ireland and the Isle of Man*. 15th annual report, 2018. 2018 Available from: http://www.njrreports.org.uk/Portals/0/PDFdownloads/NJR%2015th%20Annual%20Report%202018.pdf
2. Evans J, Evans JP, Walker RW, Blom AW, Whitehouse MR, Sayers A. How long does a hip replacement last? A systematic review and meta-analysis of case series and national registry reports with more than 15 years of follow-up. *Lancet*. 2019;393:647–54.
3. Culliford D, Maskell J, Judge A, Cooper C, Prieto-Alhambra D, Arden NK. Future projections of total hip and knee arthroplasty in the UK: Results from the UK clinical practice research datalink. *Osteoarthritis Cartilage*. 2015;23(4):594–600.
4. Inacio MCS, Graves SE, Pratt NL, Roughead EE, Nemes S. Increase in total joint arthroplasty projected from 2014 to 2046 in Australia: A conservative local model with international implications. *Clin Orthop Relat Res*. 2017;475(8):2130–7.
5. Nemes S, Rolfson O, W-Dahl A et al. Historical view and future demand for knee arthroplasty in Sweden. *Acta Orthop*. 2015;86:426–31.
6. Kurtz S, Ong K, Lau E, Mowat F, Halpern M. Projections of primary and revision hip and knee arthroplasty in the United States from 2005 to 2030. *J Bone Joint Surg Am*. 2007;89(4):780–5.
7. Hamilton DF, Howie CR, Burnett R, Simpson AH, Patton JT. Dealing with the predicted increase in demand for revision total knee arthroplasty: Challenges, risks and opportunities. *Bone Joint J*. 2015;97-b(6):723–8.
8. Bozic KJ, Kamath AF, Ong K et al. Comparative epidemiology of revision arthroplasty: Failed THA poses greater clinical and economic burdens than failed TKA. *Clin Orthop Relat Res*. 2015;473(6):2131–8.
9. Khan M, Osman K, Green G, Haddad FS. The epidemiology of failure in total knee arthroplasty: Avoiding your next revision. *Bone Joint J*. 2016;98-b (1 Suppl A):105–12.
10. Choi YJ, Ra HJ. Patient satisfaction after total knee arthroplasty. *Knee Surg Relat Res*. 2016;28(1):1–15.
11. Kahlenberg CA, Nwachukwu BU, McLawhorn AS, Cross MB, Cornell CN, Padgett DE. Patient satisfaction after total knee replacement: A systematic review. *HSS J*. 2018;14:192–201.
12. O'Brien S, Bennett D, Doran E, Beverland DE. Comparison of hip and knee arthroplasty outcomes at early and intermediate follow-up. *Orthopedics* 2009;32(3):168.

13. Aprato A, Risitano S, Sabatini L, Giachino M, Agati G, Massè A. Cementless total knee arthroplasty. *Ann Transl Med*. 2016;4(7).

14. Petersen MM, Nielsen PT, Lauritzen JB, Lund B. Changes in bone mineral density of the proximal tibia after uncemented total knee arthroplasty. A 3-year follow-up of 25 knees. *Acta Orthop Scand*. 1995;66(6):513–6.

15. Huang CC, Jiang CC, Hsieh CH, Tsai CJ, Chiang H. Local bone quality affects the outcome of prosthetic total knee arthroplasty. *J Orthop Res*. 2016;34(2): 240–8.

16. Gundry M, Hopkins S, Knapp K. A review on bone mineral density loss in total knee replacements leading to increased fracture risk. *Clin Rev Bone Miner Metab*. 2017;15(4):162–74.

17. Verstraeten A, Van Ermen H, Haghebaert G, Nijs J, Geusens P, Dequeker J. Osteoarthrosis retards the development of osteoporosis. Observation of the coexistence of osteoarthrosis and osteoporosis. *Clin Orthop Relat Res*. 1991(264):169–77.

18. Burger H, van Daele PL, Odding E et al. Association of radiographically evident osteoarthritis with higher bone mineral density and increased bone loss with age. The Rotterdam Study. *Arthritis Rheum*. 1996;39(1):81–6.

19. Hochberg MC, Lethbridge-Cejku M, Tobin JD. Bone mineral density and osteoarthritis: Data from the Baltimore Longitudinal study of aging. *Osteoarthritis Cartilage*. 2004;12(Suppl A):S45–8.

20. Kellgren JH, Lawrence JS. Radiological assessment of osteo-arthrosis. *Ann Rheum Dis*. 1957;16(4):494–502.

21. Bergink AP, van der Klift M, Hofman A et al. Osteoarthritis of the knee is associated with vertebral and nonvertebral fractures in the elderly: The Rotterdam Study. *Arthritis Rheum*. 2003;49(5):648–57.

22. Sowers M, Lachance L, Jamadar D et al. The associations of bone mineral density and bone turnover markers with osteoarthritis of the hand and knee in pre- and perimenopausal women. *Arthritis Rheum*. 1999;42(3):483–9.

23. Hart DJ, Mootoosamy I, Doyle DV, Spector TD. The relationship between osteoarthritis and osteoporosis in the general population: The Chingford Study. *Ann Rheum Dis*. 1994;53(3):158–62.

24. Hannan MT, Anderson JJ, Zhang Y, Levy D, Felson DT. Bone mineral density and knee osteoarthritis in elderly men and women. The Framingham Study. *Arthritis Rheum*. 1993;36(12):1671–80.

25. Glowacki J, Hurwitz S, Thornhill TS, Kelly M, LeBoff MS. Osteoporosis and vitamin-D deficiency among postmenopausal women with osteoarthritis undergoing total hip arthroplasty. *J Bone Joint Surg Am*. 2003;85-a(12):2371–7.

26. Zhang Y, Hannan MT, Chaisson CE et al. Bone mineral density and risk of incident and progressive radiographic knee osteoarthritis in women: The Framingham Study. *J Rheumatol*. 2000;27(4):1032–7.

27. Lingard EA, Mitchell SY, Francis RM et al. The prevalence of osteoporosis in patients with severe hip and knee osteoarthritis awaiting joint arthroplasty. *Age Ageing*. 2010;39(2):234–9.

28. Goerres GW, Hauselmann HJ, Seifert B, Michel BA, Uebelhart D. Patients with knee osteoarthritis have lower total hip bone mineral density in the symptomatic leg than in the contralateral hip. *J Clin Densitom*. 2005;8(4):484–7.

29. Im GI, Kim MK. The relationship between osteoarthritis and osteoporosis. *J Bone Miner Metab*. 2014;32(2):101–9.

30. Ishii Y, Noguchi H, Sato J, Ishii H, Todoroki K, Toyabe SI. Association between bone mineral density distribution and various radiographic parameters in patients with advanced medial osteoarthritis of the knee. *J Orthop Sci*. 2019;24(6):686–92.

31. Hopkins SJ, Toms AD, Brown M, Welsman JR, Ukoumunne OC, Knapp KM. A study investigating short- and medium-term effects on function, bone mineral density and lean tissue mass post-total knee replacement in a Caucasian female post-menopausal population: Implications for hip fracture risk. *Osteoporos Int*. 2016;27(8):2567–76.

32. Kim KK, Won YY, Heo YM, Lee DH, Yoon JY, Sung WS. Changes in bone mineral density of both proximal femurs after total knee arthroplasty. *Clin Orthop Surg*. 2014;6(1):43–8.

33. van Loon CJ, Oyen WJ, de Waal Malefijt MC, Verdonschot N. Distal femoral bone mineral density after total knee arthroplasty: A comparison with general bone mineral density. *Arch Orthop Trauma Surg*. 2001;121(5):282–5.

34. Minoda Y, Ikebuchi M, Kobayashi A, Iwaki H, Inori F, Nakamura H. A cemented mobile-bearing total knee replacement prevents periprosthetic loss of bone mineral density around the femoral component: A matched cohort study. *J Bone Joint Surg Br*. 2010;92(6):794–8.

35. van Jonbergen HP, Koster K, Labey L, Innocenti B, van Kampen A. Distal femoral bone mineral density decreases following patellofemoral arthroplasty: 1-year follow-up study of 14 patients. *BMC Musculoskelet Disord*. 2010;11:74.

36. Petersen MM, Nielsen PT, Lebech A, Toksvig-Larsen S, Lund B. Preoperative bone mineral density of the proximal tibia and migration of the tibial component after uncemented total knee arthroplasty. *J Arthroplasty*. 1999;14(1):77–81.

37. Hooper GJ, Gilchrist N, Maxwell R, March R, Heard A, Frampton C. The effect of the Oxford uncemented medial compartment arthroplasty on the bone mineral density and content of the proximal tibia. *Bone Joint J*. 2013;95-b(11):1480–3.

38. Blaty T, Krueger D, Illgen R et al. DXA evaluation of femoral bone mineral density and cortical width in patients with prior total knee arthroplasty. *Osteoporos Int*. 2018;30(2):383–90.

39. Thomas B, Binkley N, Anderson PA, Krueger D. DXA measured distal femur bone mineral density in patients after total knee arthroplasty: Method development and reproducibility. *J Clin Densitom.* 2018;22(1):67–73.

40. Prieto-Alhambra D, Javaid MK, Judge A et al. Association between bisphosphonate use and implant survival after primary total arthroplasty of the knee or hip: Population based retrospective cohort study. *BMJ* 2011;343:d7222.

41. Prieto-Alhambra D, Javaid MK, Judge A et al. Bisphosphonate use and risk of post-operative fracture among patients undergoing a total knee replacement for knee osteoarthritis: A propensity score analysis. *Osteoporos Int.* 2011;22(5):1555–71.

42. Namba RS, Inacio MC, Cheetham TC, Dell RM, Paxton EW, Khatod MX. Lower total knee arthroplasty revision risk associated with bisphosphonate use, even in patients with normal bone density. *J Arthroplasty.* 2016;31(2):537–41.

43. Shi M, Chen L, Wu H et al. Effect of bisphosphonates on periprosthetic bone loss after total knee arthroplasty: A meta-analysis of randomized controlled trials. *BMC Musculoskelet Disord.* 2018; 19(1):177.

44. Suzuki T, Sukezaki F, Shibuki T, Toyoshima Y, Nagai T, Inagaki K. Teriparatide administration increases periprosthetic bone mineral density after total knee arthroplasty: A prospective study. *J Arthroplasty.* 2018;33(1):79–85.

Rehabilitation of the osteoporotic patient

Is it different?

THEODOROS H. TOSOUNIDIS and AMY MARGOT LINDH

INTRODUCTION

Osteoporosis-related fractures most commonly occur in the proximal femur, wrist, and spine (1). These injuries are often a reflection of the patient's suboptimal physiologic state, as well as deterioration in an individual's ability to cope in his or her current environment, with osteoporosis being a contributing rather than a causative factor. Even with a low-energy insult, the consequences may be significant, with the elderly patient's capacity for recovery far inferior to that of a young patient (2). Permanent disability that often results after these injuries has been considered a factor affecting the early to medium-term mortality and morbidity in the elderly age groups (3). In a phenomenological study looking into pain and fracture-related limitation after fragility fractures of the hip, wrist, vertebrae, and multiple or other areas, Sale et al. (4) suggested that the majority of the patients report pain and other limitations at or beyond 6 months postinjury.

Rehabilitation helps patients to achieve optimal recovery of their injuries. Rehabilitation in osteroporosis-related fractures aims to the restoration of physical, psychological, and social function, with the secondary benefit of reducing these secondary complications. In this chapter, we describe the current model of fragility fracture care in the United Kingdom and the key elements in secondary prevention of these injuries, and we highlight the specific considerations for osteoporosis-related fractures of the hip and distal radius.

FRAGILITY FRACTURE CARE IN THE UNITED KINGDOM

Each year in the United Kingdom, approximately 500,000 fractures occur in patients over the age of 50 years (5). These fractures arise from a synergistic relationship between age-related bone mineral density (BMD) loss and an increasing propensity for falls among the older population. The effect of menopause on reducing BMD means that older women are most likely to suffer with this combination of problems (6). The statistics surrounding fragility fractures make for somewhat depressing reading; these fractures, in particular of the hip and the vertebrae, carry a significant burden of morbidity and mortality (5). Not only does this have serious and sometimes grave consequences for the patient, it also carries a substantial financial cost to health services. In a recent systematic review (7) that looked into the costs of hip fractures globally and identified drivers of differences in costs, a pooled estimate of the cost for the index hospitalization was $10,075 and the health and social care costs at 12 months were $43,669. In the United Kingdom every year, hip fractures alone account for 85,000 unplanned admissions, 1.8 million bed-days, and approximately £1.9 billion in hospital costs, excluding the high cost of social care (8).

In 2007, the British Orthopaedic Association (BOA), in conjunction with the British Geriatrics Society, published a guideline on the care of fragility fractures (9). The aim of the guideline was to coordinate services that were key to improving outcomes and set a gold standard for fracture care, focusing on the most costly injury (financially and clinically), which is a fractured neck of femur. In broad terms, the guideline identifies three key elements, in no particular order, of a successful outcome following an osteoporotic fracture, which can be considered essential components of successful rehabilitation: (a) multidisciplinary teamwork to address the multifactorial problems that most patients face, (b) effective secondary prevention to prevent recurrent injury, and (c) continuous feedback via audit to monitor and improve practice. It identifies points on the fragility fracture spectrum where intervention can take place and will serve to synergistically act to reduce morbidity and mortality.

The first advancement along the aforementioned spectrum should be considered as a "warning shot" based on the fact that 50% of patients who suffer a hip fracture had suffered a previous fragility fracture in the past (8). It is estimated that directed therapies can reduce the risk of refracture by 20%–70%, bringing with it significant cost savings, as well as prolonged independence and quality of life for the patient (8). Therefore, it is recommended that these patients are directed into a dedicated "fracture liaison service" at their first presentation to health services with a suspected fragility fracture, even if the management is likely to be conservative and not warrant an admission. Via this service, appropriate secondary prevention medication can be started and a thorough falls risk assessment can be carried out.

If a patient is admitted to the hospital as a consequence of a fracture, this can be considered as further progression along the spectrum. This creates another opportunity to mitigate the risk of reinjury, secondary complications, and death. The first port of call is to medically optimize the patient, which includes reducing the physiologic burden introduced by acute pain and addressing any medically reversible abnormalities (9). If operative fixation is indicated, once deemed fit for surgery, management of the fracture needs to optimize stabilization above anatomical reduction, in order to permit early functional return (10). After this acute phase is over, comprehensive orthogeriatric assessment can be undertaken. It has been demonstrated that such an assessment, which looks at a number of interrelated areas, can lead to improved rates of survival and independence (9). This is not a "one-size-fits-all" program; it involves a multidisciplinary team made up of nurses, physiotherapists, occupational therapists, and social workers. The assessment will reveal which areas are most deficient, and care planning will be designed around addressing them as effectively as possible. Some centers opt for separate orthogeriatric rehabilitation units to promote recovery to a level where they can continue to live at home rather than in social care; this may not reduce length of stay, but it may mean that an individual can return home after the hospital stay as opposed to being transferred into institutionalized care (2,9). If not already completed in the hospital, patients will be followed up for osteoporosis investigation and falls risk assessment with the fracture liaison services (8).

KEY ELEMENTS OF SECONDARY PREVENTION

In the previous section, we described the approach to fragility fracture care in the United Kingdom. Most health-care systems have adopted analogous approaches to managing fragility fractures. In this section, we look at some of the elements of secondary prevention that have robust clinical evidence for reducing future fracture risk and recommendations for how they might be used.

Drugs for bone protection

In the United Kingdom, it is recommended practice to risk assess men older than 75 years and women over 65 years for their fracture risk (11,12). The FRAX tool, developed by the World Health Organization, can be used to calculate 10-year fracture risk of any osteoporotic fracture. For hip fracture, risk assessment is recommended for both sexes older than 50 years if one of the listed risk factors is present, which includes previous fragility fracture. Measurement of BMD is recommended for anyone who has a FRAX risk score that is in the region of an intervention threshold ("consider therapy" category). In postmenopausal women who have sustained a fragility fracture, there is little indication to perform a dual-energy x-ray absorptiometry (DEXA) scan, as at this stage their refracture risk is such that drug therapy is indicated without further investigation (12).

The gold standard for measurement of BMD is DEXA scanning. If the T-score is less than −2.5, a diagnosis of osteoporosis is made. The low-cost bisphosphonate therapy tends to be the first-line drug of choice for treatment of osteoporosis; it has been shown to improve bone density and reduce new fracture risk, and it is tolerated in most individuals (12,13). The current recommended duration of treatment is 60 months (14).

Additional medications that may be prescribed to improve bone quality (but not density), based on relevant biochemistry, are vitamin D_3 and calcium supplements. The recommendation from the National Osteoporosis Society is to commence treatment with oral vitamin D_3 if the 25OHD$_2$ level is <50 nmol/L in patients with osteoporosis. This is in the form of a loading regimen, followed by a maintenance dose, with levels to be rechecked after 1 month. The National Institute for Health and Care Excellence (NICE) recommends vitamin D_3 supplementation only if dietary calcium intake is adequate, or a combined supplement of 10 micrograms of vitamin D_3 with at least 1000 mg calcium daily (20 micrograms of vitamin D_3 + 1000 mg of calcium) if the person is housebound or lives in institutionalized care (15).

Falls assessment and prevention

The NICE has published an updated guideline on the assessment and prevention of falls risk in older people (16). They have provided recommendations to guide practice based on a comprehensive assessment of the available evidence.

Of particular relevance to rehabilitation of fragility fractures, there is level I evidence to support multifactorial intervention in older people who have been injured as a result of a fall, which is in keeping with the approach recommended by the BOA. In their summary of the highest-quality available evidence, the reviewers identified the key components of successful interventions as including a medical assessment to identify the primary cause of the fall, in combination with physiotherapy and occupational therapy assessments to devise individually tailored exercise programs that addressed deficits in balance/gait, transfers, and stair climbing. These were combined with follow-up to ensure the appropriate recommendations were being followed.

The reviewers highlighted that the outcome measure of primary focus was reduction in the recurrence of falls, but in terms of important rehabilitation outcomes such as function, mobility, and psychosocial health, they were not able to appraise the evidence. They also commented on the significant crossover between secondary prevention interventions and rehabilitation; this corresponds with the model of fragility fractures as existing along a spectrum, as described in the previous section.

REHABILITATION FOR SPECIFIC FRACTURES

Hip fractures

The rehabilitation in hip fracture surgery aims to restore the preinjury functional status of the patient. Full weight-bearing should be instructed as soon as possible after surgery because it is difficult for elderly patients to follow instructions for partial weight-bearing. The outcome of surgery is multifactorial, and certain subpopulations are prone to poor recovery, including patients with poor cognitive and preexisting functional limitations, men, and nursing home residents (17). A recent Cochrane systematic review concluded that there is currently considerable uncertainty regarding the reasons why some individuals and/or groups of patients do better than others (17). The authors also suggested that research should focus on the development and testing of individual and combined treatment strategies and that more needs to be done toward the clarification of the subgroups that will benefit most from improved access to rehabilitation. Various studies (18,19) have suggested that multidisciplinary rehabilitation after hip fracture in the elderly consisting of physiotherapists, occupational therapists, dieticians, social workers, and nurses operating under the guidance of a rehabilitation physician or a geriatrician offers better results. Nevertheless, a recent Cochrane systematic review (20) of randomized controlled trials (RCTs) concluded that despite the fact that the multidisciplinary rehabilitation has superior results compared to "no treatment" (patients who received only conventional acute postsurgical care and were discharged without specific further rehabilitation) in lower extremity strength and functional status, a strong argument supporting the multidisciplinary rehabilitation cannot be made due to the high risk of bias in the included studies. The authors suggested that the research should focus on the characterization of the disciplines involved and the exact dosage/frequency of interventions required in the multidisciplinary rehabilitation mode of hip fractures (20). In the same line, another

Cochrane review (21) aiming to evaluate the effects of interventions intending to advance physical and psychosocial performance in patients with hip fractures concluded that there is insufficient evidence to suggest a change in the current practice. The authors advocated that future research should focus on patient-reported outcome measures, and attention should be drawn to the timing, duration, and administrating discipline of the rehabilitation.

Cognitive impairment is estimated to affect one-third of patients who sustain a hip fracture. Despite that, the majority of these patients are excluded from clinical studies (22). Similarly, it is well accepted that contemporary rehabilitation programs do not address the specific needs of the cognitively impaired patients who sustained a hip fracture. In a recent review, Resnick et al. (23) concluded that the implementation of a postsurgical rehabilitation program is feasible in this population of patients and that intensive rehabilitation with innovative approaches should be considered. A Cochrane review by Smith et al. (24) looking into the available evidence related to the enhanced rehabilitation programs for patients with dementia suggested that relevant research in this field should be of high priority based on the fact that the current evidence comes from small clinical trials, the population in interest is growing, and currently implementation of enhanced rehabilitation programs can be sufficiently supported by the contemporary literature.

Wrist fractures

Wrist fractures in adults can result in significant long-term functional impairment, pain, and morbidity (25–27). The basic open questions surrounding the rehabilitation of wrist fractures include the type and the duration of intervention indicated and also who should be the health professionals involved in the provision of the rehabilitation (28). Interventions described for rehabilitation of wrist fractures in adults include active and passive mobilization exercises, strengthening exercises, continuous passive motion, splints, pain management methods (heat, transcutaneous electrical nerve stimulation, massage), etc. (29). Nevertheless, significant care gaps and decreased application of screening and treatment with respect to subsequent falls/osteoporotic fracture prevention have been documented (30). Web-based educational/knowledge translation strategies to increase the engagement of hand therapists and the fall risk screening have been proposed as future research directions.

Handoll et al. (28) conducted a systematic review of RCTs or quasi-RCTs evaluating rehabilitation as part of the management of fractures of the distal radius sustained by adults and concluded that there is insufficient evidence to evaluate the effectiveness of the various rehabilitation interventions. Nevertheless, it is crucial to realize that the effect of rehabilitation is time dependent. Dewan et al. (11), in a longitudinal cohort study of 94 patients, demonstrated that after a distal radius fracture, most of the improvement related to general health status, fear of falling, and fracture-specific pain/disability takes place within the first 6 months after the injury. In a prospective cohort study, Crockett et al. (31) evaluated the changes in functional status within the first year after a distal radius fracture in women older than 50 years. The authors demonstrated that there was significantly lower functional status (patient-rated wrist evaluation) in the elderly patients across all points in time. Improvement in functional status occurred from 1 week up to 1 year, and the authors underpinned the importance of identification of the recovery pattern in patients with distal radius fractures, which might be helpful for future research and the development of preventive approaches.

REFERENCES

1. Cummings SR, Melton LJ. Epidemiology and outcomes of osteoporotic fractures. *Lancet* 2002;359(9319):1761–7.
2. Kammerlander C, Roth T, Friedman SM et al. Orthogeriatric service—A literature review comparing different models. *Osteoporos Int.* 2010;21(Suppl 4):S637–46.
3. Peterson BE, Jiwanlal A, Della Rocca GJ, Crist BD. Orthopedic trauma and aging: It isn't just about mortality. *Geriatr Orthop Surg Rehabil.* 2015;6(1):33–6.
4. Sale JEM, Frankel L, Thielke S, Funnell L. Pain and fracture-related limitations persist 6 months after a fragility fracture. *Rheumatol Int.* 2017;37(8):1317–22.
5. Svedbom A, Hernlund E, Ivergard M et al. Osteoporosis in the European Union: A compendium of country-specific reports. *Arch Osteoporos.* 2013;8:137.
6. Ikpeze TC, Omar A, Elfar JH. Evaluating problems with footwear in the geriatric population. *Geriatr Orthop Surg Rehabil.* 2015;6(4):338–40.
7. Williamson S, Landeiro F, McConnell T et al. Costs of fragility hip fractures globally: A systematic review and meta-regression analysis. *Osteoporos Int.* 2017;28(10):2791–800.
8. National Osteoporosis Society (NOS). Effective Secondary Prevention of Fragility Fractures: Clinical Standards for Fracture Liaison Services. Bath, England: NOS, 2015.
9. British Orthopaedic Association/British Geriatrics Society. *The Care of Patients with Fragility Fracture ["Blue Book"].* London, UK: British Orthopaedic Association, 2007.
10. Cornell CN. Internal fracture fixation in patients with osteoporosis. *J Am Acad Orthop Surg.* 2003;11(2):109–19.
11. Dewan N, MacDermid JC, Grewal R, Beattie K. Recovery patterns over 4 years after distal radius fracture: Descriptive changes in fracture-specific pain/disability, fall risk factors, bone mineral density, and general health status. *J Hand Ther.* 2018;31(4):451–64.
12. National Osteoporosis Guideline Group. NOGG 2017: Clinical guideline for the prevention and treatment of osteoporosis. 2017. Available from: https://www.sheffield.ac.uk/NOGG/NOGG%20Guideline%202017.pdf
13. Freemantle N, Cooper C, Diez-Perez A et al. Results of indirect and mixed treatment comparison of fracture efficacy for osteoporosis treatments: A meta-analysis. *Osteoporos Int.* 2013;24(1):209–17.
14. National Institute for Health and Care Excellence. Osteoporosis: Assessing the risk of fragility fracture. Clinical guideline [CG146]. 2012.
15. National Institute for Health and Care Excellence. Osteoporosis—Prevention of fragility fractures. Clinical Knowledge Summaries. 2016.
16. National Institute for Health and Care Excellence. *Falls in older people: Assessing risk and prevention.* Clinical guideline [CG161]. 2013.
17. Beaupre LA, Binder EF, Cameron ID et al. Maximising functional recovery following hip fracture in frail seniors. *Best Pract Res Clin Rheumatol.* 2013;27(6):771–88.
18. Cameron ID. Coordinated multidisciplinary rehabilitation after hip fracture. *Disabil Rehabil.* 2005;27(18–19):1081–90.
19. Momsen AM, Rasmussen JO, Nielsen CV, Iversen MD, Lund H. Multidisciplinary team care in rehabilitation: An overview of reviews. *J Rehabil Med.* 2012;44(11):901–12.
20. Donohue K, Hoevenaars R, McEachern J, Zeman E, Mehta S. Home-based multidisciplinary rehabilitation following Hip fracture surgery: What is the evidence? *Rehabil Res Pract.* 2013;2013:875968.
21. Crotty M, Unroe K, Cameron ID, Miller M, Ramirez G, Couzner L. Rehabilitation interventions for improving physical and psychosocial functioning after hip fracture in older people. *Cochrane Database Syst Rev.* 2010;(1):CD007624.
22. Mundi S, Chaudhry H, Bhandari M. Systematic review on the inclusion of patients with cognitive impairment in hip fracture trials: A missed opportunity? *Can J Surg.* 2014;57(4):E141–5.
23. Resnick B, Beaupre L, McGilton KS et al. Rehabilitation interventions for older individuals with cognitive impairment post-hip fracture: A systematic review. *J Am Med Dir Assoc.* 2016;17(3):200–5.
24. Smith TO, Hameed YA, Cross JL, Henderson C, Sahota O, Fox C. Enhanced rehabilitation and care models for adults with dementia following hip fracture surgery. *Cochrane Database Syst Rev.* 2015(6):CD010569.
25. Edwards BJ, Song J, Dunlop DD, Fink HA, Cauley JA. Functional decline after incident wrist fracture—Study of osteoporotic fractures: Prospective cohort study. *BMJ* 2010;341:c3324.
26. Handoll HH, Madhok R. Surgical interventions for treating distal radial fractures in adults. *Cochrane Database Syst Rev.* 2003;(3):CD003209.

27. Handoll HH, Madhok R. Conservative interventions for treating distal radial fractures in adults. *Cochrane Database Syst Rev.* 2003;(2):CD000314.

28. Handoll HH, Elliott J. Rehabilitation for distal radial fractures in adults. *Cochrane Database Syst Rev.* 2015;(9):CD003324.

29. Collins DC. Management and rehabilitation of distal radius fractures. *Orthop Clin North Am.* 1993;24;(2):365–78.

30. Dewan N, MacDermid JC, MacIntyre NJ, Grewal R. Therapist's practice patterns for subsequent fall/osteoporotic fracture prevention for patients with a distal radius fracture. *J Hand Ther.* 2019;32(4):497–506.

31. Crockett K, Farthing JP, Basran J et al. Changes in fall risk and functional status in women aged 50 years and older after distal radius fracture: A prospective 1-year follow-up study. *J Hand Ther.* 2019;32(1):17–24.

Index

Note: Page number followed by f and t indicates figure and table respectively.

A

Abaloparatide, in osteoporosis
  clinical efficacy, 78
  clinical use of, 70
  mechanism of action, 69–70, 77
    preclinical studies, 77–78
Acetabular fractures, 195–196, 196f
  acute total hip arthroplasty, 199, 199f
  classification, 195
  clinical characteristics, 195
  decision-making, 195
  nonoperative treatment of, 196–197, 196f
  operative treatment of, 197
    ORIF, 197–199, 198f
  prevalence of, 195
  radiological features of, 195, 196f
Acute total hip arthroplasty, 199, 199f
AFFs, see Atypical femoral fractures
Alendronate, 57
Alkaline phosphatase (ALP), 36–37
ALP, see Alkaline phosphatase
Alpha (α)3-integrin chain, 6
Anabolic agents, in osteoporosis, 69
  abaloparatide
    clinical use of, 70
    mechanism of action of, 69–70
  romosozumab, 70–71
  sequential therapy, 71
  teriparatide
    clinical use of, 70
    mechanism of action of, 69–70
Androgens, 15
Ankle fractures, osteoporotic, 261
  nonoperative management of, 261–262
  operative management of, 262
    arthrodesis, 263–264, 264f
    complications of, 333–334
    internal fixation, 262–263, 263f
    Steinmann pin, 264
Antagomirs, 143–145, 144f
Anterior pelvic ring, operative treatment of, 186–187
  external fixation, 187–188
  internal fixation, 188

anterior subcutaneous pelvic internal fixation, 188–189
  plate and screw osteosynthesis, 188, 189f
  retrograde transpubic screw fixation, 188
Anterior plate fixation of ilium, 183, 184f
Antiosteoporotic drugs, 92t
Arthrodesis, 129, 263–264, 264f
Arthroplasty, 129–131, 130f
Atypical femoral fractures (AFFs), 61–62, 213–214
  bisphosphonates in, 62, 97, 99–104
  criteria for, 98
    major features, 98
    minor features, 98
  denosumab, side effects, 65
  etiopathology, 97, 98f
    clinical presentation, 97–98
    radiological findings, 97–98
  incidence of, 97
  nonunion of, 100–102
  outcomes of therapy, 104, 104f
  treatment options for
    complete fracture, 98–99, 99f, 100f
    impending fracture, 99–100, 99f, 100f
    mobilization, method of, 102
    nonunion of atypical fractures, 100–102, 100f, 102f
Augmentation of fracture fixation, 128–129, 315
  anatomical indications for, 316
    calcaneal fractures, 321–322
    distal radius fractures, 321
    humeral head fractures, 317–318, 318f
    other anatomical locations, 322, 322f–323f
    proximal femoral fractures, 316–317, 317f
    spinal compressive fractures, 319–320
    tibial plateau fractures, 318–319, 319f–320f
  materials for, 315–316

calcium phosphate cement, 316
  calcium sulfate cement, 316
  polymethyl methacrylate, 316
Autograft, 128
Axin protein, 21

B

Basi-cervical neck fracture, 207
Bazedoxifene, 94
Beta (β)-catenin protein, 22
Beta (β)3-integrin chain, 6
Biochemical investigations of osteoporosis, 35–39
  ALP, 36–37
  bone formation markers, 36–37
  bone resorption markers, 37–38
  bone sialoprotein, 38
  calcium levels, 35
  clinical utility of, 39
  cortisol level, 36
  CTX, 38
  deoxypyridinoline, 38
  dexamethasone level, 36
  hydroxyproline, 37
  NTX, 38
  osteocalcin, 37
  other laboratory investigations, 36
  P1CP, 37
  P1NP, 37
  PTH analysis, 36
  pyridinoline, 38
  TRAP, 37–38
  urinary-excreted calcium, 37
  vitamin D, 35–36
Bisphosphonates, in osteoporosis, 59, 306–307
  clinical data
    adherence, 60–61
    BMD, increased, 60
    bone turnover markers, change in, 61
    fracture healing, 61–62
    glucocorticoid-induced osteoporosis, 61
    vertebral and nonvertebral fractures, 60
  mechanism, 59–60
  side effects, 62–63
    atypical fracture, 62
    cardiovascular, 63
    osteonecrosis of jaw, 62–63
    other, 63

systemic complications of treatment, 91–93
BMD, see Bone mineral density
BMPs, see Bone morphogenetic proteins
Bone cement, 174, 175f
Bone marrow mesenchymal stem cells, 142
Bone mineral density (BMD), 2, 8, 13, 16, 49, 60, 81–84
Bone morphogenetic proteins (BMPs), 6, 15, 145
Bone remodeling units (BRUs), 14
Bones, 35
  cancellous, 13–14, 43–44, 46, 114, 124, 127–128, 151, 153, 164, 178, 183–184, 277, 291, 316, 321, 329, 347
  formation, 14–15, 36–37
  loss, 13
  mechanical properties of, 107–108
  modeling, 13
  osteoporotic
    fracture fixation in, 108–109, 108f
    principles of fracture fixation in, 109–114
  peak mass, 14
  remodeling, 13, 14–15
    cycle, 14–15
    regulatory mechanisms of, 15
  resorption markers, 37–38
  Sfrps in, 23
  sialoprotein, 38
  strength, 13–14, 82
  tissue, 13
Bone sialoprotein (BSP), 38
Bone-specific alkaline phosphatase (BSAP), 61, 84
Bone turnover markers (BTMs), 60–61, 84–86
BRUs, see Bone remodeling units
BSAP, see Bone-specific alkaline phosphatase
BSP, see Bone sialoprotein
BTMs, see Bone turnover markers

C

Calciotropic hormones, 15
Calcitonin, 306
  receptors, 6, 15
  systemic complications of treatment, 93
Calcium, 15–16
  levels, 35
  urinary-excreted, 37

Calcium phosphate, 128–129, 174, 262, 316
Calcium sulfate cement, 316
CalTAD$_{AP}$, 126
Cancellous bone, 13–14, 43–44, 46, 114, 124, 127–128, 151, 153, 164, 178, 183–184, 277, 291, 316, 321, 329, 347
Cannulated screws, 124–125
Carboxyterminal telopeptide cross-linked type 1 collagen (CTX), 84
The Care of Patients with Fragility Fracture, 49
Cathepsin K, 6, 38
Closed reduction and percutaneous fixation technique, 151, 152f
"Comb" technique, 262, 263f
Complications of surgical treatment for osteoporosis, 327
  ankle fractures, 333–334
  distal humerus fractures, 329–330
  distal radius fractures, 330–331
  hip fractures, 331–333
  medical, 335–336
  proximal humerus fractures, 327–329
  spine fractures, 334–335
Computed tomography (CT)
  multidetector, 47
  quantitative, 46, 46f
Conjugation, bone, 13–14
CT, *see* Computed tomography
C-terminal cross-linking telopeptide (CTX), 61
C-terminal telopeptide of collagen type I, 38
CTX, *see* C-terminal cross-linking telopeptide
CYP17A1 gene, 17
CYP19A1 gene, 17

D

DASH (disabilities of the arm, shoulder, and hand), 171
Delayed total hip arthroplasty, 199–201, 200f
Denosumab, in osteoporosis, 141
  clinical data
    BMD, increased, 63–64
    bone turnover marker, change in, 64
    fracture healing, 64
    pharmacokinetics, 63
  long-term use concerns/ better compliance, 64–65
  mechanism, 63
  side effects
    atypical fracture, 65
    infections/immune effect, 65
    osteonecrosis of jaw, 65
    rebound effect, 65–66
    severe hypocalcemia, 65
  systemic complications of treatment, 93
Densitometry, 1
Deoxypyridinoline (DPD), 38
DEXA, *see* Dual-energy x-ray absorptiometry
DHH, *see* Distal humeral hemiarthroplasty

DIACFs, *see* Displaced intra-articular calcaneal fractures
Dickkopf-1, 70
Dickkopf-related protein 1 (Dkk-1), 38
Digital radiographs, 43
1,25-Dihydroxycholecalciferol (1,25[OH]2D3), 15
Displaced extra-articular fractures, 268
Displaced intra-articular calcaneal fractures (DIACFs), 275–276
  classification of, 276
  epidemiology of, 276
  investigation of, 276
  management of, 276–277, 277f
    avulsion fractures, 277–278, 278f
    insufficiency fractures, 278
Distal femoral fractures, 221, 235
  classification, 221
  complications, 242
  epidemiology, 235–236
  first-line arthroplasty, indications for, 236–238
    elderly osteoporotic patient, 237, 237f
    osteoporotic patient with osteoarthritis prior to fracture, 236–237
  how to fix
    anatomy, 223
    approaches, 223–224
    fixation pitfalls, 230–231, 231f
    initial management, 222–223
    intramedullary nailing surgical strategy, 224–225
    periprosthetic considerations, 225–226, 226f
    plating and nailing surgical strategy, combination of, 225
    plating surgical strategy, 224
    plating *vs.* nailing, 225
    positioning, 223
    reconstruction strategy, 226
    tips and tricks, 226–230, 227f–230f
  incidence of, 221, 235
  management, modified algorithm for, 243f
  Müller AO classification for, 236f
  ORIF of, 235
  outcome, 242
  postoperative care, 231–232, 241–242
  preoperative planning and preparation, 237
    bone conditions and fracture morphology, analysis of, 238
    logistics, 238
    patient's general health condition, analysis and management of, 237–238
    skin and vascular conditions, analysis of, 238

principles, 236
surgical technique in
  approach, 240
  bone defect filling *vs.* reconstruction implant, 240–241, 241f
  implant and constraint, choice of, 238–239, 239f, 240f
  implant fixation, principles of, 241
  implant rotation, 240
  joint-line reconstruction, 240
  patient positioning and management, 239
  primary temporary reduction, 240
  treatment algorithm for, 222f
  when to fix, 221–222, 222t
Distal humeral hemiarthroplasty (DHH), 130–131
Distal humerus fractures in elderly, 163–164, 164f
  authors' preferred treatment, 168
  complications of surgical treatment for, 329–330
  incidence of, 163
  internal fixation, primary failure mode of, 164
  open reduction with internal fixation, rationale for, 166–168
  surgeon preference, rationale for, 168
  total elbow arthroplasty, rationale for, 165–166
Distal intra-articular/extra-articular tibial fractures, 267
  classification, 267
  initial assessment of, 267, 268f
  prevalence of, 267
  surgical approaches, 269
  treatment of, 267–269, 268f
    intramedullary (IM) nailing for, 269–270, 269f–270f
    open reduction and internal fixation, 270–274, 270f–273f
    in young *vs.* elderly patients, 267
Distal radius fractures in elderly patients, 171
  complications of surgical treatment for, 330–331
  decision-making
    closed reduction, 171–172
    imaging, 171
  outcome measures, 171
  technology for
    angular stable plate and screw fixation, 173
    bone cement, 174, 175f
    bridging external fixation, 175
    dorsal bridge plating, 174–175, 175f
    dorsal plating, indications for, 173, 174f
    internal fixation, 172–173
    "Pi" plate system, 173, 173f
    volar plating, 173–174, 174f
  treatment, options for

closed treatment, 172
operative treatment, indications for, 172
Distal tibial fractures, 267
  classification, 267
  initial assessment of, 267, 268f
  prevalence of, 267
  surgical approaches, 269
  treatment of, 267–269, 268f
    intramedullary (IM) nailing for, 269–270, 269f–270f
    open reduction and internal fixation, 270–274, 270f–273f
    in young *vs.* elderly patients, 267
Dkks proteins, 23
Dorsal bridge plating, 174–175, 175f
Dorsal plating, indications for, 173, 173f
DPD, *see* Deoxypyridinoline
Dual-energy x-ray absorptiometry (DEXA), 44–46, 45f

E

Eggshell balloon cementoplasty, 287
ELISA, *see* Enzyme-linked immunosorbent assay
Enzyme-linked immunosorbent assay (ELISA), 20
Epidermal growth factor, 15
Estrogen receptor alpha (ERα), 73, 206
Estrogen receptor beta (ERβ), 73, 206
Estrogens, 15, 16–17, 93–94
  isoforms, 73
  systemic complications of treatment, 93
External fixation bridging, 175
Extra-articular proximal tibial fractures, 251–252
  case example 1, 252–255
  case example 2, 256–257
  case example 3, 257–258, 258t
  challenges in
    fracture personality, 251, 252f
    functional level and comorbidities, 251–252
    intramedullary nails, 252
    osteoporotic bone, 251

F

FGF, *see* Fibroblast growth factor
FGF2, *see* Fibroblast growth factor-2
Fibroblast growth factor (FGF), 15
Fibroblast growth factor-2 (FGF2), 9
Fibroblast growth factor 23 (FGF-23), 39
Fibular nails, 128
Fix and treat principle, 118–119
Follicle-stimulating hormone (FSH), 16–17
Fracture Reduction Evaluation of Denosumab in Osteoporosis (FREEDOM) trial, 63–65
Fracture risk assessment tool (FRAX), 50, 55–56
Fragility fracture, 1, 49–53

Fragility fractures of pelvic ring
    (FFP), 177–190
Fragility liaison service (FLS),
    development of,
    49–50, 118–119
  guidelines and models, 50
  "5IQ" model, 51–52
  practicalities, 52–53
  primary prevention, 50
  service delivery, outcomes
    and implications
    for, 53
  setup, 50–52, 51f
FRAX, see Fracture risk
    assessment tool
FSH, see Follicle-stimulating
    hormone
Fusion nails, 129
Fzd proteins, 23

G
GIOP, see Glucocorticoid-induced
    osteoporosis
Glucocorticoid-induced
    osteoporosis (GIOP),
    57, 61
Glucocorticoids, 15
GM-CSF, see Granulocyte-
    macrophage colony-
    stimulating factor
Granulocyte-macrophage colony-
    stimulating factor
    (GM-CSF), 15
Growth hormone, 15

H
Hahn-Steinthal fracture, 165
Helical blades, 128
Hemiarthroplasty, 155–156, 156f
  complications, 155
  evidence, 156
  results, 155
High-resolution peripheral
    quantitative
    computed
    tomography
    (HR-pQCT), 46
Hip
  fractures, 10, 59, 203, 331–333,
    365
  radiograph, 44f
Hot flashes, see Vasomotor
    instability syndrome
HR-pQCT, see High-resolution
    peripheral
    quantitative
    computed
    tomography
Humeral nails, 128
Humerus Block technique, 151,
    152f
Hydroxyproline, 37

I
IGF, see Insulin-like growth
    factor
Iliosacral screw fixation, 181–183,
    182f
Iliosacral screw fixation with
    cement
    augmentation, 183
Ilium, anterior plate fixation of,
    183, 184f
IMN, see Intramedullary nailing
Inability, 178
Independent geriatric syndrome,
    195
Insulin, 15
Insulin-like growth factor
    (IGF), 15

Intramedullary nailing (IMN),
    125–128, 126f–127f,
    224–225
Intramedullary osteosynthesis,
    153–155, 154f
  complications, 154
  evidence, 155
  functional results, 154
"5IQ" model, 51–52

J
Jhamaria index, 43, 44t

K
Kocher-Lorenz fracture, 165
K-wire fixation, 151

L
LDL receptor-related protein 5/6
    (LRP5/6), 21–24, 22f
Lef/Tcf transcription factors, 22
Local cell therapy in osteoporosis
    for fracture healing, 142
  reamer-irrigator-aspirator,
    142–143
Local humoral factors,
    osteoporosis, 143
  antagomirs, 143–145, 144f
  BMP-2, 145
  micro-Ribonucleicacids,
    143–145
  PTH, local release of, 143
Long bone fractures, 245
  intramedullary nailing in,
    247–248, 247f, 248t
  locking plates in, 245–246,
    246t
    features and difficulties
      of, 246, 246t
    indications for, 246t
    minimally invasive
      plate osteosynthesis,
      246–247, 247f
    principles of, 245–246,
      246t
Long nails, 126
LRP5/6, see LDL receptor-related
    protein 5/6
Lumbopelvic fixation, 185–186,
    187f

M
Macrophage colony-stimulating
    factor (M-CSF), 15
Magnetic resonance imaging
    (MRI), 47
Male osteoporosis, 2
Markov-cohort model, 3
Matrix metalloproteinase 9
    (MMP9), 6
M-CSF, see Macrophage colony-
    stimulating factor
Messenger RNA (mRNA), 8, 39
MicroRNAs (miRNAs), 8–9,
    143–145, 144f
Minimally invasive plate
    osteosynthesis
    (MIPO), 222, 224,
    232, 246–247, 256,
    258, 268
MIPO, see Minimally invasive
    plate osteosynthesis
MMP9, see Matrix
    metalloproteinase 9
Molecular mechanisms of
    osteoporosis, 13
  bone mass, 14
  bone modeling, 13
  bone remodeling, 13, 14–15
  bone strength, 13–14

bone tissue, physiology of, 13
  calcium, 15–16
  estrogen, 16–17
  FSH, 16–17
  OPG, 17, 19–21, 20f
  PTH, 15–16
  RANK, 17–21, 18t, 20f
  RANKL, 17–21, 18t, 20f
  vitamin D, 15–16
  Wnt signaling pathway, 21–24
Monitoring/surveillance
    of treatment,
    osteoporosis, 81–82
  BMD, DEXA for, 82–84
    authors' considerations,
      84
    and fracture risk, 83–84
    increase in, 82–83
    as surrogate of bone
      strength, 82
  BTM, 84–86
    adherence, 86
    authors' considerations,
      86
    efficacy, 85–86
    persistence, 86
    methods and validation for,
      82t, 86–87
    QCT, 86–87
    QUS, 86–87
MRI, see Magnetic resonance
    imaging
MRNA, see Messenger RNA
Multidetector CT, 47

N
Nailing, 125–128, 126f–127f
National Institute for Health
    and Care Excellence
    (NICE), 50
  guidelines for medical
    treatment of
    osteoporosis, 55–57
National Osteoporosis Guideline
    Group (NOGG), 56
New-generation sequencing
    (NGS) analysis, 6
NICE, see National Institute
    for Health and Care
    Excellence
NOGG, see National
    Osteoporosis
    Guideline Group
Nonsteroidal anti-inflammatory
    drugs (NSAIDs),
    305–306
NSAIDs, see Nonsteroidal anti-
    inflammatory drugs
N-terminal telopeptide of
    collagen type I, 38

O
Olerud-molander ankle score
    (OMAS), 264
OMAS, see Olerud-molander
    ankle score
"-omics" technologies, 7–8
ONJ, see Osteonecrosis of jaw
Open reduction and internal
    fixation (ORIF), 109,
    197–199, 198f, 235,
    268
OPG, see Osteoprotegerin
ORIF, see Open reduction and
    internal fixation
Osteoblasts, 6, 8–9, 13–18, 21–24,
    35, 37–38, 59, 64,
    76–77, 91, 97, 141,
    143–144, 206
Osteocalcin (OC), 37, 84

Osteoclasts, 14, 74
Osteoid, 14
Osteomalacia, 1
Osteonecrosis of jaw (ONJ),
    62–63, 65
Osteopenia, 45, 49
Osteoporosis, 1–2, 13, 35, 49, 59,
    117–118, 141, 245
  anabolic agents role in, 69
    abaloparatide, 69–70
    romosozumab, 70–71
    sequential therapy, 71
    teriparatide, 69–70
  biochemical investigations
    for, 35–39
    ALP, 36–37
    bone formation markers,
      36–37
    bone resorption markers,
      37–38
    bone sialoprotein, 38
    calcium levels, 35
    clinical utility of, 39
    cortisol level, 36
    CTX, 38
    deoxypyridinoline, 38
    dexamethasone level, 36
    hydroxyproline, 37
    NTX, 38
    osteocalcin, 37
    other laboratory
      investigations, 36
    P1CP, 37
    P1NP, 37
    PTH analysis, 36
    pyridinoline, 38
    TRAP, 37–38
    urinary-excreted calcium,
      37
    vitamin D, 35–36
  biology of, 204–205
    basic pathology, 205
    calcium, 206
    estrogen, role of,
      205–206
    PTH, 206
    vitamin D, 206
  bisphosphonates in, 59
    adherence, 60–61
    BMD, increased, 60
    bone turnover markers,
      change in, 61
    fracture healing, 61–62
    glucocorticoid-induced
      osteoporosis, 61
    mechanism, 59–60
    side effects, 62–63
    vertebral and
      nonverterbal
      fractures, 60
  complications of surgical
    treatment for, 327
    ankle fractures, 333–334
    distal humerus fractures,
      329–330
    distal radius fractures,
      330–331
    hip fractures, 331–333
    medical, 335–336
    proximal humerus
      fractures, 327–329
    spine fractures, 334–335
  definition, 1–2, 35
  denosumab in
    BMD, increased, 63–64
    bone turnover marker,
      change in, 64
    fracture healing, 64
    mechanism, 63
    pharmacokinetics, 63

Osteoporosis (*Continued*)
  safety, tolerability,
    and long-term
    monitoring, 64–65
  emerging biological markers
    of, 38–39, 38t, 39f
  epidemiology of, 2–3
  lifestyle and conditions for, 5t
  local cell therapy
    for fracture healing, 142
    reamer-irrigator-
      aspirator, 142–143
  local humoral factors, 143
    antagomirs, 143–145, 144f
    BMP-2, 145
    micro-Ribonucleicacids,
      143–145
    PTH, local release of, 143
  male, 2
  management, principle of,
    121, 122f
    aftercare, 131
    arthrodesis, 129
    arthroplasty, 129–131,
      130f
    augmentation, 128–129
    fixation, 121–122
    impaction constructs,
      124–125
    nailing, 125–128,
      126f–127f
    plating, 122–124
  molecular mechanisms
    of, 13
    bone mass, 14
    bone remodeling, 14–15
    bone strength, 13–14
    bone tissue, physiology
      of, 13
    calcium, 15–16
    estrogen, 16–17
    FSH, 16–17
    OPG, 17, 19–21, 20f
    PTH, 15–16
    RANK, 17–21, 18t, 20f
    RANKL, 17–21, 18t, 20f
    vitamin D, 15–16
    Wnt signaling pathway,
      21–24
  monitoring/surveillance of
    treatment, 81–82
    BMD, DEXA for, 82–84
    BTM, 84–86
    methods and validation
      for, 82t, 86–87
  NICE guidelines for medical
    treatment, 55–57
    assessment, risk fracture,
      56
    duration of treatments, 57
    glucocorticoid-induced
      osteoporosis, 57
    lifestyle and dietary
      measures, 56
    management algorithm
      for assessment, 56f
    postmenopausal men,
      first-line treatment
      for, 57
    postmenopausal women,
      first-line treatment
      for, 57
    risk fracture assessment,
      need for, 55–56
    therapeutic treatments,
      56–57
  patient rehabilitation,
    363–366
  pharmacological agents in
    treatment of, 73
    abaloparatide, 77–78

    raloxifene, 73–75
    romosozumab, 75–77
  physiologic *vs.* pathologic,
    2–3
  prevalence, 2–3
  primary, 6
  and proximal femur, 203–204
    fixation failure, 204
    inability to achieve
      preoperative status of
      activity, 204
    mortality, 204
    orthopedic concerns of,
      203–204
    prolonged hospital stay,
      204
    quality of life in, 204
  proximal humeral fractures,
    149–157
  radiological investigations of,
    43–47
    DEXA for, 44–46, 45f
    HR-pQCT for, 46
    MRI for, 47
    multidetector CT for, 47
    quantitative CT for, 46,
      46f
    radiography for, 43–44,
      44f, 44t
  recurrence, 118
  risks factors, 118
  risks of
    differential gene
      expression, 7–8
    epidemiological, 3–4, 3f,
      4f, 5t, 9–10
    genetic, 4–6, 6f, 9–10
    genotype, 9
    medicaments, 5t
    microRNAs (miRNAs),
      8–9
    molecular and genetic
      risk factor predictors,
      6
    molecular pathways,
      6–7, 7f
    transcriptome, 8–9
  systemic complications of
    treatment, 91
    bazedoxifene, 94
    bisphosphonates, 91–93
    calcitonin, 93
    denosumab, 93
    estrogen, 93
    parathyroid hormone-
      related protein, 94
    PTH, 94
    raloxifene, 93
    selective estrogen
      receptor modulators,
      93–94
    tamoxifen, 93
  therapy concepts for, 141–142,
    142t
  total hip replacement and,
    349–353
  total knee replacement (TKR)
    and, 357–360
  total shoulder replacement
    and, 343–347
  in women, 3
Osteoporotic bones
  fracture fixation in, 108–109,
    108f
  principles of fracture fixation
    in, 109–114
    accurate fracture
      reduction, 109–111,
      110f
    correct alignment,
      109–111, 110f

    delayed union/nonunion,
      promotion of bone
      formation and
      prevention of, 112–114
    primary stability, 109
    secondary stability,
      111–112, 112f, 113f
Osteoporotic thoracolumbar
    fractures,
    nonoperative
    treatment method
    for, 305
  comorbid management, 310
  electrotherapy, 308
  exercise and rehabilitation,
    309–310
  external support devices,
    308–309
  minimally invasive
    procedures, 308
  nonopioid analgesia, 305–306
  opioid analgesia, 305–306
  osteoporosis medication, 306
    bisphosphonates,
      306–307
    calcitonin, 306
    teriparatide, 307
  secondary prevention, 310
Osteoporotic vertebral
    compression fracture
    (OVCF), 281–282,
    282f–283f
  clinical indications, 282–285
    contraindications, 284
    imaging modalities, 283f,
      284–285
    pseudarthrosis (Kümmel
      disease), 283–284,
      284f
    for vertebroplasty, 283
  complications, 290
    adjacent vertebral
      fracture, 294–295,
      295f
    cement leakage, 291–292,
      292f
    hemodynamic, 293
    increase in pain after
      procedure, 290
    infection, 290
    neurological, 293–294
    radiation exposure, 295
    respiratory, 293
    rib and sternal fractures,
      290
  cost of treatment, 295
  kyphotic deformity, 281, 282f,
    289
  outcomes, 288
    absorbable cements
      in maintaining
      correction, effects
      of, 289
    fracture age and, 288
    kyphotic deformity, 289
    multilevel kyphoplasty,
      289–290
    postural correction *vs.*
      balloon inflation, 289
    pseudarthrotic clefts,
      effects on, 288–289
    vertebral bodies, 288
    vertebral height
      restoration, effects
      on, 289
  patient selection, 282–285
  surgical technique for,
    285–288, 286f–288f
  treatment of, 281–282
  vertebroplasty in, 281–282,
    283

Osteoprotegerin (OPG), 17,
    19–21, 20f
  genetic variation in signaling
    pathway, 21
  mechanism of action, 18f
  and RANKL, 19–20
  signaling pathway, 19
OVCF, *see* Osteoporotic vertebral
    compression fracture

P
PACS, *see* Picture archiving
    communication
    systems
Paracetamol (acetaminophen),
    305
Parathyroid hormone
    (PTH), 15–16,
    69–70, 141
  to accelerate fracture healing
    in osteoporosis, 143
  systemic complications of
    treatment, 94
Parathyroid hormone-related
    protein (PTHrP),
    69–71, 77–78, 94
Paravertebral muscle spasms, 306
Partial articular fractures,
    268–269
PASE, *see* Physical Activity Scale
    for the Elderly
Pathologic osteoporotic fractures,
    2
Patient rated wrist evaluation
    (PRWE), 171
P1CP, *see* Procollagen type
    1 C-terminal
    propeptide
PCR, *see* Polymerase chain
    reaction
Peak bone mass, 14
Pelvic fractures, 177
  aftertreatment, 189–190
  anamnesis, 177
  classification, 178–180, 179f
  clinical presentation at
    admission, 177
  decision-making in, 180
  incidence of, 177
  nonoperative
    management of,
    180–181, 180f
  operative treatment of, 181
    anterior pelvic ring,
      186–189
    posterior pelvic ring,
      181–186
  radiological examinations in
    computed tomography
    (CT) scan, 178
    conventional pelvic
      overviews, 178
    magnetic resonance
      imaging, 178
    multiplanar
      reconstructions, 178
Periostin, 38
PGF, *see* Platelet growth factor
Physical Activity Scale for the
    Elderly (PASE), 171
Picture archiving communication
    systems (PACS), 43
"Pilon" injuries, *see* Distal tibial
    fractures
"Pi" plate system, 173, 173f
Platelet growth factor (PGF), 15
Plate osteosynthesis, in proximal
    humeral fractures,
    151–153, 152f, 153f
  complications, 153
  functional results, 152–153

Plating, 122–124
PMMA, *see* Polymethyl methacrylate
P1NP, *see* Procollagen type 1 N-terminal propeptide
Polymerase chain reaction (PCR), 20
Polymethyl methacrylate (PMMA), 112, 129, 262, 316
Posterior bridging plate osteosynthesis, 184–185
Posterior pelvic ring, operative treatment of, 181–186
 anterior plate fixation of ilium, 183, 184f
 iliosacral screw fixation, 181–183, 182f
 iliosacral screw fixation with cement augmentation, 183
 lumbopelvic fixation, 185–186, 187f
 posterior bridging plate osteosynthesis, 184–185
 posterior transiliac internal fixation, 185, 186f
 sacroplasty, 183
 trans-sacral bar osteosynthesis, 183–184, 185f
Posterior transiliac internal fixation, 185, 186f
Primary osteoporosis, 6
Procollagen type 1 C-terminal propeptide (P1CP), 37
Procollagen type 1 N-terminal propeptide (P1NP), 37, 61, 84
Proximal femoral fractures
 atypical femur fractures secondary to osteoporosis treatment, 213–214
 biomechanics of, 206–207, 207f
 classification, 207
  intertrochanteric, 207–208, 208f, 208t
  subtrochanteric, 208–209, 209t
 medical treatment of antiresorptive medications, 212–213
  calcium supplementation, 212–213
  duration and monitoring of therapy, 213
  vitamin D supplementation, 212–213
 surgical treatment of, 210
  bow, mind, 211–212
  compression across fracture site, 212
  distal locking screws, use of, 212
  entry point, appropriate, 212
  lateral wall in, 211, 211f
  nail unstable fracture, 211, 211f–212f
  reduction, 210, 211f
  technical tips for, 210–212
  tip-to-apex distance in, 210–211
  varus angulation, 212

Proximal femur, osteoporosis and, 203–204
 fixation failure, 204
 inability to achieve preoperative status of activity, 204
 mortality, 204
 orthopedic concerns of, 203–204
 prolonged hospital stay, 204
 quality of life in, 204
Proximal humeral fractures
 classification, 150
 complications of surgical treatment for, 327–329
 diagnosis of, 149–150
 incidence of, 149
 management
  closed reduction and percutaneous fixation technique, 151, 152f
  hemiarthroplasty, 155–156, 156f
  intramedullary osteosynthesis, 153–155, 154f
  nonoperative treatment, 150–151
  operative treatment, 151–157
  plate osteosynthesis, 151–153, 152f
  reversed shoulder arthroplasty, 156–157, 156f
PRWE, *see* Patient rated wrist evaluation
PTH, *see* Parathyroid hormone
PTH 1 receptor (PTH1R), 69–70
PYD, *see* Pyridinoline
Pyridinoline (PYD), 38

Q
QCT, *see* Quantitative computed tomography
QFracture, 50, 55–56
QRT-PCR, *see* Quantitative real-time reverse-transcription polymerase chain reaction
Quantitative computed tomography (QCT), 86–87
Quantitative real-time reverse-transcription polymerase chain reaction (QRT-PCR), 8
Quantitative ultrasound (QUS), 86–87
QUS, *see* Quantitative ultrasound

R
Radiography, 43–44, 44f, 44t
Radiological investigations of osteoporosis, 43–47
 DEXA for, 44–46, 45f
 HR-pQCT for, 46
 MRI for, 47
 multidetector CT for, 47
 quantitative CT for, 46, 46f
 radiography for, 43–44, 44f, 44t
Raloxifene, for osteoporosis, 73, 74t, 93
 bone, effects on, 74
 clinical efficacy, 75
 mechanism of action, 73–74
 safety profile, 75

tissues, effects on, 74–75
RANK, *see* Receptor activator of nuclear factor-κB
RANKL, *see* Receptor activator of nuclear factor-κB ligand
RANK-OPG, *see* Receptor activator of nuclear factor-κB-osteo protegerin
Reamer-irrigator-aspirator (RIA), 142–143, 231
Receptor activator of nuclear factor-κB ligand (RANKL), 17–21, 18t, 20f, 70
 genetic variation in signaling pathway, 21
 mechanism of action, 18f
 and OPG, 19–20
 signaling pathway, 19
Receptor activator of nuclear factor-κB–osteoprotegerin (RANK-OPG), 6, 15
Receptor activator of nuclear factor-κB (RANK), 15
 genetic variation in signaling pathway, 21
 mechanism of action, 18f
 signaling pathway, 19
Rehabilitation of osteoporotic patient, 363–366
 fragility fracture care in United Kingdom, 363–364
 for hip fractures, 365
 secondary prevention, 364
  bone protection, drugs for, 364
  falls assessment and prevention, 364–365
 for wrist fractures, 365–366
Retrograde femoral nails, 127
Reversed shoulder arthroplasty, 156–157, 156f
 complications, 157
 evidence, 157
 results, 157
Reverse shoulder arthroplasty (RSA), 130
RIA, *see* Reamer-irrigator-aspirator
Risedronate, 57
ROC nails, 127
Romosozumab, in osteoporosis, 70–71, 75–76
 mechanism of action, 76
 preclinical studies, 76–77
 sclerostin deficiency, 76
Royal Osteoporosis Society, 50
RSA, *see* Reverse shoulder arthroplasty

S
Sacroplasty, 183
Sclerostin, 23, 39, 70
Screw augmentation with bone cement, 262
Selective estrogen receptor modulators (SERMs), 73, 74t, 93–94, 141
Sequential therapy, 71
SERMs, *see* Selective estrogen receptor modulators
Sex hormone-binding globulin (SHBG), 206
SF-36, 171
Sfrps in bones, 23
SHBG, *see* Sex hormone-binding globulin

Short nails, 126
SHS, *see* Sliding hip screw
Singh index, 43, 44t
Sliding hip screw (SHS), 124–125
Soluble Frizzled-related protein (sFRP), 38
Spinal compressive fractures, 319–320
 complications of surgical treatment for, 334–335
 kyphoplasty in, 319–320
 vertebroplasty in, 319
Staphylococcus aureus, 290
Steinmann pin, 264
Strontium, 141
Synthetic bone grafts, 128

T
Tamoxifen, 93
Tartrate-resistant acid phosphatase (TRAP), 6, 37–38
TBW, *see* Tension band wiring
TEA, *see* Total elbow arthroplasty
Tension band wiring (TBW), 124
Teriparatide, in osteoporosis, 57, 307
 clinical use of, 70
 mechanism of action of, 69–70
TGF-β, *see* Transforming growth factor β
THA, *see* Total hip arthroplasty
Thyroxine, 15
Tibio-talar calcaneal (TCC) nail, 264
TKA, *see* Total knee arthroplasty
TNF, *see* Tumor necrosis factor
TNFRSF11B gene, 21
Total elbow arthroplasty (TEA), 130, 165–166
Total hip arthroplasty (THA), 130–131, 130f
 acute, 199, 199f
 delayed, 199–201, 200f
 efficacy of, 349–353, 350f–351f, 352t
Total hip replacement, osteoporosis and, 349–353
Total knee arthroplasty (TKA), 221, 235
Total knee replacement (TKR), osteoporosis and, 357–360
 BMD changes after, 358–359
 bone quality and function after, 360
 osteoarthritis and osteoporosis, relationship between, 357–358
 pharmacologic modulation of BMD loss, 359–360
Total shoulder replacement, osteoporosis and, 343
 humeral anatomy, 344–345
 humerus
  metaphyseal fixation in, 346–347
  stem fixation in, 345–346, 345f–346f
 in trauma, 343–344
Transcriptome, 8–9
Transforming growth factor β (TGF-β), 15
Trans-sacral bar osteosynthesis, 183–184, 185f

TRAP, *see* Tartrate-resistant acid
    phosphatase
Trochanteric nails, 127
T-scores, 45–46, 45f, 49, 77,
    82–83, 118, 364
Tumor necrosis factor (TNF), 15
Type 1 collagen amino-terminal
    telopeptide (NTX), 84

U
Urinary-excreted calcium, 37

V
Vasomotor instability syndrome,
    75

VDR, *see* Vitamin D receptor
VDR-RXR, *see* Vitamin D
    receptor-retinoic acid
    x-receptor complex
Vertebral fragility fractures,
    nonoperative
    treatment method
    for, 305
    comorbid management,
        310
    electrotherapy, 308
    exercise and rehabilitation,
        309–310
    external support devices,
        308–309

minimally invasive
    procedures, 308
nonopioid analgesia, 305–306
opioid analgesia, 305–306
osteoporosis medication, 306
    bisphosphonates,
        306–307
    calcitonin, 306
    teriparatide, 307
    secondary prevention, 310
Vitamin D, 15–16, 35–36
Vitamin D receptor-retinoic acid
    x-receptor complex
    (VDR-RXR), 16
Vitamin D receptor (VDR), 16

Volar plating, 173–174, 174f

W
Wnt proteins, 6, 22
Wnt signaling pathway, 13, 21
    genetic variation in, 23–24
    key players in, 22–23
    regulation of, 23
    steps of, 21, 22f
Women, osteoporosis in, 3, 57
Wrist fractures, 365–366

Z
Zoledronate, 57
Z-score, 45